Neural Development: Beyond the Basics

Neural Development: Beyond the Basics

Editor: Stella Osborne

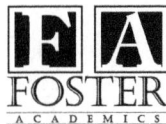

FA
FOSTER
ACADEMICS

www.fosteracademics.com

www.fosteracademics.com

FA **FOSTER** ACADEMICS

Cataloging-in-Publication Data

Neural development : beyond the basics / edited by Stella Osborne.
    p. cm.
Includes bibliographical references and index.
ISBN 978-1-63242-728-1
    1. Nervous system--Growth. 2. Developmental neurobiology. 3. Neurology. 4. Nervous system--Diseases.
5. Neurosciences. I. Osborne, Stella.
QP363.5 .N48 2019
612.8--dc23

Foster Academics,
118-35 Queens Blvd., Suite 400,
Forest Hills, NY 11375, USA

ISBN 978-1-63242-728-1 (Hardback)

Contents

Preface

In my initial years as a student, I used to run to the library at every possible instance to grab a book and learn something new. Books were my primary source of knowledge and I would not have come such a long way without all that I learnt from them. Thus, when I was approached to edit this book; I became understandably nostalgic. It was an absolute honor to be considered worthy of guiding the current generation as well as those to come. I put all my knowledge and hard work into making this book most beneficial for its readers.

The field of neural development is concerned with the study of the cellular and molecular mechanisms that are inherent to the development of the nervous system during embryonic development and throughout life. Neural development follows certain stages such as the birth and differentiation of neurons, their migration to their final positions, the growth of axons from neurons, the generation of synapses, and so on. Such neurodevelopmental processes fall within the categories of activity-dependent and activity-independent mechanisms. Defects in neural development have repercussions in terms of motor, sensory and cognitive impairments, malformations and other neurological disorders. This makes neural development an active area of study. This book includes some of the vital pieces of work being conducted across the world, on various topics related to neural development. The objective of this book is to give a general view of the different processes of neural development, and their significance. It will help the readers in keeping pace with the rapid changes in this field.

I wish to thank my publisher for supporting me at every step. I would also like to thank all the authors who have contributed their researches in this book. I hope this book will be a valuable contribution to the progress of the field.

Editor

Identification of molecular signatures specific for distinct cranial sensory ganglia in the developing chick

Cedric Patthey[2,4†], Harry Clifford[1,3†], Wilfried Haerty[1,3*], Chris P. Ponting[1,3], Sebastian M. Shimeld[2] and Jo Begbie[1*]

Abstract

Background: The cranial sensory ganglia represent populations of neurons with distinct functions, or sensory modalities. The production of individual ganglia from distinct neurogenic placodes with different developmental pathways provides a powerful model to investigate the acquisition of specific sensory modalities. To date there is a limited range of gene markers available to examine the molecular pathways underlying this process.

Results: Transcriptional profiles were generated for populations of differentiated neurons purified from distinct cranial sensory ganglia using microdissection in embryonic chicken followed by FAC-sorting and RNAseq. Whole transcriptome analysis confirmed the division into somato- versus viscerosensory neurons, with additional evidence for subdivision of the somatic class into general and special somatosensory neurons. Cross-comparison of distinct ganglia transcriptomes identified a total of 134 markers, 113 of which are novel, which can be used to distinguish trigeminal, vestibulo-acoustic and epibranchial neuronal populations. In situ hybridisation analysis provided validation for 20/26 tested markers, and showed related expression in the target region of the hindbrain in many cases.

Conclusions: One hundred thirty-four high-confidence markers have been identified for placode-derived cranial sensory ganglia which can now be used to address the acquisition of specific cranial sensory modalities.

Keywords: Cranial sensory ganglia, Viscerosensory neuron, Somatosensory neuron, Cell type markers, Chicken, FACS, Expression profiling

Background

The sensory nervous system is fundamental to perception of our body's external and internal environments. It is generally accepted that distinct types of sensation are mediated by neurons specialised in responding to specific stimuli, raising questions relating to how these distinct groups of neurons differ, both at the level of physiological function, and at the level of the acquisition of specific phenotypes during development [1]. To this end, recent publications have outlined transcriptome analysis of sensory neurons in the trunk, identifying specific subsets of somatosensory neurons [2, 3]. However, these studies provide molecular signatures specifically for trunk somatosensory neurons, and do not encompass the many other sensory modalities conveyed by cranial sensory neurons [4]. Our aim was to develop a resource which would address the paucity of markers known to distinguish between neurons characteristic of distinct cranial sensory ganglia.

The cranial sensory ganglia can be categorised as having distinct sensory modalities according to the function of their associated cranial nerve (Fig. 1A). The trigeminal ganglion (which can be subdivided into ophthalmic and maxillomandibular), associated with cranial nerve V, is

---

* Correspondence: wilfried.haerty@tgac.ac.uk; jo.begbie@dpag.ox.ac.uk
†Equal contributors
[1]Department of Physiology, Anatomy and Genetics, University of Oxford, Oxford, UK
Full list of author information is available at the end of the article

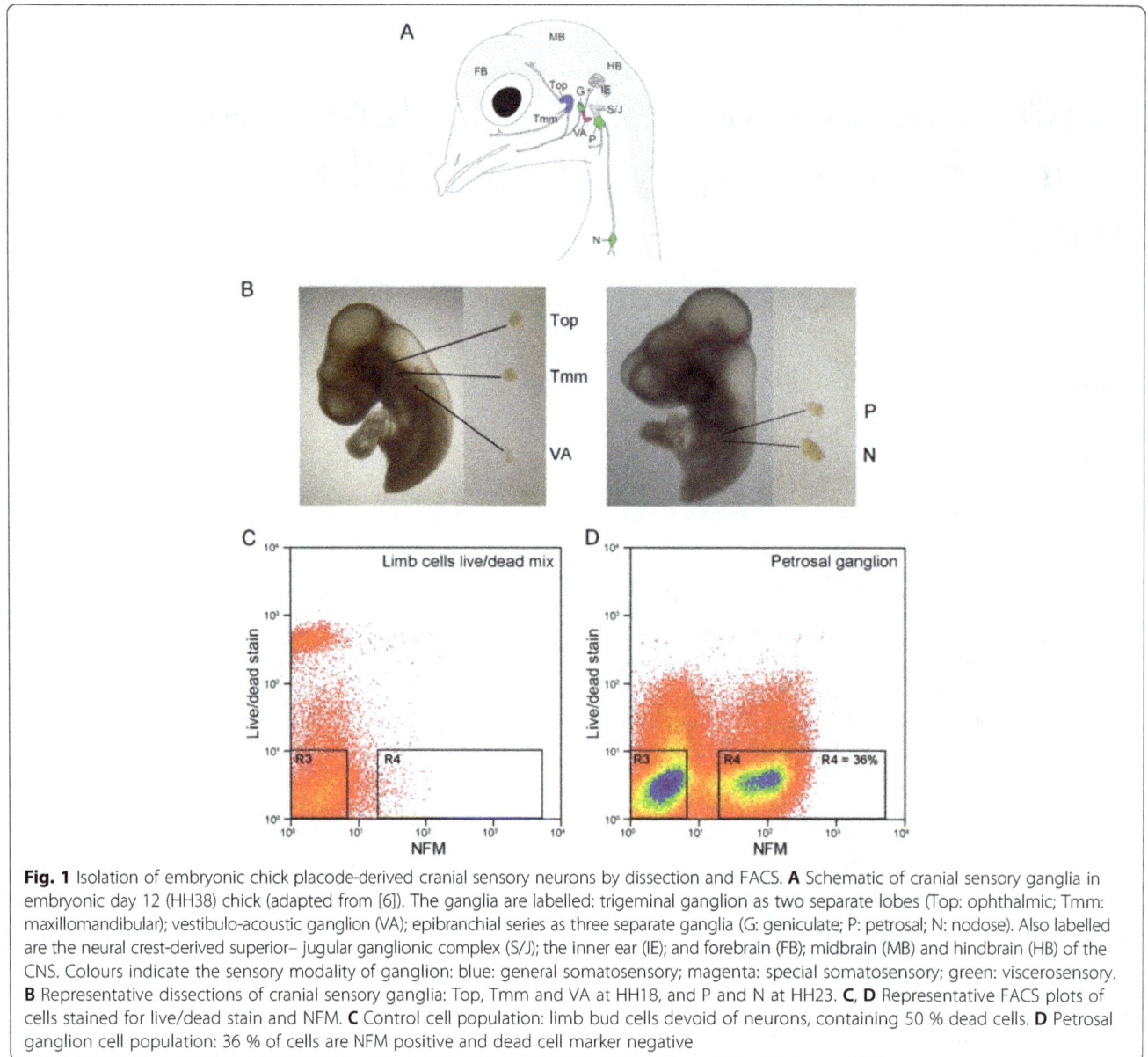

Fig. 1 Isolation of embryonic chick placode-derived cranial sensory neurons by dissection and FACS. **A** Schematic of cranial sensory ganglia in embryonic day 12 (HH38) chick (adapted from [6]). The ganglia are labelled: trigeminal ganglion as two separate lobes (Top: ophthalmic; Tmm: maxillomandibular); vestibulo-acoustic ganglion (VA); epibranchial series as three separate ganglia (G: geniculate; P: petrosal; N: nodose). Also labelled are the neural crest-derived superior– jugular ganglionic complex (S/J); the inner ear (IE); and forebrain (FB); midbrain (MB) and hindbrain (HB) of the CNS. Colours indicate the sensory modality of ganglion: blue: general somatosensory; magenta: special somatosensory; green: viscerosensory. **B** Representative dissections of cranial sensory ganglia: Top, Tmm and VA at HH18, and P and N at HH23. **C, D** Representative FACS plots of cells stained for live/dead stain and NFM. **C** Control cell population: limb bud cells devoid of neurons, containing 50 % dead cells. **D** Petrosal ganglion cell population: 36 % of cells are NFM positive and dead cell marker negative

considered most similar to the sensory dorsal root ganglia (DRG) in the trunk, being involved in touch, pain and temperature sensation. The vestibulo-acoustic ganglion, associated with cranial nerve VIII, innervates the inner ear structures involved in balance and hearing. The epibranchial ganglia, individually called geniculate, associated with cranial nerve VII; petrosal, associated with cranial nerve IX; and nodose, associated with cranial nerve X, are involved in sensing chemicals such as tastants, digestive catabolites, and blood gas levels, in addition to sensing pressure changes in blood vessels. The cranial sensory modalities thus correspond to somatosensation, which is further subdivided into general somatosensory (trigeminal)

and special somatosensory (vestibulo-acoustic), and viscerosensation (geniculate, petrosal and nodose). Our study is focused on the cranial sensory ganglia of chicken (Fig. 1A), but their organisation and function are well conserved across vertebrates [5].

The development of cranial sensory ganglia remains less well studied than that of the DRG, possibly due to their perceived complexity. Compared with the DRG, which all develop exclusively from neural crest, each individual cranial sensory ganglion develops from a distinct neurogenic placode with some neural crest contribution to the proximal cranial sensory ganglia: the proximal region of the trigeminal ganglion, small numbers of neurons in the geniculate and vestibulo-acoustic ganglia, and the entirety of the superior/jugular ganglia associated with cranial nerves IX and X [6–8]. As each different neurogenic placode utilises a distinct developmental path, they can be used to understand the acquisition of different, specific sensory modalities. Experiments addressing placode fate switching through in vivo transplantation and in vitro pathway manipulation, show that the trigeminal (somatosensory) and nodose (viscerosensory) placode are fate-restricted once neurogenesis begins [7, 9, 10]. In the mouse, expression of the transcription factor *Phox2b* underpins the fate choice between these two sensory modalities [11]. However, only a limited range of markers exist that can be used to investigate this cell type decision, and no markers are currently available to distinguish between general and special somatosensory modalities. To extend experimental analysis of cranial sensory ganglia development further, we require a broad range of markers that distinguish between differentiated neurons of different phenotypes.

Even neurons of the same sensory modality can differ depending on whether they derive from neural crest or placode. Analysis of the *Scn10a* gene promoter in the mouse has shown that a specific fragment recapitulates endogenous expression of the product $Na_v1.8$ in neural crest-derived but not placode-derived cranial sensory neurons [12]. Furthermore, nociceptive C-fibre sensory neurons innervating the lung are phenotypically distinct depending on whether they are neural crest- or placode-derived [13]. These observations reinforce the importance of producing markers that are specific for placode-derived cranial sensory neurons.

The timing and localisation of distinct placode-derived cranial sensory ganglion development have been carefully documented in the chicken [6, 9, 10, 14–19]. Here we take advantage of our knowledge of the development of the chicken system, combined with genome-wide expression profiling, to characterise ganglion-specific populations of placode-derived sensory neurons at early stages of differentiation. We present RNA-seq data generated from embryonic neurons purified from five distinct cranial sensory ganglia (namely trigeminal maxillomandibular; trigeminal ophthalmic; vestibulo-acoustic; petrosal; and nodose ganglia) separated by dissection and fluorescence-activated cell sorting (FACS). Using this gene expression data, we provide an objective and comprehensive classification of distinct populations of cranial sensory neurons. Whole transcriptome analysis confirms the dichotomy of somatosensory (somatic) versus viscerosensory (visceral) neurons, but additionally provides molecular evidence for the subdivision of the somatosensory neurons into general and special somatosensory neurons as previously described based on anatomy [11, 20]. Cross-comparison of distinct ganglia transcriptomes identifies a total of 134 markers,

113 of them novel, which can be used to distinguish trigeminal, vestibulo-acoustic and epibranchial neuronal populations. We confirm expression of 20 of these specific markers in the specific cranial sensory ganglia by in situ hybridization. Taken together, our data provides molecular signatures for distinct cranial sensory neuronal populations.

Results
Transcriptional profile analysis of cranial sensory ganglia placode-derived neurons
In all vertebrates the cranial sensory ganglia are segregated according to sensory function. In the chicken, the stereotypical localisation of the ganglia (Fig. 1A) and our detailed understanding of the timing of their development [6, 14, 18, 19, 21] make it possible to dissect the ganglia separately in order to establish expression profiles of distinct populations of developing sensory neurons. We took advantage of this to harvest the trigeminal (maxillomandibular and ophthalmic), vestibulo-acoustic, nodose and petrosal ganglia from Hamburger-Hamilton stage 18 (HH18) [22] (both trigeminal and vestibulo-acoustic) or HH23 (nodose and petrosal) chicken embryos (Fig. 1B). Collection at these embryonic stages allowed us to compensate for differences in the timing of ganglion development, thus ensuring the neurons would be investigated at a similar stage of differentiation [7, 14, 18, 19]. Furthermore, these specific timings meant that the population of collected neurons exclusively contained placode-derived neurons. This was of particular importance for the trigeminal ganglion where neural crest-derived neurons contribute directly to the ganglion at later stages, rather than forming separate ganglia [6, 8]. We confirmed that we could avoid neural crest-derived neuron contamination of our trigeminal samples in a separate experiment, specifically labelling neural crest cells with GFP and showing that these did not contribute to the neuronal pool at HH18 (Additional file 1: Figure S1). The trigeminal ganglion was collected as two separate lobes (maxillomandibular and ophthalmic) because these arise from distinct placodes with individual characteristics [14, 18, 23], and further exist as two separate ganglia in more basal vertebrates [5, 24].

In order to profile the transcriptomes of differentiated neurons rather than non-neural cell types or neural progenitors we isolated all cells positive for neurofilament medium polypeptide (NFM) antibody staining. To this aim we adapted transcription factor FACS (tfFACS) [25], a method that allows sorting of cells with antibodies raised towards intracellular epitopes. Briefly, freshly dissected ganglia were quickly dissociated to single cells and fixed, thereby freezing the cells in their transcriptional state. The cells were gently permeabilised and subjected to

NFM immunostaining, followed by FACS. Prior to fixation the cells were treated with a live/dead stain, with the gate for live/dead cells set using a control limb bud sample containing 50 % of cells killed by heat-shock (Fig. 1C). The extracted NFM positive (NFM+) neurons represented 13–41 % of the total cell population, while dead cells (4–9 % of total) were excluded (Fig. 1D). A total of 20,000 to 290,000 NFM+ neurons per sample were collected by FACS and 50-200 ng of high quality total RNA extracted (Additional file 2). Following this, RNA-sequencing returned a mean of ~77 million (~30–116 million) 100 bp reads for each of three replicates, of which an average of 88 ± 6 % mapped to the genome assembly. An average of 11,800 (10,897–12,190) genes per sample were expressed at an appreciable level (>0.3 read per kilobase per million mapped reads (RPKM), Additional file 3).

Principal Component Analysis (PCA) of gene expression across all samples revealed two distinct, unambiguous clusters indicative of two distinct categories of cranial sensory ganglia captured by the first principal component (Fig. 2A). None of the principal components significantly correlated with RNA integrity measurements (RIN values), RNA yield or sequencing depth (Additional file 2; Additional file 4: Figure S2A, B, C). The clusters reflected the known segregation of viscerosensory neurons (nodose and petrosal) and somatosensory neurons (vestibulo-acoustic and trigeminal) [11]. However, the two clusters also reflected the different embryonic stages of dissection. To test levels of neuronal maturation, we examined expression levels of six known markers of differentiated

neurons (*ELAVL4 (HUD), ISL1, MYT1, NEUROD1, RBFOX3 (NEUN)* and *TUBB3 (Tuj1)*). Levels of expression were similar across the two sets of samples, supporting the hypothesis that the clusters reflect sensory phenotype rather than maturation differences (Additional file 5: Figure S3).

The projections of the samples on PC1 and PC2 also show separation of the somatosensory cluster into a trigeminal cluster and a vestibulo-acoustic cluster (Fig. 2A): a conclusion further strengthened by analysis of the other principal components (Fig. 2B). This supports the segregation of these ganglia into general (trigeminal) and special (vestibulo-acoustic) somatosensory ganglia, terminology which has been applied largely based on the anatomy of their central projections with less known about the molecular basis [20]. Thus, our transcriptome-wide analysis supports a clear separation of cranial sensory ganglia into viscerosensory (nodose/petrosal) and somatosensory modalities (trigeminal/vestibulo-acoustic) with further subdivision of the latter into general (trigeminal) and special (vestibulo-acoustic) somatosensory modalities.

To identify ganglion-specific gene markers, differentially expressed genes were determined using both DESeq and EdgeR algorithms [26, 27], with the resultant intersect taken to ensure a robust selection. All combinations of ganglia were tested, and differentially expressed genes from both sets of analysis are available as Additional file 6. We were particularly interested in differential expression that reflected the PCA separation of the ganglia into three clusters. Accordingly our analysis identified higher expression of 1249 genes in nodose/petrosal; 447 in trigeminal

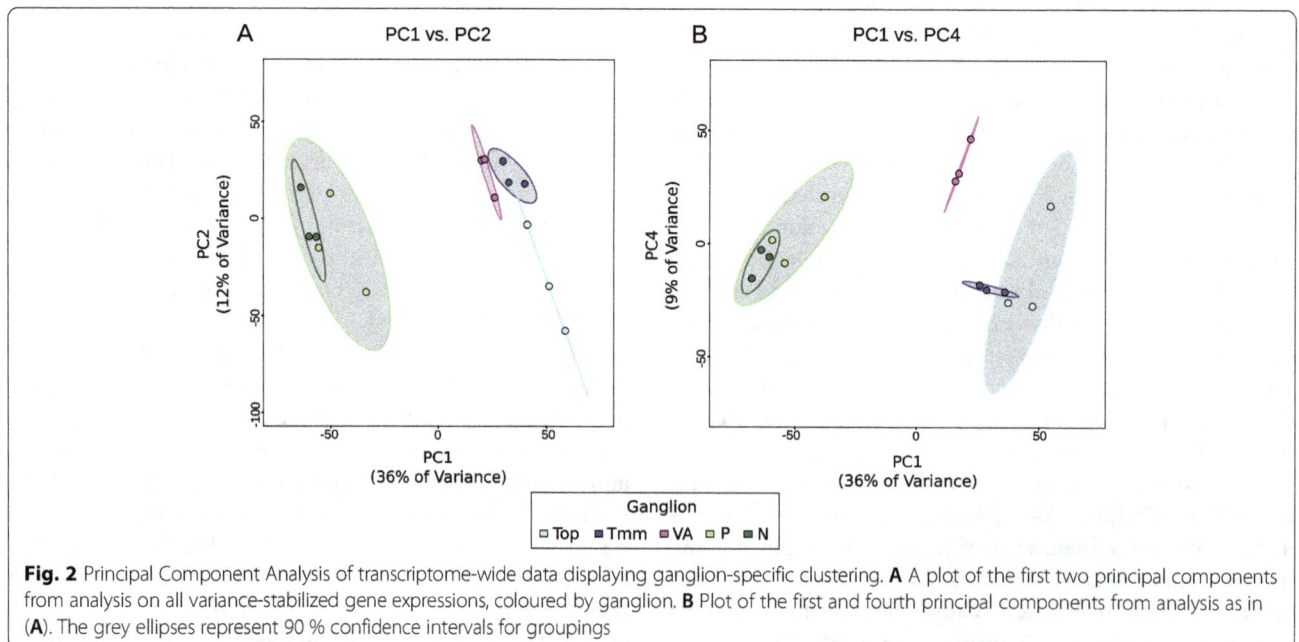

Fig. 2 Principal Component Analysis of transcriptome-wide data displaying ganglion-specific clustering. **A** A plot of the first two principal components from analysis on all variance-stabilized gene expressions, coloured by ganglion. **B** Plot of the first and fourth principal components from analysis as in (**A**). The grey ellipses represent 90 % confidence intervals for groupings

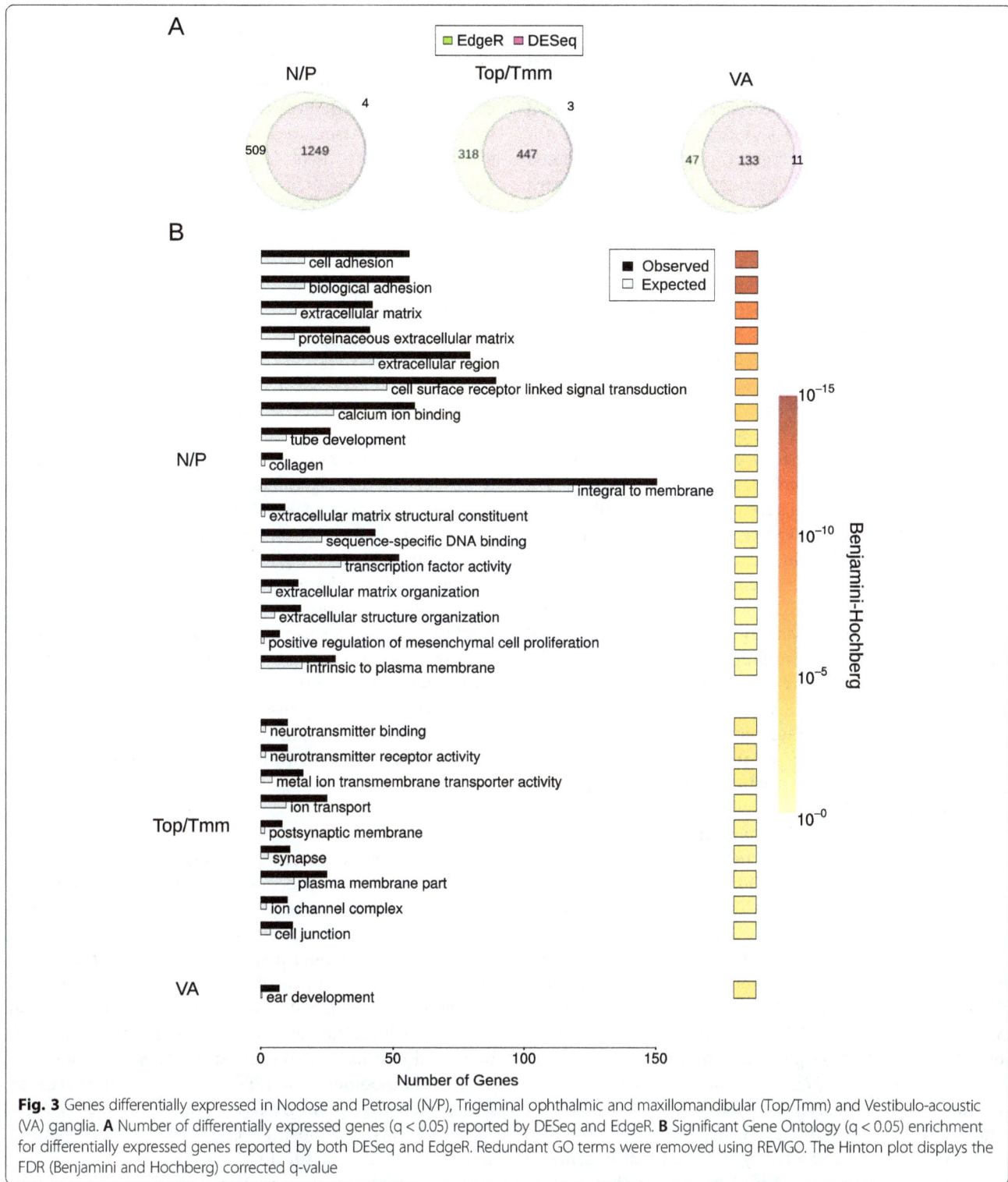

Fig. 3 Genes differentially expressed in Nodose and Petrosal (N/P), Trigeminal ophthalmic and maxillomandibular (Top/Tmm) and Vestibulo-acoustic (VA) ganglia. **A** Number of differentially expressed genes (q < 0.05) reported by DESeq and EdgeR. **B** Significant Gene Ontology (q < 0.05) enrichment for differentially expressed genes reported by both DESeq and EdgeR. Redundant GO terms were removed using REVIGO. The Hinton plot displays the FDR (Benjamini and Hochberg) corrected q-value

and 133 in vestibulo-acoustic (Fig. 3A). The numbers of up-regulated genes for other combinations of ganglia were: nodose: 169; petrosal: 7; trigeminal maxillomandibular: 60; trigeminal ophthalmic: 107; and trigeminal maxillomandibular/trigeminal ophthalmic/vestibulo-acoustic:

708 (Additional file 7: Figure S4A, Additional file 6). No differentially expressed genes were found in the remaining combinations of ganglia. Gene ontology (GO) term analysis showed that each cluster of ganglia was characterised by enrichment of a distinct set of GO categories. The

nodose/petrosal grouping showed the broadest spread of categories, with adhesion and membrane proteins being particularly enriched (Fig. 3B). The trigeminal grouping was the most overtly neuronal with neurotransmitter and ion transport activity terms enriched (Fig. 3B). Satisfyingly, the significant GO category for the vestibulo-acoustic ganglion, which is associated with the ear, was ear development (Fig. 3B). GO terms enrichments for other combinations of ganglia are listed in Additional file 7: Figure S4B.

Identification of high-confidence markers for specific cranial sensory ganglia

Genes identified as being differentially expressed using both DESeq and EdgeR were subjected to stringent selection criteria based on expression level, fold-change, and statistical significance (see Material and Methods) to generate an unbiased panel of genes that best represent individual ganglia and combinations of ganglia (Fig. 4A; Additional file 8). The hierarchical clustering of the resultant 134 markers (Fig. 4A) reflected the division of the cranial sensory ganglia demonstrated by PCA (Fig. 2). The traditional division was represented by 20 markers of the somatosensory ganglia (trigeminal/vestibulo-acoustic) and 72 markers of the viscerosensory ganglia (nodose/petrosal) were found. In addition, we found 9 markers specific for the general somatosensory (trigeminal) and 15 markers for the special somatosensory ganglia (vestibulo-acoustic).

The validity of the marker sets was confirmed by considering genes whose expression has been shown previously to be restricted to specific cranial sensory ganglia. Thus trigeminal ophthalmic expressed PAX3 [10, 28, 29]; trigeminal maxillomandibular/ophthalmic ganglia expressed DRG11 [30–32]; and nodose/petrosal ganglia expressed PHOX2B [11, 21, 33–35]. Our panel of markers included 7 genes expressed in the nodose ganglion but not in the petrosal ganglion. These included the HOX genes HOXB4, -D4, -B5, and -B6 (Fig. 4A) reflecting the well-known distribution of HOX gene expression along the rostro-caudal axis. In line with this, the more anteriorly expressed HOX genes, HOXB1 and -B2 were included in the nodose/petrosal grouping (Fig. 4A).

Surprisingly, POU4F1/BRN3A, a well-known marker of somatosensory neurons in mammals [11, 36], was not among our list of selected markers. This prompted us to verify the presence and identity of POU4 family genes in the chicken genome. We found two genes that correspond to the mammalian Pou4f1/Brn3a and Pou4f2/Brn3b, and an orthologue of amphibian Pou4f1.2 which was not found in mammals (Additional file 9: Figure S5A). Analysis of the number of reads mapping to the POU4F1 and POU4F1.2 loci (see Material and Methods) showed that the two genes collectively are expressed at higher levels

in the somatosensory than in the viscerosensory ganglia, as shown previously by in situ hybridization [14, 37] (Additional file 9: Figure S5B).

GO analysis of the panel of high-confidence marker genes as a whole demonstrated significant enrichments for categories associated with the extracellular compartment, which may be a reflection of signalling processes, and with transcription factors (Fig. 4B; Additional file 10). There were also significant enrichments in terms associated with blood vessel development, likely to reflect the known overlap between mechanisms regulating blood vessel and nerve guidance [38] (Fig. 4B).

Validation and expression pattern of selected markers

Rather than validate gene expression for each grouping of ganglia, we chose to focus on the groupings that gave us markers of distinct sensory modalities, selecting genes representative of trigeminal for general somatosensory, vestibulo-acoustic for special somatosensory, and nodose/petrosal for viscerosensory. From candidates for these ganglia, genes with the highest expression levels and fold change of differential expression were selected for in situ hybridization analysis in wholemount and on sections of chicken embryos at stage HH21 (Figs. 5, 6, 7 and 8). Priority was given to transcription factors because they are most likely to regulate the acquisition of sensory phenotype. We recognise that our validation was not comprehensive and that it does not exclude the possibility that other genes in the panel are equally good or even better markers.

Trigeminal ganglion-specific markers

The localisation of the cranial sensory ganglia in the HH21 chick can be clearly visualised by in situ hybridisation with ISL1, a marker of specific neuronal subsets including sensory neurons, which we include to allow comparison with expression in all ganglia (Fig. 5A). The trigeminal ganglion with two lobes, maxillomandibular and ophthalmic, lies at the level of the anterior hindbrain and in cross-section the ganglion can be seen adjacent to rhombomere (r)2 (Fig. 5A, A'). The transcription factor-encoding gene DRG11 (also known as DRGX, PRRXL1) was our positive control for the trigeminal ganglion [30, 32, 39, 40] (Fig. 5B-B''').

In the category of transcriptional regulators we analysed expression of PRDM12 (PR homology domain-containing member 12). PRDM12, which is essential for human pain perception, and is required for sensory neuron development in mouse and Xenopus [41–43], showed strong trigeminal expression, with little to no staining in the other cranial sensory ganglia (Fig. 5C-C''').

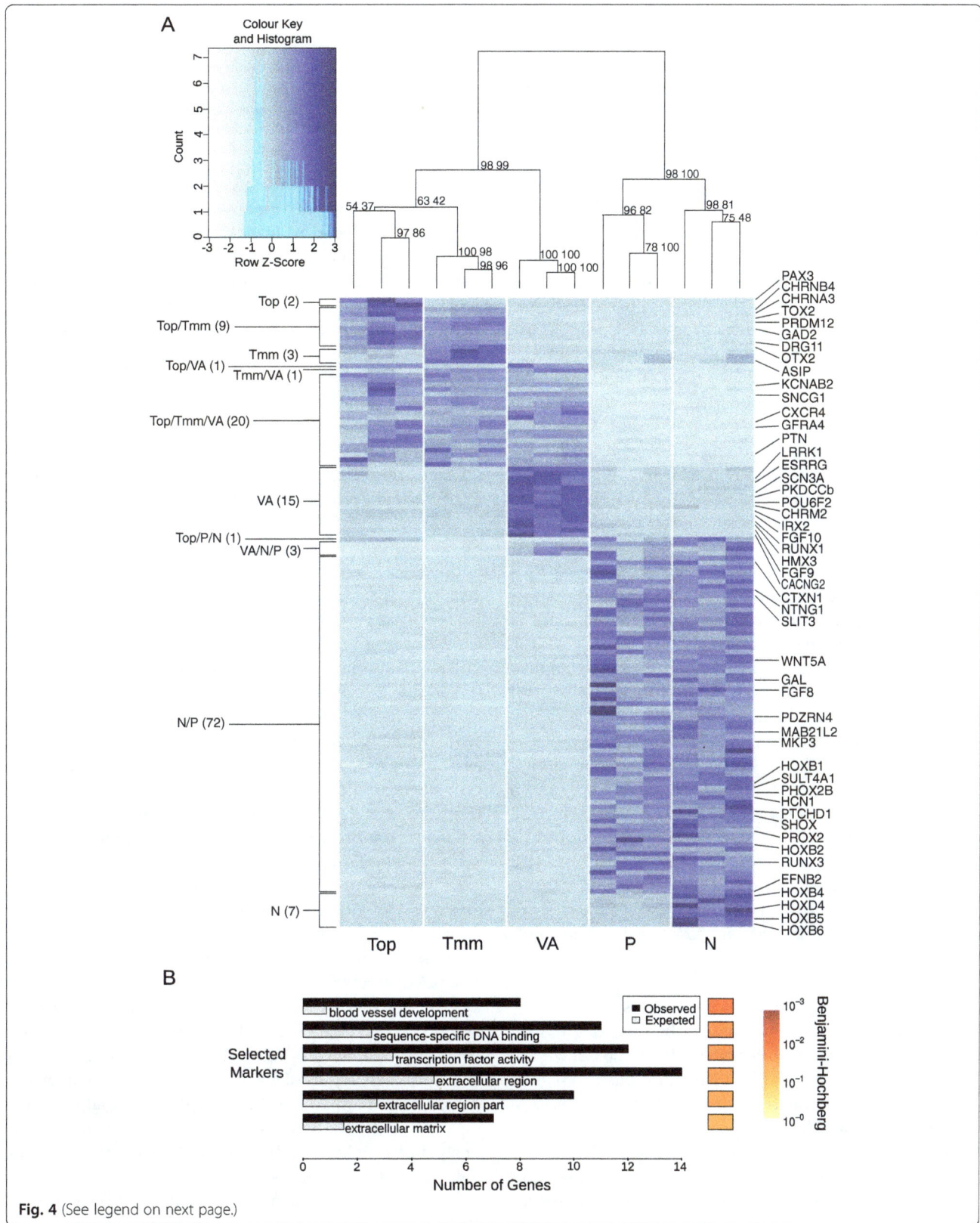

Fig. 4 (See legend on next page.)

As markers with a potential link to adult neuronal function we analysed expression of *GAD2* (GABA synthetic enzyme GAD65) and *CHRNA3* and *CHRNB4* (nicotinic acetylcholine receptor subunits alpha3 and beta4). *GAD2* expression in the PNS has been described in DRG (chick) and trigeminal ganglia (rat), and *Gad2* knockout mice are sensitised to pain [44–46]. Neuronal nicotinic receptors composed of $\alpha 3\beta 4$ subunits that are more restricted in expression than other subtypes, are present and show specific functions in the trigeminal ganglion of rat [47–49]. Our in situ hybridisation analysis showed *GAD2*, *CHRNA3* and *CHRNB4* staining in the trigeminal ganglion (Fig. 5D-F'''), which, in section, was weaker and in fewer neurons than *DRG11* and *PRDM12* (Fig. 5B'-F').

Many of the trigeminal markers were expressed elsewhere in the embryo, but importantly, expression was not seen in the other cranial sensory ganglia (Fig. 5; Table 1). We focus here on hindbrain expression as it is relevant when considering potential sensory circuits. Many of the markers showed expression at the level of r2, the entry point in the hindbrain for trigeminal axons, yet the anatomical extent of staining varied. *PRDM12* was observed in a domain of strong staining in the ventral hindbrain extending from r2 into the spinal cord, and a domain of weaker staining restricted to dorsal r2 (Fig. 5C). *DRG11* was detected in a distinct domain in dorsal r2 extending caudally to the otic vesicle (Fig. 5B). *GAD2* expression was seen to extend anteriorly into r1, but with no distinct domain in r2 (Fig. 5D). Expression of *CHRNA3* and *CHRNB4* was not observed in the hindbrain (Fig. 5E, F).

Vestibulo-acoustic ganglion-specific markers

The vestibulo-acoustic ganglion can be seen clearly with *ISL1* expression, located anterior-medial to the otic vesicle (Fig. 5A) In cross-section the vestibulo-acoustic ganglion is localised between the anterior otic vesicle and r4/r5 of the hindbrain (Fig. 5A'').

There was not a strong positive control gene for the vestibulo-acoustic ganglion because a molecular distinction between special and general somatosensory has not been described previously. However, two transcriptional regulators, *ESRRG* (estrogen-related receptor gamma) and *HMX3* (H6 family homeobox 3; also known as *NKX5.1*), have demonstrated roles in the development of inner ear structures and are important for hearing in both mice and humans [50–55]. Here our analysis showed expression of *HMX3* in the ventromedial vestibulo-acoustic ganglion and *ESRRG* in the dorsolateral vestibulo-acoustic ganglion, as well as in nascent neuronal cells migrating into the vestibulo-acoustic ganglion from the otic vesicle (Fig. 6A-B''').

In the category of transcriptional regulators, we analysed expression of *IRX2* (Iroquois homeobox gene family member 2); *POU6F2* (POU domain, class 6, transcription factor 2; also known as *RPF1*) and, *RUNX1* (*runt*-related transcription factor 1; also known as *AML1*, *Cbfa2*). Expression patterns of *IRX2* and *POU6F2* have been described in the developing chick and mouse but no role has been reported in the vestibulo-acoustic ganglion [56–59]. In mouse *RUNX1* has a role in the development of the vestibulo-acoustic ganglion [60] but is also expressed in TrkA+ nociceptive sensory neurons of the head and trunk, including a scattered population in the trigeminal ganglion [60, 61]. In our analysis *IRX2* expression was seen in the whole vestibulo-acoustic ganglion as well as the ventral otic vesicle corresponding to the location of vestibulo-acoustic ganglion neuron production (Fig. 6C''). *POU6F2* and *RUNX1* were expressed specifically in sub-divisions of the dorsolateral vestibulo-acoustic ganglion (Fig. 6D'', E'').

As markers with a potential link to signalling we analysed expression of the signalling molecule *FGF9*, and two kinases: *LRRK1* (leucine-rich repeat kinase 1) and *PKDCCB* (protein kinase domain containing, cytoplasmic b; ENSGALG00000011166: a paralogue of PKDCC also known as VLK). *FGF9* is important for development of aspects of the inner ear including the cochlear sensory cells (also known as hair cells), but weak expression has also been reported in the mouse cochlear/acoustic ganglion (part of the vestibulo-acoustic ganglion complex) [62, 63]. Neither *LRRK1* nor *PKDCCB* has previously been linked to the vestibulo-acoustic complex [64–67]. Our analysis showed expression of FGF9 in the whole vestibulo-acoustic ganglion and *LRRK* and *PKDCCB* in the dorsolateral vestibulo-acoustic ganglion (Fig. 6F-F'' and Fig. 7A-B'').

As a marker linked to adult neuronal function we analysed expression of *SCN3A* (voltage gated sodium

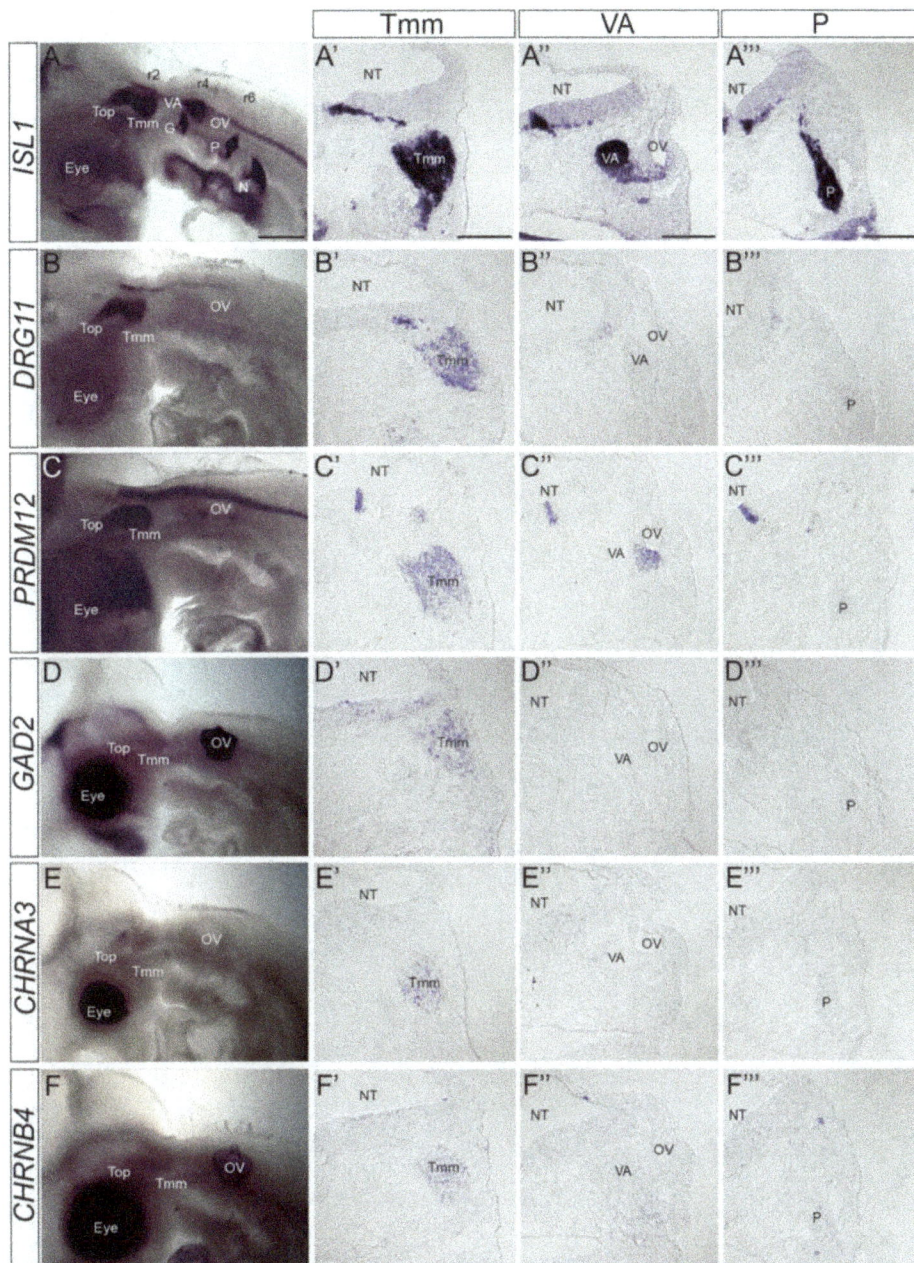

Fig. 5 Expression patterns of trigeminal ganglion-specific markers. A) Wholemount in situ hybridization of *ISL1* at HH21 to provide anatomical localisation of all cranial sensory ganglia. A'-A''') Transverse sections stained with *ISL1* at HH21 to provide comparative sections for other markers at the level of Tmm ganglion (A'); VA ganglion (A''); and P ganglion (A'''). B-F) Wholemount in situ hybridization of trigeminal ganglion specific markers at HH22. B'-F''') Transverse sections at the level of the Tmm ganglion (B'-F'), VA ganglion (B''-F'') and P ganglion (B'''-F''') stained with the named marker at HH21, showing Tmm-specific expression. B-B''') *DRG11*; C-C''') *PRDM12*; D-D''') *GAD2*; E-E''') *CHRNA3*; F-F''') *CHRNB4*. Levels of staining in the trigeminal ganglion vary, but are stronger when compared with other ganglia. Staining can be seen in the NT although specific localisation and level varies. The dark staining in the eye and OV in D-F was not observed on sections and likely represents background. Abbreviations: G: geniculate ganglion; N: nodose ganglion; NT: neural tube; OV: otic vesicle; P: petrosal ganglion; r: rhombomere; Top: trigeminal ophthalmic lobe; Tmm: trigeminal maxillomandibular lobe; VA: vestibulo-acoustic ganglion. Scalebars: A-F: 500 μm; A'-F''': 150 μm

channel type 3, alpha subunit) which in humans lies within a chromosomal locus associated with hearing loss. Expression of *SCN3A* has not been characterised in the vestibulo-acoustic ganglion in humans or mice [68].

Our analysis showed expression in the dorsolateral vestibulo-acoustic ganglion (Fig. 7C, C'').

In addition to the vestibulo-acoustic ganglion, all of the analysed genes showed expression elsewhere in the

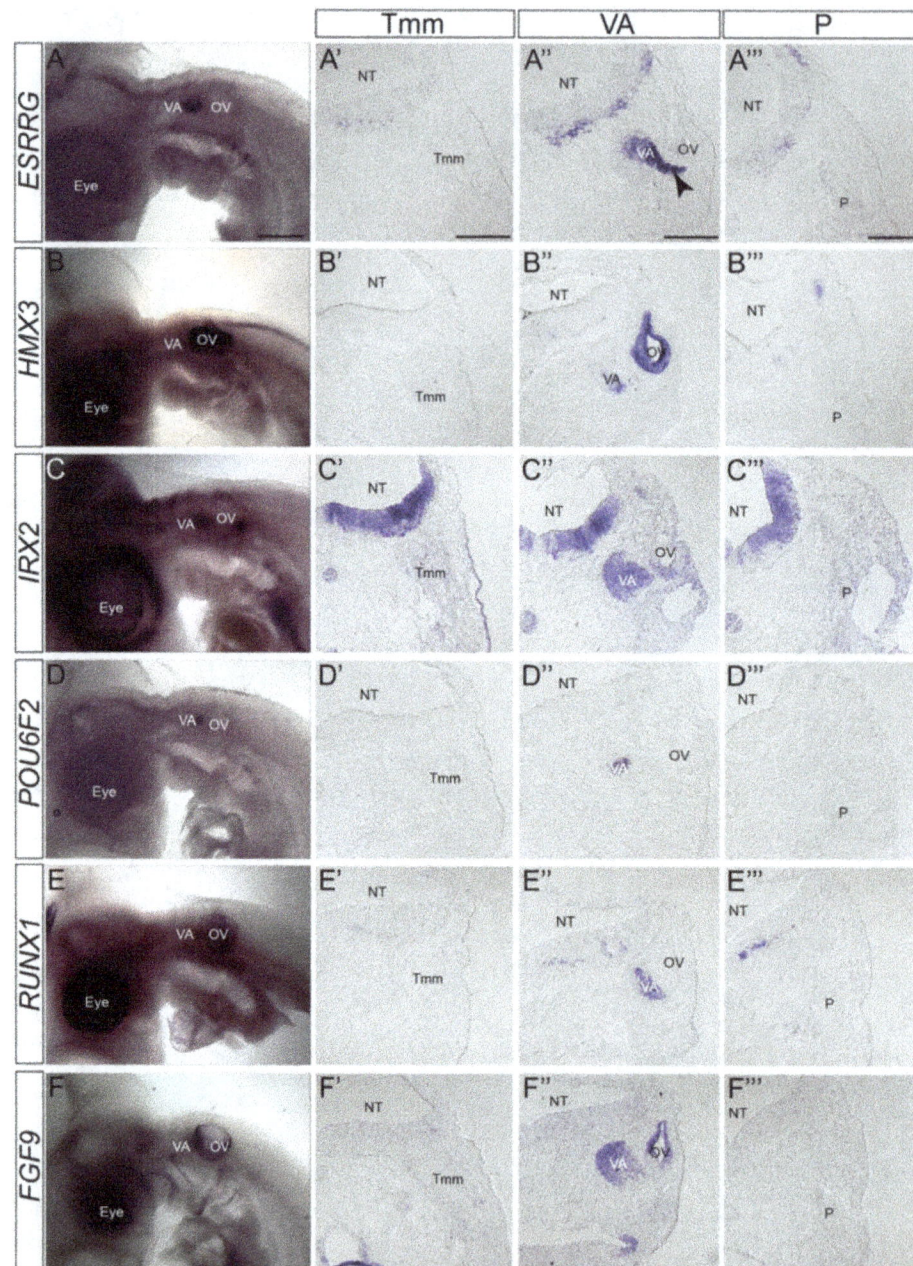

Fig. 6 Expression patterns of vestibulo-acoustic ganglion-specific markers. A-F) Wholemount in situ hybridization of vestibulo-acoustic ganglion specific markers at HH21. A'-F") Transverse sections at the level of the Tmm ganglion (A'-F'), VA ganglion (A"-F") and P ganglion (A'''-F''') stained with the named marker at HH21, showing VA-specific expression. A-A") *ESRRG*; B-B") HMX3; C-C") *IRX2*; D-D") *POU6F2*; E-E") *RUNX1*; F-F") *FGF9*. Levels of staining in the vestibulo-acoustic ganglion vary, but are stronger when compared with other ganglia. In *ESRRG* staining is also seen in nascent neurons migrating from the OV (*arrowhead*). Staining can be seen in the NT although specific localisation and level varies. The dark staining in the eye and OV in B and E was not observed on sections and likely represents background. Abbreviations: NT: neural tube; OV: otic vesicle; P: petrosal ganglion; Tmm: trigeminal maxillomandibular lobe; VA: vestibulo-acoustic ganglion; arrowhead: nascent neurons migrating from OV. Scalebars: A-I: 500 μm; A'-I": 150 μm

embryo (Figs. 6 and 7; Table 1). *SCN3A* and *LRRK1* showed weak staining in other cranial sensory ganglia, but were significantly stronger in the vestibulo-acoustic ganglion. Within the hindbrain the extent of expression varied. Analysis of sections at r4, the site of vestibulo-

acoustic ganglion axon entry, showed *ESRRG, POU6F2, PKDCCB,* and *SCN3A* staining in a similar pattern from dorsal to ventral (Fig. 6A", D" and Fig. 7B", C"). *HMX3* and *RUNX1* were expressed in discrete domains in dorsal r4 and in ventral regions extending beyond r4 (Fig. 6B",

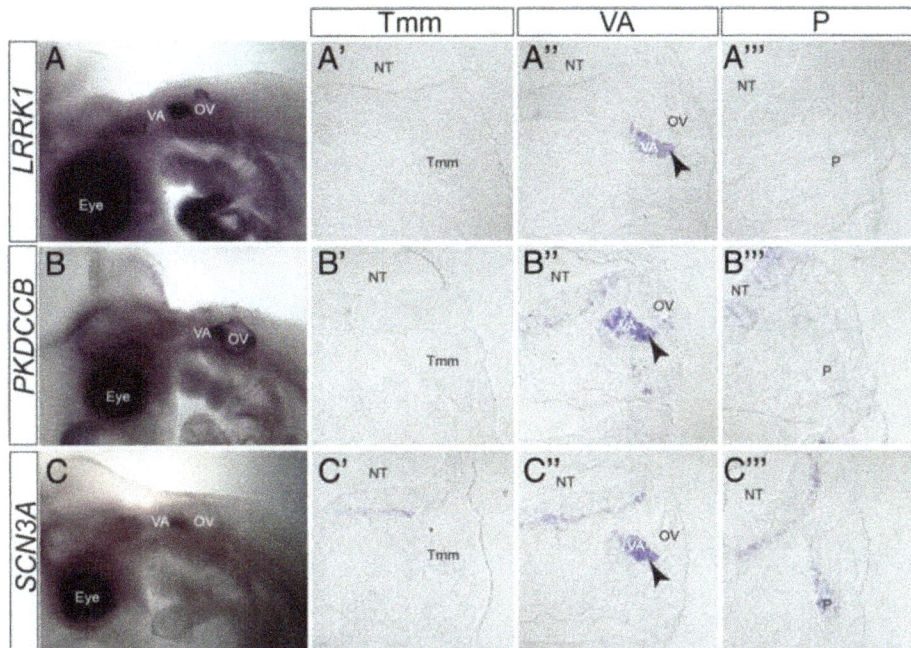

Fig. 7 Expression patterns of vestibulo-acoustic ganglion-specific markers. A-C) Wholemount in situ hybridization of vestibulo-acoustic ganglion specific markers at HH21. A'-C'') Transverse sections at the level of the Tmm ganglion (A'-C'), VA ganglion (A''-C'') and P ganglion (A'''-C''') stained with the named marker at HH21, showing VA-specific expression. A-A''') LRRK1; B-B''') PKDCCB; C-C''') SCN3A. Levels of staining in the vestibulo-acoustic ganglion vary, but are stronger when compared with other ganglia. In LRRK1, PKDCCB and SCN3A staining is also seen in nascent neurons migrating from the OV (arrowhead). Staining can be seen in the NT although specific localisation and level varies. The dark staining in the eye and OV in A-C was not observed on sections and likely represents background. Abbreviations: NT: neural tube; OV: otic vesicle; P: petrosal ganglion; Tmm: trigeminal maxillomandibular lobe; VA: vestibulo-acoustic ganglion; arrowhead: nascent neurons migrating from OV. Scalebars: A-I: 500 μm; A'-I''': 150 μm

E''). *LRRK1* signal was found in a restricted ventral domain (Fig. 7A'') while *IRX2* and *FGF9* staining was broadly distributed throughout the r4 neuroepithelium (Fig. 6C'', F'').

Epibranchial ganglia-specific markers

The petrosal and nodose ganglia represent the epibranchial series of cranial sensory ganglia which can be identified clearly in the HH21 *ISL1* stained embryo (Fig. 5A). In cross-section, we focused on the petrosal ganglion located near the pharyngeal endoderm, at a distance from r6/7 of the hindbrain (Fig. 5A'''). The transcription factor *PHOX2B* represented the positive control for the epibranchial ganglia [21, 33–35] (Fig. 8A, A''').

We analysed expression of two transcription factors-encoding genes: *PROX2* (*prospero*-related homeobox gene family, member 2) and *SHOX* (short stature homeobox transcription factor). *PROX2* expression has been described in cranial sensory ganglia in zebrafish and more specifically in the epibranchial ganglia in mouse [69, 70]. *SHOX*, important for growth in humans and zebrafish, is absent in mouse where instead the related gene *Shox2* is required for long bone growth [71–73]. Roles for mouse *Shox2* in neuronal development have been shown, and expression reported in cranial sensory ganglia [74, 75]. Our

analysis showed specific expression of *PROX2* and *SHOX* in the epibranchial ganglia (Fig. 8B-C'''). In cross section the staining for these markers was scattered throughout the ganglion, suggesting that these genes' expression may differentiate subsets of neurons (Fig. 8B''', C''').

Other genes which we identified as good markers of the epibranchial ganglia have not been well studied at either the expression or functional level. *CTXN1* (Cortexin 1), encodes a single trans-membrane domain protein identified in mouse and rat cortex [76]. *PDZRN4* (PDZ and Ring domain-containing family member 4; also known as *LNX4* (ligand of Numb protein-X)) was identified *in silico* and remains largely uncharacterised [77–79]. *SULT4A1* is a member of the sulfotransferase family, cytosolic enzymes proposed to play roles in the modulation of certain neurotransmitters, and is expressed in the human and rat brain [80, 81]. Our analysis showed expression in the epibranchial ganglia (Fig. 8D-F). As for *PROX2* and *SHOX*, the proportion of cells stained in the petrosal ganglion varied with each marker (Fig. 8E''', F''').

All of these genes showed expression elsewhere in the embryo, with the most restricted being *PROX2* (Fig. 8; Table 1). *SULT4A1* showed weak staining in the other

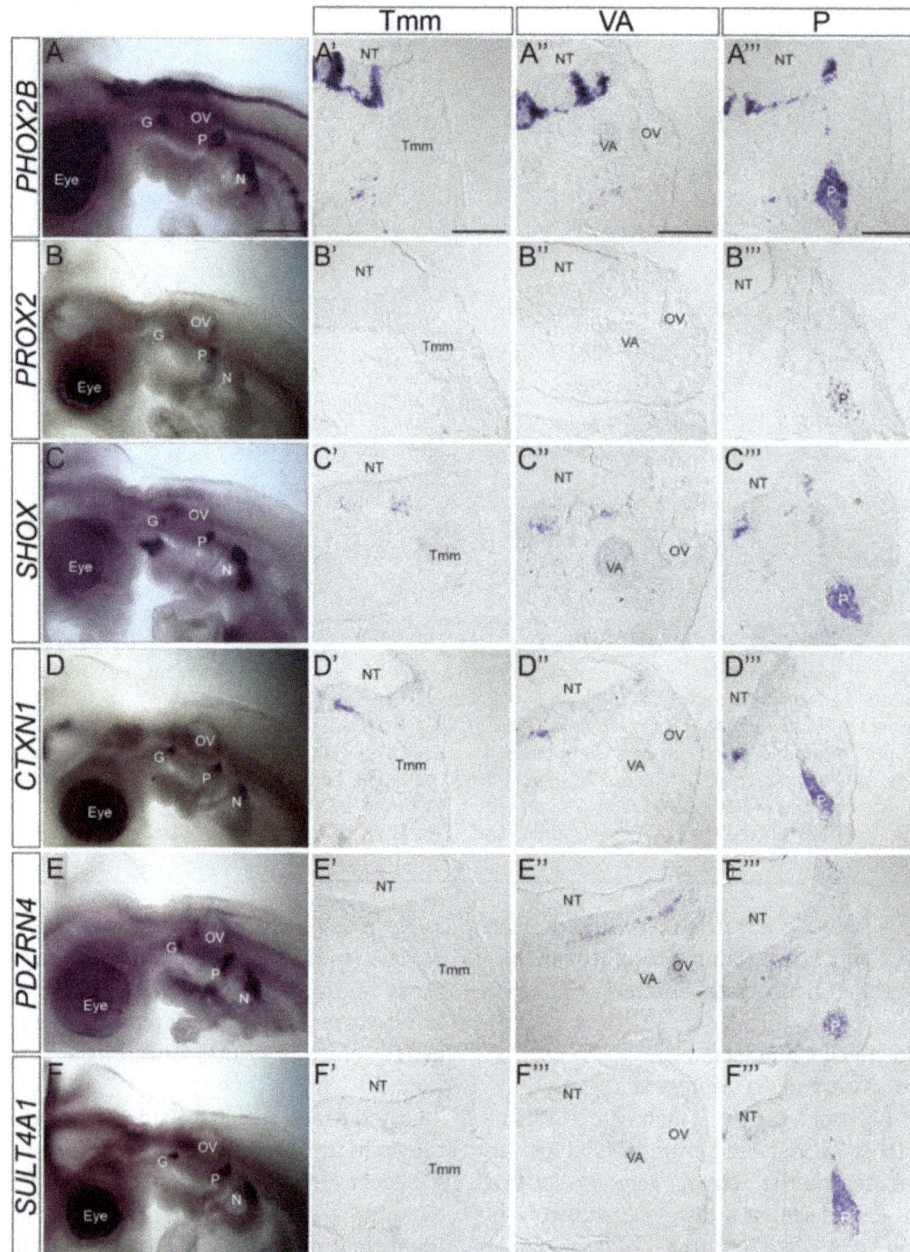

Fig. 8 Expression patterns of epibranchial ganglia-specific markers. A-F) Wholemount in situ hybridization of epibranchial ganglia-specific markers at HH21. A'-F''') Transverse sections at the level of the Tmm ganglion (A'-F'), VA ganglion (A''-F'') and P ganglion (A'''-F''') stained with the named marker at HH21, showing P-specific expression. A-A''') PHOX2B; B-B''') PROX2; C-C''') SHOX; D-D''') CTXN1; E-E''') PDZRN4; F-F''') SULT4A1. Levels of staining in the epibranchial ganglia vary, but are stronger when compared with other ganglia. Staining can be seen in the NT although specific localisation and level varies. The dark staining in the eye and OV in A, B, D and F was not observed on sections and likely represents background. Abbreviations: G: geniculate ganglion; N: nodose ganglion; NT: neural tube; OV: otic vesicle; P: petrosal ganglion; Tmm: trigeminal maxillomandibular lobe; VA: vestibulo-acoustic ganglion. Scalebars: A-F: 500 μm; A'-F''': 150 μm

cranial sensory ganglia, but was significantly stronger in the epibranchial ganglia (Fig. 8F'-F'''). In the hindbrain our analysis focused on r6, the site of entry for petrosal axons. SHOX expression resembled that of PHOX2B, with discrete staining in dorsal and ventral domains, and a small number of stained cells extending between these

two domains (Fig. 8A''', C'''). PDZRN4 also showed distinct dorsal and ventral domains of staining (Fig. 8E'''), while CTXN1 or SULT4A1 expression was restricted to a very small ventral domain (Fig. 8D'''; F''').

The expression patterns of 20 out of 26 tested markers validated the differential expression in cranial

Table 1 Summary of selected marker genes expression in the head as assessed by in situ hybridization

		Cranial sensory ganglia						Other PNS sites
		Top	Tmm	VA	G	P	N	
Trigeminal	DRG11	+++	+++	-	-	-	-	
	PRDM12	+++	+++	-	+ (distal)	+ (distal)	+ (distal)	Olfactory epithelium, ciliary ganglion, otic macular patches
	GAD2	++	++	-	-	-	-	
	CHRNB4	+	+	-	-	-	-	
	CHRNA3	+	+	-	-	-	-	
	TOX2	(+)	(+)	-	-	-	-	
	OTX2	(+)	(+)	-	-	-	-	Ventral otic vesicle
Vestibulo-acoustic	ESSRG	-	-	+++	-	-	-	
	PKDCCB	-	-	+++	-	-	-	Otic macular patches
	LRRK1	+ (distal)	+ (distal)	+++	-	-	-	
	POU6F2	+ (distal)	+ (distal)	+++	-	-	-	
	RUNX1	-	-	++	-	-	-	
	IRX2	-	-	++	-	-	-	Otic vesicle
	FGF9	-	-	++	-	-	-	
	SCN3A	+	+	+++	+	+	+	Terminal nerve ganglion
	HMX3	-	-	+	-	-	-	Dorsal otic vesicle
Epibranchial	PHOX2B	-	-	-	+++	+++	+++	Ciliary ganglion
	PROX2	-	-	-	++	++	++	Lens
	CTXN1	-	-	-	+++	+++	+++	
	SULT4A1	+ (distal)	+ (distal)	+	+++	+++	+++	Ciliary ganglion, terminal nerve ganglion
	PDZRN4	-	-	-	++	++	++	
	SHOX2	-	-	+	+++	+++	+++	
	LHX4	-	-	-	-	(+)	(+)	
	MECOM	-	-	-	-	-	-	
	PRRX1	-	-	-	-	-	-	Medial otic vesicle
	PRRX2	-	-	-	-	-	-	

Expression levels at stage HH21 are given for the cranial sensory ganglia (Top trigeminal ophthalmic, Tmm trigeminal maxillomandibular, VA vestibulo-acoustic, G geniculate, P petrosal, N nodose), as well as other sites in the PNS

sensory ganglia revealed by RNA-seq (Table 1). For each group there were exceptions where the in situ hybridisation analysis did not match expectations. These fell into two categories: i) genes which showed no, or very low, in situ signal where expected (*LHX4, OTX2, TOX2*) (Additional file 11: Figure S6A-C); and ii) genes which showed high in situ signal in surrounding tissue but not in the ganglion (*MECOM, PRRX1* and *PRRX2*) (Additional file 11: Figure S6D-F).

Discussion and conclusions

It has long been recognised that the cranial sensory ganglia represent distinct sensory functions. Nevertheless, analysis of mechanisms underlying the development of specific cranial sensory modalities has been limited by the paucity of markers for the different cell populations. To overcome this restriction we set out to identify molecular signatures for the distinct cranial sensory ganglia at early stages of neuronal differentiation. Here we report the generation of ganglion-specific expression profiles using transcriptome-wide analysis of placode-derived neurons from isolated cranial sensory ganglia in the developing chicken embryo. Differential expression analysis of the resultant data set showed differences in the profiles that correlate with distinct functions and sensory modalities. Principal component analysis revealed three separate clusters, capturing the segregation of the cranial sensory ganglia into viscerosensory epibranchial ganglia (nodose/petrosal); general somatosensory trigeminal ganglia; and special somatosensory ganglia (vestibulo-acoustic ganglion). Our study was not designed to assess the distinction between cranial and trunk sensory neurons. Using stringent selection criteria, we report a total of 134 marker genes specific for particular cranial ganglia or groups of ganglia, and show validation of 20/26 by in situ hybridization. Of our panel of marker genes, around 20 were known to have either described expression in sensory neurons, or a link to dysfunction of the relevant sensory system. However, 113 were entirely novel, with no previously described sensory neuron-specific expression. Importantly, we identify and validate several marker genes that differentiate between the trigeminal and vestibulo-acoustic neurons, providing the first molecular signature for the distinction between embryonic "general" and "special" somatosensory neurons. Our validation was restricted to a single stage (HH 21) in a single species (chick), and the observed differential expression might be a consequence of temporal differences in the onset of expression. However, we expect the markers to be generally valid across stages and vertebrate species.

The range of genes encompassed by our panel included transcriptional regulators, components of signalling pathways and ion channels (Fig. 4; Additional file 8). As a resource this panel of ganglion-specific markers will enable us to analyse experiments in greater depth to further our understanding of the acquisition of the respective sensory modality. They will be important in unambiguously determining the fate adopted by cells when extracellular signals or transcriptional regulators are modulated in experimental settings, for example in protocols aimed to derive specific sensory neurons from human pluripotent stem cells [82].

At an individual gene level, it will be interesting to investigate their roles in producing or maintaining sensory phenotype through knockdown and ectopic expression in the future. It is possible that transcription factors play a role as regulators of cell type identity, acting in concert with known genes such as *BRN3A* and *PHOX2B* [11, 83]. We also note that several ligands and receptors, all of which have a demonstrated role in cell migration and/or axon guidance, were expressed differentially between the classes of cranial sensory ganglia, such as the netrin family gene *NTNG1* and the Robo ligand *SLIT3* in nodose/petrosal viscerosensory neurons, or the chemokine receptor *CXCR4* in trigeminal (ophthalmic/maxillomandibular) and vestibulo-acoustic somatosensory neurons [84–86].

The ganglion-specific expression was readily apparent for the majority of the markers tested. Within each group we found cases which further showed expression in the target region for ganglionic projections in the hindbrain. For example, we showed expression of *ESSRG* and *POU6F2* in the dorsal-most domain

specifically at r4-5 level, where vestibulo-acoustic ganglion afferents enter the brainstem. Such co-ordinate gene expression in both sensory neurons and their target central neurons has been shown to be important for correct connectivity in both head and trunk [11, 39, 87]. Thus, our data supports the idea of a "sensory type code" aligning sensory neurons with central neurons of the same circuit. This might have functional consequences in the establishment of specific viscero- and somatosensory circuits and/or represent ancient evolutionary relationships.

Genome-wide analysis of gene expression considered pooled populations of neurons from each cranial ganglion, revealing groups of viscerosensory, general somatosensory and special somatosensory neurons. Our analysis of expression patterns by in situ hybridisation demonstrated that, as established in the trunk somatosensory population [2, 3], there are further subsets within these populations. It is recognised that the vestibulo-acoustic ganglion represents a complex of two smaller ganglia individually containing neurons involved in balance and hearing [88]. Interestingly, comparison in transverse section of all vestibulo-acoustic ganglion markers showed that they occupied different regions (Figs. 6 and 7). This may be due to expression in specific subgroups of neurons such as vestibular neurons versus auditory neurons, known to occupy separate regions within the vestibulo-acoustic ganglion complex in mouse [88]. Further analysis would have to be performed to determine the allocation to specific functions. Many of the trigeminal and epibranchial ganglia markers exhibited scattered expression rather than homogeneous staining throughout the ganglion as observed for *ISL1* or *PHOX2B* (Figs. 5, 6, 7 and 8). Thus, our markers highlight further complexity in the specific subtypes of sensory neuron.

The broad distinction between viscero- and somatosensory neurons has been more widely studied. The viscerosensory system is important in controlling the body's internal milieu including many autonomic reflexes such as baroreflex regulation of the cardiovascular system [89], hypoxia regulation of the ventilatory response [90] and nutrient-induced inhibition of food-intake [91]. The general somatosensory system is involved in response to external stimuli: in rodents the importance of touch from the whiskers can be seen in the somatotopy of the whisker barrels in the cerebral cortex [92]; in humans trigeminal involvement in pain sensation can become problematic leading to migraine and trigeminal neuralgia [93]. To date the molecular fingerprint used to recognise developing viscerosensory neurons is *Phox2a + Phox2b + Ret + Brn3a− Drg11− Runx1−*, while that for somatosensory neurons is *Phox2a− Phox2b− Ret− Brn3a + Drg11+ Runx1+*. Using this limited marker set, a seminal study found that *Phox2b* acts as a regulatory switch between the two phenotypes: in *Phox2b* mutant mice, the neurons of the epibranchial ganglia up regulate *Brn3a* leading to expression of *Drg11* and *Runx1*, and hence to the conclusion that they become somatosensory [11]. It would be interesting to re-examine this situation more closely using our data set to determine how complete this transition is, and whether the resulting somatosensory cells are more similar to trigeminal or vestibulo-acoustic neurons.

Analysis in *Brn3a* mutant mice showed changes in the subtype of somatosensory neuron specified within the trigeminal ganglion, but did not examine whether the neurons switched to a viscerosensory phenotype [83]. The studies did however, show a de-repression of genes interpreted as non-neuronal [94]. Interestingly using our panel of markers for specific cranial sensory neuronal populations, we can now identify some of these genes as markers of the viscerosensory ganglia (e.g., *ANGPTL1*; *PROX2*) or special somatosensory ganglia (e.g., *IRX2*) [94].

A complementary approach to address the generation of different cranial sensory neuron phenotypes has been to focus on the embryonic origins of the cranial sensory ganglia. There are distinct neurogenic placodes for each cranial sensory ganglion, each of which has an individual developmental profile [95, 96]. Many studies have built up our understanding of patterning the specific neurogenic placodes within the cranial ectoderm across species [97]. However, while this describes the mechanisms underlying the generation of the neurogenic placodes, it does not address how or why progenitors located in different placodes acquire distinct neuronal phenotypes. It will be interesting to interfere with aspects of neurogenic placode development, for example by transplantation or treatment with specific signalling molecules [7, 9, 10], and to use our panel of molecular markers to determine the effects on viscero- versus somatosensory neuronal differentiation.

The organisation and function of the cranial sensory ganglia is highly conserved across vertebrates. The origin of the cranial sensory ganglia from neurogenic placodes also attracts considerable interest from an evolutionary perspective. Historically neurogenic placodes have, together with neural crest cells, been suggested to be vertebrate innovations, enabling the transition to a predatory lifestyle [98], and their presence in other organisms has been examined [96, 97, 99, 100]. As with development, many of the studies to date focus on the evolution of neurogenic placodes rather than their derived sensory neurons. Provided homologous genes can be found in other organisms, our molecular profiles will be invaluable in considering the evolutionary origin of the distinct sensory neuronal phenotypes [96].

Methods
Embryonic dissection
Fertilized chicken eggs (Winter Egg Farm, UK) were incubated in a humidified chamber at 38 °C to the correct Hamburger and Hamilton (HH) stage of development [22]. To compensate for differences in the timing of migration and neuronal differentiation/maturation in the different ganglia relative to the age of the embryo, trigeminal maxillomandibular and ophthalmic and vestibulo-acoustic ganglia were dissected at HH18, while the nodose and petrosal were dissected at HH23 [7, 21]. These stages also take into account that neural crest-derived neurons differentiate at later stages in the respective ganglia [6, 8]. The cranial nerve ganglia were dissected in L15 medium (Gibco) using electrolytically sharpened 0.125 mm tungsten wire, nerve processes and mesenchyme were removed and pooled ganglia kept on ice in L15 for 0–3 h until dissociation. For each ganglion type, the left and right ganglia of 40–60 embryos were pooled. All three replicates of the different ganglia were collected independently from new individuals.

Electroporations and immunostaining on sections
Eggs were windowed at HH12 and pCAβ-EGFPm5 vector electroporated into the neural crest on one side of the embryo ($n = 4$) using an Electro Square Porator ECM 830 (BTX.Inc) by applying 5 pulses (6 V, 25 ms) at 1 s intervals. Eggs were sealed and incubated until HH18. The embryos were fixed in 4 % paraformaldehyde in phosphate buffered saline (PBS) for 2 h on ice, kept in 30 % sucrose in PBS for 3 h at 4 °C and embedded in OCT compound (Andwin Scientific) for cryosectioning. 10 µm sections were stained with anti-NFM (clone RMO270, Invitrogen, 1:5000) primary and Alexa596 anti-mouse (Life Technologies) secondary antibodies.

Antibody staining and FACS
Cells were dissociated in trypsin-EDTA (Gibco) for 5 min at 37 °C followed by inactivation with defined trypsin inhibitors (Gibco) and trituration with a 200 µl pipette tip. At all subsequent steps cells were pelleted in protein LoBind tubes (Eppendorf) at 500xg for 1 min at 4 °C and otherwise kept on ice. Live cells were treated with Near-IR fixable live/dead stain (Invitrogen) in PBS for 5 min according to the manufacturer's instructions. Cells were fixed for 10–15 min in 200 µl 4 % paraformaldehyde made in MOPS buffered saline (MBS) containing 0.1 M MOPS pH7.4, 1 mM EGTA, 2 mM $MgSO_4$ and 125 mM NaCl. Cells were permeabilized in permeabilization buffer (PB) containing 2 % BSA, 0.1 % saponin, 5 mM DTT and 100U/ml RNAse inhibitor (Roche) in MBS. Remnants of paraformaldehyde were inactivated by addition of glycine pH 8.0 to a final concentration of 100 mM. Cells were

subsequently incubated 10–15 min on ice in anti-NFM in PB (clone RMO270, Invitrogen, 1:5000). The primary antibody was replaced by anti-mouse Alexa488 secondary antibody in PB (Invitrogen, 1:1000) and cells were incubated 10 min on ice. Cells were washed briefly in MOPS-RNasin-DTT-BSA (MRDB) buffer containing 2 % BSA, 5 mM DTT and 100U/ml RNAse inhibitor (Roche) in MBS, re-suspended in 70 μl RNA-later (Ambion) and kept overnight at 4 °C. Cells were diluted by addition of 250 ml MRDB, pelleted and resuspended in 400 μl MRDB. Cells were sorted on a MoFlo Astrios sorter. Gates were set using a control sample from HH23 limb bud treated in the same way as the cranial nerve ganglia samples. The control limb sample included 50 % of cells killed by a 5 min 60 °C heat shock to set the gate for live/dead staining. Cells were sorted into 1.5 ml protein low-bind tubes containing 70 μl MRDB chilled to 4 °C during sorting. The cells were pelleted in MRDB and lyzed in RLT lysis buffer (Qiagen) containing 1 % 2-mercaptoethanol.

RNA extraction and sequencing

Total RNA was extracted using an RNeasy micro kit (Qiagen) using the modified protocol for fixed cells as per the manufacturer's instructions. Genomic DNA was eliminated by an on-column DNase-I treatment. RNA integrity was assessed using the Experion system (Biorad) and RNA quantity was measured using Qubit high-sensitivity kit. Libraries were prepared using Illumina mRNA-seq kit incorporating poly-(A) selection without further amplification and 100 bp paired-end reads were sequenced on an Illumina Hi-seq 2000 platform at the High-Throughput Genomics unit at the Wellcome Trust Centre for Human Genomics, Oxford, UK. Three biological replicates of each sample were generated and assigned to different lanes, with 5 samples multiplexed on each lane. The raw reads have been uploaded to the Short Read Archive (SRA, Accession number SRP068496).

Read mapping, quantification, and differential expression

Read quality was assessed using FASTQC. rRNA reads were identified by mapping the raw reads to chicken rRNA sequences (accession numbers: Galga 18S rRNA HQ873432.1; Galga 28S rRNA EF552813.1; Galga 5S rRNA NR046276.1; Galga 5.8S rRNA DQ018753.1) and removed from the dataset. After removal of the identified rRNA, unprocessed reads were aligned to the galGal4 chicken genome assembly (Ensembl Release 71) using the splice-aware sequence aligner Gsnap [101]. MISO [102] was used to determine an average expected insert size of 116 ± 72 bp. These values were then applied in a subsequent Gsnap iteration for more accurate paired alignment. HTseq

count [103] was used on the most conservative setting (intersection strict) to count reads mapped to gene models, which were determined using the Ensembl galGal4 reference genome, version 71. Normalization was performed with DEseq [26] and EdgeR [104]. Differential expression analysis was performed with both DESeq and EdgeR, with differentially expressed genes defined as only those returned by both of these methods of analysis, with an FDR (q-value) of 0.05 or below.

Selection of markers

Prior to estimating the gene expression of ganglia-specific markers, duplicated read pairs were identified using Picard Tools' Mark Duplicates function. Markers were selected from this pool of differentially expressed genes through the following criteria: 1) expression levels 1.5-fold higher in all samples of the high-group than all samples in the low-group; 2) minimum RPKM of 10 in the high-group; and 3) q-value < 0.05 in both DESeq and EdgeR analyses.

Functional annotation

Gene Ontology (GO) term enrichment analyses were implemented through DAVID [105]. This analysis was applied to the differentially expressed genes identified for each ganglion and groups of ganglia in turn, against a background of all expressed genes, where expressed genes are defined as those where at least one transcript of that gene had a minimum of 80 % coverage. The threshold for significance was set as below 0.05 for the Benjamini and Hochberg q-value returned by DAVID.

Analysis of POU4F1

Since no gene model for POU4F1 was included in the genome version used, reads mapped as described to the GENBANK model XM_003640558.2 were counted using HTseq with the same settings as for the Ensembl gene models as described above.

Pou4 family protein sequences were collected from GENBANK using a BLASTp approach and aligned using MAFFT with default settings. The alignment was trimmed manually in BioEdit [106]. A maximum likelihood tree was built using MEGA version 5.2 [107]. The Jones-Taylor-Thornton (JTT) amino acid substitution matrix was used and 150 bootstrap iterations were used to obtain support values at each node.

Cloning

Chick cDNA from HH18-24 heads was used for PCR cloning of the markers tested. See primers below. Products were cloned into pGEMT (Promega) or pCRII (Invitrogen).

Gene name	Forward primer	Reverse primer
CHRNA3	ATGTGACCTGGATACCCCA	CTTCATCACTGGTCGGCCTT
CHRNB4	AGTGTGAACGAACGAGAGCA	ACAGGTAGGCTGGGAGTCTT
CTXN1	GAGCTCTCGGTCTGCACAG	CATCCCTGCCCTCTACACCA
ESRRG	TCTGACGGACAGCATCAACC	AGGGTTCAGGTACGGGCTAT
FGF9	TTTGCTCAGTGACCACCTGG	TCAGGGTCCACTGGTCTAGG
GAD2	TGGTGTTGAAAGGGCCAACT	TCCTGATGAGTTGCTGCTGG
HMX3	CAAGAACCTGCTCAACGGAG	CGCTTCATGTCGAAGGTGGA
IRX2	CAGGGTTACCTCTACCAGCC	TTGCAAGCTGATCCCTTCGT
LHX4	TACCTGATGGAGGACGGGAG	CTCGGAGAGGATCTGGTCGT
LRRK1	CCTTGCCTACCTGCACAAGA	CTGCTACGAGTCCATCCGAC
MECOM	AAAGCCATGGTAACCAGCCA	ATTGGATGGCGCTGGATTCT
OTX2	CGGGCATGGATTTGTTGCAT	GGTGGTGCATAGGGGTCAAA
PDZRN4	TGGCTCTGGCCAAACTAAGG	CTCCACCTCATTGGCTGTGT
PKDCCB	ACTGCACACTTGACTTCCCC	AGCGTGGGAACAGCTAAACA
POU6F2	CCGTCATCGGCAACCAGATA	CCATAGGAACTGCTGTCGCA
PRDM12	TGATCACGTCCGACATCCTG	TGAGTTCCCGTACCAGACCA
PROX2	TCCTCGACGTGCAGTTCAGC	CGCAGCTTTGAACACTTCGG
PRRX1	TTTCCGTGAGTCACCTGCTG	ACTGTGGGCACTTGATTCCT
PRRX2	CCCTCAGAGCCGGAAAAACT	CTGGTTCTGATGCAGGCTGA
RUNX1	AACCCAGAAACACGAGGCAA	CCCTTCTGCCTCAACCACAT
SCN3A	TGGCTGGGATGGCTTGTTAG	TTGGAAGGATTGGCTGCCAT
SHOX	CGGAAGGGATCTACGAGTGC	GCTGGAGTTCTTGCTGTTGC
SULT4A1	GGCTTGCTACAGGAAGTGGT	CCACCATGGATTCCAGCTGT
TOX2	AACCTCCCTGACCCTTCACT	CCGAAGGTAGCATTGGGGTT

Other constructs were obtained: *DRG11* from Prof. J Cohen (KCL, London), *PHOX2B* from Prof. JF Brunet (ENS, Paris).

In situ hybridisation
Wholemount in situ hybridisation was carried out as described previously [8] with incubation at 65 °C. An RNAse incubation step (15mins, 37 °C) was included post-hybridisation. For in situ hybridization on section, embryos were fixed in 4 % paraformaldehyde in MOPS buffer (MB) containing 100 mM MOPS (pH 7.5), 1 mM EGTA and 2 mM MgSO$_4$ for 12 h at 4 °C. Embryos were then treated in 15 % sucrose in MB for 10 h and 30 % sucrose in MB for 2 h, and embedded in OCT compound (Andwin Scientific). 10 μm cryosections were collected and processed for in situ hybridization as previously described [108].

Additional files

Additional file 1: Figure S1. Analysis of NFM expression in neural crest-derived cells of the trigeminal ganglion at stage HH18. A-F) Immunostaining for NFM (magenta) on sections at the level of the trigeminal ophthalmic (Top, A-C) or trigeminal maxillomandibular (Tmm, D-F) ganglion in

HH18 chicken embryos in which a GFP-expressing construct was electroporated in the dorsal midbrain-hindbrain region at stage HH12. GFP expression (green) indicates origin in the cranial neural crest. GFP-positive neural crest-derived cells are NFM-negative (C and F). Scale bar: 50 μm. (PDF 6525 kb)

Additional file 2: Information for each of the 15 samples. Number of embryos dissected, number of ganglia included, proportion and number of cells sorted, quantity and integrity (RIN number) of RNA extracted, sequencing depth and proportion of reads mapped and number of genes expressed are indicated for each replicate. Genes are counted as expressed if RPKM > 0.3. (XLSX 10 kb)

Additional file 3: Normalized expression levels. Number of mapped reads per kilobase of exon per million reads (RPKM) is given for each gene and for each of the 15 replicates. (XLSX 3748 kb)

Additional file 4: Figure S2. A) Pearson coefficients of correlation between principal components 1–15 and RIN values. B) Pearson coefficients of correlation between principal components 1–15 and RNA quality. C) Pearson coefficients of correlation between principal components 1–15 and read counts. (ZIP 179 kb)

Additional file 5: Figure S3. Expression levels of neuronal differentiation markers. Expression levels as measured by RNA-seq (RPKM) for the indicated gene is shown for the 5 ganglia (Top: trigeminal ophthalmic; Tmm: trigeminal maxillomandibular; VA: vestibulo-acoustic; Pet: petrosal; Nod: nodose). Error bar: standard error of mean (s.e.m). (PDF 1432 kb)

Additional file 6: Differential expression analysis results for all pairwise comparisons between ganglia using both DESeq (i) and

EdgeR (ii). Data are available as compiled .xlsx spreadsheets (A) or individual .csv files (B). (ZIP 24942 kb)

Additional file 7: Figure S4. A) Number of genes identified as differentially expressed ($q < 0.05$) in each ganglion and in the grouped Top/Tmm/VA ganglia by DESeq and EdgeR. B) Significant Gene Ontology enrichment ($q < 0.05$) for differentially expressed genes reported by both DESeq and EdgeR in each ganglion. Redundant GO terms were removed using REVIGO. The Hinton plot displays the FDR (Benjamini and Hochberg) corrected q-value. Top: trigeminal ophthalmic; Tmm: trigeminal maxillomandibular, VA: vestibulo-acoustic, P: petrosal, N: nodose. (PDF 385 kb)

Additional file 8: Average normalized read count in ganglion of focus relative to all other ganglia, fold change and q-value (Benjamini and Hochberg) for the 134 high confidence markers computed using DESeq. (XLSX 22 kb)

Additional file 9: Figure S5. Molecular phylogenetic analysis and expression levels of POU4/BRN3 family genes. A) Maximum likelihood tree of POU4/BRN3 gene family in vertebrates. 4 paralogy groups are found across vertebrates. *POU4F1.2*, named after the *Xenopus* homologue, is present in chicken but was not found in mammals. Accession numbers are shown next to each entry and bootstrap values are shown at each node. The unique Pou4 sequence from invertebrate deuterostomes are used as an outgroup and the tree is rooted with *Lottia giantea* Pou4. Species abbreviations: Brafl: *Branchiostoma floridae*; Calmi: *Callorhynchus milii*; Chrpi: *Chrysemys picta*; Danre: *Danio rerio*; Galga: *Gallus gallus*; Homsa: *Homo sapiens*; Lotgi: *Lottia gigantea*; Sacko: Saccoglossus kowalevskii; Strpu: *Strongylocentrotus purpuratus*; Xentr: *Xenopus tropicalis*. B) Expression levels (RPKM) for chicken *POU4F1* and *POU4F1.2* across five cranial sensory ganglia assessed by RNAseq. The two genes are collectively expressed at high levels in the somatic but not visceral sensory neurons. Top: trigeminal ophthalmic; Tmm: trigeminal maxillomandibular, VA: vestibulo-acoustic, P: petrosal, N: nodose. (PDF 8575 kb)

Additional file 10: Gene Ontology annotations for the 134 high confidence ganglion-specific markers. (XLSX 13 kb)

Additional file 11: Figure S6. Expression patterns of putative ganglia-specific markers that didn't match expectations. In situ hybridization in wholemount and on sections at the level of the trigeminal maxillomandibular (Tmm), vestibulo-acoustic (VA) and petrosal (P) ganglia. A) *LHX4* expression was detected at relatively high levels in the ventral hindbrain but only at very low levels in the petrosal ganglion. B) *OTX2* staining can be observed at high levels in the rhombic lip but only slightly higher in the trigeminal than in the vestibulo-acoustic and petrosal ganglia. C) *TOX2* staining was only detected at very low levels in the ganglia in sections. D-F) *MECOM*, *PRRX1* and *PRRX2* expression was observed at high levels in the mesenchyme around, but not within, the cranial sensory ganglia. (TIF 8124 kb)

Competing interests

The authors declare they have no competing interests.

Authors' contributions

CP, JB and SMS designed experiment. CP performed all dissections, FACS and RNA preparation and section *in situs*; JB undertook cloning and wholemount *in situ*; HC performed all computational genomics analyses. WH and CPP advised HC on the computational analyses. All authors contributed to and approved the final version of the manuscript.

Acknowledgements

CP and SMS were funded by The Royal Society, EMBO, Elizabeth Hannah Jenkinson Fund, Fell Fund and the Swedish Society for Medical Research. HC, WH and CPP were funded by the MRC. Other thanks go to the Wellcome Trust Centre for Human Genetics for sequencing and to Stephen Fleenor for initial cloning and the chick cranial sensory ganglia schematic (Fig. 1A).

Author details

[1]Department of Physiology, Anatomy and Genetics, University of Oxford, Oxford, UK. [2]Department of Zoology, University of Oxford, Oxford, UK. [3]MRC Functional Genomics, University of Oxford, Oxford, UK. [4]Umeå Center for Molecular Medicine, Umeå University, Umeå, Sweden.

References

1. Le Pichon CE, Chesler AT. The functional and anatomical dissection of somatosensory subpopulations using mouse genetics. Front Neuroanat. 2014;8:21.
2. Chiu IM, Barrett LB, Williams EK, Strochlic DE, Lee S, Weyer AD, et al. Transcriptional profiling at whole population and single cell levels reveals somatosensory neuron molecular diversity. eLife. 2014;3.doi: 10.7554/eLife.04660.
3. Usoskin D, Furlan A, Islam S, Abdo H, Lonnerberg P, Lou D, et al. Unbiased classification of sensory neuron types by large-scale single-cell RNA sequencing. Nat Neurosci. 2015;18(1):145–53.
4. Bear MF, Connors BW, Paradiso MA. Neuroscience: exploring the brain. 3rd ed. Philadelphia: Lippincott Williams & Wilkins; 2007.
5. Romer AS. The vertebrate body. 3rd ed. Philadelphia: Saunders; 1962.
6. D'Amico-Martel A, Noden DM. Contributions of placodal and neural crest cells to avian cranial peripheral ganglia. Am J Anat. 1983;166(4):445–68.
7. Blentic A, Chambers D, Skinner A, Begbie J, Graham A. The formation of the cranial ganglia by placodally-derived sensory neuronal precursors. Mol Cell Neurosci. 2011;46(2):452–9.
8. Thompson H, Blentic A, Watson S, Begbie J, Graham A. The formation of the superior and jugular ganglia: insights into the generation of sensory neurons by the neural crest. Dev Dyn. 2010;239(2):439–45.
9. Baker CV, Bronner-Fraser M. Establishing neuronal identity in vertebrate neurogenic placodes. Development. 2000;127(14):3045–56.
10. Baker CV, Stark MR, Marcelle C, Bronner-Fraser M. Competence, specification and induction of Pax-3 in the trigeminal placode. Development. 1999;126(1):147–56.
11. D'Autreaux F, Coppola E, Hirsch MR, Birchmeier C, Brunet JF. Homeoprotein Phox2b commands a somatic-to-visceral switch in cranial sensory pathways. Proc Natl Acad Sci U S A. 2011;108(50):20018–23.
12. Lu VB, Ikeda SR, Puhl 3rd HL. A 3.7 kb fragment of the mouse Scn10a gene promoter directs neural crest but not placodal lineage EGFP expression in a transgenic animal. J Neurosci. 2015;35(20):8021–34.
13. Nassenstein C, Taylor-Clark TE, Myers AC, Ru F, Nandigama R, Bettner W, et al. Phenotypic distinctions between neural crest and placode derived vagal C-fibres in mouse lungs. J Physiol. 2010;588(Pt 23):4769–83.
14. Begbie J, Ballivet M, Graham A. Early steps in the production of sensory neurons by the neurogenic placodes. Mol Cell Neurosci. 2002;21(3):502–11.
15. Begbie J, Brunet JF, Rubenstein JL, Graham A. Induction of the epibranchial placodes. Development. 1999;126(5):895–902.
16. Canning CA, Lee L, Luo SX, Graham A, Jones CM. Neural tube derived Wnt signals cooperate with FGF signaling in the formation and differentiation of the trigeminal placodes. Neural Dev. 2008;3:35.
17. Freter S, Muta Y, Mak SS, Rinkwitz S, Ladher RK. Progressive restriction of otic fate: the role of FGF and Wnt in resolving inner ear potential. Development. 2008;135(20):3415–24.
18. McCabe KL, Sechrist JW, Bronner-Fraser M. Birth of ophthalmic trigeminal neurons initiates early in the placodal ectoderm. J Comp Neurol. 2009;514(2):161–73.
19. Alsina B, Abello G, Ulloa E, Henrique D, Pujades C, Giraldez F. FGF signaling is required for determination of otic neuroblasts in the chick embryo. Dev Biol. 2004;267(1):119–34.
20. Nolte J. The human brain: an introduction to its functional anatomy. 5th ed. St Louis: Mosby; 2001.
21. Smith AC, Fleenor SJ, Begbie J. Changes in gene expression and cell shape characterise stages of epibranchial placode-derived neuron maturation in the chick. J Anat. 2015;227(1):89–102.
22. Hamburger V, Hamilton HL. A series of normal stages in the development of the chick embryo. 1951. Dev Dyn. 1992;195(4):231–72.
23. Xu H, Dude CM, Baker CV. Fine-grained fate maps for the ophthalmic and maxillomandibular trigeminal placodes in the chick embryo. Dev Biol. 2008;317(1):174–86.
24. Schlosser G, Northcutt RG. Development of neurogenic placodes in Xenopus laevis. J Comp Neurol. 2000;418(2):121–46.
25. Pan Y, Ouyang Z, Wong WH, Baker JC. A new FACS approach isolates hESC derived endoderm using transcription factors. PLoS One. 2011;6(3):e17536.
26. Anders S, Huber W. Differential expression analysis for sequence count data. Genome Biol. 2010;11(10):R106.
27. Zhou X, Lindsay H, Robinson MD. Robustly detecting differential expression in RNA sequencing data using observation weights. Nucleic Acids Res. 2014;42(11):e91.

28. Dude CM, Kuan CY, Bradshaw JR, Greene ND, Relaix F, Stark MR, et al. Activation of Pax3 target genes is necessary but not sufficient for neurogenesis in the ophthalmic trigeminal placode. Dev Biol. 2009;326(2):314–26.

29. Pieper M, Eagleson GW, Wosniok W, Schlosser G. Origin and segregation of cranial placodes in Xenopus laevis. Dev Biol. 2011;360(2):257–75.

30. Jacquin MF, Arends JJ, Xiang C, Shapiro LA, Ribak CE, Chen ZF. In DRG11 knock-out mice, trigeminal cell death is extensive and does not account for failed brainstem patterning. J Neurosci. 2008;28(14):3577–85.

31. Rebelo S, Chen ZF, Anderson DJ, Lima D. Involvement of DRG11 in the development of the primary afferent nociceptive system. Mol Cell Neurosci. 2006;33(3):236–46.

32. Rhinn M, Miyoshi K, Watanabe A, Kawaguchi M, Ito F, Kuratani S, et al. Evolutionary divergence of trigeminal nerve somatotopy in amniotes. J Comp Neurol. 2013;521(6):1378–94.

33. Pattyn A, Morin X, Cremer H, Goridis C, Brunet JF. Expression and interactions of the two closely related homeobox genes Phox2a and Phox2b during neurogenesis. Development. 1997;124(20):4065–75.

34. Holzschuh J, Wada N, Wada C, Schaffer A, Javidan Y, Tallafuss A, et al. Requirements for endoderm and BMP signaling in sensory neurogenesis in zebrafish. Development. 2005;132(16):3731–42.

35. Begbie J, Graham A. Integration between the epibranchial placodes and the hindbrain. Science. 2001;294(5542):595–8.

36. Fedtsova NG, Turner EE. Brn-3.0 expression identifies early post-mitotic CNS neurons and sensory neural precursors. Mech Dev. 1995;53(3):291–304.

37. Artinger KB, Fedtsova N, Rhee JM, Bronner-Fraser M, Turner E. Placodal origin of Brn-3-expressing cranial sensory neurons. J Neurobiol. 1998;36(4):572–85.

38. Larrivee B, Freitas C, Suchting S, Brunet I, Eichmann A. Guidance of vascular development: lessons from the nervous system. Circ Res. 2009;104(4):428–41.

39. Chen ZF, Rebelo S, White F, Malmberg AB, Baba H, Lima D, et al. The paired homeodomain protein DRG11 is required for the projection of cutaneous sensory afferent fibers to the dorsal spinal cord. Neuron. 2001;31(1):59–73.

40. Rebelo S, Reguenga C, Osorio L, Pereira C, Lopes C, Lima D. DRG11 immunohistochemical expression during embryonic development in the mouse. Dev Dyn. 2007;236(9):2653–60.

41. Chen YC, Auer-Grumbach M, Matsukawa S, Zitzelsberger M, Themistocleous AC, Strom TM, et al. Transcriptional regulator PRDM12 is essential for human pain perception. Nat Genet. 2015;47(7):803–8.

42. Kinameri E, Inoue T, Aruga J, Imayoshi I, Kageyama R, Shimogori T, et al. Prdm proto-oncogene transcription factor family expression and interaction with the Notch-Hes pathway in mouse neurogenesis. PLoS One. 2008;3(12):e3859.

43. Nagy V, Cole T, Van Campenhout C, Khoung TM, Leung C, Vermeiren S, et al. The evolutionarily conserved transcription factor PRDM12 controls sensory neuron development and pain perception. Cell Cycle. 2015;14(12):1799–808.

44. Roy G, Philippe E, Gaulin F, Guay G. Peripheral projections of the chick primary sensory neurons expressing gamma-aminobutyric acid immunoreactivity. Neuroscience. 1991;45(1):177–83.

45. Hayasaki H, Sohma Y, Kanbara K, Maemura K, Kubota T, Watanabe M. A local GABAergic system within rat trigeminal ganglion cells. Eur J Neurosci. 2006;23(3):745–57.

46. Zhang Z, Cai YQ, Zou F, Bie B, Pan ZZ. Epigenetic suppression of GAD65 expression mediates persistent pain. Nat Med. 2011;17(11):1448–55.

47. Alimohammadi H, Silver WL. Evidence for nicotinic acetylcholine receptors on nasal trigeminal nerve endings of the rat. Chem Senses. 2000;25(1):61–6.

48. Flores CM, DeCamp RM, Kilo S, Rogers SW, Hargreaves KM. Neuronal nicotinic receptor expression in sensory neurons of the rat trigeminal ganglion: demonstration of alpha3beta4, a novel subtype in the mammalian nervous system. J Neurosci. 1996;16(24):7892–901.

49. Gotti C, Clementi F, Fornari A, Gaimarri A, Guiducci S, Manfredi I, et al. Structural and functional diversity of native brain neuronal nicotinic receptors. Biochem Pharmacol. 2009;78(7):703–11.

50. Feng Y, Xu Q. Pivotal role of hmx2 and hmx3 in zebrafish inner ear and lateral line development. Dev Biol. 2010;339(2):507–18.

51. Herbrand H, Guthrie S, Hadrys T, Hoffmann S, Arnold HH, Rinkwitz-Brandt S, et al. Two regulatory genes, cNkx5-1 and cPax2, show different responses to local signals during otic placode and vesicle formation in the chick embryo. Development. 1998;125(4):645–54.

52. Miller ND, Nance MA, Wohler ES, Hoover-Fong JE, Lisi E, Thomas GH, et al. Molecular (SNP) analyses of overlapping hemizygous deletions of 10q25.3 to 10qter in four patients: evidence for HMX2 and HMX3 as candidate genes in hearing and vestibular function. Am J Med Genet A. 2009;149A(4):669–80.

53. Wang W, Van De Water T, Lufkin T. Inner ear and maternal reproductive defects in mice lacking the Hmx3 homeobox gene. Development. 1998;125(4):621–34.

54. Hermans-Borgmeyer I, Susens U, Borgmeyer U. Developmental expression of the estrogen receptor-related receptor gamma in the nervous system during mouse embryogenesis. Mech Dev. 2000;97(1–2):197–9.

55. Nolan LS, Maier H, Hermans-Borgmeyer I, Girotto G, Ecob R, Pirastu N, et al. Estrogen-related receptor gamma and hearing function: evidence of a role in humans and mice. Neurobiol Aging. 2013;34(8):2077 e2071–2079.

56. Zhou H, Yoshioka T, Nathans J. Retina-derived POU-domain factor-1: a complex POU-domain gene implicated in the development of retinal ganglion and amacrine cells. J Neurosci. 1996;16(7):2261–74.

57. Yoshida S, Ueharu H, Higuchi M, Horiguchi K, Nishimura N, Shibuya S, et al. Molecular cloning of rat and porcine retina-derived POU domain factor 1 (POU6F2) from a pituitary cDNA library. J Reprod Dev. 2014;60(4):288–94.

58. Bosse A, Zulch A, Becker MB, Torres M, Gomez-Skarmeta JL, Modolell J, et al. Identification of the vertebrate Iroquois homeobox gene family with overlapping expression during early development of the nervous system. Mech Dev. 1997;69(1–2):169–81.

59. Goriely A, Diez del Corral R, Storey KG. c-Irx2 expression reveals an early subdivision of the neural plate in the chick embryo. Mech Dev. 1999;87(1–2):203–6.

60. Theriault FM, Roy P, Stifani S. AML1/Runx1 is important for the development of hindbrain cholinergic branchiovisceral motor neurons and selected cranial sensory neurons. Proc Natl Acad Sci U S A. 2004;101(28):10343–8.

61. Marmigere F, Montelius A, Wegner M, Groner Y, Reichardt LF, Ernfors P. The Runx1/AML1 transcription factor selectively regulates development and survival of TrkA nociceptive sensory neurons. Nat Neurosci. 2006;9(2):180–7.

62. Pirvola U, Zhang X, Mantela J, Ornitz DM, Ylikoski J. Fgf9 signaling regulates inner ear morphogenesis through epithelial-mesenchymal interactions. Dev Biol. 2004;273(2):350–60.

63. Huh SH, Warchol ME, Ornitz DM. Cochlear progenitor number is controlled through mesenchymal FGF receptor signaling. eLife. 2015;4. doi: 10.7554/eLife.05921.

64. Giesert F, Hofmann A, Burger A, Zerle J, Kloos K, Hafen U, et al. Expression analysis of Lrrk1, Lrrk2 and Lrrk2 splice variants in mice. PLoS One. 2013;8(5):e63778.

65. Westerlund M, Belin AC, Anvret A, Bickford P, Olson L, Galter D. Developmental regulation of leucine-rich repeat kinase 1 and 2 expression in the brain and other rodent and human organs: Implications for Parkinson's disease. Neuroscience. 2008;152(2):429–36.

66. Bordoli MR, Yum J, Breitkopf SB, Thon JN, Italiano Jr JE, Xiao J, et al. A secreted tyrosine kinase acts in the extracellular environment. Cell. 2014;158(5):1033–44.

67. Imuta Y, Nishioka N, Kiyonari H, Sasaki H. Short limbs, cleft palate, and delayed formation of flat proliferative chondrocytes in mice with targeted disruption of a putative protein kinase gene, Pkdcc (AW548124). Dev Dyn. 2009;238(1):210–22.

68. Kasai N, Fukushima K, Ueki Y, Prasad S, Nosakowski J, Sugata K, et al. Genomic structures of SCN2A and SCN3A - candidate genes for deafness at the DFNA16 locus. Gene. 2001;264(1):113–22.

69. Nishijima I, Ohtoshi A. Characterization of a novel prospero-related homeobox gene, Prox2. Mol Genet Genomics. 2006;275(5):471–8.

70. Pistocchi A, Bartesaghi S, Cotelli F, Del Giacco L. Identification and expression pattern of zebrafish prox2 during embryonic development. Dev Dyn. 2008;237(12):3916–20.

71. Cobb J, Dierich A, Huss-Garcia Y, Duboule D. A mouse model for human short-stature syndromes identifies Shox2 as an upstream regulator of Runx2 during long-bone development. Proc Natl Acad Sci U S A. 2006;103(12):4511–5.

72. Rao E, Weiss B, Fukami M, Rump A, Niesler B, Mertz A, et al. Pseudoautosomal deletions encompassing a novel homeobox gene cause growth failure in idiopathic short stature and Turner syndrome. Nat Genet. 1997;16(1):54–63.

73. Sawada R, Kamei H, Hakuno F, Takahashi S, Shimizu T. In vivo loss of function study reveals the short stature homeobox-containing (shox) gene plays indispensable roles in early embryonic growth and bone formation in zebrafish. Dev Dyn. 2015;244(2):146–56.

74. Dougherty KJ, Zagoraiou L, Satoh D, Rozani I, Doobar S, Arber S, et al. Locomotor rhythm generation linked to the output of spinal shox2 excitatory interneurons. Neuron. 2013;80(4):920–33.

75. Rosin JM, Kurrasch DM, Cobb J. Shox2 is required for the proper development of the facial motor nucleus and the establishment of the facial nerves. BMC Neurosci. 2015;16(1):39.

76. Coulter 2nd PM, Bautista EA, Margulies JE, Watson JB. Identification of cortexin: a novel, neuron-specific, 82-residue membrane protein enriched in rodent cerebral cortex. J Neurochem. 1993;61(2):756–9.

77. Flynn M, Saha O, Young P. Molecular evolution of the LNX gene family. BMC Evol Biol. 2011;11:235.

78. Rice DS, Northcutt GM, Kurschner C. The Lnx family proteins function as molecular scaffolds for Numb family proteins. Mol Cell Neurosci. 2001;18(5):525–40.

79. Katoh M, Katoh M. Identification and characterization of PDZRN3 and PDZRN4 genes in silico. Int J Mol Med. 2004;13(4):607–13.

80. Liyou NE, Buller KM, Tresillian MJ, Elvin CM, Scott HL, Dodd PR, et al. Localization of a brain sulfotransferase, SULT4A1, in the human and rat brain: an immunohistochemical study. J Histochem Cytochem. 2003;51(12):1655–64.

81. Minchin RF, Lewis A, Mitchell D, Kadlubar FF, McManus ME. Sulfotransferase 4A1. Int J Biochem Cell Biol. 2008;40(12):2686–91.

82. Dincer Z, Piao J, Niu L, Ganat Y, Kriks S, Zimmer B, et al. Specification of functional cranial placode derivatives from human pluripotent stem cells. Cell Rep. 2013;5(5):1387–402.

83. Dykes IM, Lanier J, Eng SR, Turner EE. Brn3a regulates neuronal subtype specification in the trigeminal ganglion by promoting Runx expression during sensory differentiation. Neural Dev. 2010;5:3.

84. Ratcliffe EM, Setru SU, Chen JJ, Li ZS, D'Autreaux F, Gershon MD. Netrin/DCC-mediated attraction of vagal sensory axons to the fetal mouse gut. J Comp Neurol. 2006;498(5):567–80.

85. Shiau CE, Bronner-Fraser M. N-cadherin acts in concert with Slit1-Robo2 signaling in regulating aggregation of placode-derived cranial sensory neurons. Development. 2009;136(24):4155–64.

86. Toba Y, Tiong JD, Ma Q, Wray S. CXCR4/SDF-1 system modulates development of GnRH-1 neurons and the olfactory system. Dev Neurobiol. 2008;68(4):487–503.

87. Arber S, Ladle DR, Lin JH, Frank E, Jessell TM. ETS gene Er81 controls the formation of functional connections between group Ia sensory afferents and motor neurons. Cell. 2000;101(5):485–98.

88. Lu CC, Appler JM, Houseman EA, Goodrich LV. Developmental profiling of spiral ganglion neurons reveals insights into auditory circuit assembly. J Neurosci. 2011;31(30):10903–18.

89. Davos CH, Davies LC, Piepoli M. The effect of baroreceptor activity on cardiovascular regulation. Hellenic J Cardiol. 2002;43:145–55.

90. Prabhakar NR, Joyner MJ. Tasting arterial blood: what do the carotid chemoreceptors sense? Front Physiol. 2014;5:524.

91. Ronveaux CC, Tome D, Raybould HE. Glucagon-like peptide 1 interacts with ghrelin and leptin to regulate glucose metabolism and food intake through vagal afferent neuron signaling. J Nutr. 2015;145(4):672–80.

92. Oury F, Murakami Y, Renaud JS, Pasqualetti M, Charnay P, Ren SY, et al. Hoxa2- and rhombomere-dependent development of the mouse facial somatosensory map. Science. 2006;313(5792):1408–13.

93. Lafreniere RG, Cader MZ, Poulin JF, Andres-Enguix I, Simoneau M, Gupta N, et al. A dominant-negative mutation in the TRESK potassium channel is linked to familial migraine with aura. Nat Med. 2010;16(10):1157–60.

94. Lanier J, Dykes IM, Nissen S, Eng SR, Turner EE. Brn3a regulates the transition from neurogenesis to terminal differentiation and represses non-neural gene expression in the trigeminal ganglion. Dev Dyn. 2009;238(12):3065–79.

95. Ladher RK, O'Neill P, Begbie J. From shared lineage to distinct functions: the development of the inner ear and epibranchial placodes. Development. 2010;137(11):1777–85.

96. Patthey C, Schlosser G, Shimeld SM. The evolutionary history of vertebrate cranial placodes–I: cell type evolution. Dev Biol. 2014;389(1):82–97.

97. Schlosser G, Patthey C, Shimeld SM. The evolutionary history of vertebrate cranial placodes II. Evolution of ectodermal patterning. Dev Biol. 2014;389(1):98–119.

98. Gans C, Northcutt RG. Neural crest and the origin of vertebrates: a new head. Science. 1983;220(4594):268–73.

99. Holland LZ. Chordate roots of the vertebrate nervous system: expanding the molecular toolkit. Nat Rev Neurosci. 2009;10(10):736–46.

100. Abitua PB, Gainous TB, Kaczmarczyk AN, Winchell CJ, Hudson C, Kamata K, et al. The pre-vertebrate origins of neurogenic placodes. Nature. 2015;524(7566):462–5. doi:10.1038/nature14657.

101. Wu TD, Nacu S. Fast and SNP-tolerant detection of complex variants and splicing in short reads. Bioinformatics. 2010;26(7):873–81.

102. Katz Y, Wang ET, Airoldi EM, Burge CB. Analysis and design of RNA sequencing experiments for identifying isoform regulation. Nat Methods. 2010;7(12):1009–15.

103. Anders S, Pyl PT, Huber W. HTSeq–a Python framework to work with high-throughput sequencing data. Bioinformatics. 2015;31(2):166–9.

104. Robinson MD, McCarthy DJ, Smyth GK. edgeR: a Bioconductor package for differential expression analysis of digital gene expression data. Bioinformatics. 2010;26(1):139–40.

105. da Huang W, Sherman BT, Lempicki RA. Systematic and integrative analysis of large gene lists using DAVID bioinformatics resources. Nat Protoc. 2009;4(1):44–57.

106. Hall TA. BioEdit: a user-friendly biological sequence alignment editor and analysis program for Windows 95/98/NT. Nucleic Acids Symp Sers. 1999;41:95–8.

107. Tamura K, Peterson D, Peterson N, Stecher G, Nei M, Kumar S. MEGA5: molecular evolutionary genetics analysis using maximum likelihood, evolutionary distance, and maximum parsimony methods. Mol Biol Evol. 2011;28(10):2731–9.

108. Wilkinson DG, Nieto MA. Detection of messenger RNA by in situ hybridization to tissue sections and whole mounts. Methods Enzymol. 1993;225:361–73.

2

Postnatal developmental dynamics of cell type specification genes in Brn3a/Pou4f1 Retinal Ganglion Cells

Vladimir Vladimirovich Muzyka[1*], Matthew Brooks[2] and Tudor Constantin Badea[1*] (iD)

Abstract

Background: About 20–30 distinct Retinal Ganglion Cell (RGC) types transmit visual information from the retina to the brain. The developmental mechanisms by which RGCs are specified are still largely unknown. Brn3a is a member of the Brn3/Pou4f transcription factor family, which contains key regulators of RGC postmitotic specification. In particular, Brn3a ablation results in the loss of RGCs with small, thick and dense dendritic arbors ('midget-like' RGCs), and morphological changes in other RGC subpopulations. To identify downstream molecular mechanisms underlying Brn3a effects on RGC numbers and morphology, our group recently performed a RNA deep sequencing screen for Brn3a transcriptional targets in mouse RGCs and identified 180 candidate transcripts.

Methods: We now focus on a subset of 28 candidate genes encoding potential cell type determinant proteins. We validate and further define their retinal expression profile at five postnatal developmental time points between birth and adult stage, using in situ hybridization (ISH), RT-PCR and fluorescent immunodetection (IIF).

Results: We find that a majority of candidate genes are enriched in the ganglion cell layer during early stages of postnatal development, but dynamically change their expression profile. We also document transcript-specific expression differences for two example candidates, using RT-PCR and ISH. Brn3a dependency could be confirmed by ISH and IIF only for a fraction of our candidates.

Conclusions: Amongst our candidate Brn3a target genes, a majority demonstrated ganglion cell layer specificity, however only around two thirds showed Brn3a dependency. Some were previously implicated in RGC type specification, while others have known physiological functions in RGCs. Only three genes were found to be consistently regulated by Brn3a throughout postnatal retina development – Mapk10, Tusc5 and Cdh4.

Keywords: Retinal ganglion cell, Subtype specification, Postnatal development, Brn3a, RNA sequencing, in situ hybridization, Dendrite formation, Synapse formation

Background

Retinal ganglion cells (RGCs) are the only neurons in the vertebrate retina which are directly connected to the brain. Mouse RGCs can be subdivided in ~ 30 different types with distinct specific molecular markers, dendritic arbor morphologies, synaptic partners and axonal projections [1–5]. There are several stages of RGC specification during embryonic and postnatal development. Mouse RGCs become postmitotic and start to express

selective molecular markers at embryonic day 11 (E11). RGC axons pass the optic chiasm around E12 and reach the most remote retinorecipient areas of the brain by E15 [6, 7]. Around birth (postnatal day 0, P0) RGC axons invade their target nuclei in the brain, and the first two postnatal weeks are the most intense period for synapse formation. RGC dendrites begin their development later, and the lamination within the inner plexiform layer becomes clearly visible only around P3, grossly develops by P7, and reaches nearly final state after P14 [8, 9]. Mouse eyes open at P13-P14, when synapses between RGCs and bipolar and amacrine cells are already formed, and light-driven synaptic pruning

* Correspondence: vladimir.muzyka@nih.gov; badeatc@mail.nih.gov
[1]Retinal Circuit Development & Genetics Unit, Building 6, Room 331B Center Drive, Bethesda, MD 20892–0610, USA
Full list of author information is available at the end of the article

takes place [10]. At P22 RGC axons and dendritic arbors are already "mature", and cells are completely specified into multiple subtypes [11]. Numerous screens seeking to identify RGC subpopulation specific molecules were performed [12, 13], but we still do not have a comprehensive footprint of RGC diversity in terms of unique molecular signatures.

The Brn3/Pou4f family of transcription factors (TFs) comprising Brn3a, Brn3b and Brn3c is expressed in the retina specifically in RGCs, and its members form a major part of a combinatorial code for RGC type determination [1, 2, 11, 14, 15]. The RGC specification program requires Brn3b and/or Isl1 to initiate, and these TFs are crucial for survival, correct determination of cell fate and axonal targeting of RGCs during development [11, 16–23]. Brn3a starts to be expressed in embryonic retina 1 day later than Brn3b (E12.5 vs. E11.5). It is downstream of Brn3b in the RGC developmental transcriptional cascade, and was initially thought to function redundantly with Brn3b [24, 25]. Brn3a gene ablation is perinatal lethal due to the defects in the somatosensory system and brainstem nuclei, but it does not lead to dramatic perturbations within the retina at this point of development [26, 27]. A reporter knock-in allele expressing alkaline phosphatase (AP) at the Brn3a ($Brn3a^{CKOAP}$) locus was previously used by our group to describe Brn3a cell type distribution among RGCs [2, 11], and also enabled us to identify axonal and dendrite arbor defects in RGCs missing Brn3a either alone or in combination with other Brn3s [28]. Dendrites of Brn3a-expressing RGCs are stratified in the outer laminae (~ 70%) of the inner plexiform layer (IPL) of the retina. Retina-specific Brn3a loss leads to an elimination of AP-expressing RGC arbors in a thin stripe along the border between ON and OFF layers of the IPL [11]. Retinal Brn3a loss results in a shift towards bistratified RGC dendritic arbor morphologies and overall RGC numbers reduction of around 30–40% depending on retinal region [11, 28], in part by eliminating small RGCs with dense multistratified dendritic morphology [2, 28]. The consequences of Brn3a ablation on RGC subpopulations are obvious already in the early postnatal period (P4) and associated with both cell fate change and cell number loss [11, 28]. However, the molecular mechanisms by which Brn3a controls RGC cell numbers and morphological features are still unclear. To find possible candidates of Brn3a-mediated regulation along with the novel subtype-specific markers, our group has recently performed a RNA deep sequencing screen which defined transcriptomes of Brn3a-positive RGCs and Brn3a-dependent RGC transcripts. The study found transcription factors (TFs), trans-membrane and intracellular structural molecules, that are enriched in RGC subpopulations and selectively depend on Brn3a expression. Overall, 180 transcripts were detected to be potential Brn3a targets at P3 [5].

Molecular determinants of neuronal subtypes can range from expression regulators to final-step effector molecules which provide a basis for cell-cell interactions and neuronal physiology and neuroanatomy [5]. TFs could serve as the most upstream "classifiers" of neuronal types by controlling the expression of identity-specific downstream genes which shape and modulate structural and functional characteristics of a cell [29–31]. Downstream effectors include cell-surface adhesion molecules which are crucial in definition of axon and dendritic morphologies via interaction with their partners on other cells [32–34]. Structural and cytoskeleton-associated molecules provide a mechanistic basis for morphological changes [35–38], and intracellular signaling molecules regulate those processes under transcription factor control [39–43]. Another key part of neuronal identity is provided by pre- and postsynaptic partners within the neuronal circuit. Specialized cell adhesion molecules, neurotransmitter and neurotrophin receptor subunits and other adaptors can confer specificity at both pre- and postsynaptic sites [40, 44–46]. Trophic factors and other secreted molecules are often secreted from postsynaptic sites to attract or repel presynaptic components (axons) and modulate connectivity during synaptogenesis and activity-dependent synaptic remodeling [47]. In addition to this, there are many non-secreted axon-guidance regulating molecules [48].

The goal of the current study is to identify potential Brn3a target molecules that contribute to the development and function of RGCs. Since we are interested in the terminal differentiation process – defining individual cell types – we are focusing on postnatal developmental time points. Specifically, we aim to analyze Brn3a influence on cell type determinants such as transcriptional regulators, adhesion molecules, synaptic elements and intracellular signaling/cytoskeleton apparatus. We used a Rax:Cre driver to produce retina-specific Brn3a ablation and evaluated potential targets previously identified in our P3 RNASeq screen by in situ hybridization (ISH), RT-PCR, and protein immunodetection experiments in postnatal Brn3a KO (Rax:Cre; $Brn3a^{CKOAP/KO}$) and Brn3a WT (Rax:Cre; $Brn3a^{CKOAP/WT}$) retinas. We performed our analysis over a developmental time series in order to correlate the expression dynamics of our target molecules to the postnatal stages of RGC development. We find that RNASeq and ISH data are in good agreement with regard to RGC enrichment and only to some extent to Brn3a regulation of our target genes at P3, but that many of the tested targets exhibit significant changes in expression profile between P0 and P22. For many of our target genes, multiple transcripts are expressed coincidentally in the retina with clearly distinct cell specificity. Finally, predicted intron-exon structures from genome annotation are not always accurate, and novel exon splicing sequences can be detected upon closer scrutiny. Nevertheless, multiple targets exhibit interesting patterns consistent with expression in one or a few RGC types, and regulation by Brn3a.

Methods
Mouse strains and crosses
Mouse lines carrying alleles Rax:Cre and $Brn3a^{CKOAP}$ were previously described [11, 49]. To obtain Cre-mediated recombination in RGCs, the following cross was set up: Rax:Cre; $Brn3a^{KO/WT}$ male x $Brn3a^{CKOAP/CKOAP}$ female, to generate two types of progeny: Rax:Cre; $Brn3a^{CKOAP/WT}$ and Rax:Cre; $Brn3a^{CKOAP/KO}$. RGCs/retinas of these mice were either Brn3a heterozygotes, which are phenotypically wild type ($Brn3a^{AP/WT}$, WT) or Brn3a knock-outs ($Brn3a^{AP/KO}$, KO). All mice were on C57/Bl6-SV129 mixed background. All animal procedures were approved by the National Eye Institute (NEI) Animal Care and Use Committee under protocol NEI640.

In situ hybridization (ISH)
ISH experiments were performed on P0, P3, P7, P14 and P22 eyes using an adapted Schaeren-Wiemers protocol [5]. Probes had a length between 160 and 900 bp (Table 1), a melting temperature between 77 °C and 94 °C, and were devoid of low-complexity regions, GC-rich or repetitive sequences. Probes for the main screen (experiments in Figs. 2, 3, 4, 5, 6, 7, 8, 9, 10, 11, 12 and 13) were targeted to 3'-UTRs of studied genes. Transcript-specific probes were designed for Pnkd and Clcc1 by targeting probes to unique exons as indicated in Figs. 14 and 15. The specific regions of the mRNA chosen for probes were in the areas highly covered by RNASeq reads, as determined from our data using IgViewer [50]. DNA templates for probes were derived by PCR from mouse genomic ES cell DNA (SV129 strain). All primers are provided in Table 1. A T3 promoter consensus sequence (GGAG CAAATTAACCCTCACTAAAGGG) was added to each reverse primer. Purified PCR products were used as templates for RNA probe synthesis, using T3 polymerase. Quality and concentration of the resulting RNA was assessed by 260/280 spectrometry or micro-electrophoretic analysis on a Bioanalyzer instrument (Thermo Scientific). Eyes for ISH were enucleated, cornea and lens removed, and the resulting eyecups were fixed for 1 h at RT in 4% paraformaldehyde (PFA). For each age, 4–8 eyes including Brn3a WT and KO genotypes were embedded in one OCT block, cryoprotected and sectioned at 14 μm thickness. ISH procedure was then performed as recently described [5], with two significant differences: 200 ng of probe were used for each hybridization, and the anti-DIG-AP antibody was used at 1:2000 (Fab fragments; Roche). The colorimetric reaction was developed between 2 and 9 h, individual incubation times for each probe are provided in Table 1.

All images were acquired using the 20× objective of a Zeiss Axio Imager.Z2 at bright-field settings and Axiovision software. For each probe, genotype and age, six or more images derived from 2 to 3 animals were collected.

Quantitation: For each genotype and age 2–3 images were used. From each image for P7-P22 ages we picked 3 areas (ROIs) in each of GCL (ganglion cell layer), IPL (inner plexiform layer), INL (inner nuclear layer) and ONL (outer nuclear layer) and quantitated mean gray value of the pixels. The areas of ROIs from same retina layer were similar. For each measurement, GCL, INL, ONL and IPL ROIs of same length were registered along the section plane. At P3 we were restricted only to 3 layers (GCL, IPL and NBL - neuroblast layer), at P0 – only two – GCL and NBL. For P7-P22 measurements, we subtracted the GCL, the INL and the ONL values from the respective IPL ROI value to acquire normalized values. In case of P3 we subtracted the GCL and the NBL values from the IPL ones. Finally, in case of P0 we were not able to provide IPL normalization because at this age there are no visible IPL. Normalized (P3-P22) and un-normalized (P0) values we then used for representation on the plots.

There are certain limitations to our quantitation method especially in the case of sparsely expressed genes. Even if sparsely located cells have extremely high expression levels, after averaging to the whole area, this could be hidden by the non-expressing or low-expressing majority of cells (for example, in case of Gabra1 expression in WT GCL at P14).

Reverse transcription – Polymerase chain reaction (RT-PCR)
Total RNA from P3 WT retinas was extracted as previously described. Reverse transcription was performed according to manufacturer's instructions using SuperScript II RT (Invitrogen) and PCR amplification using Taq DNA polymerase (New England Biolabs), using a touch-down protocol. Forward and reverse primers for PCR are shown in Table 1, and primer combinations used for transcript-specific identification are presented in Table 2. PCR products were assessed in 1.5% agarose gel electrophoresis, extracted from gel, eluted in TE buffer, and inserted by T-A cloning into the pGEM-T Easy Vector System (Promega). After transformation, 4 colonies for each inserted PCR product were recovered, and analyzed by restriction digestion. All insert diagnostic digests resulted in DNA fragments of expected length. For each predicted product, identity was confirmed by sequencing plasmid DNA from two of the recovered colonies.

Indirect immunofluorescence (IIF)
For IIF, eyecups were fixed in 2% PFA for 30 min at RT, and cryoprotected in OCT. Slides were blocked (PBS,

Table 1 Primers for ISH probes and RT-PCR

Gene	Forward Primer Sequence	Reverse Primer Sequence	Product Size, bp	Incubation (P0-P7), h	Incubation (P14-P22), h
For 3'-UTR probes					
Ankrd13b	TCCAAGGGCGGAGGCAGGT	ATCAGGGAAGGGAAGAGGAAG	821 + (26)	5	6
Cdh4	AAGTCCCAGCACTGATGAAAAA	CACCACCCGAATTGTTTGC	501 + (26)	6	6
Elfn1	CCTGCGCAAGAAGGTTCAGTT	CTTGCTTGCTTGCACCAGGC	367 + (26)	6	6
Eml1	CACTGTGATTTCTGTTTTGTCTA	GCCAGCCTCCCAAAGGGAG	473 + (26)	6	3
Fam19a4	AACTTTATGAACCTTGGAGAATG	TGAAATTGGAGGCAAGATGACT	498 + (26)	6	3
Foxp2	CTGTGCTGTTAGTGTAAAGATGT	GTTGCTTTCTAGAGTGTCATAAC	503 + (26)	3	3
Gabra1	GTTCTTTTAGTCGTATTCTGTTG	GAGCTTGCAAAATAGATTTGCC	900 + (26)	6	6
Grm4	GCCACACAGGCCTTCCTTCC	CTTCGAAACACACTCAAGATTAG	433 + (26)	6	5
Hpca	CCTCTCCCTCGTGTCTATCC	GAGCTGGGACAAGAAGTGTTC	443 + (26)	6	3
Plppr3	CAGTGCCAGCTCCGACTCTT	TTGCCAGGCTTAGTCCTGGTA	469 + (26)	6	6
Mapk10	GTCACAACGCACTCACGAAAG	ATCTGTATCTACATCCATCTGAC	364 + (26)	6	5
Nptx1	GGGGCTGAGAGCTCACTTG	ACCACTTCGAGCCACGCTC	600 + (26)	6	5
Nptx2	TCTCCGTCCCAGAGGCCAC	CAGTTCCCTCAGACGGAAAG	486 + (26)	6	6
Ntrk1	ATCGAGTGTATCACGCAGGGC	TATGATGGATGCTGGCCATGAA	328 + (26)	6	5
Pcdh20	GACGAGTTTCCTACTTCTTGGG	TTATCGTTGATGTCCAGAAGAAG	511 + (26)	6	9
Pick1	ACCACTGTAGGACAGCGAAGG	TTATTCAATACAGGCCCAGCTTC	393 + (26)	6	9
Pip5kl1	ACAAGGTGTGTCGAAGTCGAAG	TAAGGGTTGGGGTCAGGGTC	458 + (26)	6	6
Pnkd	CTTCACCATCCTCTTCATCACT	GAAGGTGGAAGATAGACTAGCC	360 + (26)	6	6
Rims1	CACCCTCCTCTGGAGTCCAG	TGTGTCTGCAGTTTATACCAATG	500 + (26)	2	3
Tmem25	TGCCTGTCCCTGTTGTGACC	GTACAAAACGATGCAGAGCTAC	687 + (26)	6	6
Tmem91	CAACAAGGCTTGGGCCAAGG	GGGTATCTTTAATTTCTCACATTG	348 + (26)	6	5
Tshz2	GCAGAAAGAAAGGGAAATATGTG	CATCACCTATTTGTTCTCTTCG	418 + (26)	6	6
Tusc5	CTGGAGATCTCCGAACCTACAT	ATGGAGGATTTCCGTATGGCC	492 + (26)	6	5
Pou4f1 (control)	TGTGTAGAAGATCCCCTTTGG	GCACAGAAATGGTTCTGATG	519 + (26)	3	3
For transcript-specific probes					
Clcc1 (pr.1 + pr.9) ^	CACAGCTGCGGGCCGAGC	CTGAGATTTCCTCATCGTTCCT	208 + (26)		
Clcc1 (pr.2 + pr.9)	AGTCCGCTCGGGACTCCAG	CTGAGATTTCCTCATCGTTCCT	181/252 + (26)	7	7
Clcc1 (pr.3 + pr.9) ^	TGTTTGAGGTAGGCGGCTCG	CTGAGATTTCCTCATCGTTCCT	220 + (26)		
Clcc1 (pr.4 + pr.9) ^	TCGGCGTCTTCCGCGGCC	CTGAGATTTCCTCATCGTTCCT	203 + (26)		
Clcc1 (pr.5 + pr.9) ^	TCCCTCTGAAAGAGCAGGCAG	CTGAGATTTCCTCATCGTTCCT	172 + (26)		

Table 1 Primers for ISH probes and RT-PCR *(Continued)*

Gene	Forward Primer Sequence	Reverse Primer Sequence	Product Size, bp	Incubation (P0-P7), h	Incubation (P14-P22), h
Clcc1 (pr.6 + pr.9) ^*	TGAGTGGGCGCTCTTCGGTG	CTGAGATTTCCTCATCGTTCCT	293 + (26)		
Clcc1 (pr.7 + pr.9) ^	CGTTTCCAGGATACACCGAGA	CTGAGATTTCCTCATCGTTCCT	300 + (26)		
Clcc1 (pr.2 + pr.8) ^*	AGTCCGCTCGGGACTCCAG	CGGGTTAAGGGAAGTCAAATTC	199/270 + (26)		
Clcc1(pr.7 + pr.8) ^^	CGTTTCCAGGATACACCGAGA	CGGGTTAAGGGAAGTCAAATTC	159 + (26)	4	3
Clcc1(pr.10 + pr.11)^	GTGAGGTCTGGAACATCAGAG	CATAAACACATTATATGGATCTA	432 + (26)		
Pnkd (pr.1 + pr.2)	TGGGACCCGAACATGGCGG	GGCTAGCCCCACGGCTTTC	246 (+ 26)	2	3
Pnkd (pr.3 + pr.4) *	TGTGGTATCCTCTTCTTCGTC	CTCCTTCCACGGTGTGGAAG	289 + (26)	2	3
Pnkd (pr.5 + pr.6)	CCCAGCATGGCTTGGCAGG	CCGATTCGGAAGAGCAGCCG	167 (+ 26)	2	3
Pnkd (pr.5 + pr.7) ^	CCCAGCATGGCTTGGCAGG	ATTGAAGAGGCGGGGCTGAG	282 (+ 26)		

Left column represents gene name, or gene name together with primer combination for transcript-specific probes. Second and third columns show primer sequences, fourth column shows product length, fifth and sixth columns represent ISH probe incubation times for P0-P7 and P14-P22 retinas. Some of the primer combinations could give rise to two different DNA fragments depending on splice variants. ^ - primer combination used for RT-PCR not ISH. ^^ - primer combination used for ISH not RT-PCR. * - primer combination gave negative result in RT-PCR. Primer combinations pr.3 + pr.8, pr.4 + pr.8, pr.6 + pr.8 for Clcc1 not shown in this table also gave negative results (for predicted fragment sizes see Table 2). Numbers in parenthesis refer to T3 promoter extension, as required for ISH probe generation

Table 2 Predicted and confirmed splicing variants for Clcc1 and Pnkd

Primer Pair	fragment size, bp	Predicted transcripts	Confirmed splice junctions
Clcc1			
pr.1 + pr.9	208 + (26)	NM_145543^	ex.1a_ex.3
pr.2 + pr.9	181+ (26), 252 + (26)	NM_145543^, NM_001177771, XM_006501416^, XM_011240107	ex.1a/1b_ex.3
pr.3 + pr.9	220 + (26)	NM_001177771, XM_006501416^, XM_011240107	ex.1b_ex.3
pr.4 + pr.9	203 + (26)	NM_001177771, NM_001177770, XM_006501416^, XM_011240107	ex.1b_ex.3
pr.5 + pr.9	172 + (26)	NM_001177771, NM_001177770, XM_006501416^, XM_011240107	ex.1b_ex.3
pr.6 + pr.9*	293 + (26)	NM_001177770, XM_011240107	none
pr.7 + pr.9	300 + (26)	NM_001177771, novel uncharacterized	ex.2_ex.3
pr.2 + pr.8*	199 + (26) 270 + (26)	NM_001177771	none
pr.3 + pr.8*	238 + (26)	NM_001177771	none
pr.4 + pr.8*	221 + (26)	NM_001177771	none
pr.6 + pr.8*	453 + (26)	none	none
pr.7 + pr.8	159 + (26)	NM_001177771, novel uncharacterized	ex.2
pr.10 + pr.11	432 + (26)	all transcripts	ex.4_ex.5_ex.6
Pnkd			
pr.1 + pr.2	246 + (26)	NM_025580, NM_001039509^	ex.2_ex.3
pr.3 + pr.4*	289 + (26)	NM_025580	none
pr.5 + pr.6	167 + (26)	NM_019999^	ex.5
pr.5 + pr.7	282 + (26)	NM_019999^	ex.5_ex.6
pr.8 + pr.9	360 + (26)	all transcripts	3'-UTR

Column 1 represents primer combinations, column 2 – DNA fragment size after RT-PCR. Some of the primer combinations could give rise to two different DNA fragments from two different splice variants. Column 3 shows transcript variants predicted to be recognized by the respective primer combination. Column 4 demonstrates exon-to-exon splicing junction which were experimentally confirmed by RT-PCR using respective primer combination. ^ - transcripts detected by RT-PCR. * - primer combination which gave negative result in RT-PCR. Numbers in parenthesis refer to T3 promoter extension, as required for ISH probe generation (Table should appear after *"Clcc1 transcripts detected in the retina"* section in "Results")

10% bovine serum albumin (BSA), 10% normal donkey serum (NDS) and 0.5% Triton) for 1 h at RT and incubated at 4 °C overnight in primary antibody mixes (PBS, 10% BSA, 3% NDS, 0.5% Triton, and primary antibodies). Antibodies used were 1:100 rat anti-Cdh4 (MRCD5, provided by M. Takeichi and H. Matsunami to DSHB; dshb.biology.uiowa.edu; [51]), 1:200 rabbit anti-Elfn1 (gift from Dr. K. Martemyanov, The Scripps Research Institute, Jupiter, USA), 1:200 sheep anti-AP (American Research products, 13–2355), 1:20 mouse anti-Brn3a (MAB1585; Chemicon-Millipore). After washes, secondary antibody solutions were applied for 1 h RT (150 μl per slide - PBS, 10% BSA, 3% NDS, 0.5% Triton, 0.5 μl of 1000× DAPI and secondary antibodies). All secondaries were Alexa conjugated Donkey sera from Molecular Probes. Images were captured with a 40× lens on a Zeiss Imager.Z2 fitted with an Apotome for fluorescent imaging and Axiovision software. For each probe, genotype and age, eight or more images derived from at least 3 animals were collected.

Statistical analysis

We used Kolmogorov-Smirnov (KS2) test for statistical assessment of ISH quantitation results. Sample numbers, means, medians and significance levels for KS2 and student t tests are provided in Additional file 1: Table S1.

Results

Screening strategy

To identify genes that could be responsible for RGC type specification in Brn3a-knockout retinas, we performed an in situ hybridization screen using a set of potential Brn3a-specific target genes recently identified in our RGC-specific RNASeq screening [5].

In order to achieve complete ablation of *Brn3a* from RGCs, we crossed females homozygote for the previously reported $Brn3a^{CKOAP/CKOAP}$ allele [9] with Rax:Cre; $Brn3a^{KO/WT}$ males. Rax:Cre is a BAC transgenic allele [49] that provides essentially complete Cre recombination beginning at early stages of eye development (Embryonic day 9, E9). Offspring were either Rax:Cre; $Brn3a^{CKOAP/WT}$ resulting in Brn3a heterozygote RGCs (henceforth $Brn3a^{AP/WT}$ RGCs) or Rax:Cre; $Brn3a^{CKOAP/KO}$ resulting in Brn3a knockout RGCs (henceforth $Brn3a^{AP/KO}$ RGCs). As previously reported, Brn3a protein is expressed in a large fraction of Ganglion Cell Layer (GCL) nuclei, and dendrites of $Brn3a^{AP/WT}$ RGCs occupy the outer two-thirds of the Inner Plexiform Layer (IPL, Fig. 1a, c). However, in Rax:Cre; $Brn3a^{CKOAP/KO}$ retinas there are essentially no Brn3a positive cells, and the dendrites of $Brn3a^{AP/KO}$ RGCs show a gap in AP-positive lamination (Fig. 1b, d). This gap, which extends between the characteristic positions of Choline-Acetyl-Transferase (ChAT) positive Starburst

Amacrine cells, is largely due to loss of RGCs with small and dense dendritic arbor (midget-like cells) (Fig. 1b, d) [2, 9, 28]. In order to capture the essential events in RGC type specification (dendrite formation, axon invasion into retinorecipient nuclei, synaptogenesis, and functional maturation) we prepared retinal sections from Rax:Cre; $Brn3a^{CKOAP/KO}$ and Rax:Cre; $Brn3a^{CKOAP/WT}$ littermate controls at five postnatal ages – P0, P3, P7, P14 and P22.

The genes screened in this study represent a subset of potential Brn3a target genes identified by comparing transcript level RNASeq data from $Brn3a^{AP/KO}$ and $Brn3a^{AP/WT}$ postnatal day 3 RGCs [5]. Genes selected in our ISH analysis had to have at least one transcript with more than 2 FPKM (fragments per million reads per gene kilobase) expression level in RGCs, and at least a two-fold differential in $Brn3a^{AP/WT}$ versus $Brn3a^{AP/KO}$ RGCs (Brn3a regulated or dependent). In addition, the Brn3a dependent transcript should show no Brn3b regulation (less than two-fold differential in P3 $Brn3b^{AP/WT}$ versus $Brn3b^{AP/KO}$ RGCs). From the set of 180 differentially expressed transcripts that had these criteria (identified in [5]), we focused on genes whose products had potential functional association with gene regulation, synapse formation, cell adhesion, vesicle transport, cytoskeleton changes, intracellular signaling, or secreted molecules. These molecular classes should be particularly important during RGC type specification.

In Figs. 2, 3, 4, 5, 6, 7, 8, 9, 10, 11, 12 and 13, we provide RNASeq data for transcript and gene expression and ISH results together with its quantitation for all target genes, organized by molecular class. ISH quantitation results are summarized in Additional file 1: Table S1. RNASeq data for transcript expression are derived from the Sajgo et al. [5] data set and gene level analysis is based on the same dataset (however it takes into account all possible transcript isoforms, not only RefSeq ones). RNASeq data for transcript expression represent all RefSeq transcripts that had at least 1 FPKM expression level in at least one retinal or RGC sample and including the ones that passed the above selection criteria. Note that the x scales for each plot are different, depending on the range of FPKM/CPM (counts per million reads) values in the individual samples. The ISH panels show the gene level analysis, with riboprobes directed against the 3'-Untranslated Regions (3'-UTR), which are shared by all transcripts.

Transcriptional and translational regulators (Figures 2 and 3)

Two transcription factors (Foxp2 and Tshz2) and one RNA processing factor (Rbfox1) passed our selection criteria. Two Rbfox1 (RNA binding protein, fox-1 homolog 1) RefSeq transcripts were significantly expressed in P3 Brn3a+ RGCs compared to the retina (NM_021477 and

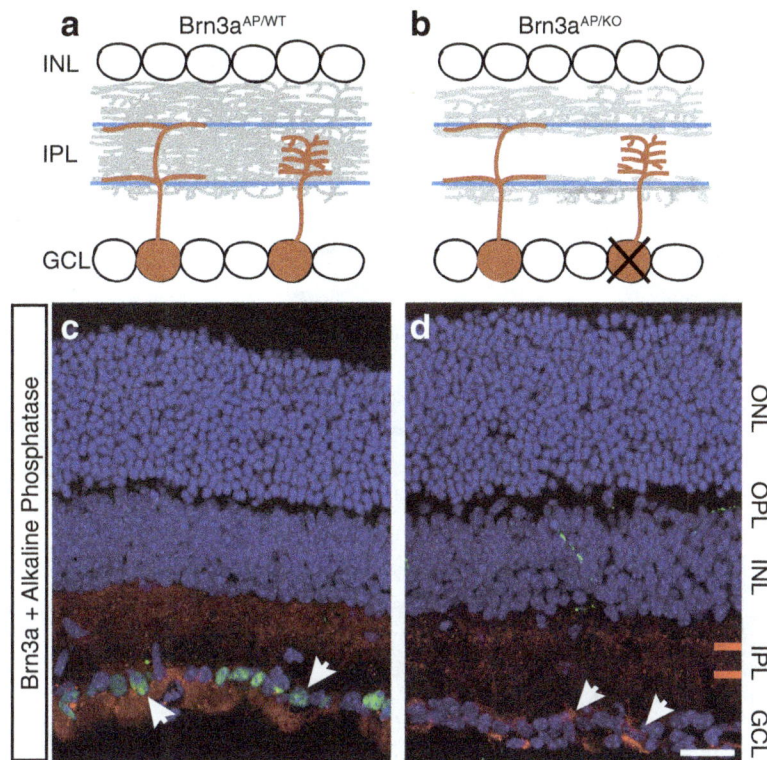

Fig. 1 Retinal Brn3a ablation results in specific RGC defects. **a-b** Summary of Brn3a RGC phenotype, based on previous work [2, 9, 28]. Distribution of dendritic arbors for Brn3a heterozygote (**a**, Brn3a$^{AP/WT}$) and Brn3a knock-out (**b**, Brn3a$^{AP/KO}$) RGCs. **a** Dendrites of Brn3a$^{AP/WT}$ RGCs, including ON-OFF-DS bistratified (left) and midget-like (right) cells, occupy the outer two-thirds of the Inner Plexiform Layer (IPL, gray). **b** Midget-like cells are absent from Brn3a$^{AP/KO}$ RGCs, and the dendrites of remaining cells are co-stratifying with the inner and outer Starburst Amacrine cell dendritic arbors (blue lines). **c-d** Indirect immunofluorescence illustrating Brn3a^{AP} RGC arbors and cell bodies (red), and Brn3a transcription factor expression (green) in Rax:Cre; Brn3a$^{CKOAP/WT}$ (**c**) and Rax:Cre; Brn3a$^{CKOAP/KO}$ (**d**) adult retinas. Note the gap of Brn3a^{AP} staining in **d**, and the absence of Brn3a TF positive cell bodies in the GCL. ONL = Outer Nuclear Layer; OPL = Outer Plexiform Layer; INL = Inner Nuclear Layer; IPL = Inner Plexiform Layer; GCL = Ganglion Cell Layer. Red bars in IPL of (**d**) indicate the position of inner and outer ChAT bands. Arrowheads are showing AP-expressing cells. Scale bar in D, 25 μm

NM_183188, Fig. 3a^{II}-a^{III}), but only NM_021477 showed significant Brn3a dependence. Gene level RNASeq analysis for Rbfox1 also revealed both RGC-enrichment as well as tendency towards Brn3a-mediated regulation of expression (Fig. 3a^{I}). The in situ time series (Fig. 2a) confirmed relative GCL enrichment for Rbfox1 from P0-P7 (P0 WT and KO – $p < 0.001$; P3 KO, P7 WT and KO – $p < 0.05$, Additional file 1: Table S1 A-C), however beginning with P7, the INL and eventually the ONL turned positive (Figs. 2a, 3a). Differential expression between Brn3aWT and KO retinas was not observed. Both Foxp2 (forkhead box P2) transcripts expressed in the retina (NM_212435 and NM_053242) were selectively enriched in Brn3a RGCs and appeared regulated by Brn3a (Fig. 3b^{II}-b^{III}). Gene level RNASeq analysis also showed strong differential expression in Brn3a WT RGCs compared to Brn3a KO RGCs. Enrichment of Foxp2 expression in the GCL was confirmed by ISH in early time-points (P0-P3) and in the adult, while the significant ($p < 0.001$) regulation by Brn3a in the GCL

was observed at P7 and P22 (Figs. 2b, 3b, Additional file 1: Table S1). Tshz2 (teashirt zinc finger homeobox 2) showed enrichment in RGCs vs. retina as well as Brn3a dependency at both gene and transcript level (Fig. 3c^{I}-c^{II}). ISH confirms modest but significant GCL enrichment from P0-P14 and Brn3a regulation at P3 ($p < 0.05$) and P22 ($p < 0.001$, Figs. 2c, 3c, Additional file 1: Table S1). Note that Brn3a signal can still be detected in the GCL of Rax:Cre; Brn3a$^{CKOAP/KO}$ (KO) retinas (Fig. 2d), since the ISH probe is directed against the 3'UTR region which is not ablated in the recombined conditional knock-in allele (Brn3a^{AP}) and Brn3a ablation results in only 30–40% reduction in total Brn3a$^+$ RGC numbers [5, 9, 28].

Intracellular signaling and cytoskeleton-associated proteins (Figures 4 and 5)

Eml1 (echinoderm microtubule associated protein like 1) has 3 transcripts (NM_001286347, NM_001043335 and NM_001286346, Fig. 5a^{II}-a^{IV}), and only one of them (NM_001286347) shows Brn3a RGC enrichment and

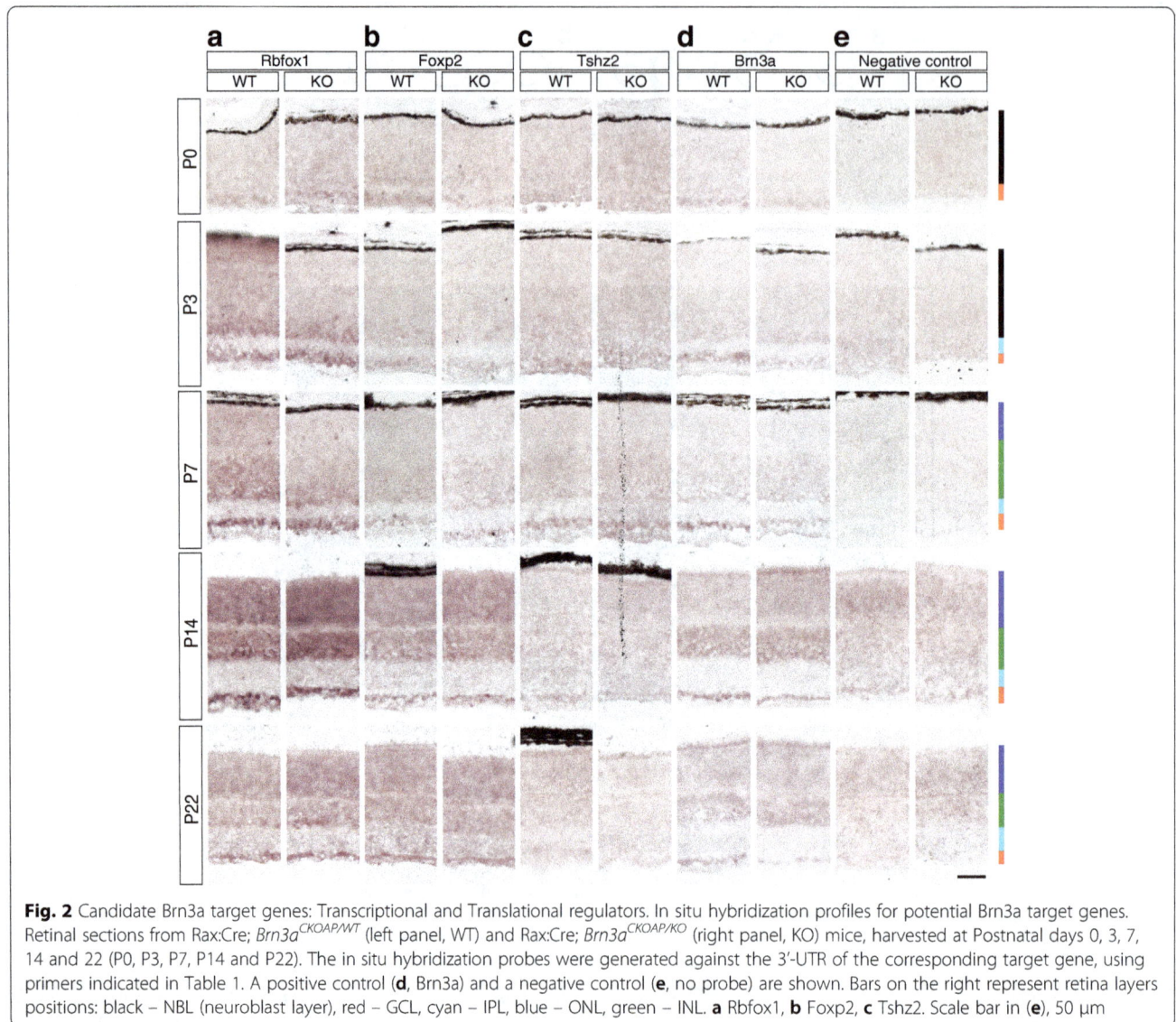

Fig. 2 Candidate Brn3a target genes: Transcriptional and Translational regulators. In situ hybridization profiles for potential Brn3a target genes. Retinal sections from Rax:Cre; *Brn3a^CKOAP/WT* (left panel, WT) and Rax:Cre; *Brn3a^CKOAP/KO* (right panel, KO) mice, harvested at Postnatal days 0, 3, 7, 14 and 22 (P0, P3, P7, P14 and P22). The in situ hybridization probes were generated against the 3'-UTR of the corresponding target gene, using primers indicated in Table 1. A positive control (**d**, Brn3a) and a negative control (**e**, no probe) are shown. Bars on the right represent retina layers positions: black – NBL (neuroblast layer), red – GCL, cyan – IPL, blue – ONL, green – INL. **a** Rbfox1, **b** Foxp2, **c** Tshz2. Scale bar in (**e**), 50 µm

Brn3a dependence. Gene level analysis shows even distribution of expression between RGC and retina samples at P3 (Fig. 5a^I). ISH (Fig. 4a) demonstrates that Eml1 is significantly GCL enriched in both WT and Brn3a KO from P0-P7, however beginning with P14, the INL and later the ONL become positive (Fig. 5a, Additional file 1: Table S1). Eml1 is not differentially expressed between Brn3a WT and KO retinas throughout studied postnatal developmental period. Hpca (hippocalcin) has 4 transcripts expressed in the retina (NM_001130419, NM_010471, NM_001286081 and NM_001286083). First three of them were highly expressed in P3 Brn3a^{AP} RGCs compared to the retina (Fig. 5b^{II}-b^{IV}), while NM_001286083 (Fig. 5b^V) was selectively enriched in Brn3a^{KO} retina. Only NM_001130419 appeared regulated by Brn3a (Fig. 5b^{II}). Gene level analysis revealed enrichment in both Brn3aWT and Brn3aKO RGCs (Fig. 5b^I). Strong and significant GCL enrichment was

confirmed by ISH from P0-P7, however beginning with P14 Hpca is highly expressed in both GCL and inner INL. A modest reduction in Hpca level is apparent in the GCL of Brn3a^{KO} retinas at P0 ($p < 0.01$), P14 ($p < 0.01$) and P22 ($p < 0.05$, Figs. 4b, 5b, Additional file 1: Table S1). The only expressed Plppr3 (phospholipid phosphatase related 3) transcript shows a moderate enrichment in P3 RGCs vs. retina (Fig. 5c^{II}), while RNASeq gene level analysis does not reveal any strong signs of GCL enrichment or Brn3a dependency (Fig. 5c^I). ISH time series confirms the transcript RNASeq results in terms of GCL enrichment from P0-P14 (Figs. 4c, 5c, Additional file 1: Table S1 A-D). The expression of Plppr3 decreases towards adult and this gene is not affected by Brn3a loss at P0-P7, while at P14 we found significant differential expression between Brn3a WT and KO ($p < 0.01$, Fig. 5c, Additional file 1: Table S1 A-D). Both Mapk10 (mitogen-activated protein

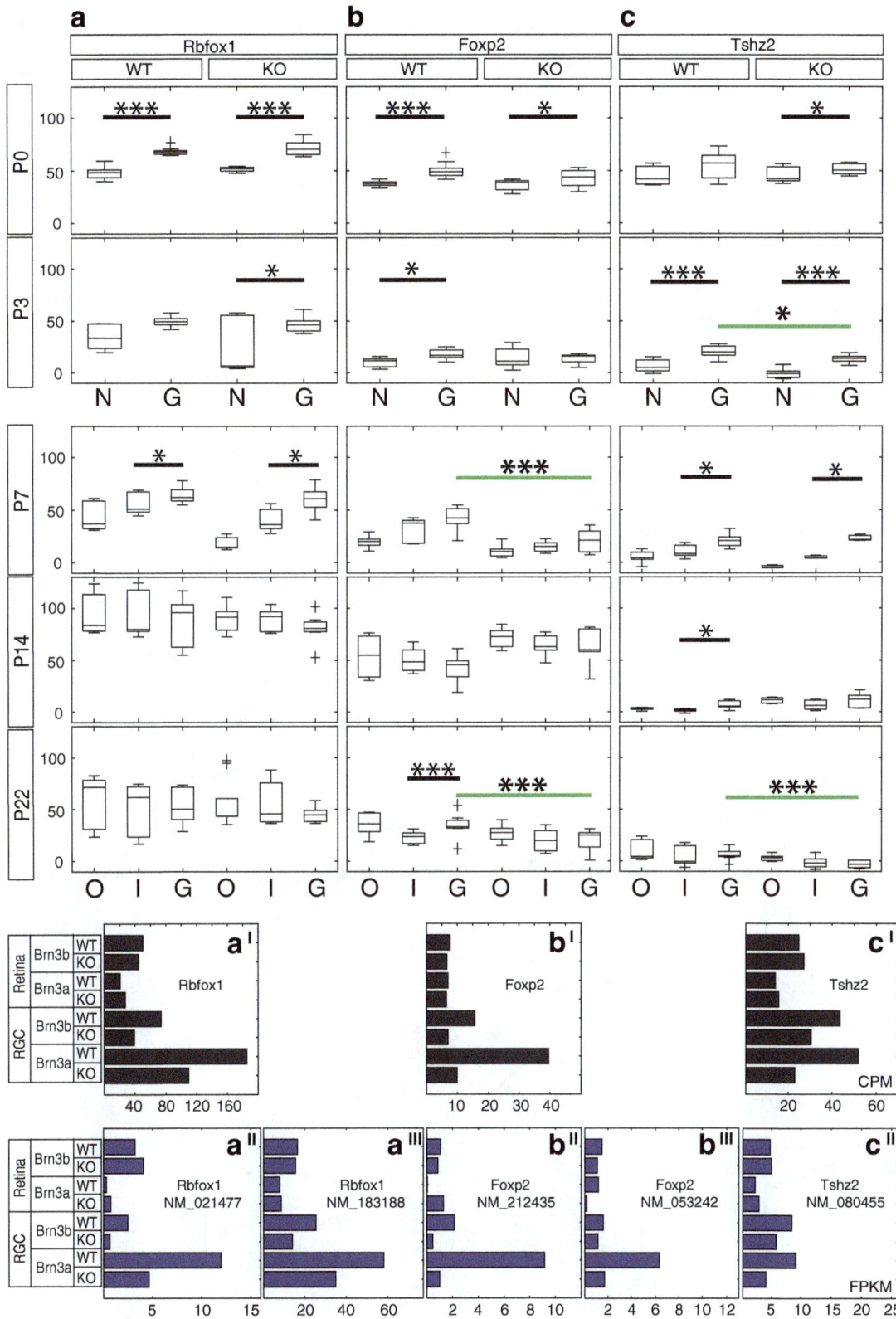

Fig. 3 (See legend on next page.)

(See figure on previous page.)

Fig. 3 Candidate Brn3a target genes: Transcriptional and Translational regulators. RNASeq and ISH quantitation. In situ hybridization quantitation (**a-c**), and gene (d^l- c^l) and transcript (d^{ll}- c^{ll}) level RNASeq profiles for potential Brn3a target genes. **a-c** Box-whiskers plots for NBL and GCL of P0 and P3, and ONL, INL and GCL for P7-P22 retinas from Rax:Cre; $Brn3a^{CKOAP/WT}$ (left panel, WT) and Rax:Cre; $Brn3a^{CKOAP/KO}$ (right panel, KO) mice, harvested at P0, P3, P7, P14 and P22 show normalized (all except P0) mean intensity values from images of retinal sections (Y axis). Individual values for each layer are normalized to the respective IPL value in P3-P22 cases. X axis represents retinal layers: N – NBL, G – GCL, O – ONL, I – INL. Horizontal bars in panels denote observation pairs showing significant expression differences (Kolmogorov-Smirnov - KS2 test) between INL/NBL and GCL (black bar) and Brn3a-dependency by comparing respective WT and KO GCL values (green bar; significance levels * $p < 0.05$, ** $p < 0.01$, *** $p < 0.001$). All values and KS2 test outcomes are provided in Additional file 1: Table S1. d^l-c^l Gene level RNASeq profiles from affinity purified Brn3^{AP} RGCs (RGC) and retinal supernatants (Retina) derived from P3 mice with the following genotypes: Pax6α:Cre; $Brn3a^{CKOAP/WT}$ (Brn3a-WT), Pax6α:Cre; $Brn3a^{CKOAP/KO}$ (Brn3a-KO), Pax6α:Cre; $Brn3b^{CKOAP/WT}$ (Brn3b-WT), and Pax6α:Cre; $Brn3b^{CKOAP/KO}$ (Brn3b-KO) (Sajgo et al. 2017). Values on the x axis are in CPM (counts per million reads), and bars represent mean values for two replicates (RGC samples) and single samples (retina supernatants). d^{ll}-c^{ll} Transcript level RNASeq profiles from the same samples as in d^l-c^l Values on the x axis are in FPKM, and bars represent mean values for two replicates (RGC samples) and single samples (retina supernatants). For each gene, only transcripts having detectable (> 1 FPKM values) in at least one of the samples are presented. The transcript (NM) number is indicated under the gene name. d^l-a^{lll} Rbfox1, b^l-b^{lll} Foxp2, c^l-c^{ll} Tshz2

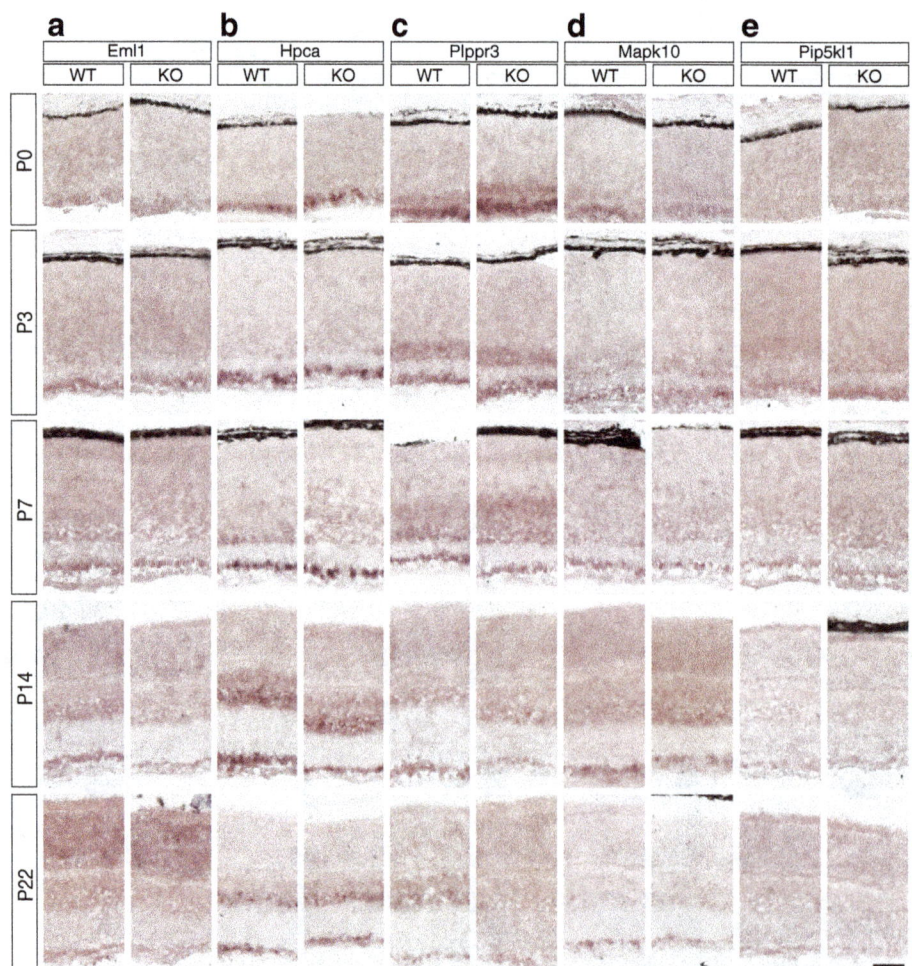

Fig. 4 Candidate Brn3a target genes: Intracellular signaling and cytoskeleton-associated proteins. **a-e** In situ hybridization analysis in WT and Brn3a-KO mouse retinas at 5 postnatal ages. **a** Eml1, **b** Hpca, **c** Plppr3, **d** Mapk10, **e** Pip5kl1. All samples were collected, imaged and formatted as in Fig. 2. Scale bar – 50 μm

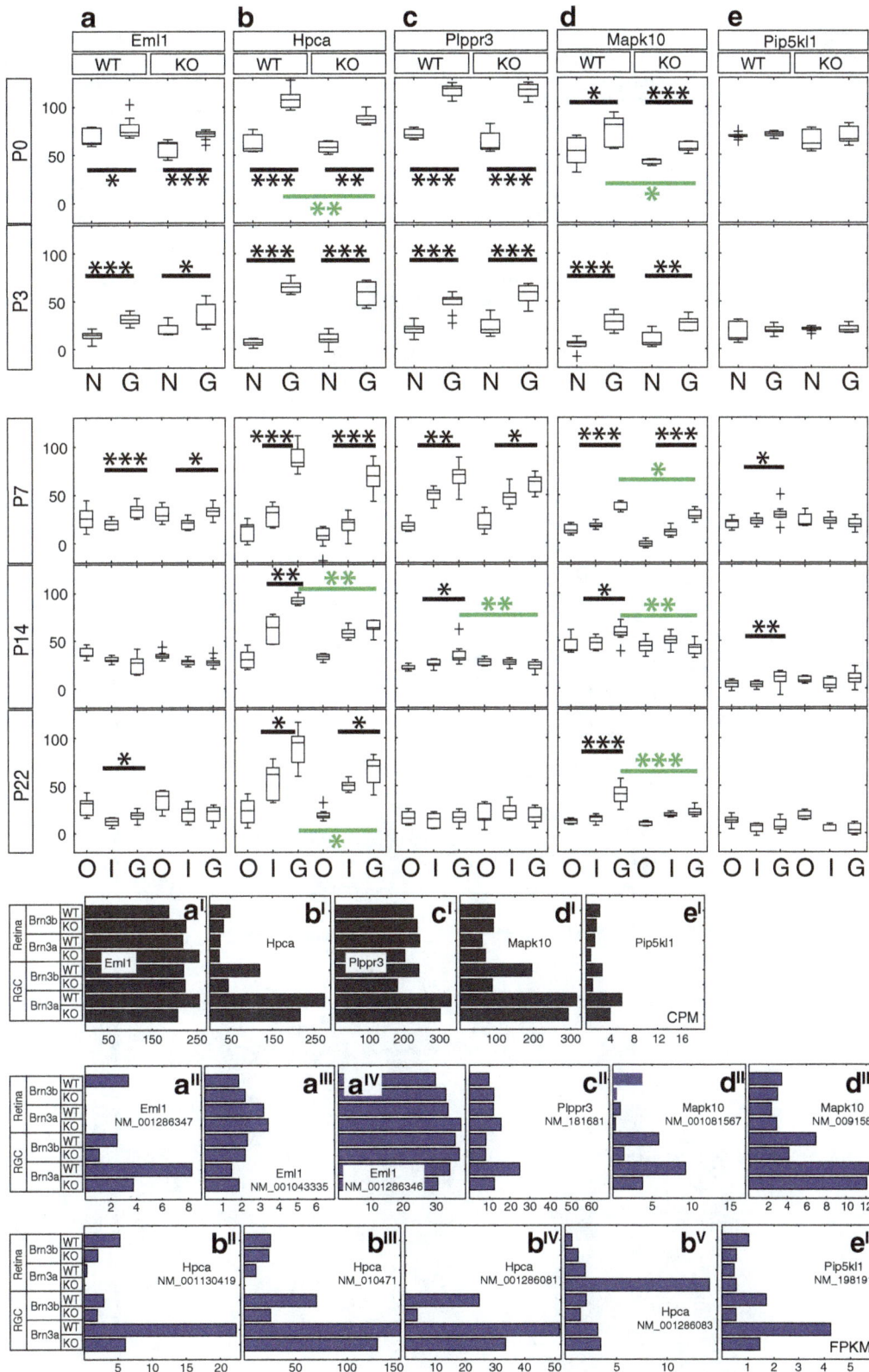

Fig. 5 (See legend on next page.)

(See figure on previous page.)

Fig. 5 Candidate Brn3a target genes: Intracellular signaling and cytoskeleton-associated proteins. RNASeq and ISH quantitation. **a-e** In situ hybridization quantitation analysis in WT and Brn3a-KO mouse retinas at 5 postnatal ages. a^I-e^I RNASeq gene level profiles at P3 (expressed in CPM). a^{II}-e^{II} RNASeq transcript level profiles expressed in FPKM for all transcripts of the five genes detected at more than 1 FPKM in at least one P3 retinal sample. a-a^{IV} Eml1, b-b^V Hpca, c-c^{II} Plppr3, d-d^{III} Mapk10, e-e^{II} Pip5kl1. Plot formatting and annotations as in Fig. 3

kinase 10) isoforms (NM_001081567 and NM_009158, Fig. $5d^{II}$-d^{III}) are enriched in RGCs compared to the retina. Only one of them (NM_001081567) appears to be regulated by Brn3a (and also Brn3b) at P3. Gene level analysis confirms only enrichment in Brn3a WT and KO samples, and differential expression between Brn3b WT and KO (Fig. $5d^I$). ISH reveals significant Mapk10 GCL enrichment throughout postnatal development (P0-P22, Figs. 4d, 5d, Additional file 1: Table S1). Beginning with P7, Mapk10+ cell bodies sparsely label the GCL, and their number appears to be reduced in Brn3a^{KO} retinas compared to the WT at the majority of studied ages (P0 $p < 0.05$, P7 $p < 0.05$, P14 $p < 0.01$, P22 $p < 0.001$, Additional file 1: Table S1). Transcript and gene RNASeq profiles show enrichment, and in case of a transcript – Brn3a dependency of Pip5kl1 (phosphatidylinositol-4-phoshate 5-kinase like 1) expression in P3 RGCs vs. retina (Fig. $3e^I$-e^{II}). However, in situ time series confirms GCL enrichment only at P7 ($p < 0.05$) and P14 ($p < 0.01$), and it does not reveal a considerable Brn3a regulation of Pip5kl1 (Figs. 4e, 5e, Additional file 1: Table S1).

Vesicle-associated proteins (Figures 6 and 7)

Transcript level RNASeq shows that the only expressed Ankrd13b (ankyrin repeat domain 13b) RefSeq transcript is strongly enriched in Brn3a$^{AP/WT}$ RGCs compared to

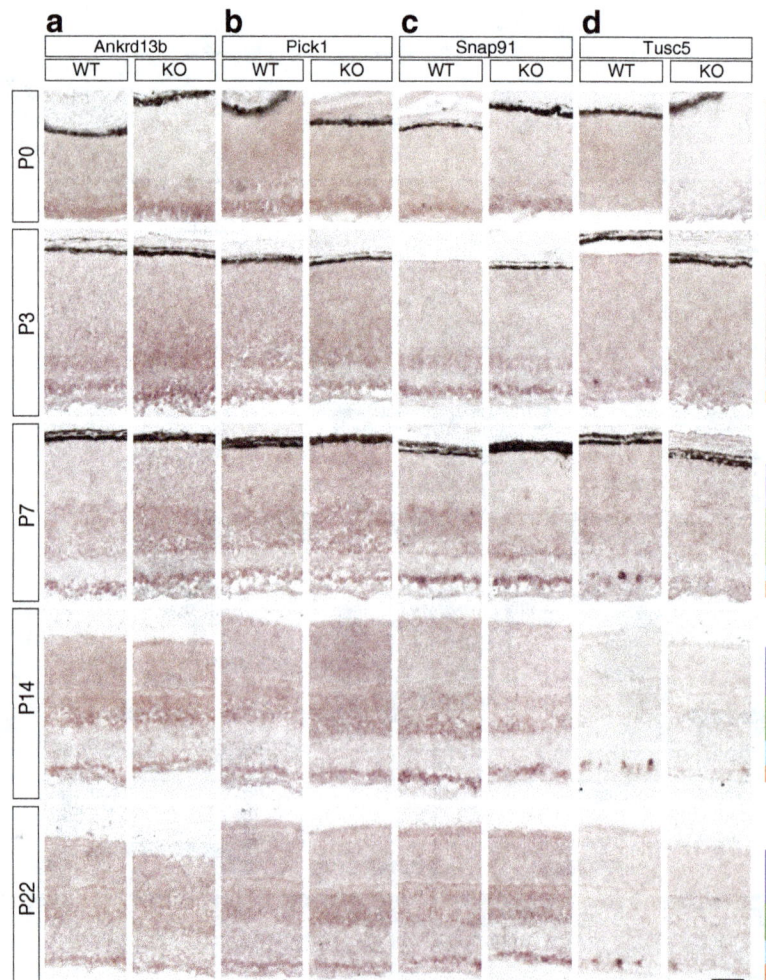

Fig. 6 Candidate Brn3a target genes: Vesicle-associated proteins. **a-d** In situ hybridization analysis in WT and Brn3a-KO mouse retinas at 5 postnatal ages. **a** Ankrd13b, **b** Pick1, **c** Snap91, **d** Tusc5. All samples were collected, imaged and formatted as in Fig. 2. Scale bar – 50 μm

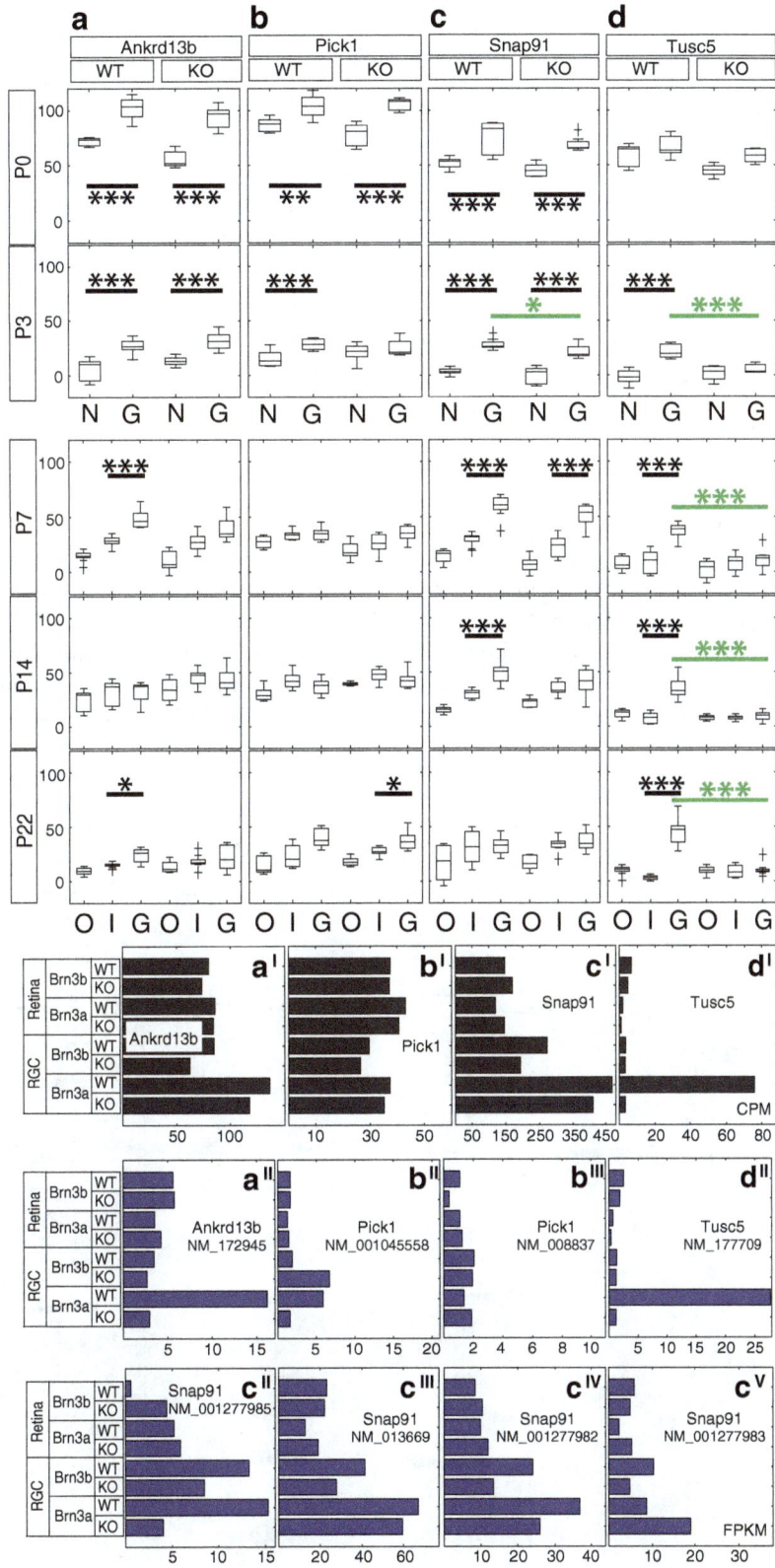

Fig. 7 (See legend on next page.)

(See figure on previous page.)
Fig. 7 Candidate Brn3a target genes: Vesicle-associated proteins. RNASeq and ISH quantitation. **a-d** In situ hybridization quantitation analysis in WT and Brn3a-KO mouse retinas at 5 postnatal ages. a^I-d^I RNASeq gene level profiles at P3 (expressed in CPM). a^{II}-d^{II} RNASeq transcript level profiles expressed in FPKM for all transcripts of the four genes detected at more than 1 FPKM in at least one P3 retinal sample. a-a^{II} Ankrd13b, b-b^{III} Pick1, c-c^V Snap91, d-d^{II} Tusc5. Plot formatting and annotations as in Fig. 3

the retina and other RGC samples (Fig. 7a^{II}). At the same time, gene level analysis revealed only the enrichment in Brn3a WT and KO samples but not the dependency on Brn3a (Fig. 7a^I). ISH confirms strong enrichment in the GCL from P0-P7, which decreases towards adult (Fig. 7a). There is no significant Brn3a regulation in the GCL at any of the studied ages (Additional file 1: Table S1). Two Pick1 (protein interacting with C kinase 1) transcripts (NM_001045558 and NM_008837, Fig. 7b^{II}-b^{III}) demonstrated a modest enrichment in RGCs vs. retina at P3, while gene expression RNASeq analysis did not show any signs of it (Fig. 7b^I). One of the transcripts (NM_001045558) was enriched in Brn3a$^{AP/WT}$ and Brn3b$^{AP/KO}$ RGCs, suggesting positive regulation by Brn3a and negative regulation by Brn3b (Fig. 7b^{II}). ISH confirms GCL enrichment from P0-P3, however it does not show a significant Brn3a-dependent differential expression (Figs. 6b and 7b, Additional file 1:

Table S1). Snap91 (synaptosome associated protein 91) gene has 4 retinally expressed isoforms (NM_001277985, NM_013669, NM_001277982 and NM_001277983, Fig. 7c^{II}-c^V), all of which showed enrichment in RGCs compared to the retina. However only NM_001277985 shows a strong dependency on Brn3a expression in RGCs (Fig. 7c^{II}). Gene level analysis confirms RGC enrichment, especially in Brn3a RGC samples, but it does not show Brn3a-dependent differential expression (Fig. 7c^I). ISH time series confirms a significant enrichment in the GCL from P0-P14, and shows the only time point (P3) with significant ($p < 0.05$) Brn3a dependency of expression (Figs. 6c, 7c, Additional file 1: Table S1). According to P3 RNA-Seq data (Fig. 7d^I-d^{II}), Tusc5 (tumor suppressor candidate 5) is highly enriched in Brn3a$^{AP/WT}$ RGCs, compared to the retina and other RGC samples, and strongly regulated by Brn3a. ISH reveals intensely stained sparse cell bodies in the GCL of Brn3a WT retinas, which are nearly completely

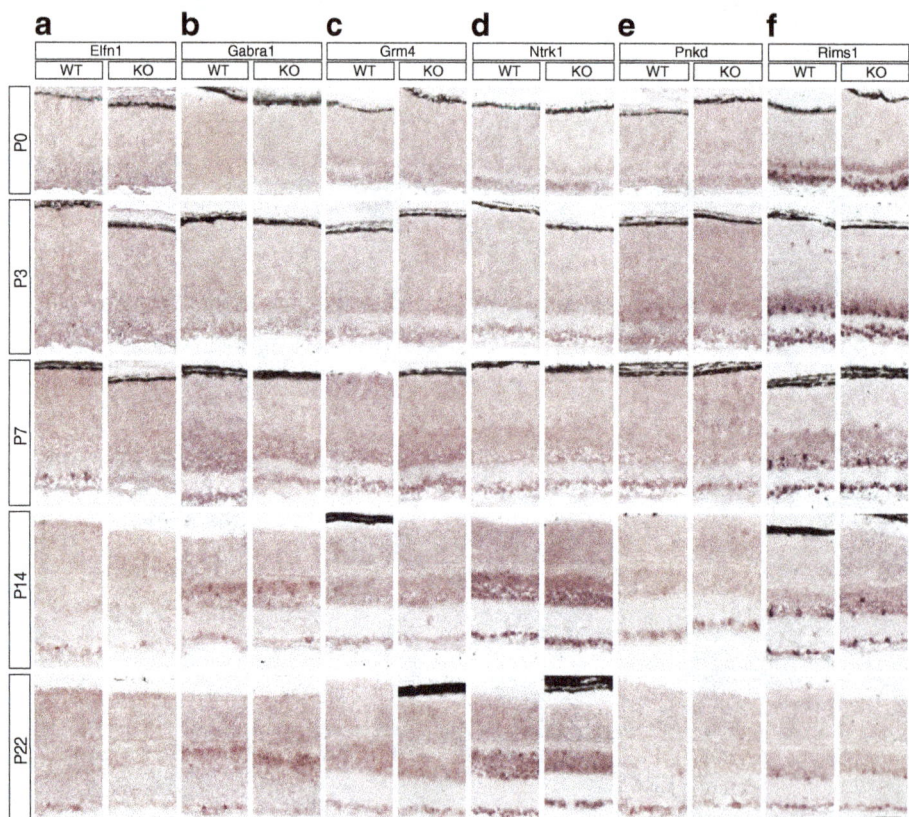

Fig. 8 Candidate Brn3a target genes: Synapse-associated proteins. **a-f** In situ hybridization analysis in WT and Brn3a-KO mouse retinas at 5 postnatal ages. **a** Elfn1, **b** Gabra1, **c** Grm4, **d** Ntrk1, **e** Pnkd, **f** Rims1. All samples were collected, imaged and formatted as in Fig. 2. Scale bar – 50 μm

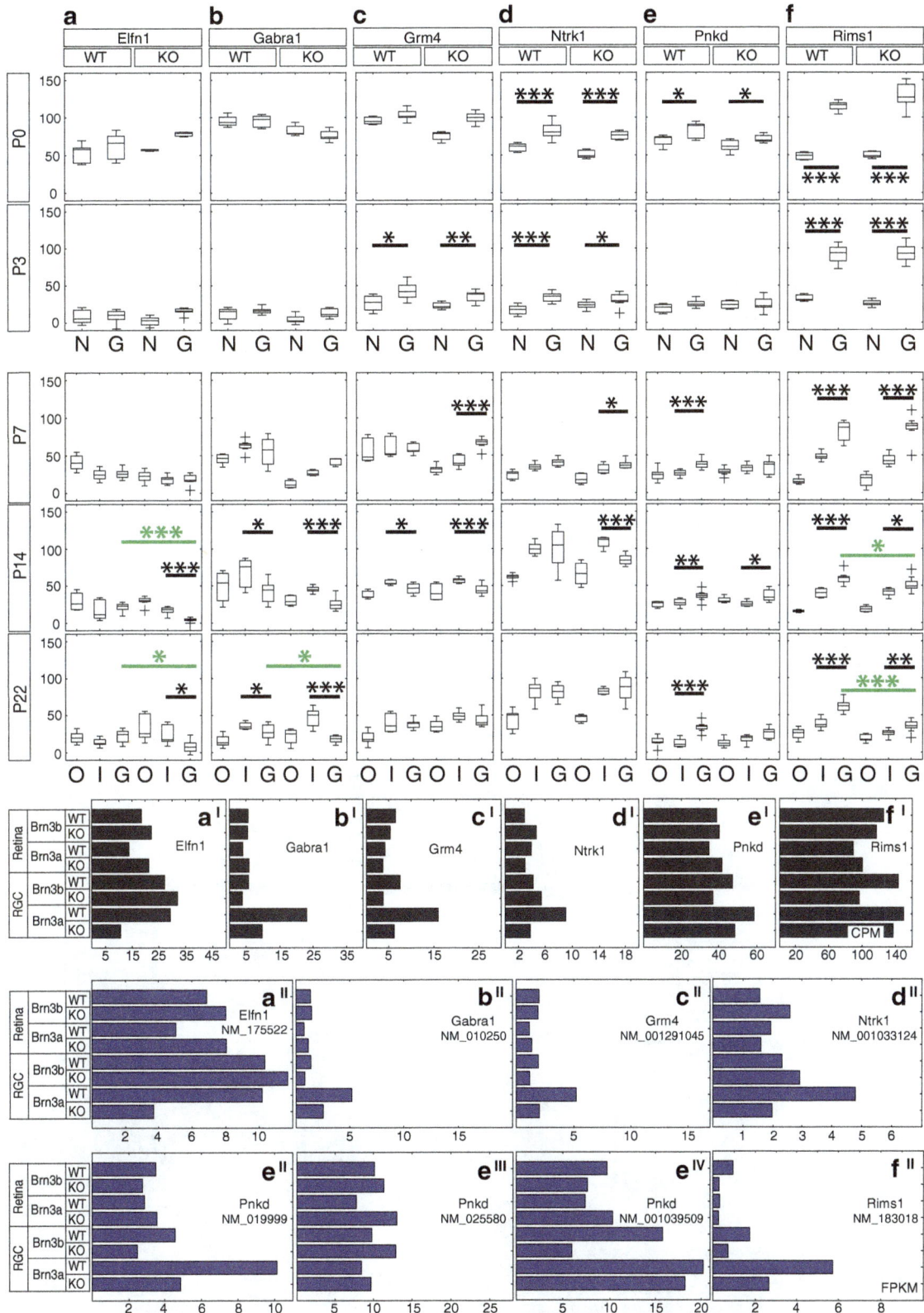

Fig. 9 (See legend on next page.)

(See figure on previous page.)

Fig. 9 Candidate Brn3a target genes: Synapse-associated proteins. RNASeq and ISH quantitation. **a-f** In situ hybridization quantitation analysis in WT and Brn3a-KO mouse retinas at 5 postnatal ages. a^I-f^I RNASeq gene level profiles at P3 (expressed in CPM). a^{II}-f^{II} RNASeq transcript level profiles expressed in FPKM for all transcripts of the six genes detected at more than 1 FPKM in at least one P3 retinal sample. a-a^{II} Elfn1, b-b^{II} Gabra1, c-c^{II} Grm4, d-d^{II} Ntrk1, e-e^{IV} Pnkd, f-f^{II} Rims1. Plot formatting and annotations as in Fig. 3

lost in Brn3a^{KO} (Fig. 6d). ISH quantitation results confirm strong GCL enrichment in the Brn3a WT retinas, and almost absolute dependency of GCL expression on Brn3a (Fig. 7d, Additional file 1: Table S1).

Synapse-associated proteins (Figures 8 and 9)

A single expressed Elfn1 (leucine rich repeat and fibronectin type III, extracellular 1) transcript is expressed in both retina and RGCs, and RNASeq demonstrated its profound differential between Brn3a$^{AP/WT}$ and Brn3a$^{AP/KO}$ RGCs (Fig. 9a^{II}), and gene level analysis confirms this result (Fig. 9a^I). ISH reveals intense sparse labelling in the GCL beginning with P3, peaking around P7 but

persisting in the adult (Fig. 8a). Due to the sparseness of expression the quantitation does not allow to capture significant GCL enrichment (Fig. 9a, Additional file 1: Table S1). Starting at P14, Elfn1 expression can also be seen in the INL and ONL. Beginning with P7, the number of intensely labelled GCL cell bodies declines in the Brn3a KO retinas (Fig. 8a), and this reduction reaches significant levels at P14 ($p < 0.001$) and persists in adult stage ($p < 0.05$, Fig. 9a, Additional file 1: Table S1 D-E). Surprisingly, due to downregulation in Brn3a KO GCL, we also can see a significant enrichment of expression in the INL compared to the GCL at P14 ($p < 0.001$) and adult age ($p < 0.05$). Gabra1 (gamma-aminobutyric acid

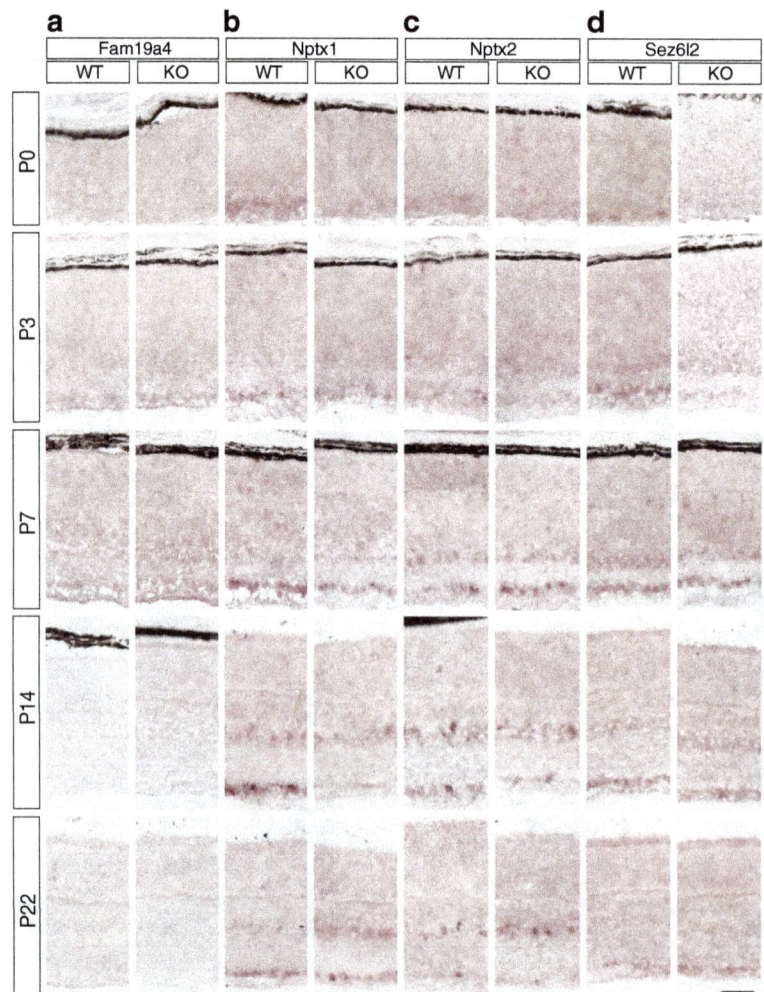

Fig. 10 Candidate Brn3a target genes: Secreted proteins. **a-d** In situ hybridization analysis in WT and Brn3a-KO mouse retinas at 5 postnatal ages. **a** – Fam19a4, **b** – Nptx1, **c** – Nptx2, **d** – Sez6l2. All samples were collected, imaged and formatted as in Fig. 2. Scale bar – 50 μm

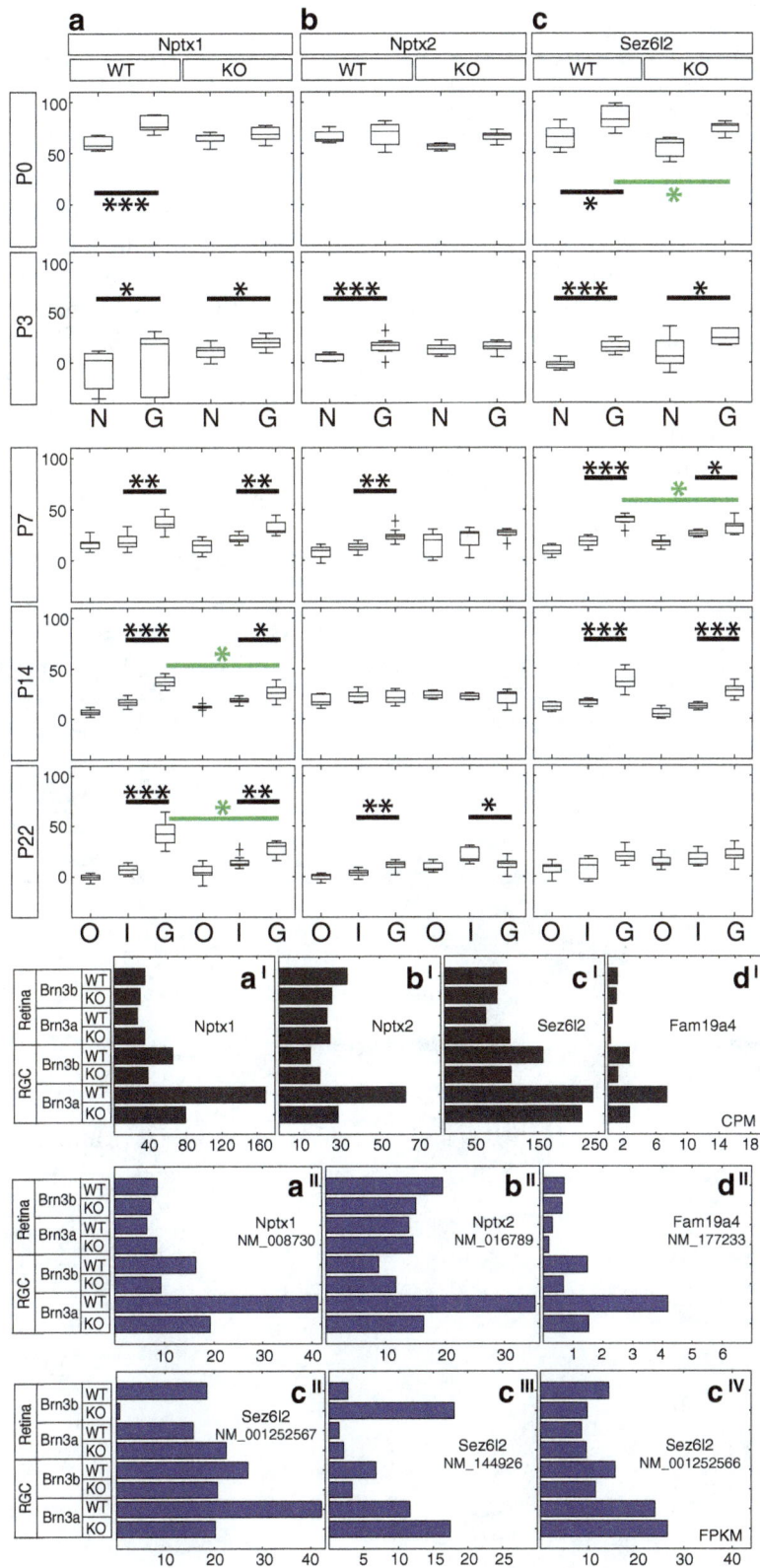

Fig. 11 (See legend on next page.)

(See figure on previous page.)
Fig. 11 Candidate Brn3a target genes: Secreted proteins. RNASeq and ISH quantitation. **a-c** In situ hybridization quantitation analysis in WT and Brn3a-KO mouse retinas at 5 postnatal ages. d^I-d^I RNASeq gene level profiles at P3 (expressed in CPM). a^{II}-d^{II} RNASeq transcript level profiles expressed in FPKM for all transcripts of the four genes detected at more than 1 FPKM in at least one P3 retinal sample. a-a^{II} Nptx1, b-b^{II} Nptx2, c-c^{IV} Sez6l2, d-d^{II} Fam19a4. Plot formatting and annotations as in Fig. 3.

A receptor) has one transcript that is enriched in Brn3a$^{AP/WT}$ RGCs compared to the retina and downregulated in Brn3a$^{AP/KO}$ RGCs (Fig. 9b^{II}), which is confirmed by gene level RNASeq analysis (Fig. 9b^I). ISH reveals the start of the expression at P3 in the GCL and P7 in the INL with progressive increase of the signal towards P14 and P22 (Fig. 8b). There are sparse intensely labelled cells in both INL and GCL of P14 and P22 Brn3a WT retina. And due to the sparseness of expression in the GCL but not as much in the INL, the INL levels are significantly higher compared to GCL level in both Brn3a WT and KO at P14 and P22 (Fig. 9b, Additional file 1: Table S1 D-E). Moreover, P22 Brn3a

KO retinas lack positive signal in the GCL but not the INL, suggesting a strong Brn3a dependency of Gabra1 in RGCs but not INL cells (likely Bipolar and/or Amacrine cells). Both transcript and gene level RNASeq analysis suggests that Grm4 (glutamate metabotropic receptor 4) – is enriched in Brn3a$^{AP/WT}$ RGCs and regulated by Brn3a (Fig. 9c^I-c^{II}). ISH reveals Grm4 expression in both GCL and INL (NBL) beginning with P0-P7 and continuing towards adult with no visible downregulation in Brn3a KO retinas (Fig. 8c). ISH quantitation shows a significant level of GCL enrichment at P3 (WT $p < 0.05$, KO < 0.01), which later reverts into INL enrichment (P14 WT $p < 0.05$, KO < 0.001, Fig. 9c). ISH results

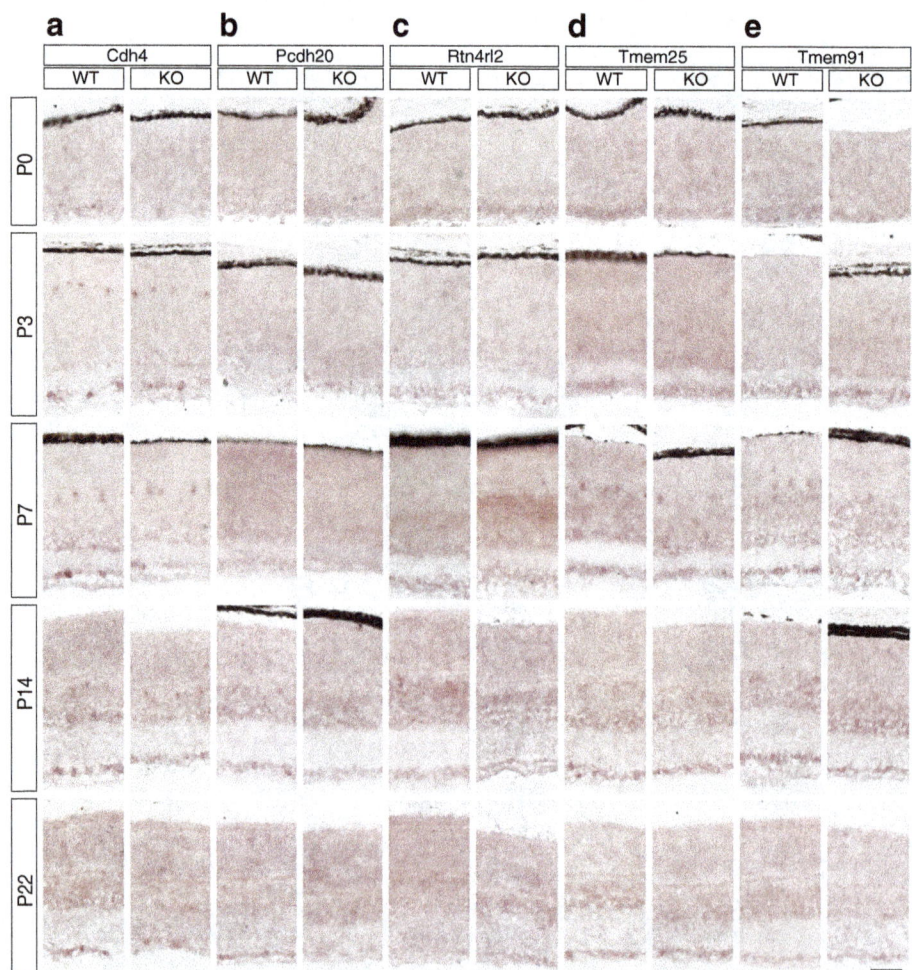

Fig. 12 Candidate Brn3a target genes: Adhesion molecules and other transmembrane proteins. **a-e** In situ hybridization analysis in WT and Brn3a-KO mouse retinas at 5 postnatal ages. **a** Cdh4, **b** Pcdh20, **c** Rtn4rl2, **d** Tmem25, **e** Tmem91. All samples were collected, imaged and formatted as in Fig. 2. Scale bar – 50 μm.

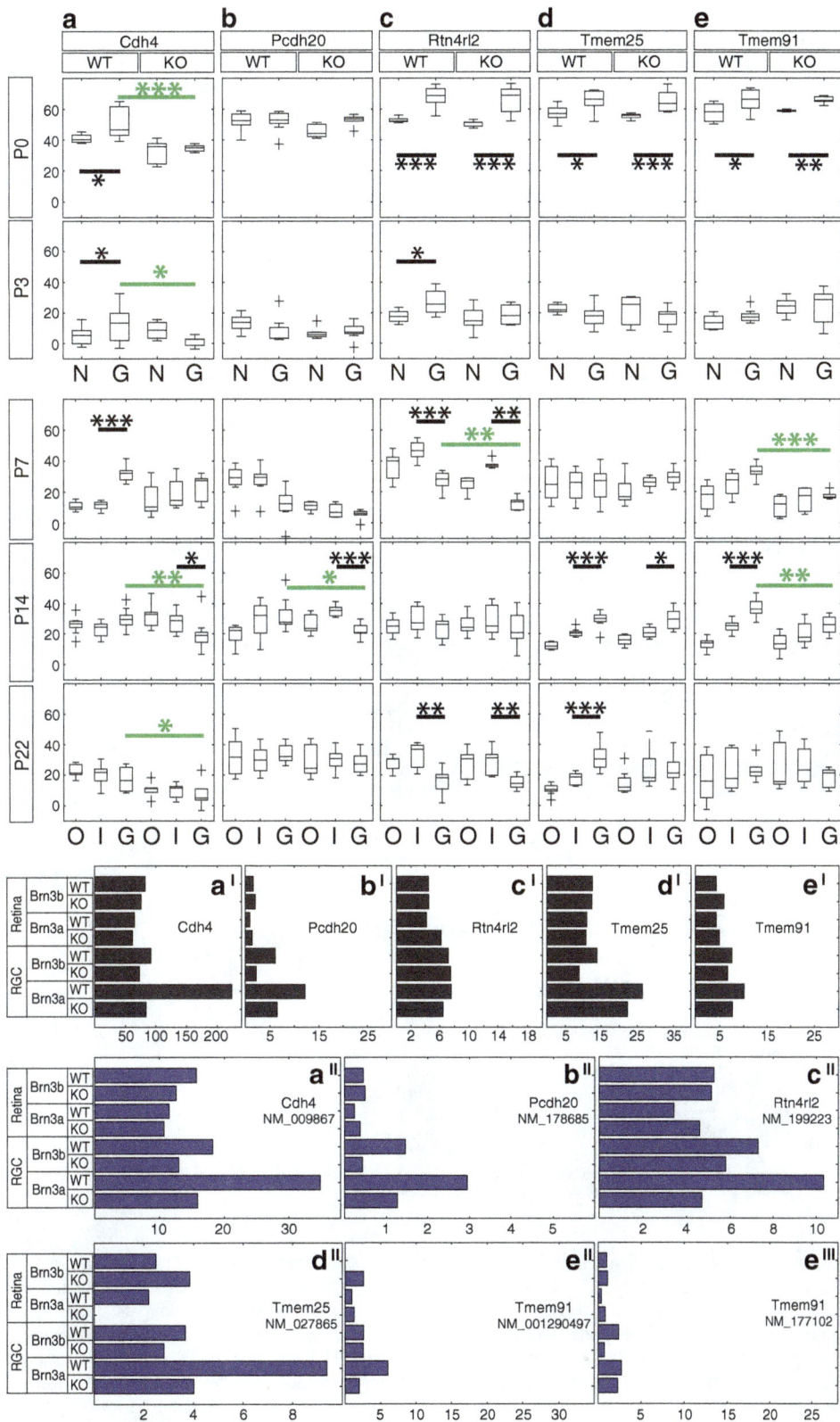

Fig. 13 (See legend on next page.)

(See figure on previous page.)

Fig. 13 Candidate Brn3a target genes: Adhesion molecules and other transmembrane proteins. RNASeq and ISH quantitation. **a-e** In situ hybridization quantitation analysis in WT and Brn3a-KO mouse retinas at 5 postnatal ages. d^I-e^I RNASeq gene level profiles at P3 (expressed in CPM). a^{II}-e^{III} RNASeq transcript level profiles expressed in FPKM for all transcripts of the five genes detected at more than 1 FPKM in at least one P3 retinal sample. a-a^{II} Cdh4, b-b^{II} Pcdh20, c-c^{II} Rtn4rl2, d-d^{II} Tmem25, e-e^{III} Tmem91. Plot formatting and annotations as in Fig. 3

do not support dependency of Grm4 expression on Brn3a (Additional file 1: Table S1). Ntrk1 (neurotrophic tyrosine kinase, receptor, type 1) is expressed both in retina and RGCs and differentially regulated by Brn3a (Fig. $9d^I$-d^{II}). ISH confirms significant Ntrk1 GCL enrichment at P0 and P3 (Figs. 8d, 9d, Additional file 1: Table S1 A-B). The INL expression starts at P3, catches up with the GCL at P7-P14, and they both proceed into adult age. Ntrk1 is expressed exceptionally highly at P14 and P22, however no differential between Brn3a WT and KO retinas is apparent at any age (Figs. 8d, 9d, Additional file 1: Table S1). Pnkd (paroxysmal non-kinesigenic dyskinesia) has three RefSeq isoforms (NM_019999, NM_025580 and NM_001039509, Fig. $9e^{II}$-e^{IV}), all of them seem to be

expressed in both RGCs and retina, but only one of them is regulated by Brn3a (NM_019999, Fig. $9e^{II}$). Gene level analysis demonstrates broad expression in both RGCs and retina with no apparent regulation by Brn3a (Fig. $9e^I$). The 3'-UTR in situ probe common for all 3 isoforms allows to find Pnkd expression in the GCL and other retinal layers beginning with P0-P3 (Fig. 9e). We find significant enrichment of Pnkd expression in the GCL of Brn3a WT retinas at most of studied ages (P0 $p < 0.05$, P7 $p < 0.001$, P14 $p < 0.01$, P22 $p < 0.001$), but no confirmation of potential Brn3a-mediated regulation (Fig. 9e, Additional file 1: Table S1). Selective expression of Pnkd transcripts will be described below (Fig. 14). Rims1 (regulating synaptic membrane exocytosis 1) transcript and gene expression is

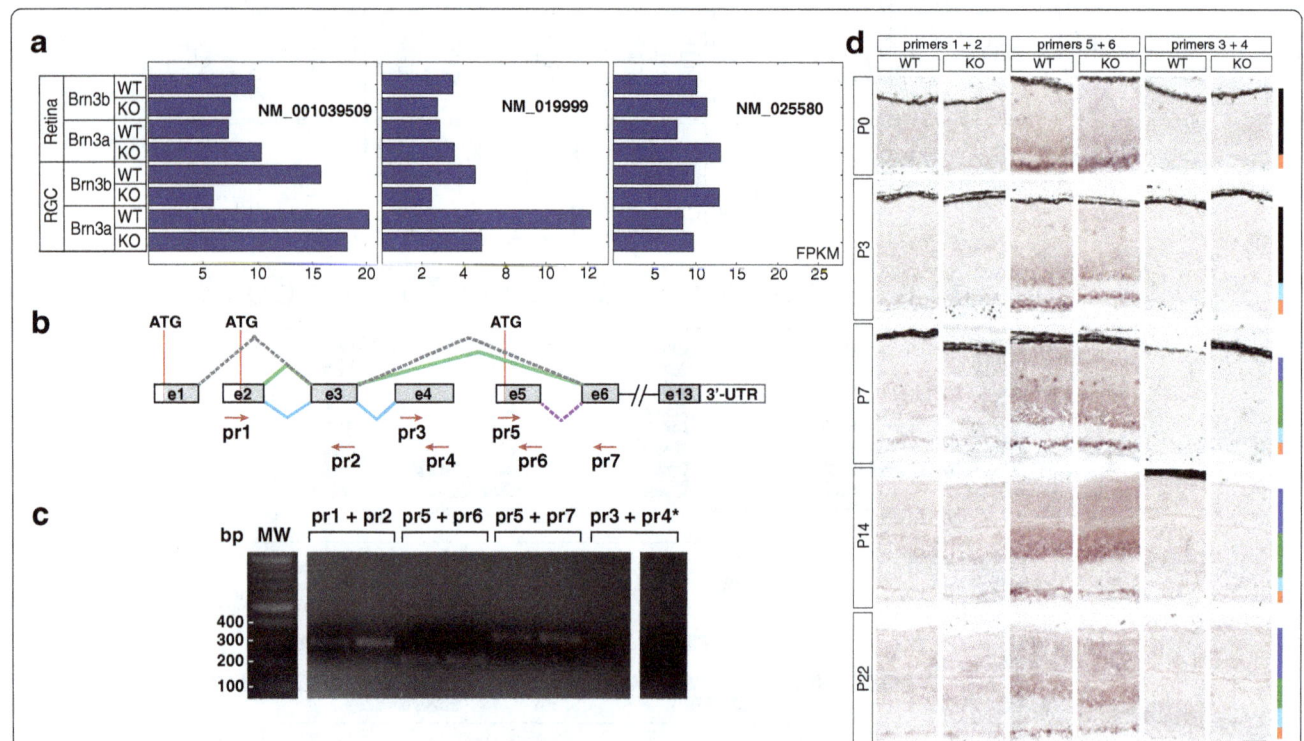

Fig. 14 Pnkd transcripts detected in the retina. **a** RNAseq profiles expressed in FPKM of three expressed Pnkd RefSeq transcripts from retinal and RGC-derived samples of Brn3a and Brn3b WT and KO mice at P3. **b** Predicted Pnkd splicing variants. Exons are represented as boxes and numbered. White boxes are untranslated regions, gray boxes are coding regions. Splicing sequences for alternative transcripts are indicated above or below the exons. Green lines indicate connected exons for transcript NM_001039509, blue – for NM_025580, purple – for NM_019999. Gray lines represent a putative transcript (XM_006496167) that was not detected by RNAseq. Exons 6–13 are common to NM_001039509 and NM_019999. Red arrows show the positions of primers made to check the presence of each predicted variant (see also Table 2). **c** Agarose-gel electrophoresis showing RT-PCR reactions from P3 retina RNA. Indicated primer pairs refer to B. Duplicates are shown for each primer combination. The expected sizes for all primer combinations are indicated in Table 2. All bands generated by RT-PCR were gel-extracted, subcloned and sequenced for confirmation. **d** in situ hybridization analysis in WT and Brn3a-KO mouse retinas at 5 postnatal ages. RNA probes were designed to detect transcript-specific exons: primers 1 and 2 for NM_001039509 (green) and NM_025580 (blue) isoforms, primers 5 and 6 specifically for NM_019999 (purple), and primer 3 and 4 –specifically for NM_025580. Scale bar – 50 μm

enriched in RGCs vs. retina, but only transcript-specific RNASeq analysis reveals Brn3a-dependent differential expression (Fig. 9f^I-f^{II}) . ISH confirms strong and significant GCL enrichment throughout postnatal development (WT retinas $p < 0.001$, Additional file 1: Table S1) and reveals some high-expressing cells in both the INL and GCL (Figs. 8f, 9f). Expression of Rims1 is high from P0-P14, and slightly decreases in the adult. Its dependency on Brn3a was apparent at P14 ($p < 0.05$) and becomes more significant in the adult ($p < 0.001$) (Fig. 9f, Additional file 1: Table S1 D-E).

Secreted proteins (Figures 10 and 11)

RNASeq results predicted Brn3a$^{AP/WT}$ RGCs enrichment and Brn3a regulation for Fam19a4 (family with sequence similarity 19, member A4) (Fig. 11d^I-d^{II}), however ISH showed only low level of GCL staining exclusively at P3-P7 without visible regulation by Brn3a (Fig. 10a). The only detectable Nptx1 (neuronal pentraxin 1) RefSeq transcript (Fig. 11a^{II}) is expressed in all retina samples however it is significantly enriched in Brn3a$^{AP/WT}$ RGCs and regulated by Brn3a, which is in agreement with RNASeq gene level analysis (Fig. 11a^I). ISH largely confirms these findings, showing intense GCL staining beginning with P0 and persisting into the adult (Figs. 10b, 11a). Starting at P14 intense signal also appears in the INL, in a position consistent with Amacrine cell expression (Fig. 10b), but the significant GCL enrichment persists (P14 and P22 WT retinas $p < 0.001$, Fig. 11a). The GCL signal appears to be Brn3a dependent at the later ages (P14 and P22, $p < 0.05$), as it is significantly reduced in Brn3a KO retinas (Figs. 10b and 11a, Additional file 1: Table S1 D-E). Nptx2 (neuronal pentraxin 2) is GCL enriched and Brn3a-regulated according to transcript and gene level RNASeq (Fig. 11b^I-b^{II}). In ISH (Fig. 10c) Nptx2 labels fewer cell bodies in the GCL compared to Nptx1, however it is also GCL enriched in the Brn3a WT at P3 ($p < 0.001$), P7 ($p < 0.01$) and adult ($p < 0.01$) but not regulated significantly by Brn3a (Figs. 10c and 11b, Additional file 1: Table S1). Sez6l2 (seizure related 6 homolog-like 2) has 3 transcripts with very diverse profiles of expression at P3 (NM_001252567, NM_144926 and NM_001252566, Fig. 11c^{II}-c^{IV}). NM_001252567 is highly expressed in both RGCs and retina, except Brn3b KO retina, and it is the only Brn3a-dependent isoform (Fig. 11c^{II}). NM_144926 is strongly represented in Brn3a RGCs and, surprisingly, in Brn3b KO retina, and is not regulated by Brn3a (Fig. 11c^{III}). NM_001252566 expression is evenly distributed between RGCs and retina, with some enrichment in Brn3a RGCs (Fig. 11c^{IV}). Gene level analysis does reveal Brn3a RGC enrichment, but it does not demonstrate any Brn3a dependency (Fig. 11c^I). ISH using a 3'-UTR probe common for all three isoforms shows GCL enrichment

throughout the larger part of postnatal development (P0-P14, Figs. 10d, 11c, Additional file 1: Table S1) and significant signs of Brn3a regulation in the GCL at P0 and P7 ($p < 0.05$). However, in the adult the GCL signal in Brn3a WT and KO retinas is indistinguishable (Figs. 10d, 11c).

Adhesion molecules and other transmembrane proteins (Figures 12 and 13)

Both transcript and gene level RNASeq analyses demonstrated that Cdh4 (cadherin 4) is significantly enriched in Brn3a$^{AP/WT}$ RGCs in comparison to all other retinal and RGC samples, including Brn3a$^{AP/KO}$ RGCs, suggesting regulation by Brn3a in specific RGC populations (Fig. 13a^I-a^{II}). ISH reveals that Cdh4 is already expressed and GCL enriched at P0 (Figs. 12a, 13a), the expression increases at P3, and it is sparse in both GCL as well as INL. The distribution of INL staining is consistent with horizontal cell and amacrine cell expression (Fig. 12a). The number of Cdh4$^+$ cells in the Brn3a KO GCL is consistently smaller compared to Brn3a WT throughout postnatal development, and the quantitation confirms it for the majority of studied ages (P0 $p < 0.001$, P3 $p < 0.05$, P14 $p < 0.01$, P22 $p < 0.05$, Additional file 1: Table S1). According to our RNASeq results Pcdh20 (protocadherin 20) is enriched in Brn3a$^{AP/WT}$ RGCs relative to other RGC and retina samples, although its general level of expression is comparatively low (Fig. 13b^I-b^{II}). It is decreased in both Brn3a$^{AP/KO}$ and Brn3b$^{AP/KO}$ RGCs, suggesting regulation by both transcription factors, although, due to its low expression level (< 2 FPKM for the transcript) in Brn3b$^{AP/WT}$ RGCs Pcdh20 was not selected as a Brn3b regulated gene in the screen. ISH showed very low levels of expression from P0 to P7, and a modest GCL enrichment (KO $p < 0.001$, WT not significant) and differential regulation by Brn3a ($p < 0.05$) at P14 (Figs. 12b, 13b, Additional file 1: Table S1 D). Both gene and transcript RNASeq analyses show that Rtn4rl2 (reticulon 4 receptor-like 2) is rather homogeneously distributed between RGCs and the retina (Fig. 13c^I-1c^{II}). Transcript analysis also reveals a high differential between Brn3a WT and KO RGCs (Fig. 13c^{II}). ISH shows that Rtn4rl2 is GCL enriched early (P0-P3), and then the distribution changes after P7 and the level in the INL becomes significantly higher than in the GCL (P7 WT $p < 0.001$, KO $p < 0.01$, Figs. 12c, 13c, Additional file 1: Table S1 C). Tmem25 (transmembrane protein 25) has only one RefSeq transcript expressed in the retina. Despite both transcript and gene level RNASeq analyses show enrichment in Brn3a WT RGCs, the gene level diagram does not show regulation by Brn3a in RGCs probably due to the contribution of non-RefSeq transcripts (Fig. 13d^I-d^{II}). In situ developmental profile shows GCL enrichment of the expression at P0 (WT $p < 0.05$), P14 (WT $p < 0.001$) and

P22 (WT p < 0.001), but no considerable signs of Brn3a-mediated regulation (Figs. 12d, 13d, Additional file 1: Table S1). Tmem91 (transmembrane protein 91) has two transcript isoforms (NM_001290497 and NM_177102, Fig. 13e^{II}-e^{III}), both of them show a modest expression in retina and RGCs. NM_001290497 is differentially expressed in Brn3a$^{AP/WT}$ RGCs compared to Brn3a$^{AP/KO}$ RGCs, NM_177102 is not, and probably because of this gene level analysis does not reveal differential regulation by Brn3a (Fig. 13e^{I}). ISH confirms expression of Tmem91 starting at P0-P3, increasing through P7-P14, and diminishing in P22 (Fig. 12e). It also shows a significant differential between Brn3a WT and Brn3a KO GCL expression at P7 (p < 0.001) and P14   (p < 0.01) (Figs. 12e, 13e, Additional file 1: Table S1 C-D).

Combined RNASeq, RT-PCR and ISH analysis for specific transcript isoform expression

Many of the described candidate genes (Figs. 2, 3, 4, 5, 6, 7, 8, 9, 10, 11, 12 and 13), selected based on the presence of at least one transcript enriched in Brn3a^{AP} RGCs and regulated by Brn3a, had several transcript isoforms expressed in the retina, often showing distinct expression patterns. The ISH tests performed with 3'-UTR probes common to all transcripts (Table 1) did therefore report a combination of the expression patterns and levels of these different transcripts, thus reflecting essentially a "gene level" expression profile. Whereas it is important to understand the expression pattern of our candidates at gene level, some biologically relevant functions could be dependent on the expression of specific isoforms. We therefore decided to further investigate the differential expression for transcripts of two genes predicted to have multiple retina-specific isoforms, Pnkd and Clcc1.

Pnkd transcripts detected in the retina

According to RNASeq data, 3 Pnkd transcripts are expressed broadly among retina and Brn3^{AP} RGC samples (Fig. 14a-b). The long isoform (NM_001039509), initiated at exon 2, and skipping exons 4 and 5 (green splicing sequence, Fig. 14b) is enriched in both Brn3a$^{AP/WT}$ and Brn3b$^{AP/WT}$ RGCs, but only regulated by Brn3b. The "medium" transcript (NM_019999), predicted to start at exon 5 (purple splicing sequence, Fig. 14b), is enriched in RGCs but regulated by Brn3a. The "short" transcript isoform (NM_025580), spans three exons (e2, e3 and e4, blue splicing sequence, Fig. 14b), and shows no enrichment in RGCs. A further putative transcript, initiating at exon 1, was not detected by RNASeq in the retina or RGCs (gray splicing sequence, Fig. 14b). We sought to confirm the existence of these alternative transcripts by using RT-PCR analysis from P3 retina RNA

(Fig. 14b, c; Tables 1 and 2). Bands for all positive reactions were cloned and confirmed by sequencing.

The reaction of primers 1 and 2, common to the short (NM_025580) and long (NM_001039509) transcripts, resulted in the expected product length, equal to combined exons 2 and 3. However, primers 3 + 4, recognizing exon 4, specific for the short isoform, did not produce any RT-PCR fragment, suggesting that this transcript (NM_025580) is not present in P3 retina. Primer combinations 5 + 6, and 5 + 7, specific for the exon 5 or the sum of exons 5 and 6 respectively, are selective for the medium isoform (NM_019999). Both reactions resulted in the correct product sizes (Tables 1 and 2, Fig. 14b, c). In summary, the RT-PCR analysis suggests that the long (NM_001039509) and medium (NM_019999) transcripts are expressed at detectable levels in the retina, while the short (NM_025580) transcript is not. Finally, to look at the temporal and spatial distribution of Pnkd isoforms in the retina, we generated isoform specific probes covering the long (Pr1 + Pr2), medium (Pr5 + Pr6) and short (Pr3 + Pr4) transcripts and screened our panel of postnatal retina sections (Fig. 14b, d). The long isoform is expressed at low levels in a GCL-specific manner beginning with P3 and continuing into adult (Fig. 14d, left). The medium transcript is highly expressed in the GCL from P0 to P22, but INL expression picks up at P3 and persists into the adult (Fig. 14d, middle). There is little or no Brn3a regulation for either the long or medium isoform. The short isoform was not observed in either Brn3a WT or KO retinas from P0 to P22, right column. It should be noted that the signal intensity for the medium isoform is much stronger than the one seen for the 3'-UTR probe (Fig. 8e), that should be common for both long and medium (but not short) isoforms, but the differential between signal intensity in GCL and other retinal layers is conserved between these two probes. Taken together these results suggest that Pnkd is expressed in the retina, predominantly in the GCL, but also in the INL. Whereas the enrichment of long and medium isoforms in the GCL, predicted by RNASeq data, is confirmed, the relative level of expression of the transcripts, as judged by ISH, is not entirely consistent with the RNASeq predictions. Moreover, the ubiquitous retinal expression of the short isoform, predicted by RNA-Seq, is not confirmed by either RT-PCR or ISH.

Clcc1 transcripts detected in the retina

GeneBank annotation predicts that Clcc1 has five transcript isoforms, consisting mostly of alternative, partially overlapping sequences for exon 1, resulting from 4 alternative transcription start sites and three different exon1 3' ends: NM_145543 – exon 1a, XM_006501416 – exon 1b, NM_001177771 – exon 1c, XM_011240107 – exon 1d, NM_001177770 – exon 1e. Exon 2 is included only in transcript NM_001177771 (Fig. 15b). Our RNASeq data predicted three retinally expressed Clcc1 transcripts: NM_145543, NM_001177771 and NM_001177770 (Fig. 15a, b). NM_145543 (Fig. 15b, green splicing sequence) is highly expressed in RGCs and retina, with lowest expression levels in Brn3a$^{AP/WT}$ and Brn3a$^{AP/KO}$ RGCs (Fig. 15a, left). In contrast, NM_001177771 (Fig. 15b, blue splicing sequence) is considerably expressed only in Brn3a$^{AP/WT}$ RGCs (Fig. 15a, middle), predicting both specificity for Brn3a RGCs and regulation by Brn3a. Finally, NM_001177770 (Fig. 15b, gray

splicing sequence) is expressed moderately in both retina and RGCs (Fig. 15a, right). Given the large degree of overlap between Clcc1 isoforms, and the presence of potential alternative open reading frames, we were interested to map out the precise boundaries of exon 1 variants. We performed RT-PCR from P3 retina samples using primers targeted to specific exon regions of each transcript (Tables 1 and 2, Fig. 15b-d). All positive bands were subcloned and confirmed by sequencing. Primers 10 and 11 were used to diagnose a product

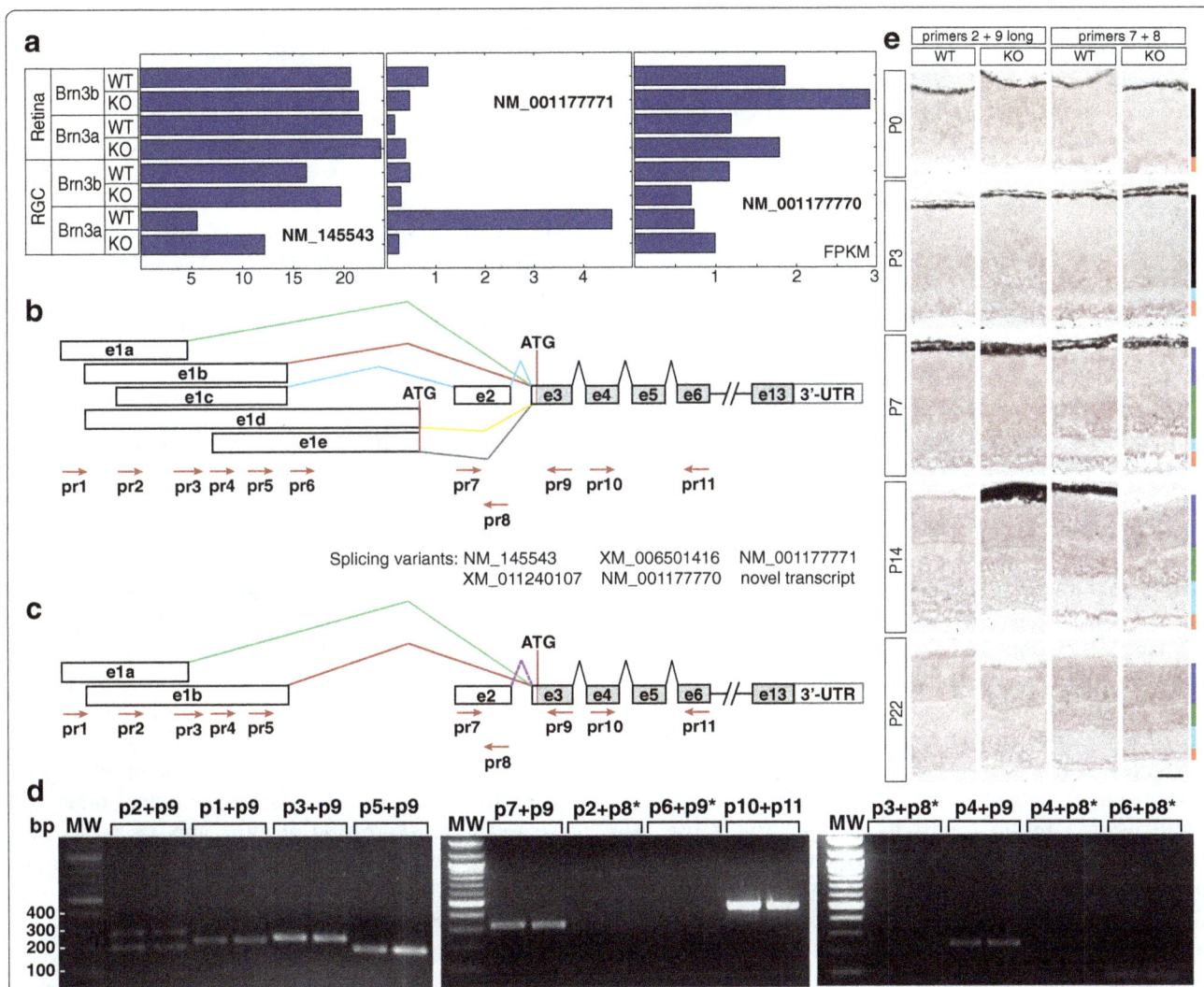

Fig. 15 Clcc1 transcripts detected in the retina. **a** RNAseq profiles expressed in FPKM of the three Clcc1 transcripts detected in retinal and RGC-derived samples of Brn3a and Brn3b WT and KO mice at P3. **b** Predicted Clcc1 splicing variants. Exon and splicing connection annotations (labelled as in Fig. 14), for five distinct transcript variants are annotated: NM_145543, NM_001177771, NM_001177770, XM_006501416, XM_011240107. Red arrows show the positions of diagnostic primers (see also Table 2). Translation start sites are in exons e1d, e1e and e3 (ATGs indicated). **c** Confirmed Clcc1 splicing variants. Purple line indicates a novel transcript suggested by our RT-PCR analysis. **d** RT-PCR reactions from P3 retina RNA. Primer pairs as in **b**. Pairs marked with a star indicate negative or nonspecific (weak bands of incorrect size) reactions. Duplicates are shown for each primer combination. For expected product sizes, see Table 2. All bands generated by RT-PCR were gel-extracted, subcloned and sequenced for confirmation. **e** in situ hybridization in retinal sections from WT and Brn3a-KO retinas at five developmental stages. RNA probes were targeted against exons that are specific for different transcript variants. For pr2 + pr9, the probe was generated from the longer product (see panel **d**), and is predicted to detect both NM_145543 (green) and XM_006501416 (red) isoforms. Probe generated from pr7 + pr8 targets exon2 and therefore detects the newly identified transcript. Scale bar – 50 μm

spanning exons 4, 5 and 6, common to all transcript variants (~ 400 bp, Fig. 15b-d).

Forward primers Pr1 to Pr6, tilling all possible exon 1 variants, were individually paired with reverse primer Pr9, placed in exon 3, the first common exon for all splicing isoforms. Combinations of Pr1 to Pr5 with Pr9 resulted in product lengths consistent with the presence of exon variants 1a, and 1b, and excluding variants 1c, 1d and 1e (Fig. 15b-d, and see Table 2 for product lengths). E.g., the primer combination Pr2 + Pr9 gave 2 bands corresponding to XM_006501416 (exon e1b, longer fragment, ~ 300 bp) and NM_145543 (exon 1a, shorter fragment, ~ 200 bp), while combination Pr1 + Pr9 gave only one band ~ 200 bp for NM_145543 as expected. The combination of Pr6 + Pr9 showed only nonspecific bands (small amount and incorrect size), thus excluding isoforms XM_011240107 and NM_001177770 (exons 1d or 1e spliced to exon 3). All primer combinations detecting splicing sequences including exons 1 and 2 (forward Pr2, Pr3, Pr4, Pr6 combined with reverse Pr8) failed to give a positive reaction. However, splicing of exon 2 onto exon 3 is occurring, since the combination of forward primer Pr7 (5′ end of exon 2) and reverse Pr9 gave a positive reaction of expected length and sequence. Pr7 + Pr8 produced the expected size product (see below). In summary, our RT-PCR analysis narrows the number of Clcc1 transcripts expressed in the retina to NM_145543 and XM_006501416, and proposes a new alternative transcript initiating at exon 2. This novel transcript would explain the reads assigned to NM_00117771, that follows the splicing sequence e1 – e2 – e3, which we could not detect in the retina. We next determined the cellular distribution and developmental profile of the retinally expressed Clcc1 isoforms by ISH. The combined expression pattern of NM_145543 and XM_006501416 was determined using a probe that spans the exon 1b to exon 3 splicing event (Pr2 + Pr9, long product), while the novel transcript variant was tested using a probe against its unique exon 2 (Pr7 + Pr8). We find that the exon 2-containing transcript is expressed in the GCL starting with P3 and the INL beginning with P7. The GCL signal persists into the adult age and shows only a modest differential in Brn3a KO vs. WT retinas (Fig. 15e, right column), while ISH signal generated by the combined expression level of NM_145543 and XM_006501416 was relatively low throughout postnatal development (Fig. 15e, left column). In summary, only three Clcc1 transcript isoforms are present in retina: NM_145543, XM_006501416, and a novel uncharacterized transcript containing exons 2 and 3. The three isoforms are predicted to encode the same protein, with the translation initiation site located in exon 3, however, they have three distinct transcription start sites.

Immunohistochemical analysis of two potential Brn3a targets – Elfn1 and Cdh4

We have focused so far on validating expression of potential Brn3a target molecules at the mRNA level. However, we are ultimately interested in the potential roles played by the encoded proteins in RGC cell type formation. We therefore sought to determine the cell type distribution and cellular localization of some of our targets. We show here results for two adhesion molecules playing potential roles in dendrite lamination and synaptic development, Cdh4 and Elfn1, during one developmental time point (P7) and in the adult (P22).

At P7, Elfn1 expression is found in RGCs, Amacrine, Horizontal cells and Photoreceptors (Fig. 16a-b). Some Elfn1$^+$ RGCs (identified by co-labelling with AP generated from the recombined $Brn3a^{AP}$ allele) show intense staining in proximal dendrites. By P22, intense and punctate Elfn1$^+$ staining is visible in the OPL (Fig. 16c-d). A distinct Elfn1$^+$ lamina is visible in the IPL of Brn3a WT retinas, but essentially absent in Brn3a KO retinas. This suggests that at least one Elfn1$^+$ cell type, presumably an RGC, is either deleted or has an altered morphology in Brn3a KO retinas. Alternatively, Elfn1 could be under Brn3a transcriptional control (Fig. 16c, d, i, j).

Cdh4 is expressed at P7 in RGCs, Amacrine and Horizontal cells. Strongly labeled Cdh4$^+$ cell bodies in the INL most likely belong to Amacrine and Horizontal cells and are observed at both P7 and P22 (Fig. 16e-h). RGC staining does not seem to persist in the adult Brn3a WT retina (Fig. 16g) One Cdh4$^+$ lamina is present in the IPL at P7 (Fig. 16e-f), while two laminae appear intensely Cdh4$^+$ in the adult (Fig. 16g-h). None of these laminae is significantly affected by Brn3a ablation at either P7 or P22 (Fig. 16g, h, k, l). Unlike for Elfn1, a strong OPL Cdh4$^+$ positive staining emerges already at P7. In conclusion, whereas both Elfn1 and Cdh4 were somewhat enriched in RGC during early postnatal development, adult patterns of expression include multiple other cell types, and RGC expression of Elfn1 appears profoundly regulated by Brn3a in the adult stage, while Cdh4 RGC expression levels decline to undetectable levels in both WT and Brn3aKO GCL.

Discussion

We report here the results of a screen for genes potentially involved in mediating the effects of transcription factor Brn3a in RGC type specification. The screen covered 5 postnatal ages, between P0 and adult, and employed ISH, RT-PCR, and immunohistochemistry. The genes were selected using data from a previously published RNASeq screen for Brn3a candidate target genes in P3 RGCs [5], and had to have at least one transcript satisfying the following three criteria: 1) expression of at least 2 FPKM in Brn3a^{AP} RGCs; 2) expression

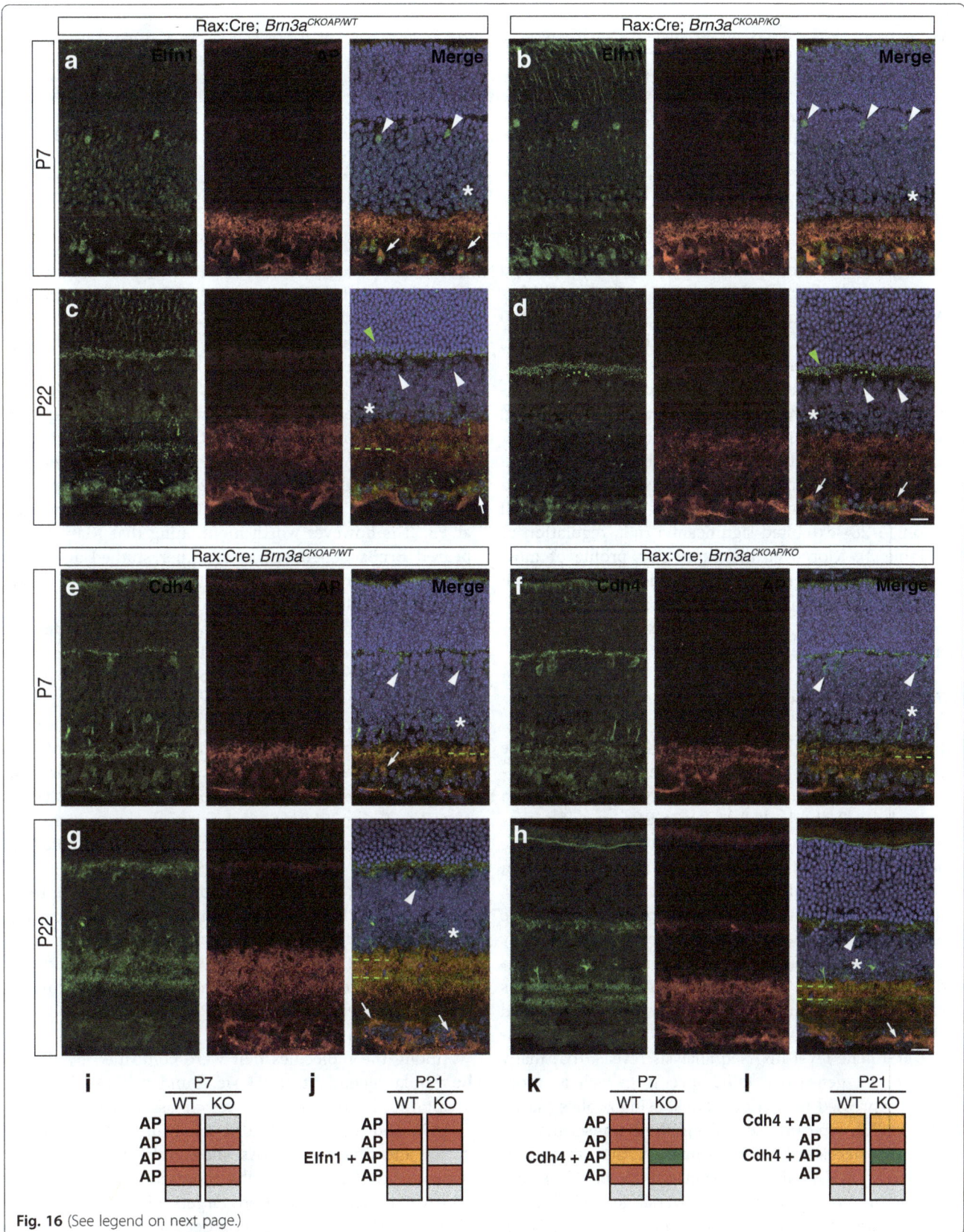

Fig. 16 (See legend on next page.)

(See figure on previous page.)

Fig. 16 Distinct Brn3a effects on the expression of two adhesion molecules – Elfn1 and Cdh4. Retinal sections were prepared from either Rax:Cre; Brn3a$^{CKOAP/WT}$ (**a, c, e, g**) or Rax:Cre; Brn3a$^{CKOAP/KO}$ (**b, d, f, h**) mice at P7 (**a, b, e, f**) or P22 (**c, d, g, h**). Immunostaining for either Elfn1 (green, **a-d**) or Cdh4 (green, **e-h**) was performed in conjunction with immunostaining for Brn3a^{AP} RGCs (red, AP) and nuclear layers counterstain (DAPI, in blue, in merge channel). For every immunostaining Elfn1 (left), AP (middle) and merge (right) channels are shown. White arrowheads, asterisks and arrows indicate Horizontal Cells, Amacrine Cells and RGCs. Green arrowheads in C and D reveal synaptic staining in the OPL, as previously reported [81]. Green stippled lines in the merge channel indicate lamination of Elfn1$^+$ or Cdh4$^+$ neurites in the IPL, if present. Scale bar in H = 50 μm. **i-l** Schematics of Brn3a^{AP} RGCs dendrites (red) and Elfn1 (orange, I, J) and Cdh4 (green or orange, K, L) lamination in the IPL, at P7 (I, K) or P22 (J, L), in Rax:Cre; Brn3a$^{CKOAP/WT}$ (left, WT) or Rax:Cre; Brn3a$^{CKOAP/KO}$ (right, KO) retinas. Elfn1 stains only a few diffuse dendrites at P7, however a sharp lamina is labelled in P22, and this lamina is absent from Brn3a null retinas. Cdh4$^+$ dendrites form one clear lamina at P7 and two distinct laminae at P22, however the lamination pattern is not affected by Brn3a ablation

enrichment of two-fold in Brn3a$^{AP/WT}$ RGCs compared to the retina; 3) downregulation of at least two-fold between Brn3a$^{AP/WT}$ and Brn3a$^{AP/KO}$ RGCs. From the 180 transcripts satisfying these criteria in the original screen, we narrowed our search to genes whose molecular structure suggested potential functions in cell type specification, i.e. transcription, translation, intracellular signaling, synapse formation and function, vesicular transport or release, secreted and cell surface molecules. Of the 28 selected genes, a majority (20/28) showed increased GCL signal compared to the retina, but only a small fraction (4/28) exhibited significant Brn3a regulation at P3 (Table 3). Moreover, the expression profile of most candidate genes was extremely dynamic during postnatal development, and only a handful exhibited RGC enrichment and/or Brn3a regulation throughout all developmental ages.

Differential expression: RNASeq, ISH and developmental dynamics

What molecules with potential to influence RGC type specificity are Brn3a targets? The gene expression profiling screen at the origin of this study was focused on postnatal day 3 and looked at Brn3a RGC specific transcripts. Our reasoning was that P3 is a particularly active time point for neurite branching and synapse formation for both RGC dendrites and axons. However, RGCs, which become postmitotic beginning with E12.5, are probably amongst the most mature neurons in the early postnatal retina. Thus, by selecting genes that had transcripts with higher expression levels in Brn3a RGCs versus retina supernatants, it is likely that we included molecules enriched in mature neurons. In addition, transcript and gene level RNAseq analysis reveals that many of our target genes had RGC specific as well as more broadly expressed transcripts. Thus, using probes placed in the 3'UTR, typically recognizing most transcripts of a gene, will necessarily miss some of the differences predicted by RNASeq at the transcript level. Nevertheless, it is important to know the overall gene expression levels for any given gene in the retina and RGCs, in order to better predict and understand phenotypic changes upon loss of function manipulations. Taken all

these considerations into account, it is rewarding to find that gene-level ISH confirmed RGC enrichment for about two thirds of the targets (20 of 28, 71% accuracy), and slightly more than half for Brn3a dependent RGC expression at any given age (16 of 28, 57% accuracy). A subset of our targets, (Rbfox1, Eml1, Hpca, Mapk10, Pick1, Pnkd, Sez6l2, Tmem91) had multiple RefSeq transcripts, some of which were not Brn3a dependent; with gene level RNASeq analysis did not show Brn3a dependency. This could explain why, for all these genes, ISH using the 3'UTR did not show differences of expression at P3. It is however worth mentioning that Mapk10 appeared Brn3a dependent at all other studied ages. Another 16 targets (Foxp2, Plppr3, Pip5kl1, Pak6, Ankrd13b, Elfn1, Gabra1, Grm4, Ntrk1, Rims1, Fam19a4, Nptx1, Nptx2, Pcdh20, Rtn4rl2, Tmem25) have only one expressed transcript each, predicted to be Brn3a-dependent. Exactly half of those genes (8 of 16) seem to be significantly regulated at postnatal ages other than P3 (Foxp2 – P7, P22; Plppr3 – P14; Elfn1 – P14-P22; Gabra1 – P22; Rims1 – P14-P22; Nptx1 – P14-P22; Pcdh20 – P14; Rtn4rl2 – P7), but another half (Pip5kl1, Pak6, Ankrd13b, Grm4, Ntrk1, Fam19a4, Nptx2, Tmem25) do not reveal any signs of Brn3a-mediated regulation at any stage of postnatal development. Of note, the presence of Brn3a independent transcripts was a strong predictor of lack of Brn3a regulation at gene level. However the presence of only one, Brn3a dependent RefSeq transcript was not necessarily linked with gene level regulation, or confirmation by ISH, most likely suggesting the existence of further, non-RefSeq transcripts (e.g. Pip5kl1, Ankrd13b and Tmem25).

Among the molecules that were confirmed by ISH to be Brn3a-dependent at P3 we found mRNAs for transcription factor Tshz2, vesicle-associated proteins Snap91 and Tusc5, and adhesion protein Cdh4. While Tshz2 and Snap91 mRNAs show only transient Brn3a dependency, Tusc5 and Cdh4 represent developmentally consistent Brn3a regulation targets (Table 3). Mapk10 showed fairly consistent Brn3a-dependency (with the exception of P3, Figs. 4d, 5d). Brn3a regulation could be hidden by Brn3a-negative RGC types, or by non-RGC

Table 3 The expression of Brn3a target genes: ISH and RNASeq results comparison

Gene	Known function	GCL P3	GCL P0-P22	Brn3a target P3	Brn3a target any age	Postnatal GCL Expression			GCL Sparse	Brn3a-independ. Transcripts	Brn3a-regulation Gene level
						Onset	Peak	Offset			
Transcriptional and translational regulators											
Foxp2	TF	yes	no	no	yes	P0	P7	no	no	no	yes
Tshz2	TF	yes	yes	yes	yes	P3	P7	no	no	no	yes
Rbfox1	Splicing of neuronal genes	yes	no	no	no	P0	P14	no	no	yes	no
Intracellular signaling and cytoskeleton-associated genes											
Eml1	Microtubule-binding protein	yes	no	no	no	P0	P7	no	no	yes	no
Hpca	Calcium sensor	yes	yes	no	yes	P0	P7-P14	no	no	yes	no
Plppr3	Neurite growth and regeneration	yes	yes	no	yes	P0	P0	no	no	no	no
Mapk10	Axonal growth and neuronal survival	yes	yes	no	yes	P0	P7-P14	no	yes	yes	no
Pip5kl1	Cell morphology and adhesion	no	no	no	no	P3	P7	no	no	no	no
Pak6	Signaling kinase	no	no	no	no	no	no	no	no	no	na
Vesicle-associated proteins											
Ankrd13b	Caveolin- mediated endosomal traffick	yes	yes	no	no	P0	P7	no	no	no	no
Pick1	Glutamate receptor trafficking	yes	no	no	no	P0	no	no	no	yes	no
Snap91	Clathrin-mediated endocytosis	yes	yes	yes	yes	P0	P7-P14	no	yes	yes	no
Tusc5	Insulin-stimulated glucose transport	yes	yes	yes	yes	P3	P14	no	yes	no	yes
Synapse-associated proteins											
Elfn1	Synaptic adhesion protein	yes	no	no	yes	P3	P7	no	yes	no	yes
Gabra1	GABA receptor alpha1 subunit	no	no	no	yes	P3	no	no	yes	no	yes
Grm4	Metabotropic glutamate receptor	yes	no	no	no	P0	P7	no	no	no	yes
Ntrk1	Neurotrophin receptor	yes	no	no	no	P0	P14-P22	no	no	no	yes
Pnkd	Synaptic vesicle release	no	yes	no	no	P0	P7-P14	no	yes	yes	no
Rims1	Synaptic vesicle release & recycling	yes	yes	no	yes	P0	P0-P3	no	yes	no	no
Secreted proteins											
Fam19a4	Unknown	no	no	no	no	P3	P3-P7	P7	no	no	yes
Nptx1	Trans-synaptic, excitatory synapse	yes	yes	no	yes	P0	P14	no	yes	no	yes
Nptx2	Trans-synaptic, excitatory synapse	yes	no	no	no	P3	P7-P14	no	yes	no	yes
Sez6l2	Synapse formation	yes	yes	no	yes	P3	P7	no	no	yes	no
Adhesion molecules and other transmembrane proteins											
Cdh4	Cell adhesion molecule	yes	no	yes	yes	P0	no	no	yes	no	yes
Pcdh20	Cell adhesion molecule	no	no	no	yes	P14	no	no	no	no	yes
Rtn4rl2	Axon guidance molecule	yes	yes	no	yes	P0	no	P22	no	no	no
Tmem25	Unknown	no	no	no	no	P0	P7-P14	no	no	no	no
Tmem91	Unknown	no	no	no	yes	P0	P7-P14	no	no	yes	no

Column 1 represents gene name, column 2 – known function of the gene, column 3 – GCL enrichment at P3, column 4 – consistent GCL enrichment (at least at 4 out of 5 ages) from P0-P22. Fifth column shows whether the gene is regulated by Brn3a at P3, 6th – regulated by Brn3a at any of 5 studied ages. Columns 7, 8 and 9 represent the onset, the peak and the offset respectively of postnatal gene expression in the GCL. Column 10 shows whether the gene is highly and sparsely expressed in the GCL at any of studied ages. Columns 11 and 12 identify the genes that had unregulated transcripts or exhibited gene level regulation by RNASeq

expression in the ganglion cell layer which derives from Amacrine cells. In case of genes regulated by Brn3a early (P3-P7), but not late (P14-P22) (for instance, Snap91), delayed expression could occur in Brn3a-independent RGC subtypes or in Amacrine cells. A subset of targets (Elfn1, Gabra1, Rims1, Nptx1 and Pcdh20) which are GCL-expressed and Brn3a-regulated at later ages (P14-P22), are potentially more important during RGC synapse maturation in the retina after eye-opening and for Brn3a-expressing RGC function. Our findings suggest that patterns revealed by RNA sequencing may only partially be reproduced by other detection techniques. In addition, many genes may change their pattern of expression over time, especially when samples are derived from rapidly developing tissues, such as early postnatal retina. These dynamic expression profiles could also suggest the developmental steps at which the various target genes might be involved, as described below.

Transcript level analysis of cell type specificity

Many of the candidate genes identified in our RNAseq screen had two or more transcripts, with mixed patterns of RGC enrichment and/or Brn3a regulation. We therefore tested the accuracy of transcript level analysis and its influence on diagnosing cell type specificity of gene expression for two candidate genes – Pnkd and Clcc1, using transcript-specific RT-PCR reactions and ISH probes. We chose Pnkd since it has three previously characterized transcripts, encoding different protein isoforms, with the long version, Pnkd-L (long transcript) thought to be CNS-specific [52]. For Pnkd (3 predicted retinal transcripts - long, medium and short), only one transcript was predicted by RNASeq to be Brn3a-dependent. Both RT-PCR and ISH confirmed the RGC enrichment of the Pnkd medium transcript suggested by RNAseq for P3 retina. However, there was a strong discrepancy between the relative abundance of the long and medium size transcripts as reported by RNASeq and ISH, and the third, short isoform was undetectable by either RT-PCR or ISH. Furthermore, the ISH signal intensity was far stronger for the medium transcript specific probe compared to the 3'UTR probe detecting all isoforms, although hybridization strength based on base pair composition and probe length (360 bases for 3'-UTR and 167 bases for medium transcript) favor the 3'UTR probe. Clcc1 has an unusually large number of exon 1 variants – based on different transcription start sites and exon 1 splice donor sites. Also, Clcc1 transcript NM_001177771 was predicted to be highly expressed specifically in Brn3a WT and not in Brn3a KO RGCs or other parts of retina. Clcc1 has 5 alternative transcripts, mostly based on alternative transcription start sites at exon 1. Of the three predicted retina specific variants, one (NM_001177771) was supposed to be highly differentially expressed in Brn3a$^{AP/WT}$ RGCs and regulated by Brn3a. Our RT-PCR analysis with transcript-specific primers did not confirm the expression of this isoform, but rather suggests the presence of a novel, closely related transcript initiated at exon 2, and splicing onto exon 3. This novel isoform was found to be GCL-enriched by ISH at P3 but expanded its expression to the INL from P7 to P22. The encoded protein should be the same for NM_001177771 and the novel isoform since the open reading frame starts at exon 3, shared by both. Moreover, long exon 1 variants (NM_001177770 and XM_011240107) were not confirmed in our experiments, suggesting that there is no basis for existence of alternative protein variants with an open reading frame start at exon 1. Taken together, the outcomes of the transcript level analyses for Pnkd and Clcc1 raise several points to be considered when evaluating RNASeq predictions of cell type specificity. Transcript level analysis by RNASeq is constrained to aligning reads onto the existing transcript annotations, and hence relies on their quality. In addition, it could misrepresent the relative abundance of existing transcripts if it relies on reduced read numbers that do not span exon boundaries. In the case of Clcc1, the challenge was particularly steep given the large number of annotated alternative transcription start sites and splice donor sites at exon 1. Since most RNASeq data are derived from mRNA by using poly-dT capture of the polyA at the 3' end, this last issue could be particularly severe at the 5' end of the mRNA, as seen for both Pnkd and Clcc1. RNASeq results could be biased by amplification artefacts, while ISH detection could be influenced by the specific sequence properties of the used probes, as seen for the Pnkd medium isoform. Although, for both tested genes, a careful transcript level analysis did explain the RNASeq predictions, our data argues for using the deep sequencing predictions as a starting point for more careful transcript characterization.

Transcription and translation – related targets

The two identified transcription factors, Foxp2 and Tshz2 [53, 54] are expressed and GCL-enriched early in postnatal development (P0-P7), however at P14 – P22 Tshz2 expression is reduced but limited to the GCL, while Foxp2 expression extends to include both INL and GCL. This is somewhat surprising since recent reports suggest that retinal Foxp2 expression is restricted to a subset of RGC types [55, 56]. However, a transiently broader pattern of expression is suggested by using a Foxp2^{Cre} crossed into a general reporter [55]. Although Foxp2 missense mutations are associated with speech impairment in humans, the gene has clearly a broader developmental role, as mouse loss of function alleles result in lethality at 3–4 weeks of age [57]. Tshz2 is one of the three homologues of the Drosophila transcription factor teashirt, a gene involved in the homeotic control of body segment and imaginal disc formation that cooperates with eyeless (Pax6) in establishing fly retina identity [54]. Tshz2 has not been studied in great detail, however, mouse ISH data reveals cell type specific localization in several brain regions [58], suggesting a role in cell type specification. Thus, both identified TFs are good candidates for mediating Brn3a roles in RGC type specification. The splicing regulator Rbfox1 is enriched but not restricted to the GCL beginning with P3, and eventually expands to the whole retina by adult age. This could reflect a role in neuronal maturation, by regulating splicing of mRNAs for proteins implicated in synapse transmission and plasma membrane potential formation [59], especially during the period of active synaptogenesis (P3-P14) when its level is high according to our data.

Intracellular signaling components

We characterized the expression of five genes involved in intracellular signaling cascades. Eml1 is a microtubule-binding protein, and its disruption results in the generation of ectopic neuronal progenitors in the cerebral cortex of both mouse and human [60]. Interestingly, the fish homologue of Eml1 is expressed in photoreceptors and mediates Ca^{2+} modulation of the cyclic GMP gated channel [61, 62]. Hpca is a calcium sensor protein modulating slow afterhyperpolarization in the brain [63], but with many other suggested functions in morphogenesis. Mapk10 encodes the signaling molecule Jnk3 implicated in axonal growth and regeneration and neuronal survival [39, 64]. Plppr3 is a member of the lipid phosphate phosphatase-related protein family, which share sequence homology with known phosphatases but are catalytically inactive due to substitutions in known key aminoacids in the catalytic domains. They are five pass transmembrane proteins, were shown to stimulate membrane protrusions and neurite growth in cell lines and primary neuron culture and facilitate axonal outgrowth and regenerative sprouting [65, 66]. Pip5kl1 is a brain-specific, kinase-dead isoform of phosphatidil-inositol-(4)-phosphate 5-kinase, operating as a scaffold for recruitment of other phosphatidil inositol 5 – kinases, and implicated in cell morphology control and adhesion foci [67]. Eml1, Hpca, and Mapk10 were all expressed in the GCL beginning with P0 with a peak around P7-P14, and persistence into the adult. Their early and persistent pattern of expression is consistent with participation in both molecular and activity dependent processes, beyond the period of eye-opening (~P14) [68, 69]. The two molecules involved in phospholipid signaling, Plppr3 and Pip5kl1, follow different trends. Plppr3 expression is strong already at P0, and decreases dramatically towards adult, while Pip5kl1 is expressed in the GCL, although transiently (P3-P7) and at low levels. This expression profile suggest roles in the early stages of dendrite formation and/or axon branching.

Three of the genes encoding vesicle-associated proteins – Ankrd13b, Pick1 and Snap91 – also showed early expression in the GCL (P0 – P3), with gradual expansion of the signal in both the GCL and the INL from P3 till adult age. Ankrd13b participates in caveolin-1 mediated endosomal trafficking [70]. Pick1 is involved in glutamate receptor trafficking [71], while Snap91 is implicated in clathrin-mediated endocytosis, and participates in axogenesis and dendritic growth in hippocampal neurons [72]. Tusc5 is the only gene from this group showing strong and sparse GCL signal that is Brn3a dependent, beginning with P3. It was shown before to regulate insulin-stimulated glucose transport in adipocytes [73], but it is also expressed in peripheral neurons [74] and olfactory receptors [75].

Synapse associated molecules

The expression dynamic observed for intracellular signaling and vesicle associated proteins is largely followed by most synapse-associated genes explored in our screen, i.e. Gabra1, Grm4, Ntrk1 and Pnkd. Early (P0 or P3) GCL enrichment is followed by expansion of the expression domain into the INL towards the adult ages. Later the expression patterns diversify. Gabra1 becomes highly but sparsely expressed in the INL and GCL, and exhibits Brn3a regulation in the GCL, while Grm4 and Ntrk1 expression is broad in the INL and the GCL. The expression for both Grm4 (encoding the metabotropic glutamate receptor mGluR4 [76]) and Gabra1 (encoding the GABA (gamma amino butyric acid) receptor alpha 1 subunit) [77, 78] have been previously characterized in the retina at the protein level. Both receptors exhibit characteristic lamination profiles in the IPL. Our in situ data now shows that mGluR4 (Grm4) and Gabra1 are expressed in Bipolar, Amacrine and Ganglion cells, and thus could participate in Bipolar-Amacrine-RGC triad synapses at both pre-and postsynaptic sites, as suggested for the cerebellum [79]. The recently characterized synaptic molecule Elfn1 is also expressed pre- and post-synaptically in multiple neuronal cell types [80–82]. It presumably acts as a trans-synaptic adhesion molecule, and regulates presynaptic release probability of certain hippocampal neurons [82]. In the retina, Elfn1 was shown to participate in establishment of Photoreceptor-Bipolar Cell contacts via trans-synaptic interaction with metabotropic glutamate receptor mGluR6 [81]. Our ISH reveals high levels of Elfn1 expression in a subpopulation of RGCs beginning with P3 and through adult age, while IIF reveals Elfn1 positive cell bodies in the GCL and a narrowly stratified band in adult but not P7 IPL. Both the intensely labelled GCL cell bodies and the Elfn1 positive IPL sublamina are under Brn3a control, as they are absent from the Brn3a KO retina. In addition, immuno-detection of Elfn1 protein confirmed the previously described punctate (synaptic) pattern in the OPL [81], but also revealed expression in Photoreceptors, Horizontal, Amacrine and RGCs beginning at P7 and into the adult age. A similar pattern is revealed by Cao et al. [81] in supplementary material. These results are distinct from the ISH pattern, which confirms widespread retinal expression of Elfn1 only in the adult. This may be due to distinctions in sensitivity between ISH probe and antibody, or different stability of the mRNA versus protein.

The broad expression of Ntrk1 (encoding the neurotrophin receptor TrkA) in Bipolar, Amacrine and RGCs raises some interesting questions regarding the role of neurotrophic support in the inner retina. Whereas a role of TrkA as a RGC receptor for target derived neurotrophins originating in the retinorecipient areas has been proposed [83], the expression in many inner retina neurons after eye opening may suggest a broader role in establishing and maintaining synaptic communication in the IPL.

Pnkd exhibits a significant differential between GCL and INL especially in the adult, when the GCL pattern becomes sparse, while Rims1 is highly expressed in sparse populations in the adult, combined with lower expression level in the rest of the INL and GCL. Pnkd could be implicated in presynaptic vesicle release, by interacting with the protein encoded by Rims1 [52], a major component of the vesicle release machinery in multiple neuronal types [84, 85]. Thus Pnkd and/or Rims1 could potentially cooperate in modulating the synaptic release properties for distinct RGC subtypes.

Three genes from the secreted proteins group are also associated with synaptic function. Nptx1 (neuronal pentraxin 1, NP1) is a trans-synaptic factor for glutamate receptor subunit GluR4 recruitment to synapses, and it is secreted from presynaptic neurons [47]. The product of Nptx2 gene – Narp (neuronal activity regulated protein) is also synaptically released [86], and it is crucial for excitatory synapse maturation in hippocampus [87]. Both Narp and Nptx1 participate in synaptic refinement in developing visual system [88]. In our ISH screen, mRNAs of those two genes are sparsely and highly expressed in both the INL and the GCL, but Nptx1 seems more GCL-enriched and Brn3a-dependent compared to Nptx2 during postnatal development. Sez6l2 is a member of the "Brain-Specific Receptor-Like" family of proteins which contains single-pass transmembrane receptors whose extracellular domain can be cleaved [89, 90]. Knock-out mice for the three members of this family exhibit synapse formation abnormalities in the cerebellum, and autoantibodies against Sez6l2 are implicated in an autoimmune syndrome comprising ataxia and retinopathy [90, 91]. Sez6l2 seems to maintain a level of enrichment in the GCL from P3 to P14 in our ISH and the related Sez6l is expressed in subpopulations of RGCs and Amacrine cells [92].

The final group contains genes encoding cell surface molecules potentially involved in cell-cell communication

and/or axon/dendrite growth. Cdh4 (R-cadherin) is a cell adhesion molecule which was previously shown to be expressed in the retina in RGCs, Amacrine and Horizontal cells, findings which were largely confirmed in our ISH and IIF data [93–95]. Although our ISH data also shows a modest regulation of Cdh4 by Brn3a at late postnatal ages, the two IPL laminae typically marked by Cdh4 protein [94] are not affected in Brn3a KO mice, suggesting that they are generated by Amacrine cells or Brn3a independent RGCs. We also find late developmental GCL enrichment and Brn3a regulation for Pcdh20, a protocadherin expressed in several other neuronal cell types [96, 97]. In contrast, Rtn4rl2, encoding the Nogo receptor 2, is GCL enriched only early (P0-P3), and then gets upregulated in the INL. Its exact function in neuronal development, including the visual system is still unclear [98–100]. Finally, not much is known about the two transmembrane proteins Tmem25 and Tmem91.

Our screen also revealed several molecules that are associated with neuronal activity. Several genes (e.g. Hpca and Rbfox1) have a peak of expression at P14, with decreasing abundance in the adult. This could represent the changes in almost mature retina after eye-opening, when the amounts of gene and protein expression required for arbor formation and growth are substituted with the amounts needed for maintenance of the structure and functionality.

According to our data, Brn3a regulates constitutively expressed partner of the immediate early gene Nptx2 – Nptx1 [47, 86, 87, 101, 102], as well as the GABA receptor subunit Gabra1 [103] around and after eye-opening (P14, P22), when synaptic maturation in retinal circuits occurs [104]. Assuming that this is not caused by specific, late RGC cell loss, it would argue for a role of Brn3a in functional maturation of RGCs. Those changes take place during the period of light-driven dendritic refinement, and they are morphologically subtle compared to events during first 2 postnatal weeks [10].

Conclusions

Brn3a controls the expression of several GCL-enriched genes which encode synaptic, cell-surface and intracellular proteins. However, the extent and temporal dynamics of this regulation for molecules within different groups could vary, potentially depending on their molecular roles during specific stages of RGC subtype development (Table 3). The candidates identified by RNA sequencing of purified RGCs at a particular developmental time point have to be assessed using transcript-level analysis and throughout development, in order to identify potential RGC type markers. Most of the studied genes show GCL-enriched pattern of expression, and more than a half of them show Brn3a dependency during particular postnatal developmental time points. However, only

Mapk10, Tusc5 and Cdh4 represent a developmentally consistent targets of Brn3a-mediated regulation in the mouse retina. According to Brn3a KO GCL pattern, while Mapk10 and Cdh4 expression are not entirely controlled by Brn3a, Tusc5$^+$ cell bodies are almost completely eliminated from Brn3a KO retinas. Tusc5 thus could be a marker of one or a few Brn3a-expressing and -dependent RGC subtypes.

Abbreviations

AP: Alkaline phosphatase; BAC: Bacterial artificial chromosome; BSA: Bovine serum albumin; ChAT: Choline acetyl transferase; CPM: Counts per million reads; ES cell: Embryonic stem cell; FPKM: Fragments per million reads per gene kilobase; GCL: ganglion cell layer; IIF: Indirect immunofluorescence; INL: Inner nuclear layer; IPL: Inner plexiform layer; ISH: in situ hybridization; NBL: Neuroblast layer; NDS: Normal donkey serum; ONL: Outer nuclear layer; OPL: Outer plexyform layer; PBS: Phosphate buffered saline; PFA: paraformaldehyde; RGC: Retinal ganglion cell; RNASeq: RNA sequencing; RT: Room temperature; RT-PCR: Reverse transcription–polymerase chain reaction; TF: Transcription factor; 3'-UTR: 3'-untranslated region

Acknowledgements

We would like to thank Dr. Kirill Martemyanov from The Scripps Research Institute, Jupiter, USA for providing primary anti-Elfn1 antibody, National Eye Institute IRTA-fellow Nadia Parmhans for the help with animal genotyping and Zbynek Kozmik, Institute of Molecular Genetics of the ASCR, Prague, Czech Republic for Rax:Cre mice.

Funding

The funding was obtained from the NIH Intramural Program. NIH funding body did not have any role in the design of the study and collection, analysis and interpretation of data, and in writing the manuscript.

Authors contributions

V.M. performed all experiments and participated in planning the experiments and writing the manuscript. M.B. performed RNASeq transcript and gene level expression analysis. T.B. participated in planning the experiments and writing the manuscript. All authors read and approved the final manuscript.

Competing interests

The authors declare that they have no competing interests.

Author details

^{1}Retinal Circuit Development & Genetics Unit, Building 6, Room 331B Center Drive, Bethesda, MD 20892–0610, USA. ^{2}Genomics Core, Neurobiology-Neurodegeneration & Repair Laboratory, National Eye Institute, NIH, Building 6, Room 331B Center Drive, Bethesda, MD 20892–0610, USA.

References

1. Badea TC, Nathans J. Quantitative analysis of neuronal morphologies in the mouse retina visualized by using a genetically directed reporter. J Comp Neurol. 2004;480(4):331–51.
2. Badea TC, Nathans J. Morphologies of mouse retinal ganglion cells expressing transcription factors Brn3a, Brn3b, and Brn3c: Analysis of wild type and mutant cells using genetically-directed sparse labeling. Vision Res. 2011;51(2):269–79.
3. Coombs J, van der List D, Wang G-Y, Chalupa LM. Morphological properties of mouse retinal ganglion cells. Neuroscience. 2006;140(1):123–36.
4. Sumbul U, Song S, McCulloch K, Becker M, Lin B, Sanes JR, Masland RH, Seung HS. A genetic and computational approach to structurally classify neuronal types. Nat Commun. 2014;5:3512.
5. Sajgo S, Ghinia MG, Brooks M, Kretschmer F, Chuang K, Hiriyanna S, Wu Z, Popescu O, Badea TC. Molecular codes for cell type specification in Brn3 retinal ganglion cells. Proc Natl Acad Sci U S A. 2017;114(20):E3974–83.
6. Godement P, Salaun J, Imbert M. Prenatal and postnatal development of retinogeniculate and retinocollicular projections in the mouse. J Comp Neurol. 1984;230(4):552–75.
7. Marcus RC, Mason CA. The first retinal axon growth in the mouse optic chiasm: axon patterning and the cellular environment. J Neurosci. 1995;15(10):6389–402.
8. Coombs JL, Van Der List D, Chalupa LM. Morphological properties of mouse retinal ganglion cells during postnatal development. J Comp Neurol. 2007;503(6):803–14.
9. Diao L, Sun W, Deng Q, He S. Development of the mouse retina: emerging morphological diversity of the ganglion cells. J Neurobiol. 2004;61(2):236-49. PubMed PMID: 15389605.
10. Liu X, Robinson ML, Schreiber AM, Wu V, Lavail MM, Cang J, Copenhagen DR. Regulation of neonatal development of retinal ganglion cell dendrites by neurotrophin-3 overexpression. J Comp Neurol. 2009;514(5):449–58.
11. Badea TC, Cahill H, Ecker J, Hattar S, Nathans J. Distinct Roles of Transcription Factors Brn3a and Brn3b in Controlling the Development, Morphology, and Function of Retinal Ganglion Cells. Neuron. 2009;61(6):852–64.
12. Siegert S, Cabuy E, Scherf BG, Kohler H, Panda S, Le YZ, Fehling HJ, Gaidatzis D, Stadler MB, Roska B. Transcriptional code and disease map for adult retinal cell types. Nat Neurosci. 2012;15(3):487–95. S481–482
13. Wang Q, Marcucci F, Cerullo I, Mason C. Ipsilateral and Contralateral Retinal Ganglion Cells Express Distinct Genes during Decussation at the Optic Chiasm. eNeuro. 2016;3(6)
14. Xiang M, Zhou L, Macke JP, Yoshioka T, Hendry SH, Eddy RL, Shows TB, Nathans J. The Brn-3 family of POU-domain factors: primary structure, binding specificity, and expression in subsets of retinal ganglion cells and somatosensory neurons. J Neurosci. 1995;15(7 Pt 1):4762–85.
15. Quina LA, Pak W, Lanier J, Banwait P, Gratwick K, Liu Y, Velasquez T, O'Leary DDM, Goulding M, Turner EE. Brn3a-expressing retinal ganglion cells project specifically to thalamocortical and collicular visual pathways. J Neurosci. 2005;25(50):11595–11,604.
16. Gan L, Wang SW, Huang Z, Klein WH. POU domain factor Brn-3b is essential for retinal ganglion cell differentiation and survival but not for initial cell fate specification. Dev Biol. 1999;210(2):469–80.
17. Erkman L, Yates PA, McLaughlin T, McEvilly RJ, Whisenhunt T, O'Connell SM, Krones AI, Kirby MA, Rapaport DH, Bermingham JR, et al. A POU domain transcription factor-dependent program regulates axon pathfinding in the vertebrate visual system. Neuron. 2000;28(3):779–92.
18. Wang SW, Gan L, Martin SE, Klein WH. Abnormal polarization and axon outgrowth in retinal ganglion cells lacking the POU-domain transcription factor Brn-3b. Mol Cell Neurosci. 2000;16(2):141–56.
19. Mu X, Beremand PD, Zhao S, Pershad R, Sun H, Scarpa A, Liang S, Thomas TL, Klein WH. Discrete gene sets depend on POU domain transcription factor Brn3b/Brn-3.2/POU4f2 for their expression in the mouse embryonic retina. Development. 2004;131(6):1197–210.
20. Qiu F, Jiang H, Xiang M. A comprehensive negative regulatory program controlled by Brn3b to ensure ganglion cell specification from multipotential retinal precursors. J Neurosci. 2008;28(13):3392–403.

21. Mu X, Fu X, Beremand PD, Thomas TL, Klein WH. Gene regulation logic in retinal ganglion cell development: Isl1 defines a critical branch distinct from but overlapping with Pou4f2. Proc Natl Acad Sci U S A. 2008;105(19):6942–7.

22. Elshatory Y, Deng M, Xie X, Gan L. Expression of the LIM-homeodomain protein Isl1 in the developing and mature mouse retina. J Comp Neurol. 2007;503(1):182–97.

23. Elshatory Y, Everhart D, Deng M, Xie X, Barlow RB, Gan L. Islet-1 controls the differentiation of retinal bipolar and cholinergic amacrine cells. J Neurosci. 2007;27(46):12707–12,720.

24. Liu W, Khare SL, Liang X, Peters MA, Liu X, Cepko CL, Xiang M. All Brn3 genes can promote retinal ganglion cell differentiation in the chick. Development. 2000;127(15):3237–47.

25. Pan L, Yang Z, Feng L, Gan L. Functional equivalence of Brn3 POU-domain transcription factors in mouse retinal neurogenesis. Development. 2005; 132(4):703–12.

26. McEvilly RJ, Erkman L, Luo L, Sawchenko PE, Ryan AF, Rosenfeld MG. Requirement for Brn-3.0 in differentiation and survival of sensory and motor neurons. Nature. 1996;384(6609):574–7.

27. Xiang M, Gan L, Zhou L, Klein WH, Nathans J. Targeted deletion of the mouse POU domain gene Brn-3a causes selective loss of neurons in the brainstem and trigeminal ganglion, uncoordinated limb movement, and impaired suckling. Proc Natl Acad Sci U S A. 1996;93(21):11950–11,955.

28. Shi M, Kumar SR, Motajo O, Kretschmer F, Mu X, Badea TC. Genetic interactions between Brn3 transcription factors in retinal ganglion cell type specification. PLoS one. 2013;8(10):e76347.

29. Patel T, Hobert O. Coordinated control of terminal differentiation and restriction of cellular plasticity. Elife. 2017;6.

30. Guillemot F. Spatial and temporal specification of neural fates by transcription factor codes. Development. 2007;134(21):3771–80.

31. Jessell TM. Neuronal specification in the spinal cord: inductive signals and transcriptional codes. Nat Rev Genet. 2000;1(1):20–9.

32. Halbleib JM, Nelson WJ: Cadherins in development: cell adhesion, sorting, and tissue morphogenesis. Genes Dev 2006, 20(23):3199–3214.

33. Sakurai T. The role of cell adhesion molecules in brain wiring and neuropsychiatric disorders. Mol Cell Neurosci. 2017;81:4–11.

34. Hirano S, Takeichi M. Cadherins in brain morphogenesis and wiring. Physiol Rev. 2012;92(2):597–634.

35. Chang JD, Field SJ, Rameh LE, Carpenter CL, Cantley LC. Identification and characterization of a phosphoinositide phosphate kinase homolog. J Biol Chem. 2004;279(12):11672–11,679.

36. Conde C, Caceres A. Microtubule assembly, organization and dynamics in axons and dendrites. Nat Rev Neurosci. 2009;10(5):319–32.

37. Dent EW, Gupton SL, Gertler FB. The growth cone cytoskeleton in axon outgrowth and guidance. Cold Spring Harb Perspect Biol. 2011;3(3)

38. Georges PC, Hadzimichalis NM, Sweet ES, Firestein BL. The yin-yang of dendrite morphology: unity of actin and microtubules. Mol Neurobiol. 2008; 38(3):270–84.

39. Barnat M, Enslen H, Propst F, Davis RJ, Soares S, Nothias F. Distinct roles of c-Jun N-terminal kinase isoforms in neurite initiation and elongation during axonal regeneration. J Neurosci. 2010;30(23):7804–16.

40. Barford K, Deppmann C, Winckler B. The neurotrophin receptor signaling endosome: Where trafficking meets signaling. Dev Neurobiol. 2017;77(4):405–18.

41. Huber AB, Kolodkin AL, Ginty DD, Cloutier JF. Signaling at the growth cone: ligand-receptor complexes and the control of axon growth and guidance. Annu Rev Neurosci. 2003;26:509–63.

42. Luo L. Rho GTPases in neuronal morphogenesis. Nat Rev Neurosci. 2000; 1(3):173–80.

43. Villarroel-Campos D, Gastaldi L, Conde C, Caceres A, Gonzalez-Billault C. Rab-mediated trafficking role in neurite formation. J Neurochem. 2014;129(2):240–8.

44. Sudhof TC. The presynaptic active zone. Neuron. 2012;75(1):11–25.

45. Sudhof TC. Synaptic Neurexin Complexes: A Molecular Code for the Logic of Neural Circuits. Cell. 2017;171(4):745–69.

46. Zipursky SL, Sanes JR. Chemoaffinity revisited: dscams, protocadherins, and neural circuit assembly. Cell. 2010;143(3):343–53.

47. Sia GM, Beique JC, Rumbaugh G, Cho R, Worley PF, Huganir RL. Interaction of the N-terminal domain of the AMPA receptor GluR4 subunit with the neuronal pentraxin NP1 mediates GluR4 synaptic recruitment. Neuron. 2007; 55(1):87–102.

48. Schwab ME. Functions of Nogo proteins and their receptors in the nervous system. Nat Rev Neurosci. 2010;11(12):799–811.

49. Klimova L, Lachova J, Machon O, Sedlacek R, Kozmik Z. Generation of mRx-Cre transgenic mouse line for efficient conditional gene deletion in early retinal progenitors. PloS one. 2013;8(5):e63029.

50. Thorvaldsdottir H, Robinson JT, Mesirov JP. Integrative Genomics Viewer (IGV): high-performance genomics data visualization and exploration. Brief Bioinform. 2013;14(2):178–92.

51. Matsunami H, Takeichi M. Fetal brain subdivisions defined by R- and E-cadherin expressions: evidence for the role of cadherin activity in region-specific, cell-cell adhesion. Dev Biol. 1995;172(2):466–78.

52. Shen Y, Ge WP, Li Y, Hirano A, Lee HY, Rohlmann A, Missler M, Tsien RW, Jan LY, Fu YH, et al. Protein mutated in paroxysmal dyskinesia interacts with the active zone protein RIM and suppresses synaptic vesicle exocytosis. Proc Natl Acad Sci U S A. 2015;112(10):2935–41.

53. Carlsson P, Mahlapuu M. Forkhead transcription factors: key players in development and metabolism. Dev Biol. 2002;250(1):1–23.

54. Pan D, Rubin GM. Targeted expression of teashirt induces ectopic eyes in Drosophila. Proc Natl Acad Sci U S A. 1998;95(26):15508–15,512.

55. Rousso DL, Qiao M, Kagan RD, Yamagata M, Palmiter RD, Sanes JR. Two Pairs of ON and OFF Retinal Ganglion Cells Are Defined by Intersectional Patterns of Transcription Factor Expression. Cell Rep. 2016;15(9):1930–44.

56. Sato C, Iwai-Takekoshi L, Ichikawa Y, Kawasaki H. Cell type-specific expression of FoxP2 in the ferret and mouse retina. Neurosci Res. 2017; 117:1–13.

57. French CA, Fisher SE. What can mice tell us about Foxp2 function? Curr Opin Neurobiol. 2014;28:72–9.

58. Caubit X, Tiveron MC, Cremer H, Fasano L. Expression patterns of the three Teashirt-related genes define specific boundaries in the developing and postnatal mouse forebrain. J Comp Neurol. 2005;486(1):76–88.

59. Gehman LT, Stoilov P, Maguire J, Damianov A, Lin CH, Shiue L, Ares M Jr, Mody I, Black DL. The splicing regulator Rbfox1 (A2BP1) controls neuronal excitation in the mammalian brain. Nat Genet. 2011;43(7):706–11.

60. Kielar M, Tuy FP, Bizzotto S, Lebrand C, de Juan Romero C, Poirier K, Oegema R, Mancini GM, Bahi-Buisson N, Olaso R, et al. Mutations in Eml1 lead to ectopic progenitors and neuronal heterotopia in mouse and human. Nat Neurosci. 2014;17(7):923–33.

61. Korenbrot JI, Mehta M, Tserentsoodol N, Postlethwait JH, Rebrik TI. EML1 (CNG-modulin) controls light sensitivity in darkness and under continuous illumination in zebrafish retinal cone photoreceptors. J Neurosci. 2013; 33(45):17763–17,776.

62. Rebrik TI, Botchkina I, Arshavsky VY, Craft CM, Korenbrot JI. CNG-modulin: a novel Ca-dependent modulator of ligand sensitivity in cone photoreceptor cGMP-gated ion channels. J Neurosci. 2012;32(9):3142–53.

63. Tzingounis AV, Kobayashi M, Takamatsu K, Nicoll RA. Hippocalcin gates the calcium activation of the slow afterhyperpolarization in hippocampal pyramidal cells. Neuron. 2007;53(4):487–93.

64. Yang DD, Kuan CY, Whitmarsh AJ, Rincon M, Zheng TS, Davis RJ, Rakic P, Flavell RA. Absence of excitotoxicity-induced apoptosis in the hippocampus of mice lacking the Jnk3 gene. Nature. 1997;389(6653):865–70.

65. Yu P, Agbaegbu C, Malide DA, Wu X, Katagiri Y, Hammer JA, Geller HM. Cooperative interactions of LPPR family members in membrane localization and alteration of cellular morphology. J Cell Sci. 2015;128(17):3210–22.

66. Brauer AU, Nitsch R. Plasticity-related genes (PRGs/LRPs): a brain-specific class of lysophospholipid-modifying proteins. Biochim Biophys Acta. 2008; 1781(9):595–600.

67. Shi L, Wang K, Zhao M, Yuan X, Huang C. Overexpression of PIP5KL1 suppresses the growth of human cervical cancer cells in vitro and in vivo. Cell Biol Int. 2010;34(3):309–15.

68. Blankenship AG, Feller MB. Mechanisms underlying spontaneous patterned activity in developing neural circuits. Nat Rev Neurosci. 2010;11(1):18–29.

69. Sanes JR, Zipursky SL. Design principles of insect and vertebrate visual systems. Neuron. 2010;66(1):15–36.

70. Burana D, Yoshihara H, Tanno H, Yamamoto A, Saeki Y, Tanaka K, Komada M. The Ankrd13 Family of Ubiquitin-interacting Motif-bearing Proteins Regulates Valosin-containing Protein/p97 Protein-mediated Lysosomal Trafficking of Caveolin 1. J Biol Chem. 2016;291(12):6218–31.

71. Lu W, Ziff EB. PICK1 interacts with ABP/GRIP to regulate AMPA receptor trafficking. Neuron. 2005;47(3):407–21.

72. Bushlin I, Petralia RS, Wu F, Harel A, Mughal MR, Mattson MP, Yao PJ. Clathrin assembly protein AP180 and CALM differentially control axogenesis and dendrite outgrowth in embryonic hippocampal neurons. J Neurosci. 2008;28(41):10257–10,271.

73. Fazakerley DJ, Naghiloo S, Chaudhuri R, Koumanov F, Burchfield JG, Thomas KC, Krycer JR, Prior MJ, Parker BL, Murrow BA, et al. Proteomic Analysis of GLUT4 Storage Vesicles Reveals Tumor Suppressor Candidate 5 (TUSC5) as a Novel Regulator of Insulin Action in Adipocytes. J Biol Chem. 2015;290(39):23528–42.

74. Oort PJ, Warden CH, Baumann TK, Knotts TA, Adams SH. Characterization of Tusc5, an adipocyte gene co-expressed in peripheral neurons. Mol Cell Endocrinol. 2007;276(1–2):24–35.

75. Kanageswaran N, Demond M, Nagel M, Schreiner BS, Baumgart S, Scholz P, Altmuller J, Becker C, Doerner JF, Conrad H, et al. Deep sequencing of the murine olfactory receptor neuron transcriptome. PloS one. 2015;10(1):e0113170.

76. Quraishi S, Gayet J, Morgans CW, Duvoisin RM. Distribution of group-III metabotropic glutamate receptors in the retina. J Comp Neurol. 2007;501(6):931–43.

77. Bleckert A, Parker ED, Kang Y, Pancaroglu R, Soto F, Lewis R, Craig AM, Wong RO. Spatial relationships between GABAergic and glutamatergic synapses on the dendrites of distinct types of mouse retinal ganglion cells across development. PloS one. 2013;8(7):e69612.

78. Haverkamp S, Wassle H. Immunocytochemical analysis of the mouse retina. J Comp Neurol. 2000;424(1):1–23.

79. Antflick JE, Hampson DR. Modulation of glutamate release from parallel fibers by mGlu4 and pre-synaptic GABA(A) receptors. J Neurochem. 2012;120(4):552–63.

80. Dolan J, Mitchell KJ. Mutation of Elfn1 in mice causes seizures and hyperactivity. PloS one. 2013;8(11):e80491.

81. Cao Y, Sarria I, Fehlhaber KE, Kamasawa N, Orlandi C, James KN, Hazen JL, Gardner MR, Farzan M, Lee A, et al. Mechanism for Selective Synaptic Wiring of Rod Photoreceptors into the Retinal Circuitry and Its Role in Vision. Neuron. 2015;87(6):1248–60.

82. Sylwestrak EL, Ghosh A. Elfn1 regulates target-specific release probability at CA1-interneuron synapses. Science. 2012;338(6106):536–40.

83. Zanellato A, Comelli MC, Dal Toso R, Carmignoto G. Developing rat retinal ganglion cells express the functional NGF receptor p140trkA. Dev Biol. 1993;159(1):105–13.

84. Kaeser PS, Deng L, Wang Y, Dulubova I, Liu X, Rizo J, Sudhof TC. RIM proteins tether Ca2+ channels to presynaptic active zones via a direct PDZ-domain interaction. Cell. 2011;144(2):282–95.

85. Schoch S, Castillo PE, Jo T, Mukherjee K, Geppert M, Wang Y, Schmitz F, Malenka RC, Sudhof TC. RIM1alpha forms a protein scaffold for regulating neurotransmitter release at the active zone. Nature. 2002;415(6869):321–6.

86. Tsui CC, Copeland NG, Gilbert DJ, Jenkins NA, Barnes C, Worley PF. Narp, a novel member of the pentraxin family, promotes neurite outgrowth and is dynamically regulated by neuronal activity. J Neurosci. 1996;16(8):2463–78.

87. Pelkey KA, Barksdale E, Craig MT, Yuan X, Sukumaran M, Vargish GA, Mitchell RM, Wyeth MS, Petralia RS, Chittajallu R, et al. Pentraxins coordinate excitatory synapse maturation and circuit integration of parvalbumin interneurons. Neuron. 2015;85(6):1257–72.

88. Bjartmar L, Huberman AD, Ullian EM, Renteria RC, Liu X, Xu W, Prezioso J, Susman MW, Stellwagen D, Stokes CC, et al. Neuronal pentraxins mediate synaptic refinement in the developing visual system. J Neurosci. 2006;26(23):6269–81.

89. Boonen M, Staudt C, Gilis F, Oorschot V, Klumperman J, Jadot M. Cathepsin D and its newly identified transport receptor SEZ6L2 can modulate neurite outgrowth. J Cell Sci. 2016;129(3):557–68.

90. Miyazaki T, Hashimoto K, Uda A, Sakagami H, Nakamura Y, Saito SY, Nishi M, Kume H, Tohgo A, Kaneko I, et al. Disturbance of cerebellar synaptic maturation in mutant mice lacking BSRPs, a novel brain-specific receptor-like protein family. FEBS Lett. 2006;580(17):4057–64.

91. Yaguchi H, Yabe I, Takahashi H, Okumura F, Takeuchi A, Horiuchi K, Kano T, Kanda A, Saito W, Matsumoto M, et al. Identification of anti-Sez6l2 antibody in a patient with cerebellar ataxia and retinopathy. J Neurol. 2014;261(1):224–6.

92. Gunnersen JM, Kuek A, Phipps JA, Hammond VE, Puthussery T, Fletcher EL, Tan SS. Seizure-related gene 6 (Sez-6) in amacrine cells of the rodent retina and the consequence of gene deletion. PloS one. 2009;4(8):e6546.

93. Duan X, Krishnaswamy A, De la Huerta I, Sanes JR. Type II cadherins guide assembly of a direction-selective retinal circuit. Cell. 2014;158(4):793–807.

94. Honjo M, Tanihara H, Suzuki S, Tanaka T, Honda Y, Takeichi M. Differential expression of cadherin adhesion receptors in neural retina of the postnatal mouse. Invest Ophthalmol Vis Sci. 2000;41(2):546–51.

95. Inuzuka H, Miyatani S, Takeichi M. R-cadherin: a novel Ca(2+)-dependent cell-cell adhesion molecule expressed in the retina. Neuron. 1991;7(1):69–79.

96. Kim SY, Mo JW, Han S, Choi SY, Han SB, Moon BH, Rhyu IJ, Sun W, Kim H. The expression of non-clustered protocadherins in adult rat hippocampal formation and the connecting brain regions. Neuroscience. 2010;170(1):189–99.

97. Lee W, Cheng TW, Gong Q. Olfactory sensory neuron-specific and sexually dimorphic expression of protocadherin 20. J Comp Neurol. 2008;507(1):1076–86.

98. Wills ZP, Mandel-Brehm C, Mardinly AR, McCord AE, Giger RJ, Greenberg ME. The nogo receptor family restricts synapse number in the developing hippocampus. Neuron. 2012;73(3):466–81.

99. Baumer BE, Kurz A, Borrie SC, Sickinger S, Dours-Zimmermann MT, Zimmermann DR, Bandtlow CE. Nogo receptor homolog NgR2 expressed in sensory DRG neurons controls epidermal innervation by interaction with Versican. J Neurosci. 2014;34(5):1633–46.

100. Dickendesher TL, Baldwin KT, Mironova YA, Koriyama Y, Raiker SJ, Askew KL, Wood A, Geoffroy CG, Zheng B, Liepmann CD, et al. NgR1 and NgR3 are receptors for chondroitin sulfate proteoglycans. Nat Neurosci. 2012;15(5):703–12.

101. O'Brien RJ, Xu D, Petralia RS, Steward O, Huganir RL, Worley P. Synaptic clustering of AMPA receptors by the extracellular immediate-early gene product Narp. Neuron. 1999;23(2):309–23.

102. Xu D, Hopf C, Reddy R, Cho RW, Guo L, Lanahan A, Petralia RS, Wenthold RJ, O'Brien RJ, Worley P. Narp and NP1 form heterocomplexes that function in developmental and activity-dependent synaptic plasticity. Neuron. 2003;39(3):513–28.

103. Ponomarev I, Maiya R, Harnett MT, Schafer GL, Ryabinin AE, Blednov YA, Morikawa H, Boehm SL 2nd, Homanics GE, Berman AE, et al. Transcriptional signatures of cellular plasticity in mice lacking the alpha1 subunit of GABAA receptors. J Neurosci. 2006;26(21):5673–83.

104. Tian N. Synaptic activity, visual experience and the maturation of retinal synaptic circuitry. J Physiol. 2008;586(18):4347–55.

3

In vivo functional analysis of *Drosophila* Robo1 immunoglobulin-like domains

Marie C. Reichert[1,2], Haley E. Brown[1] and Timothy A. Evans[1]* (iD)

Abstract

Background: In animals with bilateral symmetry, midline crossing of axons in the developing central nervous system is regulated by Slit ligands and their neuronal Roundabout (Robo) receptors. Multiple structural domains are present in an evolutionarily conserved arrangement in Robo family proteins, but our understanding of the functional importance of individual domains for midline repulsive signaling is limited.

Methods: We have examined the functional importance of each of the five conserved immunoglobulin-like (Ig) domains within the *Drosophila* Robo1 receptor. We generated a series of Robo1 variants, each lacking one of the five Ig domains (Ig1-5), and tested each for their ability to bind Slit when expressed in cultured *Drosophila* cells. We used a transgenic approach to express each variant in *robo1's* normal expression pattern in wild-type and *robo1* mutant embryos, and examined the effects of deleting each domain on receptor expression, axonal localization, regulation, and midline repulsive signaling in vivo.

Results: We show that individual deletion of Ig domains 2–5 does not interfere with Robo1's ability to bind Slit, while deletion of Ig1 strongly disrupts Slit binding. None of the five Ig domains (Ig1-5) are individually required for proper expression of Robo1 in embryonic neurons, for exclusion from commissural axon segments in wild-type embryos, or for downregulation by Commissureless (Comm), a negative regulator of Slit-Robo repulsion in *Drosophila*. Each of the Robo1 Ig deletion variants (with the exception of Robo1ΔIg1) were able to restore midline crossing in *robo1* mutant embryos to nearly the same extent as full-length Robo1, indicating that Ig domains 2–5 are individually dispensable for midline repulsive signaling in vivo.

Conclusions: Our findings indicate that four of the five Ig domains within *Drosophila* Robo1 are dispensable for its role in midline repulsion, despite their strong evolutionary conservation, and highlight a unique requirement for the Slit-binding Ig1 domain in the regulation of midline crossing.

Keywords: *Drosophila*, Slit, Robo, Axon guidance, Midline crossing, Immunoglobulin-like domain

Abbreviations: CNS, Central nervous system; Comm, Commissureless; Fn, Fibronectin type III repeat; Ig, Immunoglobulin-like domain; Robo, Roundabout

Background

Slits and Robos regulate midline crossing in bilaterian animals

The proper establishment of connectivity across the midline of the central nervous system (CNS) is essential for bilateral coordination in a wide variety of animal groups [1]. During embryonic development, CNS axons must choose whether or not to cross the midline in response to attractant and repellant cues produced by midline cells. Axon guidance receptors of the Roundabout (Robo) family regulate midline crossing by signaling midline repulsion in response to their canonical ligand Slit [2]. While the core components of the Slit-Robo pathway (one or more Slits signaling through one or more Robo receptors) are evolutionarily conserved across bilaterian phyla [3–13], the number and identity of pathway components varies, and distinct regulatory mechanisms have appeared in different animal groups [14–16].

* Correspondence: evanst@uark.edu
[1]Department of Biological Sciences, University of Arkansas, Fayetteville, AR 72701, USA
Full list of author information is available at the end of the article

Slit-Robo signaling in *Drosophila*

Robo1 is the primary Slit receptor in *Drosophila*, and normally non-crossing axons ectopically cross the midline in every segment of the embryonic CNS in *robo1* null mutants [3, 17]. Robo1 is broadly expressed in the *Drosophila* embryonic CNS, yet the majority of CNS axons will cross the midline [3, 18]. Two regulatory mechanisms have been identified which prevent premature Slit-Robo1 repulsion in pre-crossing commissural axons in *Drosophila*. The endosomal sorting receptor Commissureless (Comm) prevents newly synthesized Robo1 proteins from reaching the growth cone surface as commissural axons are growing towards and across the midline [14, 19–21], and Robo2 acts non-autonomously to antagonize repulsive signaling by the remaining surface-localized Robo1, facilitating midline crossing [15]. Comm also appears to regulate Robo1 through an additional mechanism that is independent of endosomal sorting, but this role is not well understood [22]. Orthologs of Comm and Robo2 have not been identified outside of insects, and vertebrates have acquired distinct regulatory mechanisms to prevent premature Slit-Robo repulsion in commissural axons [16, 23].

Conserved structure of Robo receptors and functional modularity of Ig domains

Nearly all Robo family receptors in insects, mammals, nematodes, and planarians share a conserved protein structure, with five immunoglobulin-like (Ig) domains and three fibronectin type III (Fn) repeats making up each receptor's ectodomain [3, 5, 8, 10, 24–26]. The exceptions to this rule are mammalian Robo4/Magic Roundabout, which lacks Ig3, Ig4, Ig5, and Fn1 [27], and Robo1a/Robo1b from the silkworm *Bombyx mori*, which lack Ig5 and Fn1 [11].

In vitro biochemical interaction and co-crystallization studies have shown that the N-terminal Ig1 domain is the primary Slit-binding region in both insect and mammalian Robo receptors [28–33], and in vivo studies demonstrate the functional importance of Ig1 for midline repulsive activity of both *Drosophila* Robo1 and Robo2 [15, 34]. Functional roles for other extracellular Robo domains in contexts other than Slit-dependent midline repulsion have been described. For example, *Drosophila* Robo2's Ig2 domain contributes to its role in promoting midline crossing [15, 35], while Robo2's Ig3 domain has been implicated in regulating longitudinal pathway formation in the *Drosophila* embryonic CNS [35]. In mammals, the divergent Robo3/Rig-1 receptor does not bind Slit [33], but interacts with the novel ligand Nell2 in an Fn-dependent manner to steer commissural axons towards the midline of the embryonic mouse spinal cord [36].

An in vivo structure/function analysis of all five Robo1 Ig domains

Although it is clear that the various axon guidance activities of Robo family members depend on individual functional domains within the receptor, or combinations thereof, we do not yet have a clear picture of how each domain contributes to individual axon guidance events. Apart from Ig1, which of the other domains in *Drosophila* Robo1 are required for midline repulsion, if any? Are any of the other Robo1 Ig or Fn domains required for receptor expression, protein stability, axonal localization, or Slit binding? Here, we address these questions by individually deleting each of the five Robo1 Ig domains and examining the effects of these deletions on Slit binding as well as in vivo protein expression, localization, and Slit-dependent midline repulsive signaling. We use a previously-established genetic rescue assay [34, 37] to remove endogenous *robo1* function and systematically replace it with *robo1* variants from which individual Ig domain coding sequences have been deleted. We find that Ig domains 2–5 of Robo1 are individually dispensable for Slit binding, receptor expression and axonal localization, regulation by Comm, and midline repulsive signaling activity. Our results indicate that the Slit-binding Ig1 domain is the only immunoglobulin-like domain that is individually required for Robo1's role in midline repulsion during development of the *Drosophila* embryonic CNS.

Methods

Molecular biology

Robo1 Ig domain deletions

Individual Robo1 Ig domain deletions were generated via site-directed mutagenesis using Phusion Flash PCR MasterMix (Thermo Scientific), and completely sequenced to ensure no other mutations were introduced. Robo1 deletion variants include the following amino acid residues, relative to Genbank reference sequence AAF46887: Robo1ΔIg1 (L153-T1395); Robo1ΔIg2 (P56-V152/V253-T1395); Robo1ΔIg3 (P56-Q252/P345-T1395); Robo1ΔIg4 (P56-P344/E441-T1395); Robo1ΔIg5 (P56-D440/G535-T1395).

pUAST cloning

Robo1 coding sequences were cloned as BglII fragments into p10UASTattB for S2R+ cell transfection. All *robo1* p10UASTattB constructs include identical heterologous 5′ UTR and signal sequences (derived from the Drosophila *wingless* gene) and an N-terminal 3xHA tag. To make *P{10UAS-Comm}86FB*, the entire *comm* coding sequence (plus 163 bp of the 5′ untranslated region) was cloned as an EcoRI-XbaI fragment into p10UASTattB without heterologous leader sequences or epitope tags.

robo1 rescue construct cloning

Construction of the *robo1* genomic rescue construct was described previously [34]. Full-length and variant Robo1 coding sequences were cloned as BglII fragments into the BamHI-digested backbone. Robo1 proteins produced from this construct include the endogenous Robo1 signal peptide, and the 4xHA tag is inserted directly upstream of the first Ig domain (Ig2 in Robo1ΔIg1; Ig1 in all other constructs).

Genetics

The following *Drosophila* mutant alleles were used: *robo1¹* (also known as *robo^GA285*). The following *Drosophila* transgenes were used: P{GAL4-elav.L}3 (elavGAL4), P{10UAS-Comm}86FB, P{robo1::HArobo1} [34], P{robo1::HArobo1ΔIg1} [34], P{robo1::HArobo1ΔIg2}, P{robo1::HArobo1ΔIg3}, P{robo1::HArobo1ΔIg4}, P{robo1::HArobo1ΔIg5}. Transgenic flies were generated by BestGene Inc (Chino Hills, CA) using ΦC31-directed site-specific integration into attP landing sites at cytological position 86FB (for UAS-Comm) or 28E7 (for *robo1* genomic rescue constructs). *robo1* rescue transgenes were introduced onto a *robo1¹* chromosome via meiotic recombination, and the presence of the *robo1¹* mutation was confirmed in all recombinant lines by DNA sequencing. All crosses were carried out at 25 °C.

Slit binding assay

Drosophila S2R+ cells were cultured at 25 °C in Schneider's media plus 10 % fetal calf serum. To assay Slit binding, cells were plated on poly-L-lysine coated coverslips in six-well plates (Robo-expressing cells) or 75 cm^2 cell culture flasks (Slit-expressing cells) at a density of 1-2 × 10^6 cells/ml, and transfected with pRmHA3-GAL4 [38] and HA-tagged p10UAST-Robo or untagged pUAST-Slit plasmids using Effectene transfection reagent (Qiagen). GAL4 expression was induced with 0.5 mM CuSO$_4$ for 24 h, then Slit-conditioned media was harvested by adding heparin (2.5 ug/ml) to Slit-transfected cells and incubating at room temperature for 20 min with gentle agitation. Robo-transfected cells were incubated with Slit-conditioned media at room temperature for 20 min, then washed with PBS and fixed for 20 min at 4 °C in 4 % formaldehyde. Cells were permeabilized with PBS + 0.1 % Triton X-100, then stained with antibodies diluted in PBS + 2 mg/ml BSA. Antibodies used were: mouse anti-SlitC (Developmental Studies Hybridoma Bank [DSHB] #c555.6D, 1:50), rabbit anti-HA (Covance #PRB-101C-500, 1:2000), Cy3-conjugated goat anti-mouse (Jackson Immunoresearch #115-165-003, 1:500), and Alexa 488-conjugated goat anti-rabbit (Jackson #111-545-003, 1:500). After antibody staining, coverslips with cells attached were mounted in Aqua-Poly/Mount (Polysciences, Inc.). Confocal stacks were collected using a Leica SP5 confocal microscope and processed by Fiji/ImageJ [39] and Adobe Photoshop software.

Immunohistochemistry

Drosophila embryo collection, fixation and antibody staining were carried out as previously described [40]. The following antibodies were used: FITC-conjugated goat anti-HRP (Jackson #123-095-021, 1:100), mouse anti-Fasciclin II (DSHB #1D4, 1:100), mouse anti-βgal (DSHB #40-1a, 1:150), mouse anti-Robo1 (DSHB #13C9, 1:100), rabbit anti-GFP (Invitrogen #A11122, 1:1000), mouse anti-HA (Covance #MMS-101P-500, 1:1000), Cy3-conjugated goat anti-mouse (Jackson #115-165-003, 1:1000), Alexa 488-conjugated goat anti-rabbit (Jackson #111-545-003, 1:500). Embryos were genotyped using balancer chromosomes carrying *lacZ* markers, or by the presence of epitope-tagged transgenes. Ventral nerve cords from embryos of the desired genotype and developmental stage were dissected and mounted in 70 % glycerol/PBS. Fluorescent confocal stacks were collected using a Leica SP5 confocal microscope and processed by Fiji/ImageJ [39] and Adobe Photoshop software.

Results

Robo1 Ig domains 2–5 are individually dispensable for Slit binding in cultured *Drosophila* cells

The Roundabout (Robo) receptor family is an evolutionarily conserved group of transmembrane axon guidance receptors that regulate midline crossing of axons in many bilaterian species. Nearly all Robo receptors share a conserved arrangement of five immunoglobulin-like (Ig) domains and three fibronectin type III (Fn) repeats in their extracellular region. We have recently demonstrated that deletion of the Ig1 domain from *Drosophila* Robo1 prevents it from binding to Slit, and abolishes its ability to prevent midline crossing of axons in vivo [34]. To determine whether Ig domains 2–5 of Robo1 contribute to Slit binding we generated a series of Robo1 variants, each lacking one of the five extracellular Ig domains, and assayed their ability to bind Slit when expressed in cultured *Drosophila* cells. While deletion of the Ig1 domain reduced Slit binding to background levels [34], we found that Robo1ΔIg2, Robo1ΔIg3, Robo1ΔIg4, and Robo1ΔIg5 bound Slit as effectively as full-length Robo1 (Fig. 1). All of the variant receptors were expressed at similar levels and properly localized to the plasma membrane, as assayed by anti-HA staining of transfected cells. Thus, individual deletion of Ig2, Ig3, Ig4, or Ig5 does not affect membrane localization of Robo1 or its ability to interact with Slit.

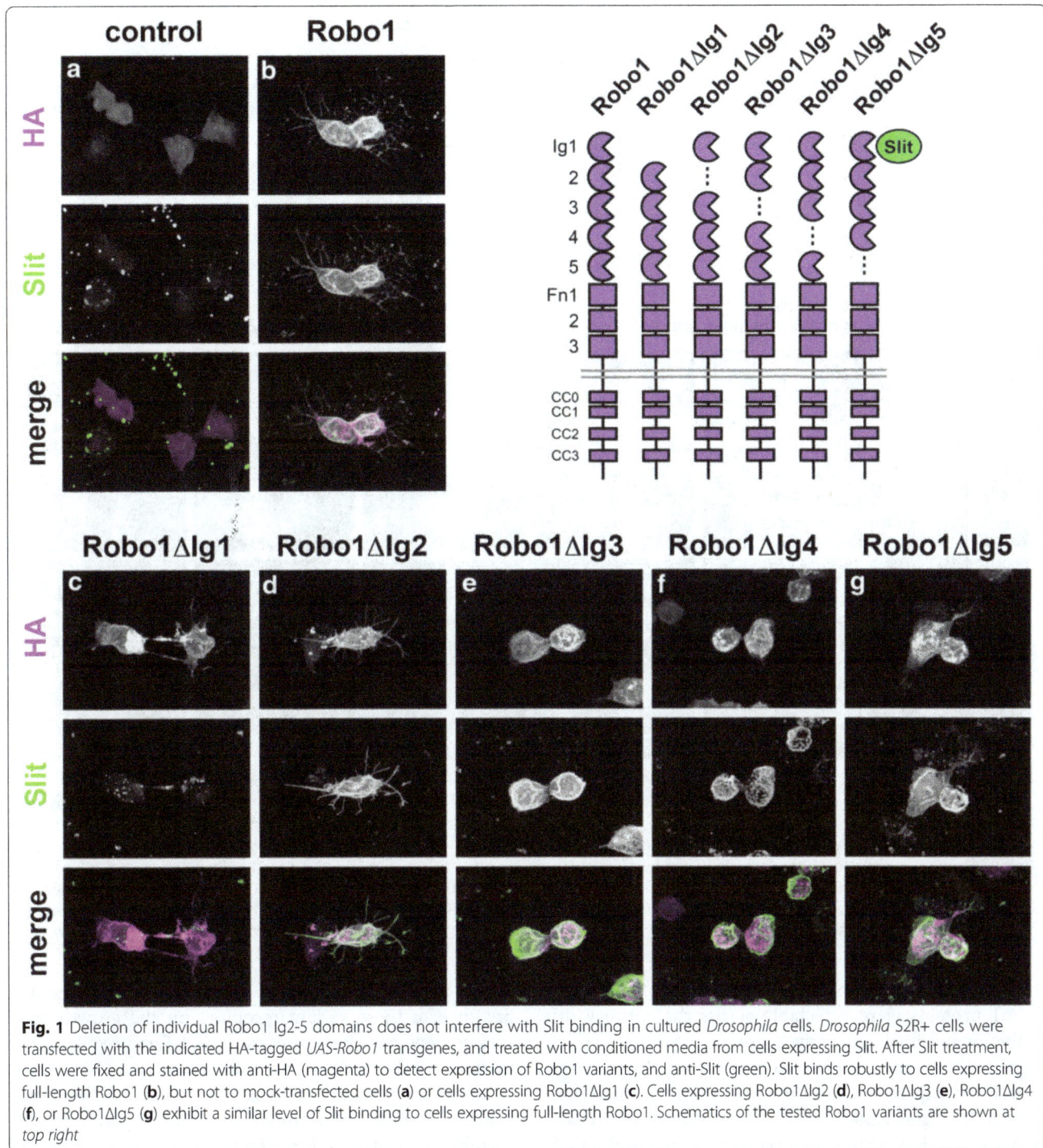

Fig. 1 Deletion of individual Robo1 Ig2-5 domains does not interfere with Slit binding in cultured *Drosophila* cells. *Drosophila* S2R+ cells were transfected with the indicated HA-tagged *UAS-Robo1* transgenes, and treated with conditioned media from cells expressing Slit. After Slit treatment, cells were fixed and stained with anti-HA (magenta) to detect expression of Robo1 variants, and anti-Slit (green). Slit binds robustly to cells expressing full-length Robo1 (**b**), but not to mock-transfected cells (**a**) or cells expressing Robo1ΔIg1 (**c**). Cells expressing Robo1ΔIg2 (**d**), Robo1ΔIg3 (**e**), Robo1ΔIg4 (**f**), or Robo1ΔIg5 (**g**) exhibit a similar level of Slit binding to cells expressing full-length Robo1. Schematics of the tested Robo1 variants are shown at *top right*

Robo1 Ig domains are not individually required for expression and localization in vivo

To compare the expression, localization, and activity of our Robo1 domain deletion variants in vivo, we used a *robo1* genomic rescue construct in which regulatory sequences derived from the endogenous *robo1* locus control expression of HA-tagged cDNAs encoding full-length Robo1 or each of our Robo1 Ig deletion variants (Fig. 2) [34, 37]. All rescue constructs contain identical upstream and downstream regulatory sequences, and all transgenes were inserted into the same genomic location to ensure equivalent expression levels (insertion site 28E7).

We found that all five Robo1 variants were expressed at similar levels to full-length Robo1 and localized to axons in the embryonic ventral nerve cord. Similar to

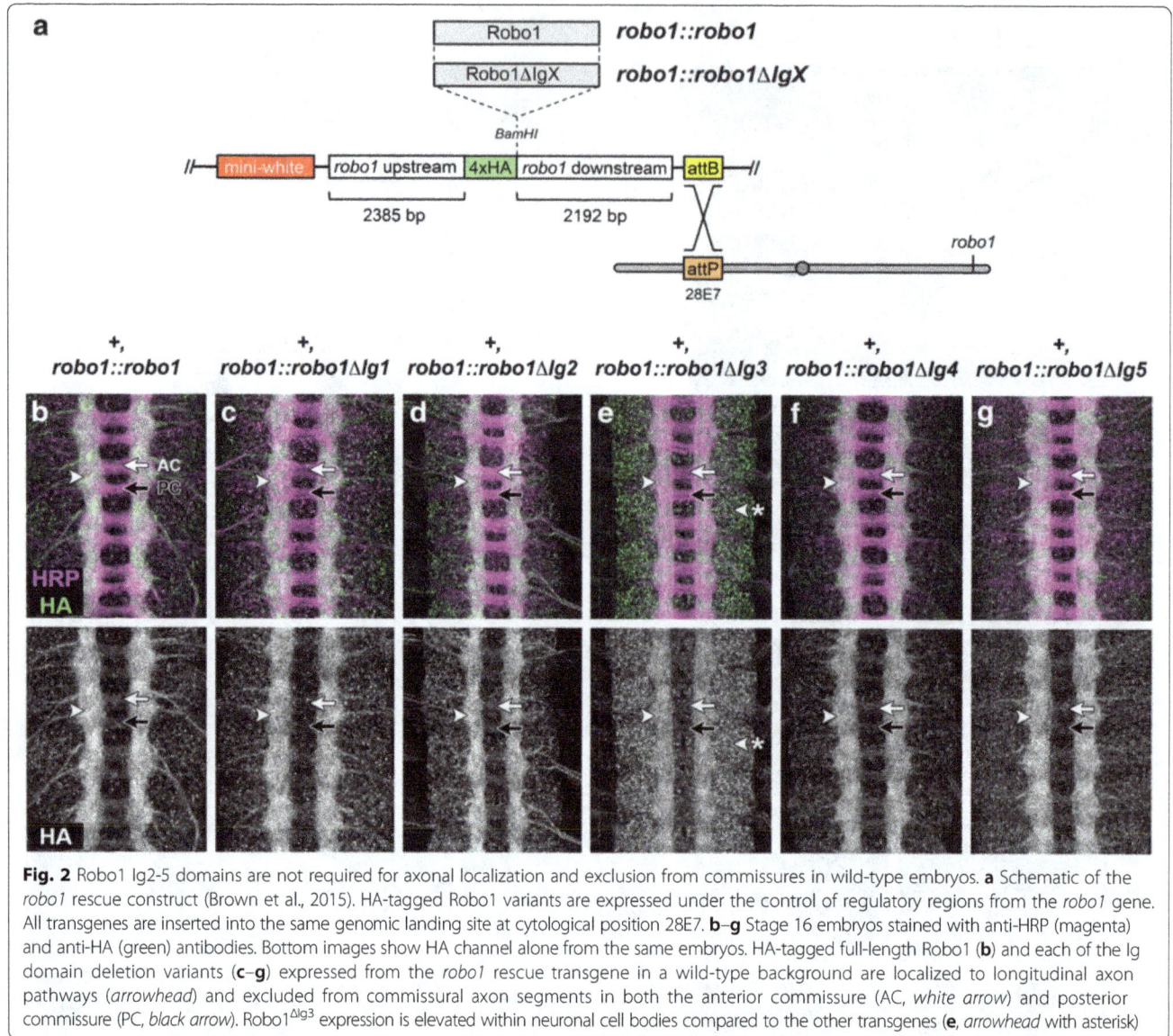

Fig. 2 Robo1 Ig2-5 domains are not required for axonal localization and exclusion from commissures in wild-type embryos. **a** Schematic of the *robo1* rescue construct (Brown et al., 2015). HA-tagged Robo1 variants are expressed under the control of regulatory regions from the *robo1* gene. All transgenes are inserted into the same genomic landing site at cytological position 28E7. **b–g** Stage 16 embryos stained with anti-HRP (magenta) and anti-HA (green) antibodies. Bottom images show HA channel alone from the same embryos. HA-tagged full-length Robo1 (**b**) and each of the Ig domain deletion variants (**c–g**) expressed from the *robo1* rescue transgene in a wild-type background are localized to longitudinal axon pathways (*arrowhead*) and excluded from commissural axon segments in both the anterior commissure (AC, *white arrow*) and posterior commissure (PC, *black arrow*). Robo1$^{\Delta Ig3}$ expression is elevated within neuronal cell bodies compared to the other transgenes (**e**, *arrowhead* with asterisk)

the wild-type Robo1 expression pattern, all five variant Robo1 proteins were detectable across the entire width of the longitudinal connectives, and were strongly down-regulated on commissural axon segments (Fig. 2b–g). Indeed the expression patterns of all variants tested here were indistinguishable from the endogenous Robo1 pattern or the HA expression pattern in the full-length Robo1 genomic rescue transgene, with the exception of Robo1ΔIg3. While this variant displayed axonal localization and commissural down-regulation within the neuropile, it also displayed elevated expression in a punctate pattern in the neuronal cell bodies in the cortex (Fig. 2e).

We did not observe any apparent dominant negative effects of expressing any of our Robo1 Ig deletion variants in an otherwise wild-type background, even when present in two copies in homozygous embryos, suggesting that the presence of these variant receptors on the growth cone surface does not alter endogenous Slit-Robo regulation of midline repulsion. Similarly, embryos carrying two copies of any of the rescue transgenes along with two functional copies of endogenous *robo1* did not display any discernible gain-of-function effects (i.e. thinning or loss of commissures indicating increased midline repulsion). This, together with their clearance from commissural axon segments, suggests that the Robo1 Ig deletion variants are subject to the same regulation as endogenous Robo1.

Regulation of Robo1 Ig deletion variants by Comm

Commissureless (Comm) is an important negative regulator of Slit-Robo1 repulsion in *Drosophila* [14, 19–22]. We have previously reported that the Ig1 domain of

Robo1 is not required for regulation of Robo1 by Comm in vivo [34]. To determine whether the other Ig domains of Robo1 are required for Comm-dependent regulation, we examined the effect of Comm misexpression on the expression levels and localization of our Robo1 Ig deletion variants in embryonic neurons. Forced expression of Comm in all embryonic neurons strongly reduces the levels of Robo1 protein on neuronal axons, as Comm is an endosomal sorting receptor that prevents Robo1 protein from reaching the surface of axonal growth cones. We found that for each of our variants,

the levels of HA-tagged Robo1 protein on axons were strongly reduced in embryos carrying *elav-GAL4* and *UAS-Comm* compared to embryos carrying *elav-GAL4* alone (Fig. 3). Consistent with down-regulation of both the transgenic and endogenous Robo1 protein, these embryos also displayed a strongly *slit*-like phenotype reflecting high levels of ectopic midline crossing (Fig. 3e–h). These results demonstrate that individually deleting any of the Ig domains from Robo1 does not disrupt Comm-dependent regulation in embryonic neurons.

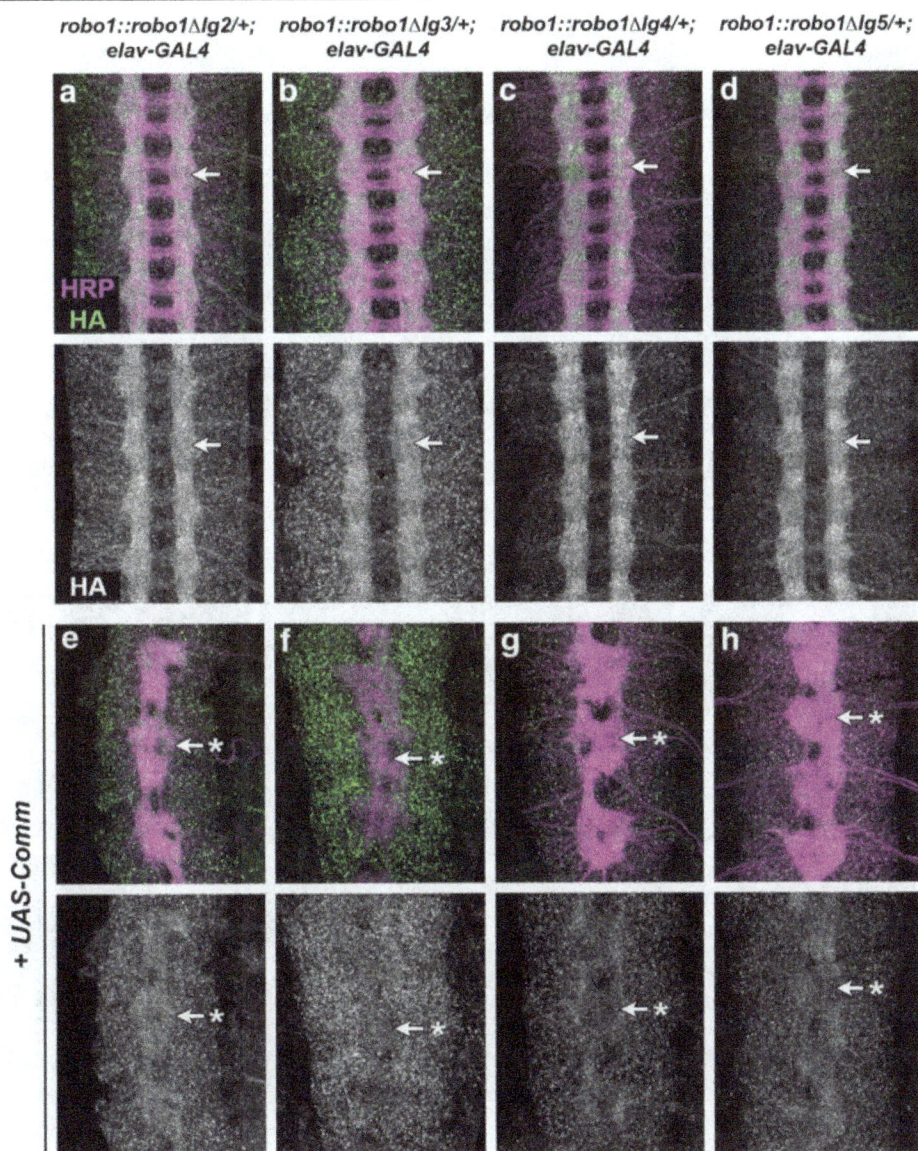

Fig. 3 Robo1 Ig domains are not required for regulation by Comm. **a–h** Stage 16 embryos stained with anti-HRP (magenta) and anti-HA (green) antibodies. Lower images show HA channel alone from the same embryos. Embryos carrying one copy of the indicated *robo1* transgenes along with *elav-GAL4* display normal expression of the HA-tagged Robo1 variants (**a-d**, *arrows*). Embryos carrying one copy of the indicated *robo1* transgenes along with *elav-GAL4* and *UAS-Comm* display strong reduction in axonal HA expression and a *slit*-like midline collapse phenotype reflecting increased midline crossing (**e-h**, *arrows* with asterisk). Pairs of sibling embryos shown here (**a** and **e**; **b** and **f**; **c** and **g**; **d** and **h**) were stained in the same tube and imaged using identical confocal settings to allow an accurate comparison of HA levels between embryos

Robo1's Ig2-5 domains are not individually required for midline repulsion in vivo

The Slit-binding Ig1 domain of Robo1 is required for its in vivo role in midline repulsion [34]. To test whether Ig domains Ig2-Ig5 are individually required for midline repulsion in vivo, we introduced our robo1::robo1ΔIgX rescue transgenes into a robo1 null mutant background and measured their ability to rescue midline repulsion in the absence of endogenous robo1 activity. Homozygous null robo1 embryos carrying two copies of our full-length Robo1 rescue transgene exhibited a wild-type axon scaffold, and transgenic HA-tagged Robo1 protein was properly localized to axons and excluded from commissural segments (Fig. 4a), while robo1 mutant embryos expressing Robo1ΔIg1 phenocopied the robo1 null phenotype, and transgenic Robo1ΔIg1 protein was detectable on axons as they crossed the midline (Fig. 4b), as previously described [34]. We found that expression of any of our Ig2-5 deletion transgenes in robo1 null mutants was able to restore the wild-type appearance of the axon scaffold, as measured by anti-HRP staining (Fig. 4c–f). Further, each of the transgenic Robo1 proteins was properly expressed and excluded from commissures in this background, indicating that endogenous robo1 is not required for proper expression, commissural clearance, or midline repulsive signaling of Robo1ΔIg2, Robo1ΔIg3, Robo1ΔIg4, or Robo1ΔIg5 (Fig. 4c–f). As in a wild-type

background, we detected elevated levels of Robo1ΔIg3 in neuronal cell bodies in addition to its axonal expression (Fig. 4d; compare to Fig. 2e).

To more closely examine the ability of our rescue transgenes to restore midline repulsion in the absence of endogenous robo1, we quantified ectopic midline crossing of FasII-positive longitudinal axons in each of our robo1 rescue backgrounds. In wild-type embryos or robo1 null mutants rescued with a full-length Robo1 transgene, FasII-positive axons rarely crossed the midline (Fig. 5a, c), but they crossed the midline in 100 % of segments in robo1 mutants (Fig. 5b). As we have previously reported [34], Robo1ΔIg1 was completely unable to rescue midline repulsion in robo1 mutant embryos, reflecting the critical role of Robo1 Ig1 in midline repulsion (Fig. 5d). In contrast, we could restore midline repulsion to near-wild-type levels by similarly expressing Robo1ΔIg2, Robo1ΔIg3, Robo1ΔIg4, or Robo1ΔIg5 (Fig. 5e–h). In segments where ectopic crossing was observed in these rescue backgrounds, it was typically less severe than in robo1 mutants (Fig. 5e, arrow with asterisk).

Discussion

In this paper, we have examined the functional importance of each of the five immunoglobulin-like (Ig) domains of the Drosophila Robo1 axon guidance receptor. We deleted each Ig domain individually and examined

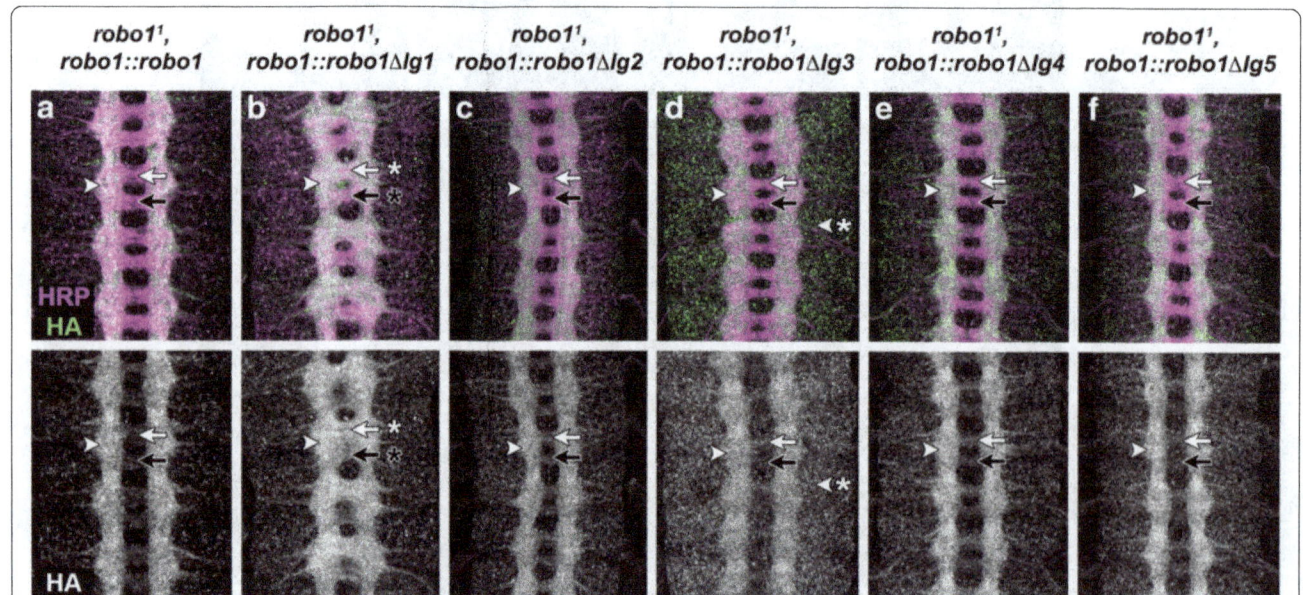

Fig. 4 Expression of Robo1 Ig2-5 deletion proteins in robo1 mutant embryos. a–f Stage 16 robo1 mutant embryos carrying indicated robo1 rescue transgenes, stained with anti-HRP (magenta) and anti-HA (green) antibodies. Lower images show HA channel alone from the same embryos. Expression of full-length Robo1 via the robo1 rescue transgene in a robo1 null mutant (a) restores the wild-type structure of the axon scaffold, but expression of Robo1ΔIg1 does not (b; compare to robo1 null mutant shown in Fig. 5b). Each of the Ig2-5 deletion variants restore axon scaffold morphology to a similar extent as full-length Robo1 (c–f). In the absence of endogenous robo1, all of the variants are localized to the longitudinal pathways as in wild-type embryos (arrowheads) and excluded from the anterior and posterior commissures (arrows in a, c-f), with the exception of Robo1ΔIg1 (b, arrows with asterisks). As in wild-type embryos, Robo1ΔIg3 displays elevated expression levels in neuronal cell bodies compared to the other Robo1 variants (d, arrowhead with asterisk)

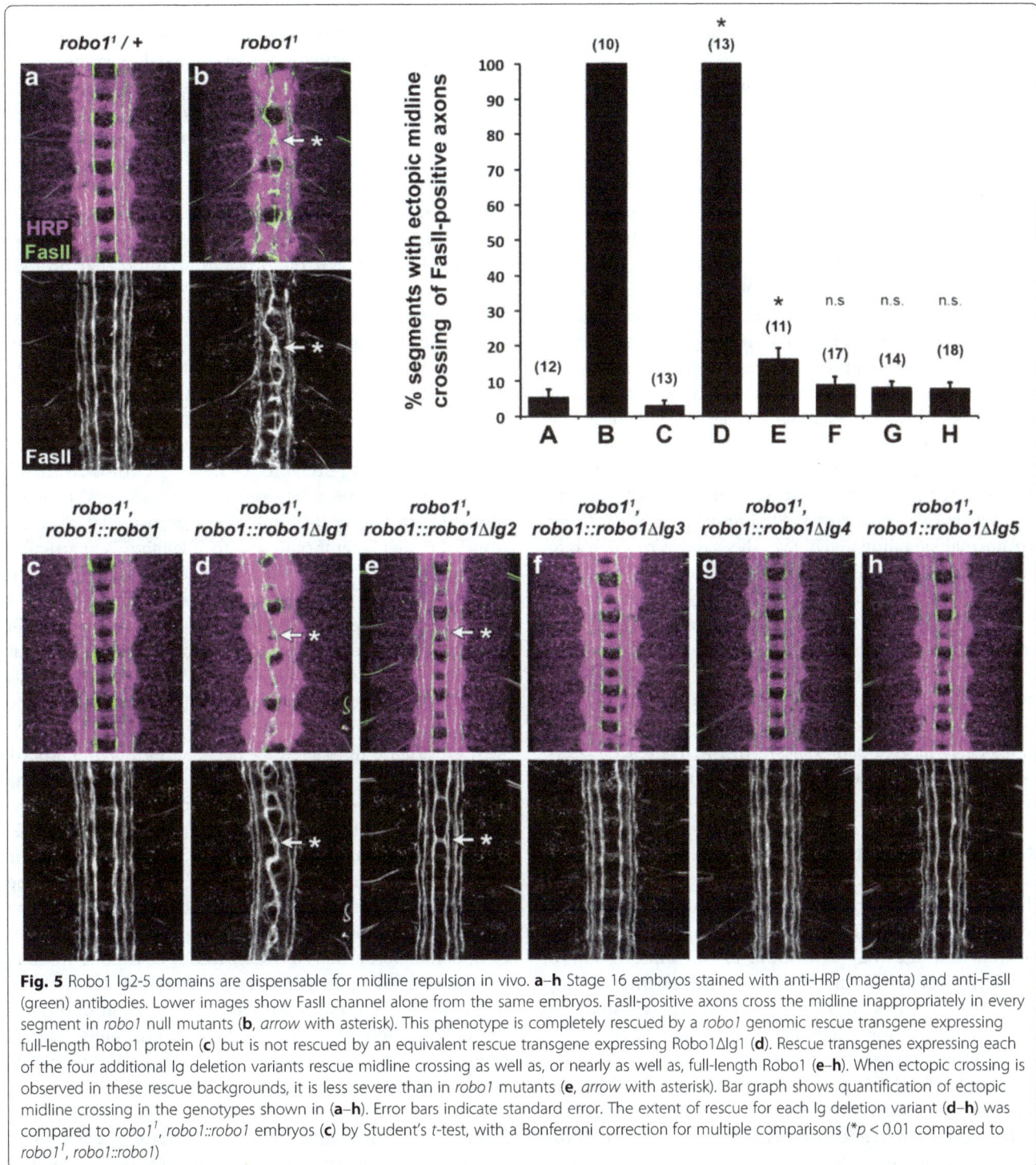

Fig. 5 Robo1 Ig2-5 domains are dispensable for midline repulsion in vivo. **a–h** Stage 16 embryos stained with anti-HRP (magenta) and anti-FasII (green) antibodies. Lower images show FasII channel alone from the same embryos. FasII-positive axons cross the midline inappropriately in every segment in *robo1* null mutants (**b**, *arrow* with asterisk). This phenotype is completely rescued by a *robo1* genomic rescue transgene expressing full-length Robo1 protein (**c**) but is not rescued by an equivalent rescue transgene expressing Robo1ΔIg1 (**d**). Rescue transgenes expressing each of the four additional Ig deletion variants rescue midline crossing as well as, or nearly as well as, full-length Robo1 (**e–h**). When ectopic crossing is observed in these rescue backgrounds, it is less severe than in *robo1* mutants (**e**, *arrow* with asterisk). Bar graph shows quantification of ectopic midline crossing in the genotypes shown in (**a–h**). Error bars indicate standard error. The extent of rescue for each Ig deletion variant (**d–h**) was compared to *robo1¹, robo1::robo1* embryos (**c**) by Student's *t*-test, with a Bonferroni correction for multiple comparisons (*$p < 0.01$ compared to *robo1¹, robo1::robo1*)

the effects on Robo1's ability to bind its ligand Slit, on expression and localization of Robo1 in the embryonic CNS, and on Robo1's ability to regulate midline repulsion in vivo. Our results suggest that Ig1 is the only immunoglobulin-like domain in *Drosophila* Robo1 that is indispensable for its midline repulsive activity. Deleting any of the other four Ig domains individually does not

alter the structure or confirmation of Robo1 in a way that interferes with Slit binding in vitro or repulsive signaling in vivo. This is consistent with recent evidence that deleting Ig2 from Robo2 does not interfere with its ability to bind Slit or signal midline repulsion [15], and supports a modular view of Robo1 ectodomains wherein individual Ig domains can function independently to promote distinct molecular events (e.g. ligand binding) and cellular outcomes (e.g. axon repulsion) [35].

Robo1 Ig domains are not individually required for protein stability or axonal localization

Deleting any of the five Ig domains did not significantly disrupt the expression or axonal localization of Robo1 in embryonic neurons, suggesting no large effects on protein stability or folding (Fig. 2b–g). HA expression in wild-type embryos carrying each of the Ig deletion variants was largely indistinguishable from full-length HA-tagged Robo1, or endogenous Robo1 protein expression, with the exception of Robo1ΔIg3. This variant displayed axonal expression levels that were roughly equivalent to full-length Robo1 and the other Ig deletion variants, but was also detectable at increased levels within neuronal cell bodies (Fig. 2e). Notably, Robo1ΔIg3 did not appear to localize to the cell body plasma membrane, but remained within intracellular puncta, presumably vesicles within the protein synthesis and transport pathway. The levels of axonal Robo1ΔIg3 appear to be sufficient for normal signaling activity, as this variant rescued midline repulsion equally as well as the other Ig deletion variants (Fig. 5f).

All five Robo1 Ig deletion variants were cleared from commissures when expressed in otherwise wild-type embryos, and we did not observe any obvious gain of function or dominant negative effects caused by their expression, as the axon scaffold appeared normal in embryos carrying two copies of any of the five rescue transgenes when visualized with anti-HRP antibody staining (Fig. 2c–g).

Does Ig2 contribute to Slit binding or midline repulsion?

Notably, Robo1ΔIg2 was the only deletion variant (other than Robo1ΔIg1) whose ability to rescue robo1 mutants was significantly different than full-length Robo1, suggesting that Ig2 may contribute to Slit binding and/or repulsive signaling, though to a lesser extent than Ig1 (Fig. 5e). Previous in vitro experiments suggested that Ig2 is required for Slit binding by human Robo1 [29], while other experiments suggested that Ig2 does not contribute to Slit binding [32, 41]. While we did not detect any qualitative differences in Slit binding between full-length Robo1 and Robo1ΔIg2 in our cell culture-based experiments (Fig. 1b, d), perhaps a quantitative difference in Slit affinity might be detected using more sensitive assays [30–32, 35]. Even if Ig2 does not directly contribute to Slit binding, it may help to stabilize or enhance interactions with Slit or heparin, which forms a ternary complex with Slit and Robo and contributes to Slit-Robo signaling [42–45]. In previous studies, site-specific mutations of evolutionarily conserved residues in Ig2 of Drosophila Robo1 had minor effects on binding

of Slit or heparin to Robo1 in vitro [32]; perhaps this could account for the slight but significant reduction in midline repulsive activity of our Robo1ΔIg2 variant.

Signaling mechanisms of Robo family receptors

Robo family receptors are transmembrane proteins which lack intracellular catalytic domains, and the mechanisms through which they signal axon repulsion are not well characterized. Although it is known that cytoplasmic effector proteins are recruited to the Robo1 cytodomain upon Slit binding [46, 47] and that proteolytic processing and endocytosis of Robo1 are necessary for repulsive signaling [48, 49], it is unknown whether ligand binding induces a change in multimerization state, or some other type of conformational change in order to trigger downstream signaling events. It is also unknown how (or even whether) the extracellular domains apart from Ig1 contribute to the signaling mechanism(s). Perhaps Ig domains 2–5, though not individually required for midline repulsion, serve as "spacers" to position the Slit-binding Ig1 domain at a particular distance from the cell membrane or to facilitate a particular conformational change within the ectodomain upon Slit binding. If this is the case, the requirement must not be a strict one because we can delete any single Ig domain in between Ig1 and the transmembrane region without severely compromising Robo1's ability to signal. In this context, it is worthwhile to note that Ig1 and Ig2 are the most strongly conserved in terms of sequence identity, with 58 % and 48 % identity between Drosophila Robo1 and human Robo1 for Ig1 and Ig2, respectively [3]. The sequences of Ig 3–5 are less highly conserved (35 % identity for each of the three domains between Drosophila Robo1 and human Robo1), perhaps indicating that their three-dimensional structure or arrangement might be more important than their amino acid sequence. It will be interesting to determine how many, or what combination of Ig domains can be removed without disrupting midline repulsive signaling. In vitro structural studies will likely be required (for example, a structural comparison of the entire Robo1 ectodomain in liganded and unliganded states) to fully understand how each domain contributes to Slit-dependent signaling.

Evolutionary conservation of Robo receptor Ig domains

Nearly all Robo family receptors share Drosophila Robo1's 5 Ig + 3 Fn ectodomain structure. The Ig1 domain of Drosophila Robo1 is absolutely required for Slit binding and midline repulsive activity in vivo [34]; Ig1 domains in other Robo receptors appear to have equally important roles in Slit binding [15, 31, 32]. In contrast, Ig domains 2–5 appear to be individually dispensable for Slit binding and midline repulsive activity, at least in the case of Drosophila Robo1 (this study). If the other four

Ig domains are dispensable for midline repulsion, why is their number and arrangement so strongly evolutionarily conserved? One possibility is that they are required for signaling by Robo1 in contexts other than midline repulsion of axons, for example embryonic muscle migration [50], migration of embryonic chordotonal sensory neurons [51], or guidance and targeting of dendrites [52–56], or for midline repulsion of axons in other developmental stages or tissues not examined here, for example gustatory receptor neurons in the adult [57]. Another possibility is that one or more of these domains are required for regulation by Robo2, which inhibits Slit-Robo1 repulsion to promote midline crossing [15]. Robo2-dependent defects in midline crossing are evident only when attractive Netrin-Frazzled signaling is also compromised in *robo2* mutants [15, 37], so we would not necessarily expect to observe a decrease in midline crossing if any of our Robo1 Ig deletion variants were insensitive to Robo2. Future studies will examine the effects of misexpressing Robo2 or removing *fra* function in each of the rescue backgrounds described here, which may provide further insight into how Robo2 inhibits Robo1 to promote midline crossing of commissural axons.

Conclusions

We have described here a systematic functional analysis of all five immunoglobulin-like domains in the *Drosophila* Robo1 axon guidance receptor. This work is the first in vivo study of the functional importance of Robo1 Ig domains other than the Slit-binding Ig1 domain. We have shown that Ig domains 2–5 are not required for Slit binding, and that despite their strong evolutionary conservation, Ig 2–5 are individually dispensable for *Drosophila* Robo1's in vivo role in regulating midline repulsion in the embryonic CNS. These observations indicate that Ig1 is the only Ig domain in *Drosophila* Robo1 that is uniquely required for midline repulsion, and suggest that the mechanism by which Robo1 signals axon repulsion is not strictly dependent on the evolutionarily conserved 5 Ig + 3 Fn ectodomain structure that is characteristic of Robo family receptors.

Acknowledgements

We thank Elise Arbeille for providing the *Drosophila comm* cDNA. We acknowledge the two anonymous reviewers, who provided helpful comments on the manuscript. Stocks obtained from the Bloomington *Drosophila* Stock Center (NIH P40OD018537) were used in this study. Monoclonal antibodies were obtained from the Developmental Studies Hybridoma Bank, created by the NICHD of the NIH and maintained at The University of Iowa, Department of Biology, Iowa City, IA 52242.

Funding

This work was supported by funds from the University of Arkansas. The funders had no role in the design of the study, collection, analysis, and interpretation of data, decision to publish, or preparation of the manuscript.

Authors' contributions

MCR contributed to the generation of Robo1 deletion constructs and genetic strains, performed the Slit binding and Comm downregulation assays, and contributed to data acquisition and analysis. HEB contributed to the generation of Robo1 deletion constructs and genetic strains, and scored and analyzed midline crossing defects. TAE conceived and designed the study, contributed to data acquisition and analysis, and wrote the initial draft of the paper. All authors read and approved the final manuscript.

Competing interests

The authors declare that they have no competing interests.

Author details

[1]Department of Biological Sciences, University of Arkansas, Fayetteville, AR 72701, USA. [2]Present address: Intramural Research Training Program, National Human Genome Research Institute, Bethesda, MD 20892, USA.

References

1. Evans TA, Bashaw GJ. Axon guidance at the midline: of mice and flies. Curr Opin Neurobiol. 2010;20:79–85.
2. Dickson BJ, Gilestro GF. Regulation of commissural axon pathfinding by slit and its Robo receptors. Annu Rev Cell Dev Biol. 2006;22:651–75.
3. Kidd T, Brose K, Mitchell KJ, Fetter RD, Tessier-Lavigne M, Goodman CS, et al. Roundabout controls axon crossing of the CNS midline and defines a novel subfamily of evolutionarily conserved guidance receptors. Cell. 1998;92:205–15.
4. Kidd T, Bland KS, Goodman CS. Slit is the midline repellent for the robo receptor in Drosophila. Cell. 1999;96:785–94.
5. Zallen JA, Yi BA, Bargmann CI. The conserved immunoglobulin superfamily member SAX-3/Robo directs multiple aspects of axon guidance in C. elegans. Cell. 1998;92:217–27.
6. Fricke C, Lee JS, Geiger-Rudolph S, Bonhoeffer F, Chien CB. astray, a zebrafish roundabout homolog required for retinal axon guidance. Science. 2001;292:507–10.
7. Long H, Sabatier C, Ma L, Plump AS, Yuan W, Ornitz DM, et al. Conserved roles for Slit and Robo proteins in midline commissural axon guidance. Neuron. 2004;42:213–23.
8. Cebrià F, Newmark PA. Morphogenesis defects are associated with abnormal nervous system regeneration following roboA RNAi in planarians. Development. 2007;134:833–7.
9. Cebrià F, Guo T, Jopek J, Newmark PA. Regeneration and maintenance of the planarian midline is regulated by a slit orthologue. Dev Biol. 2007;307: 394–406.
10. Evans TA, Bashaw GJ. Slit/Robo-mediated axon guidance in Tribolium and Drosophila: Divergent genetic programs build insect nervous systems. Dev Biol. 2012;363:266–78.
11. Li X-T, Yu Q, Zhou Q-S, Zhao X, Liu Z-Y, Cui W-Z, et al. BmRobo1a and BmRobo1b control axon repulsion in the silkworm Bombyx mori. Gene. 2016;577:215–20.
12. Li X-T, Yu Q, Zhou Q-S, Zhao X, Liu Z-Y, Cui W-Z, et al. BmRobo2/3 is required for axon guidance in the silkworm Bombyx mori. Gene. 2015
13. Yu Q, Li X-T, Liu C, Cui W-Z, Mu Z-M, Zhao X, et al. Evolutionarily conserved repulsive guidance role of slit in the silkworm bombyx Mori. PLoS ONE. 2014;9:e109377.
14. Keleman K, Ribeiro C, Dickson BJ. Comm function in commissural axon guidance: cell-autonomous sorting of Robo in vivo. Nat Neurosci. 2005;8:156–63.

15. Evans TA, Santiago C, Arbeille E, Bashaw GJ. Robo2 acts in trans to inhibit Slit-Robo1 repulsion in pre-crossing commissural axons. Elife. 2015;4:e08407.

16. Jaworski A, Long H, Tessier-Lavigne M. Collaborative and specialized functions of robo1 and robo2 in spinal commissural axon guidance. J Neurosci. 2010;30:9445–53.

17. Seeger M, Tear G, Ferres-Marco D, Goodman CS. Mutations affecting growth cone guidance in Drosophila: genes necessary for guidance toward or away from the midline. Neuron. 1993;10:409–26.

18. Rickert C, Kunz T, Harris K-L, Whitington PM, Technau GM. Morphological characterization of the entire interneuron population reveals principles of neuromere organization in the ventral nerve cord of Drosophila. J Neurosci. 2011;31:15870–83.

19. Kidd T, Russell C, Goodman CS, Tear G. Dosage-sensitive and complementary functions of roundabout and commissureless control axon crossing of the CNS midline. Neuron. 1998;20:25–33.

20. Keleman K, Rajagopalan S, Cleppien D, Teis D, Paiha K, Huber LA, et al. Comm sorts robo to control axon guidance at the Drosophila midline. Cell. 2002;110:415–27.

21. Tear G, Harris R, Sutaria S, Kilomanski K, Goodman CS, Seeger MA. commissureless controls growth cone guidance across the CNS midline in Drosophila and encodes a novel membrane protein. Neuron. 1996;16:501–14.

22. Gilestro GF. Redundant mechanisms for regulation of midline crossing in Drosophila. PLoS ONE. 2008;3:e3798.

23. Chen Z, Gore BB, Long H, Ma L, Tessier-Lavigne M. Alternative splicing of the Robo3 axon guidance receptor governs the midline switch from attraction to repulsion. Neuron. 2008;58:325–32.

24. Simpson JH, Kidd T, Bland KS, Goodman CS. Short-range and long-range guidance by slit and its Robo receptors. Robo and Robo2 play distinct roles in midline guidance. Neuron. 2000;28:753–66.

25. Rajagopalan S, Vivancos V, Nicolas E, Dickson BJ. Selecting a longitudinal pathway: Robo receptors specify the lateral position of axons in the Drosophila CNS. Cell. 2000;103:1033–45.

26. Yuan SS, Cox LA, Dasika GK, Lee EY-HP. Cloning and functional studies of a novel gene aberrantly expressed in RB-deficient embryos. Dev Biol. 1999;207:62–75.

27. Huminiecki L, Gorn M, Suchting S, Poulsom R, Bicknell R. Magic roundabout is a new member of the roundabout receptor family that is endothelial specific and expressed at sites of active angiogenesis. Genomics. 2002;79:547–52.

28. Chen JH, Wen L, Dupuis S, Wu JY, Rao Y. The N-terminal leucine-rich regions in Slit are sufficient to repel olfactory bulb axons and subventricular zone neurons. J Neurosci. 2001;21:1548–56.

29. Liu Z, Patel K, Schmidt H, Andrews W, Pini A, Sundaresan V. Extracellular Ig domains 1 and 2 of Robo are important for ligand (Slit) binding. Mol Cell Neurosci. 2004;26:232–40.

30. Howitt JA, Clout NJ, Hohenester E. Binding site for Robo receptors revealed by dissection of the leucine-rich repeat region of Slit. EMBO J. 2004;23:4406–12.

31. Morlot C, Thielens NM, Ravelli RBG, Hemrika W, Romijn RA, Gros P, et al. Structural insights into the Slit-Robo complex. Proc Natl Acad Sci U S A. 2007;104:14923–8.

32. Fukuhara N, Howitt JA, Hussain S-A, Hohenester E. Structural and functional analysis of slit and heparin binding to immunoglobulin-like domains 1 and 2 of Drosophila Robo. J Biol Chem. 2008;283:16226–34.

33. Zelina P, Blockus H, Zagar Y, Péres A, Friocourt F, Wu Z, et al. Signaling switch of the axon guidance receptor Robo3 during vertebrate evolution. Neuron. 2014;84:1258–72.

34. Brown HE, Reichert MC, Evans TA. Slit binding via the Ig1 domain is essential for midline repulsion by drosophila Robo1 but dispensable for receptor expression, localization, and regulation in vivo. G3 (Bethesda). 2015;5:2429–39.

35. Evans TA, Bashaw GJ. Functional diversity of robo receptor immunoglobulin domains promotes distinct axon guidance decisions. Curr Biol. 2010;20(6):567–72.

36. Jaworski A, Tom I, Tong RK, Gildea HK, Koch AW, Gonzalez LC, et al. Operational redundancy in axon guidance through the multifunctional receptor Robo3 and its ligand NELL2. Science. 2015;350:961–5.

37. Spitzweck B, Brankatschk M, Dickson BJ. Distinct protein domains and expression patterns confer divergent axon guidance functions for drosophila robo receptors. Cell. 2010;140:409–20.

38. Klueg KM, Alvarado D, Muskavitch MAT, Duffy JB. Creation of a GAL4/UAS-coupled inducible gene expression system for use in Drosophila cultured cell lines. Genesis. 2002;34:119–22.

39. Schindelin J, Arganda-Carreras I, Frise E, Kaynig V, Longair M, Pietzsch T, et al. Fiji: an open-source platform for biological-image analysis. Nat Methods. 2012;9:676–82.

40. Patel NH. Imaging neuronal subsets and other cell types in whole-mount Drosophila embryos and larvae using antibody probes. Methods Cell Biol. 1994;44:445–87.

41. Morlot C, Hemrika W, Romijn RA, Gros P, Cusack S, McCarthy AA. Production of Slit2 LRR domains in mammalian cells for structural studies and the structure of human Slit2 domain 3. Acta Crystallogr D Biol Crystallogr. 2007;63:961–8.

42. Hussain S-A, Piper M, Fukuhara N, Strochlic L, Cho G, Howitt JA, et al. A molecular mechanism for the heparan sulfate dependence of slit-robo signaling. J Biol Chem. 2006;281:39693–8.

43. Smart AD, Course MM, Rawson JM, Selleck SB, Van Vactor D, Johnson KG. Heparan sulfate proteoglycan specificity during axon pathway formation in the Drosophila embryo. Dev Neurobiol. 2011;71:608–18.

44. Steigemann P, Molitor A, Fellert S, Jäckle H, Vorbrüggen G. Heparan sulfate proteoglycan syndecan promotes axonal and myotube guidance by slit/robo signaling. Curr Biol. 2004;14:225–30.

45. Johnson KG, Ghose A, Epstein E, Lincecum J, O'Connor MB, Van Vactor D. Axonal heparan sulfate proteoglycans regulate the distribution and efficiency of the repellent slit during midline axon guidance. Curr Biol. 2004;14:499–504.

46. Yang L, Bashaw GJ. Son of sevenless directly links the Robo receptor to rac activation to control axon repulsion at the midline. Neuron. 2006;52:595–607.

47. Fan X, Labrador J-P, Hing H, Bashaw GJ. Slit stimulation recruits Dock and Pak to the roundabout receptor and increases Rac activity to regulate axon repulsion at the CNS midline. Neuron. 2003;40:113–27.

48. Coleman HA, Labrador J-P, Chance RK, Bashaw GJ. The Adam family metalloprotease Kuzbanian regulates the cleavage of the roundabout receptor to control axon repulsion at the midline. Development. 2010;137:2417–26.

49. Chance RK, Bashaw GJ. Slit-dependent endocytic trafficking of the robo receptor is required for Son of sevenless recruitment and midline axon repulsion. PLoS Genet. 2015;11:e1005402.

50. Kramer SG, Kidd T, Simpson JH, Goodman CS. Switching repulsion to attraction: changing responses to slit during transition in mesoderm migration. Science. 2001;292:737–40.

51. Kraut R, Zinn K. Roundabout 2 regulates migration of sensory neurons by signaling in trans. Curr Biol. 2004;14:1319–29.

52. Godenschwege TA, Simpson JH, Shan X, Bashaw GJ, Goodman CS, Murphey RK. Ectopic expression in the giant fiber system of Drosophila reveals distinct roles for roundabout (Robo), Robo2, and Robo3 in dendritic guidance and synaptic connectivity. J Neurosci. 2002;22:3117–29.

53. Furrer M-P, Vasenkova I, Kamiyama D, Rosado Y, Chiba A. Slit and Robo control the development of dendrites in Drosophila CNS. Development. 2007;134:3795–804.

54. Dimitrova S, Reissaus A, Tavosanis G. Slit and Robo regulate dendrite branching and elongation of space-filling neurons in Drosophila. Dev Biol. 2008;324:18–30.

55. Mauss A, Tripodi M, Evers JF, Landgraf M. Midline signalling systems direct the formation of a neural map by dendritic targeting in the Drosophila motor system. PLoS Biol. 2009;7:e1000200.

56. Brierley DJ, Blanc E, Reddy OV, VijayRaghavan K, Williams DW. Dendritic targeting in the leg neuropil of Drosophila: the role of midline signalling molecules in generating a myotopic map. PLoS Biol. 2009;7:e1000199.

57. Mellert DJ, Knapp J-M, Manoli DS, Meissner GW, Baker BS. Midline crossing by gustatory receptor neuron axons is regulated by fruitless, doublesex and the Roundabout receptors. Development. 2010;137:323–32.

4

The emergence of mesencephalic trigeminal neurons

Marcela Lipovsek[1], Julia Ledderose[2,3], Thomas Butts[1,4], Tanguy Lafont[1], Clemens Kiecker[1], Andrea Wizenmann[2] and Anthony Graham[1]* (iD)

Abstract

Background: The cells of the mesencephalic trigeminal nucleus (MTN) are the proprioceptive sensory neurons that innervate the jaw closing muscles. These cells differentiate close to the two key signalling centres that influence the dorsal midbrain, the isthmus, which mediates its effects via FGF and WNT signalling and the roof plate, which is a major source of BMP signalling as well as WNT signalling.

Methods: In this study, we have set out to analyse the importance of FGF, WNT and BMP signalling for the development of the MTN. We have employed pharmacological inhibitors of these pathways in explant cultures as well as utilising the electroporation of inhibitory constructs in vivo in the chick embryo.

Results: We find that interfering with either FGF or WNT signalling has pronounced effects on MTN development whilst abrogation of BMP signalling has no effect. We show that treatment of explants with either FGF or WNT antagonists results in the generation of fewer MTN neurons and affects MTN axon extension and that inhibition of both these pathways has an additive effect. To complement these studies, we have used in vivo electroporation to inhibit BMP, FGF and WNT signalling within dorsal midbrain cells prior to, and during, their differentiation as MTN neurons. Again, we find that inhibition of BMP signalling has no effect on the development of MTN neurons. We additionally find that cells electroporated with inhibitory constructs for either FGF or WNT signalling can differentiate as MTN neurons suggesting that these pathways are not required cell intrinsically for the emergence of these neurons. Indeed, we also show that explants of dorsal mesencephalon lacking both the isthmus and roof plate can generate MTN neurons. However, we did find that inhibiting FGF or WNT signalling had consequences for MTN differentiation.

Conclusions: Our results suggest that the emergence of MTN neurons is an intrinsic property of the dorsal mesencephalon of gnathostomes, and that this population undergoes expansion, and maturation, along with the rest of the dorsal midbrain under the influence of FGF and WNT signalling.

Keywords: Mesencephalic trigeminal nucleus, MTN, MesV, Jaw proprioception, Midbrain, FGF, WNT BMP

Background

The routes through which cranial primary sensory neurons are generated are complex. In contrast to the trunk, where sensory neurons are formed exclusively by neural crest cells, those in the head have disparate embryonic origins. The majority of the cranial sensory neurons are derived from the neurogenic placodes, which are transient focal thickenings of the cranial ectoderm [1–3]. This includes all of those contributing to the epibranchial ganglia: the geniculate, petrosal and nodose, the cells of the vestibuloacoustic ganglion, and many of the neurons of the trigeminal ganglion, and in some vertebrate clades neurons associated with the spiracular/paratympanic organ [4]. Additionally, there are neural crest derived sensory neurons in the head and these will form the proximal ganglia of the IXth and Xth nerves, the Superior and Jugular, as well as contributing to the trigeminal ganglion [1, 3, 5]. Finally, there is one last significant population of sensory neurons in the head which do not lie in a peripheral ganglion but which are

* Correspondence: anthony.graham@kcl.ac.uk
[1]Centre for Developmental Neurobiology, Kings College London, London SE1 1UL, UK
Full list of author information is available at the end of the article

situated within the central nervous system (CNS), the cells of the Mesencephalic Trigeminal Nucleus (MTN), (also sometimes abbreviated as MesV), which relay information about the position of the jaw [6, 7].

We know much about how neural crest derived sensory neurons are formed [8, 9] and, over the last two decades, we have developed an increasing understanding of how placodally derived sensory neurons arise [10]. However, we have very little understanding of how the MTN forms, despite the importance of these cells; they are the proprioceptive neurons that innervate the jaw closing muscles and they thus play a central role in co-ordinating biting and mastication [11, 12]. Furthermore, the evolution of this population is generally believed to have been concomitant with the evolution of jawed vertebrates, the gnathostomes, and to have facilitated that transition [13, 14]. The appearance of jaws necessitated the emergence of novel sensory systems to co-ordinate jaw movement and this need was met by the MTN.

MTN neurons emerge during comparatively early periods, and these are the first born neurons of the mesencephalon in amniotes. They are generated either side of the dorsal midline forming first posteriorly close to the isthmus but then later across the anteroposterior extent of the midbrain [13, 15]. Indeed, the production of these cells occurs over a protracted period, between stages (HH) 14 and 25 in chick [7, 13, 16]. MTN cells differentiate as unipolar neurons that then project axons away from the dorsal midline ventrally towards the sulcus limitans, at which point they make a caudal turn and contribute to the forming lateral longitudinal fasciculus (LLF) [7]. They further extend their axons along this tract crossing the isthmus to enter the hindbrain before their axons bifurcate and one branch exits through rhombomere two and then projects along the mandibular ramus of the trigeminal nerve towards the mandibular arch.

Importantly, there has been controversy over the embryonic origin of these neurons. It was proposed that these cells are neural crest derived [17] and as such would share a common embryonic origin with other proprioceptive sensory neurons such as those found in the dorsal root ganglia at limb levels. However, other studies failed to find support for this view and it was argued that MTN neurons have a CNS origin [13]. More recently genetic fate-mapping in mice has provided definitive proof for this. MTN cells are part of the Wnt3a lineage which is restricted to cells derived from the dorsal midline of the midbrain and does not include neural crest cells [18]. Given that the embryonic origin of these neurons has now been resolved, it is important that we gain an understanding of how these cells are generated.

As with other regions of the developing CNS, cell type specification within the mesencephalon is likely to involve positional cues emanating from signalling centres, which pattern the anteroposterior (AP) and dorsoventral (DV) axes [19, 20]. In the case of the MTN, these cues would include signals from the isthmus for the AP axis, FGF and WNT, and from the dorsal midline for the DV axis, primarily BMP, but also WNT signalling [21]. However, from the few studies that have been reported to date, it is far from clear how, or if, isthmic and dorsal signals act to specify MTN neurons and what the actual roles of these signalling pathways are during the development of this population. Thus, while a previous study of ours found evidence to suggest that FGF signalling from the isthmus promotes MTN formation in chick [13] a more recent study in zebrafish found that FGF activity had a negative effect whilst WNT signalling had a positive effect on MTN differentiation [22]. Other work has shown that dorsal midbrain development involves signals from the roof plate and that positional identity is set at periods just after the onset of MTN formation [23]. However, it is unclear how the generation of these cells fits with this process and whether or not it is impacted by BMP signalling.

In this study, we have set out to analyse the importance of signals derived from the isthmus and dorsal midline for the development of the MTN. We find that, in cultured explants, interfering with either FGF or WNT signalling results in the generation of fewer MTN neurons, and that these pathways have additive effects. However, this population was still present. Contrastingly, abrogation of BMP signalling has no effect. We also find that inhibition of FGF and WNT signalling affects MTN neuronal axonal extension. To complement these studies, we have used electroporation to inhibit BMP, FGF and WNT signalling within dorsal midbrain cells in vivo prior to, and during, their differentiation as MTN neurons. We found that in all cases cells electroporated with any of these inhibitory constructs can differentiate as MTN neurons suggesting that none of these pathways are required cell intrinsically for the emergence of these neurons. Again, we find that inhibition of BMP signalling has no effect on the development of MTN neurons, while inhibition of FGF or WNT signalling has consequences for MTN differentiation. Double electroporation to inhibit both FGF and WNT signalling suggests that these pathways are additive. Finally, we conducted a series of explant studies to determine if the isthmus or the dorsal midline are at all required for the emergence of MTN neurons at stages after the specification of AP and DV identities. We find that MTN neurons are still generated in cultured explanted dorsal midbrains from stage 12 embryos without the isthmus and roof plate. Thus, although MTN neurons are born close to both the isthmus and the roof plate the emergence of these neurons per se does not directly involve ongoing signalling from these structures. Here, we provide evidence suggesting that the generation of MTN neurons is an intrinsic property of the dorsal mesencephalon, with these being the first cohort of neurons to be born here. This population then undergoes expansion along with the rest of the dorsal midbrain under the influence of FGF and WNT signalling. Furthermore, we uncover an additional role for FGF and WNT signalling in supporting extension of MTN axons.

Methods
Explant cultures
Fertilised hen's eggs were incubated at 38 °C until HH stage 11 or stage 13 [24]. Embryos were dissected and extra-embryonic tissue removed. For the pharmacological manipulation of signalling pathways, embryos were cut anterior to the midbrain/diencephalon border and posterior of the otic vesicle. For the midbrain tissue explant cultures, the midbrain region was first dissected and the isthmus or roof plate regions removed using fine tungsten needles. Explant pieces were embedded in type I collagen (Roche), dorsal side up and cultured overnight, at 37 °C in F12 medium (Sigma) supplemented with 10% fetal calf serum (Life Technologies) and penicillin/streptomycin (Sigma). All drugs were dissolved in DMSO to the following stock concentrations: dorsomorphin, 5 mM; SU5402, 34 mM; IWP-2; 1 mM. Stock solutions were stored at −20 °C. Drugs, or equal volume of DMSO (1-9ul /ml depending on the corresponding concertation of the drug) for the controls, were added to the culture medium. Explants were fixed in formaldehyde for subsequent immunostaining.

In ovo electroporations
Fertilised hen's eggs were incubated at 38 °C. Eggs were windowed using sharp surgical scissors. The midbrain neural tube was injected with ~100–200 nl of the corresponding plasmid DNA at a concentration of 2 μg/μl. Plasmid constructs used were: CAGGS-GFP, pCAβ-Smad6-IRES-GFP [25], pCAβ-dnFGFR1-IRES-GFP [26] and pCAβ-GSK3-IRES-GFP (this construct was generated by inserting full-length human GSK3 into the pCAβ-IRES-eGFPm5 plasmid) [27]. Three 20 ms/10 V square waveform electrical pulses were passed between electrodes placed on either side of the midbrain with a slight sideways inclination so as to direct the current on a ventral to dorsal and left to right angle, targeting the dorsal midbrain. Approximately 1 ml of Tyrode's solution with penicillin/streptomycin was added before the eggs were resealed and incubated for a further day at 38 °C. Embryos were collected at stage 18–20, the midbrain and rostral hindbrain regions dissected and fixed with 4% paraformaldehyde (in phosphate-buffered saline). Wholemount midbrains were either processed for immunostaing or cryosectioning.

Immunofluorescence
Previously fixed explant cultures, electroporated whole midbrains or cryosections were washed three times 30 min in PBS/1% TritonX-100 (PBSTx) before being washed in a blocking solution of 10% goat serum in PBSTx twice for 1 h at room temperature. The relevant primary antibodies were diluted in blocking solution and the tissues incubated at 4 °C for 4 days. Samples were then rinsed in blocking solution and washed three times for 1 h in blocking solution before adding the secondary antibody diluted in blocking solution, and incubated at 4 °C for a further 2–3 days. The primary antibodies used were mouse anti-Isl1/2 at 1:100 (DSHB 39.4D5 created by Jessell, T.M. / Brenner-Morton, S) kindly supplied by Dr. Ivo Lieberam, KCL) rabbit anti-NFM at 1:500 (Abcam) and rabbit anti-phospho-SMAD1/5/8 at 1:100 (Cell Signalling). Secondary antibodies used were Alexa 633-conjugated goat anti-mouse IgG, and Alexa 568 goat anti-rabbit IgG, both at 1:500 (Molecular Probes).

Imaging, cell counting and statistical analysis
Images were acquired by laser scanning confocal microscopy (Olympus AX70). Image analysis and processing was performed in ImageJ and Photoshop. The cell counting of MTN cells on explant cultured midbrains was performed on z stack pictures from a dorsal view. Images were thresholded for unbiased detection of ISL1/2+ nuclei. The total number of cells in each explant was counted manually, at the dorsal midbrain region, using a cell counting plugin on imageJ. Absolute numbers were then averaged for each experimental condition and normalised to the corresponding mean control value. Bar graphs show normalised mean ± S.E.M. values. Statistical analysis was performed on GraphPad Prism version 6.00 for Windows (GraphPad Software, La Jolla California USA, www.graphpad.com). Pairwise comparisons against the corresponding DMSO controls were performed using the two-tailed Mann Whitney test. Multiple comparisons were performed using Kruskal-Wallis test with Dunn's correction.

Results
MTN neurons are generated close to the dorsal midline and in many jawed vertebrates they first appear in the posterior midbrain, close to the isthmus, before spreading anteriorly [13, 15]. Thus, their formation may be controlled by the isthmus and the dorsal midline, and involve signals secreted by these territories. Much is known about the role of the isthmus in early neural development and it has been shown that FGF and WNT signalling from this structure play a key role in midbrain

patterning [19, 28–30]. Contrastingly, comparatively little is known about dorsal patterning in the midbrain. However, it has been shown that dorsalising signals are produced by the roof plate and that dorsal and ventral identities are fixed in the chick from HH stage 15 onwards, which is after the initial production of MTN neurons [23].

We therefore sought to assess the roles of key signalling pathways emanating from the isthmus and dorsal midline in the emergence of MTN cells. To achieve this we used two independent and complementary approaches. We performed pharmacological inhibition of signalling pathways on explant cultures of chick embryos, and additionally, analysed the cell intrinsic role of signalling pathways by expression of inhibitory constructs through *in ovo* electroporation of the embryonic dorsal midbrain.

Pharmacological inhibition of signalling pathways reveals a role for FGF and WNT, but not BMP, signalling in MTN development

We established an ex vivo system that allowed for the controlled application of pharmacological reagents. Embryos were isolated and cut anteriorly at the mesencephalic/diencephalic junction and posteriorly of the otic vesicle, at the middle of the hindbrain. These pieces were then embedded in collagen and cultured overnight. The explanted tissue comprised the normal environment in which MTN cells are generated. After incubation, the explant cultures displayed normal morphology. We performed these experiments at two developmental stages: stage 13, just before the first postmitotic MTN neurons are produced [13], and DV identity is in the process of being fixed; and stage 11, when DV identity in the midbrain is completely labile [23]. After incubation, we assessed the presence of MTN neurons by immunostaining for ISL1/2 and NFM [13]. These neurons are the first born in the midbrain, and remain the only differentiated neurons in the dorsal midbrain for an extended period of time. Consequently, the analysis of early axonal extensions is straightforward.

To inhibit BMP signalling we used dorsomorphin [31], which selectively inhibits the BMP type I receptors ALK2, ALK3 and ALK6 and thus blocks BMP-mediated SMAD1/5/8 phosphorylation. In explant cultures performed at stage 13, which is just prior to emergence of the first MTN neurons [7, 13], we observed no effect of BMP signalling inhibition. Both the number of MTN cells generated (identified as ISL1/2$^+$ cells) and their position within the midbrain showed no differences between control (DMSO treated) explants and dorsomorphin treated explants. Moreover, the initial axon extension also appeared unaffected by dorsomorphin treatment (Fig. 1 a-b). To confirm the effectiveness of the dorsomorphin treatment we performed immunostainings for p-SMAD 1/5/8. While DMSO controls showed strong p-SMAD labelling, this was completely lost in explants treated with dorsomorphin (Fig. 1 a, DMSO and Dorsomorphin panels).

In explant cultures performed at stage 11, we also observed no effects of blocking BMP signalling on MTN development. Both the number of MTN cells generated and their position within the midbrain were indistinguishable from DMSO treated controls (Fig. 2a-b). These results suggest that MTN neuronal development is not under the control of BMP signalling.

To study the effects of FGF signalling from the isthmus on MTN neuronal development, we treated explant cultures with SU5402, which selectively blocks FGFRs by inhibiting their kinase activity [32]. Treatment of stage 13 explant cultures with SU5402 resulted in a significant dose dependent reduction in the number of MTN cells produced, when compared with DMSO treated controls; at the highest concentration of SU5402 tested we observed a 50% reduction in the number of ISL1/2$^+$ cells produced. However, we observed no effect on the position of ISL1/2$^+$ cells within the midbrain. Yet, axon extension was greatly impaired (Fig. 1a-b).

To further evaluate whether any FGF dependent specification of MTN neurons occurred prior to this stage, we performed explant culture experiments on stage 11 embryos and treated them with SU5402. Here we observed a greater reduction in the number of MTN neurons produced, with SU5402 treated explants showing on average 20% of the number of ISL1/2$^+$ cells when compared to DMSO treated controls (Fig. 2 a-b). However, MTN neurons still differentiated.

In order to analyse the role of WNT signalling in MTN neuronal development, we treated explant cultures with IWP-2, an inhibitor of porcupine, the enzyme responsible for the palmitoylation of WNT proteins, which is essential for their secretion [33]. In stage 13 explants inhibition of WNT signalling caused a 50% reduction in the number of MTN neurons, but did not affect the distribution of MTN neurons within the midbrain. The remaining neurons showed abnormal extension of axons (Fig. 1a-b). In explants performed at stage 11 we also observed a tendency towards a reduction in the number of ISL1/2$^+$ neurons, albeit not statistically significant (Fig. 2a-b).

To evaluate whether FGF and WNT signalling interact during the development of MTN neurons, we treated explant cultures with SU5402 and IWP-2, to inhibit both pathways. In explant cultures of both stage 13 or stage 11 embryos, we observed an additive effect on the reduction of MTN neurons produced on treated explants when compared to explants treated with each drug individually and DMSO treated controls (Figs. 1 and 2).

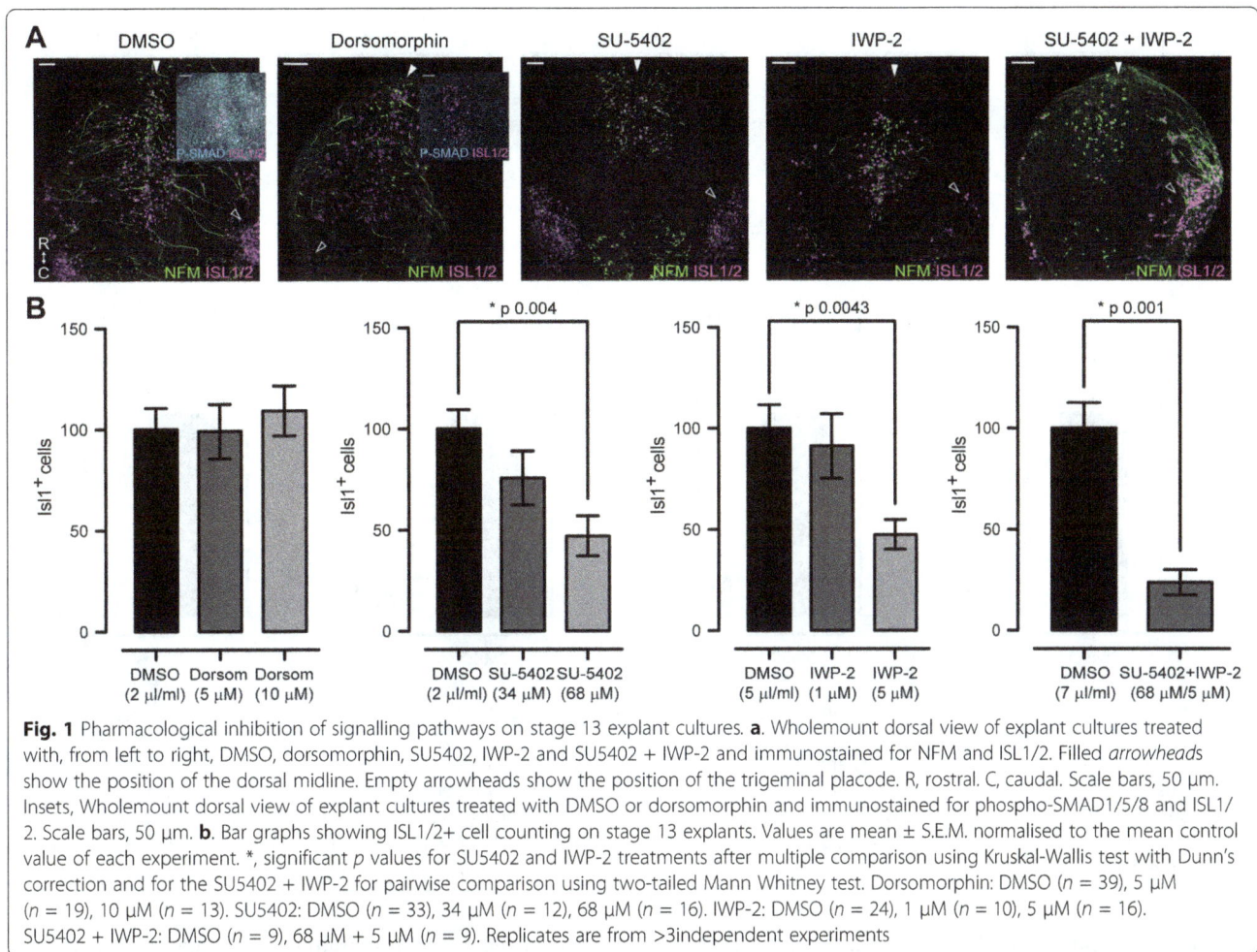

Fig. 1 Pharmacological inhibition of signalling pathways on stage 13 explant cultures. **a**. Wholemount dorsal view of explant cultures treated with, from left to right, DMSO, dorsomorphin, SU5402, IWP-2 and SU5402 + IWP-2 and immunostained for NFM and ISL1/2. Filled *arrowheads* show the position of the dorsal midline. Empty arrowheads show the position of the trigeminal placode. R, rostral. C, caudal. Scale bars, 50 μm. Insets, Wholemount dorsal view of explant cultures treated with DMSO or dorsomorphin and immunostained for phospho-SMAD1/5/8 and ISL1/2. Scale bars, 50 μm. **b**. Bar graphs showing ISL1/2+ cell counting on stage 13 explants. Values are mean ± S.E.M. normalised to the mean control value of each experiment. *, significant *p* values for SU5402 and IWP-2 treatments after multiple comparison using Kruskal-Wallis test with Dunn's correction and for the SU5402 + IWP-2 for pairwise comparison using two-tailed Mann Whitney test. Dorsomorphin: DMSO (*n* = 39), 5 μM (*n* = 19), 10 μM (*n* = 13). SU5402: DMSO (*n* = 33), 34 μM (*n* = 12), 68 μM (*n* = 16). IWP-2: DMSO (*n* = 24), 1 μM (*n* = 10), 5 μM (*n* = 16). SU5402 + IWP-2: DMSO (*n* = 9), 68 μM + 5 μM (*n* = 9). Replicates are from >3 independent experiments

Inhibition of both FGF and WNT pathways simultaneously did not affect the position of the MTN neurons within the midbrain; however, it greatly affected axon formation. In spite of the observed reduction in the number of neurons produced and their abnormal axonal projections, postmitotic, ISL1/2+ MTN neurons were still generated in the absence of FGF and WNT signalling.

Inhibition of BMP, FGF and WNT signalling via expression of inhibitory constructs in vivo

Our analysis of the role of BMP, FGF and WNT signalling pathways using pharmacological inhibitors highlighted the involvement of FGF and WNT signalling pathways in aspects of early MTN differentiation. To complement these systemic inhibitory approaches, and to further clarify the possible ongoing roles of these pathways in MTN development, we used in vivo electroporation of pathway manipulation constructs. This approach allows us to assess the cell intrinsic role of signalling pathways on MTN development and, in particular, their initial differentiation and subsequent axon

extension. In all cases embryos were electroporated between stages 10 and 13, which is prior to the fixation of dorsal identity and before the formation of any MTN neurons. The embryos were fixed at stages 18–20, by which point MTN neurons have differentiated and have extended axons ventrally and posteriorly.

Figure 3a shows a representative picture of the targeting of the dorsal mesencephalon using a GFP expression construct (the same phenotype was seen in all embryos (*n* = 25)). Labelling was focussed along the dorsal midline (Fig. 3a – filled arrowhead) and the GFP+ cells included both differentiated ISL1+/NFM+ post-mitotic MTN neurons (Fig. 3 a-b, thin arrows) as well as mesencephalic neuroepithelial cells. MTN neurons were also identified by their large somas, lack of dendrites and superficial (pial) location. More importantly, labelling via in vivo electroporation enabled us to scrutinise the axon trajectories of individual cells that carry the construct of interest. A hallmark of MTN neurons is the extension of ventral axonal projections, along the pial surface and with a slight caudal angle. These MTN axons turn sharply caudally at the sulcus limitans where they

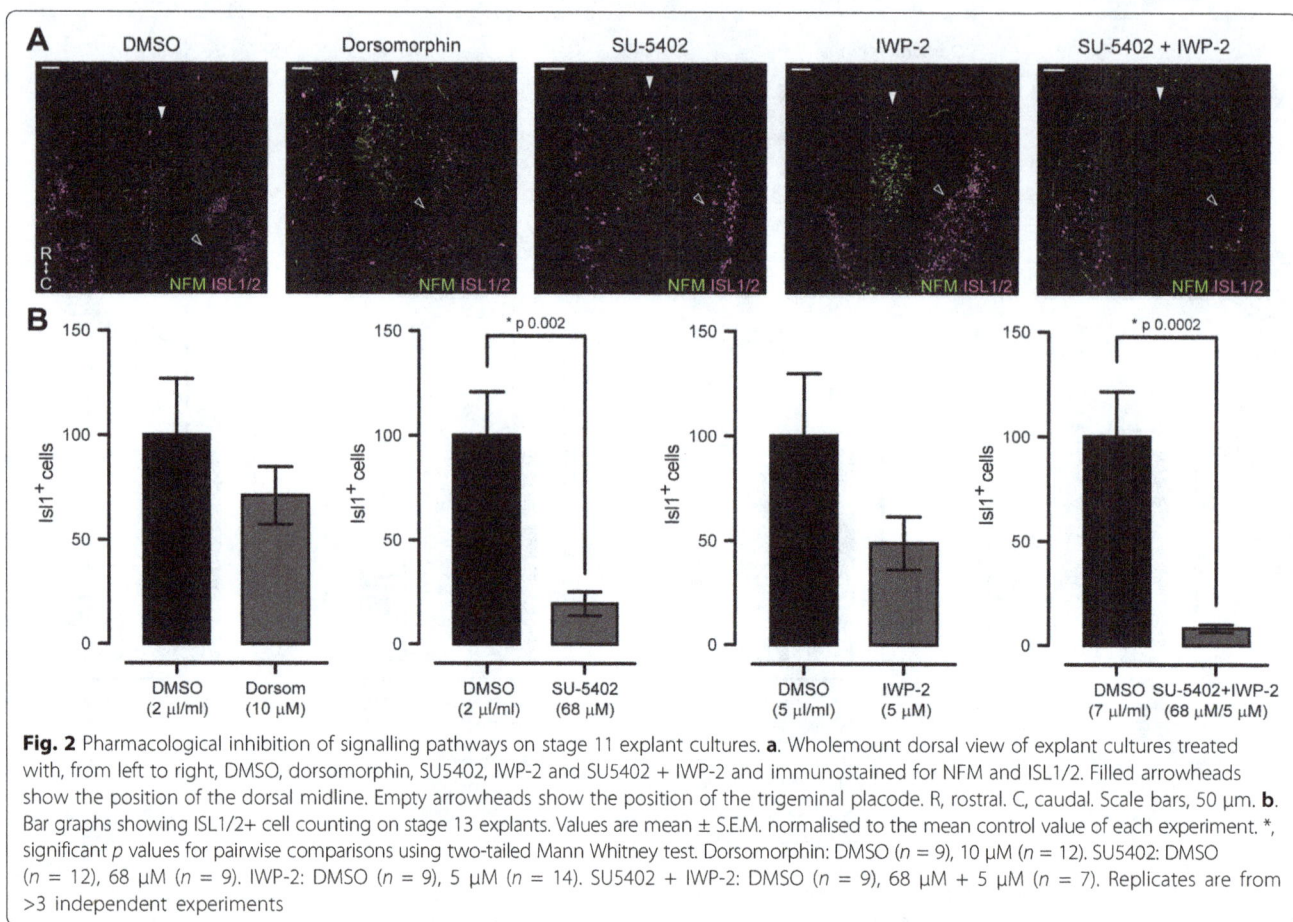

Fig. 2 Pharmacological inhibition of signalling pathways on stage 11 explant cultures. **a.** Wholemount dorsal view of explant cultures treated with, from left to right, DMSO, dorsomorphin, SU5402, IWP-2 and SU5402 + IWP-2 and immunostained for NFM and ISL1/2. Filled arrowheads show the position of the dorsal midline. Empty arrowheads show the position of the trigeminal placode. R, rostral. C, caudal. Scale bars, 50 µm. **b.** Bar graphs showing ISL1/2+ cell counting on stage 13 explants. Values are mean ± S.E.M. normalised to the mean control value of each experiment. *, significant p values for pairwise comparisons using two-tailed Mann Whitney test. Dorsomorphin: DMSO (n = 9), 10 µM (n = 12). SU5402: DMSO (n = 12), 68 µM (n = 9). IWP-2: DMSO (n = 9), 5 µM (n = 14). SU5402 + IWP-2: DMSO (n = 9), 68 µM + 5 µM (n = 7). Replicates are from >3 independent experiments

converge to populate the LLF (Fig. 3a, big arrows) along which they cross the isthmus and head into the hindbrain. Figure 3c shows a representative picture of a transverse cryosection of a GFP electroporated midbrain. On this plane of view the labelling of mesencephalic neuroepithelial cells and differentiated ISL1/2+ neurons (thin arrows) was clearly distinguishable. MTN neurons were identified by their location around the dorsal midline (filled arrowhead) and at the pial surface, ISL1/2 expression, large somas and the characteristic ventrally projecting axon, coursing along the pial surface. These experiments also showed that electroporation per se does not impair MTN development.

Inhibition of BMP signalling via SMAD6 over-expression has no effect on MTN development

To assess the requirement for BMP signalling in the generation of MTN neurons and their subsequent early development, chick embryos were electroporated at the dorsal midline with a SMAD6 expression construct, as overexpression of this gene has been shown to block BMP signalling [25]. Electroporations were performed at stages 10–13 and embryos were fixed at stage 18–20 (the same result was seen in all embryos (n = 8)). We observed no

noticeable effects on midbrain morphology and general distribution of ISL1/2+ cells when comparing SMAD6-IRES-GFP electroporated midbrains against GFP electroporated control midbrains. Figure 4 shows that cells carrying the SMAD6 construct exhibit normal MTN development, which is consistent with our in vitro analyses. GFP+ cells differentiate into postmitotic ISL1/2+ neurons (Fig. 4 a – thin arrows) and were appropriately positioned both along the AP axis and relative to the dorsal midline. Furthermore, these neurons project their axons ventrally towards the LLF in a manner similar to GFP controls. On transverse cryosections we observe that GFP+ MTN neurons were correctly positioned at the pial surface of the neuroepithelium, have the characteristic big somas and extended their axons ventrally coursing right at the pial surface (Fig. 4b – thin arrows). Thus, as with our explant studies, we found no requirement for BMP signalling for the generation and normal early development of MTN neurons.

Inhibition of FGF signalling via dn-FGFR1 over-expression has no effect on MTN generation but affects axon projection and apicobasal positioning

We have previously used electroporation of a dominant negative form of FGFR1 to render neural crest cells

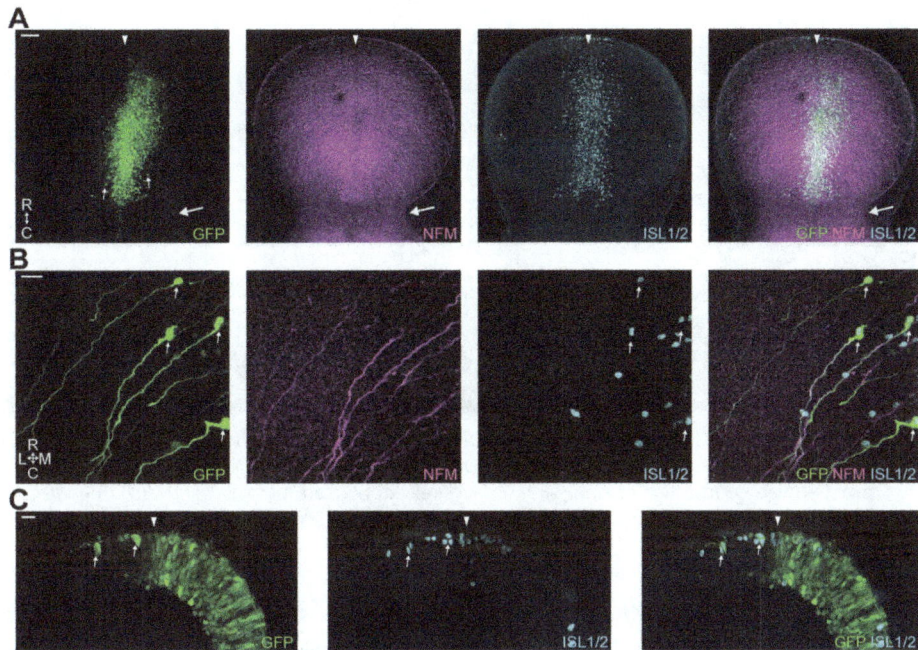

Fig. 3 *In ovo* electroporation of the dorsal midbrain. **a.** Representative wholemount dorsal view of a midbrain electroporated with CAGGS-GFP (*n* = 25). *Arrowhead* denotes the position of the dorsal midline. *Thin arrows*, typical MTN neurons. *Big arrow*, right side LLF. Scale bar, 50 μm. **b.** Higher magnification image of GFP-electroporated cells. *Thin arrows*, typical MTN neurons. Scale bar, 20 μm. **c.** Transverse cryosection of a GFP electroporated midbrain. *Arrowhead* denotes the position of the dorsal midline. Thin arrows, typical MTN neurons. Scale bar, 20 μm. R, rostral. C, caudal. M, medial. L, lateral

insensitive to FGF signalling [26]. We employed the same approach here to assess the requirement for FGF signalling in the differentiation and early development of MTN neurons. Electroporations were performed at stages 10–13 and embryos were fixed at stage 18–20 (the same phenotypes was seen in all embryos (*n* = 18)). We observed no noticeable effects on midbrain morphology and general distribution of ISL1/2+ cells when comparing dnFGFR1-IRES-GFP electroporated midbrains

against GFP electroporated control midbrains. Moreover, we found that MTN neurons bearing this construct were produced, as observed by the presence of numerous GFP+/ISL1/2+ cells (Fig. 5 - thin arrows), suggesting that FGF signalling is not required on a cell intrinsic level for their differentiation from dorsal mesencephalic precursors. However, cells carrying the dnFGFR1 construct displayed abnormal axonal projections. Axons often showed a dwindling trajectory with

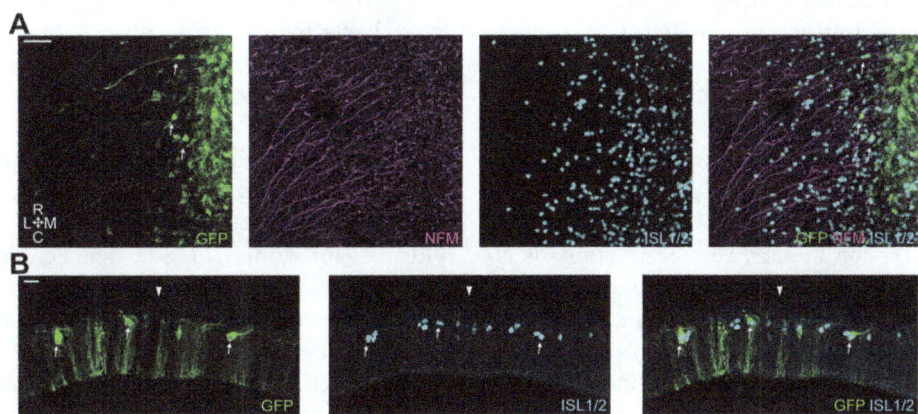

Fig. 4 Inhibition of BMP signalling via *in ovo* electroporation of the dorsal midbrain. **a.** Representative high magnification image of Smad6-IRES-GFP electroporated cells. *Thin arrows*, typical MTN neurons. Scale bar, 25 μm (*n* = 8). **b.** Transverse cryosection of a Smad6-IRES-GFP electroporated midbrain. *Arrowhead* denotes the position of the dorsal midline. *Thin arrows*, typical MTN neurons. Scale bar, 20 μm

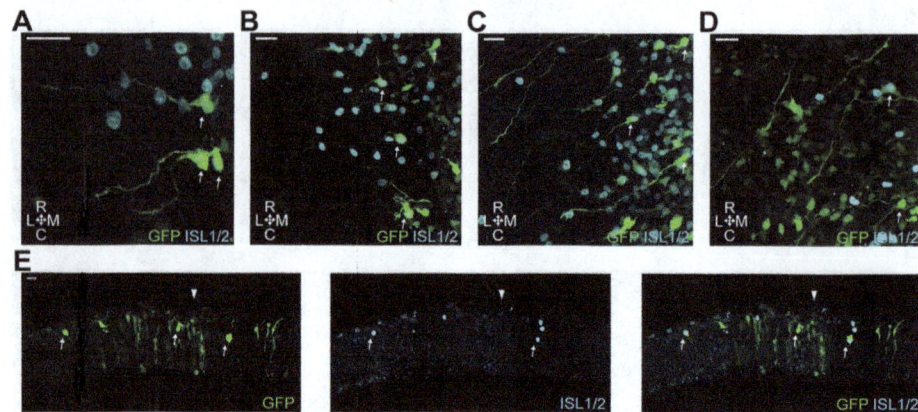

Fig. 5 Inhibition of FGF signalling via *in ovo* electroporation of the dorsal midbrain. **a, b, c** and **d**. Representative high magnification images of dnFGFR1-IRES-GFP electroporated cells illustrating the different morphologies observed (*n* = 18). *Thin arrows*, typical dnFGFR1 electroporated MTN neurons. Scale bars, 20 μm. **e**. Transverse cryosection of a dnFGFR1-IRES-GFP electroporated midbrain. *Arrowhead* denotes the position of the dorsal midline. *Thin arrows*, typical dnFGFR1 electroporated MTN neurons. Scale bar, 20 μm

numerous small branchings (Fig. 5a, c and c) or stopped short after a deviated trajectory (Figs. 5a, b and d). In many cases we observed GFP+ and ISL1/2 + cells with a stubby morphology and a high number of very short projections with no apparent general direction (Fig. 5b). Overall, even though we have occasionally observed dnFGFR1 electroporated cells projecting towards the LLF many of these cells showed random projections. Additionally, on transverse cryosections, we observed that the ISL1+/GFP+ MTN cells were often mislocalised and could be found away from the pial surface projecting an axon from this abnormal position (Fig. 5e – thin arrows).

Inhibition of WNT signalling via GSK3 over-expression has no effect on MTN generation but perturbs axon projection and apicobasal positioning

To assess the requirement for WNT signalling in cells of the dorsal midbrain for early aspects of MTN development, chick embryos were electroporated with a glycogen synthase kinase-3 (GSK3) over-expression construct. GSK3 is a known antagonist of the canonical WNT signalling pathway that forms a complex with, and phosphorylates, the WNT signal transducer β-catenin, thereby marking it for proteasomal degradation. Although GSK3 has many cellular targets (reviewed in [34]), its over-expression in early vertebrate embryos affects the canonical WNT pathway with high specificity [35, 36]. Unlike the WNT inhibitors of the SFRP and DKK families, GSK3 allows blocking of WNT signalling intracellularly, in a cell-autonomous manner. Electroporations were performed at stages 10–13 and embryos were fixed at stage 18–20. All embryos showed the same phenotype (*n* = 19). We observed no noticeable effects on midbrain size and general distribution of ISL1/2+

cells when comparing GSK3-IRES-GFP electroporated midbrains against GFP electroporated control midbrains. We observed the presence of ISL1+/GFP+ MTN neurons (Fig. 6a – thin arrow) indicating that interfering with WNT signalling does not result in a failure of dorsal mesencephalic cells to generate MTN neurons. Also, we noted no difference in the AP position of these neurons, nor their location relative to the dorsal midline. We further found that the axons extended by electroporated neurons were relatively normal; they projected towards the LLF but occasionally exhibited small branches (Fig. 6a – thin arrow). However, transverse cryosections showed that GFP+ MTN neurons were misplaced within the apicobasal axis of the neuroepithelium. Many of the ISL1+/GFP+ cells had not reached the pial surface (Fig. 6b – thin arrows). In line with this observation, we could observe GFP+/ISL1+ cells extending axons ventrally, but positioned one on top of the other (dorsal view of Fig. 6a). While the axon of the cell on top (thin arrow) was most likely following the normal MTN route along the pial surface, the axon of the second cell (asterisk) headed ventrally embedded in the neuroepithelium.

Combinatorial inhibition of FGF and WNT signalling has no effect on MTN generation but affects axon projection and apicobasal positioning

Our explant studies suggest that FGF and WNT signalling may have an additive effect during MTN differentiation. We therefore sought to analyse how these signalling pathways may affect MTN development in vivo on a cell intrinsic level via a combined electroporation with the dnFGFR1-IRES-GFP and GSK3-IRES-GFP constructs. Electroporations were performed at stages 10–13 and embryos were fixed at stages 18–20. The same phenotype was seen in all embryos (*n* = 11).

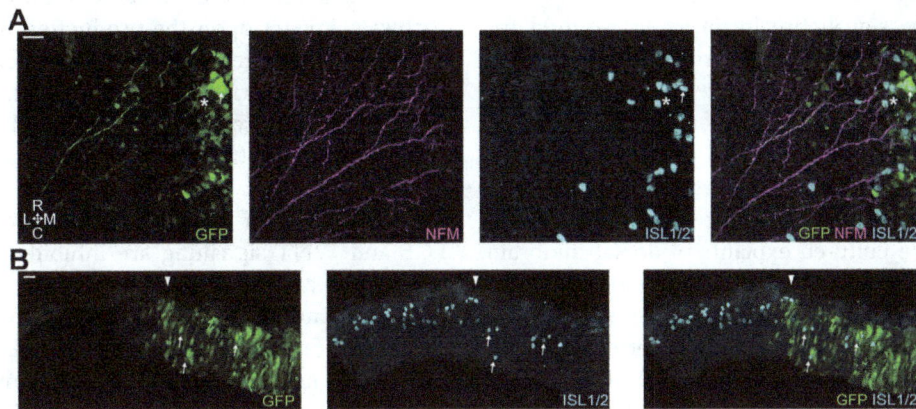

Fig. 6 Inhibition of WNT signalling via *in ovo* electroporation of the dorsal midbrain. **a**. Representative high magnification image of GSK3-IRES-GFP electroporated cells (*n* = 19). *Thin arrow*, typical GSK3 electroporated MTN neuron. *Asterisk*, deeper MTN neuron. Scale bar, 20 μm. **b**. Transverse cryosection of a GKS3-IRES-GFP electroporated midbrain. *Arrowhead* denotes the position of the dorsal midline. *Thin arrows*, typical GSK3 electroporated MTN neurons. Scale bar, 20 μm

We observed no noticeable effects on midbrain size and general distribution of ISL1/2+ cells when comparing dnFGFR1-IRES-GFP + GSK3-IRES-GFP electroporated midbrains against GFP electroporated control midbrains, or between electroporated and non electroporated areas of each individual midbrain. Moreover, we found that MTN neurons were generated, as depicted by the numerous GFP+ and ISL1/2+ cells observed (Fig. 7a – thin arrows), and correctly positioned on the AP and DV axes. The axonal phenotypes displayed by the ISL1+/GFP+ cells resembled those associated with cells electroporated with either construct alone (see Figs. 5 and 6). Thus, axons from ISL1+/GFP+ neurons often showed branchings, dwindling trajectories, numerous small branchings and axons coursing underneath other MTN

cells (Fig. 7a – thin arrows). Once again we also observed GFP+ cells with a stubby morphology depicting a high number of very short projections with no apparent general direction (Fig. 7a – asterisk). On transverse cryosections we observed many GFP+ and ISL1/2+ cells misplaced within the neuroepithelium, positioned away from the pial surface (Fig. 7b – thin arrows).

MTN formation does not depend on ongoing isthmus or roof plate signalling

MTN neurons emerge close to the isthmus and the dorsal midline, two major signalling centres in the developing midbrain. Consequently, it might be anticipated that these would act to direct the formation of MTN neurons. However, our analysis of the requirement for BMP,

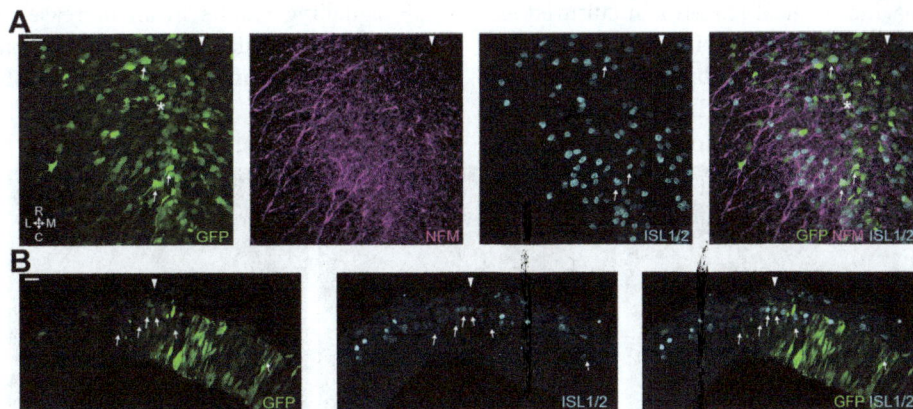

Fig. 7 Inhibition of FGF and WNT signalling via *in ovo* electroporation of the dorsal midbrain. **a**. Representative high magnification image of dnFGFR1-IRES-GFP and GSK3-IRES-GFP electroporated cells (*n* = 11). *Thin arrow*, typical dnFGFR1 + GSK3 electroporated MTN neurons. *Asterisk*, Stubby GFP+ cell. *Arrowhead* denotes the position of the dorsal midline. Scale bar, 20 μm. **b**. Transverse cryosection of a dnFGFR1-IRES-GFP and GKS3-IRES-GFP electroporated midbrain. *Arrowhead* denotes the position of the dorsal midline. *Thin arrows*, typical GSK3 electroporated MTN neurons. Scale bar, 20 μm

FGF and WNT signalling in MTN generation suggests that none of these signals are intrinsically required for the initial generation of these neurons, although FGF and WNT signalling are important for increasing the size of this population and initial extension of axonal projections. We have therefore used explants studies to directly test if these signalling centres, the isthmus and/or the roof plate, are required for the production of MTN neurons. We cultured explants of dorsal midbrain neural tube from embryos at stage 11/12 with and without the isthmus and the roof plate. Explants were embedded in collagen gel and cultured overnight. In all control explants we found that many ISL1/2+ MTN neurons were generated in all explants analysed ($n = 6/6$) (Fig. 8). However, we also found many ISL1/2 neurons in explants cultured without the isthmus ($n = 22/22$) (Fig. 8). Finally, we found that explants lacking both the isthmus and the roof plate also generated ISL1/2+ MTN neurons ($n = 30/38$) (Fig. 8). Overall, our results show that the generation of MTN neurons is intrinsic to dorsal midbrain tissues from stage 10 onwards and does not involve isthmic or roof plate signals.

Discussion

Mesencephalic trigeminal neurons form in close proximity to the signalling centres of the dorsal midbrain, the isthmus and the roof plate. In this study, we have analysed the importance of key signalling pathways emanating from these organising centres on the development of these cells. These pathways include FGF and WNT signalling, which are involved in mediating isthmic patterning along the AP axis, and BMP signalling which is primarily associated with the dorsal midline and the patterning of dorsal neuronal populations of the developing CNS, although a role for WNT signalling from the dorsal midline is also possible [20, 21]. We inhibited these pathways using pharmacological reagents in cultured explants and via expression of inhibitory constructs of these pathways in vivo. Systemic inhibition of FGF and

WNT signalling in explants demonstrated that these pathways impact upon the production of MTN neurons. When inhibited the number of MTN cells is significantly reduced. However, we also find that dorsal midbrain cells rendered insensitive to FGF and WNT signalling still progress to differentiate as MTN neurons. Nonetheless, we show that these signalling pathways are important for aspects of MTN neuronal development. When FGF and WNT signalling are inhibited the early axonal projections are abnormal; they are shorter, exhibit more processes and show more random projection patterns, and MTN neurons are often apicobasally misplaced within the neuroepithelium. Perhaps most surprisingly, we find no evidence for a role for BMP signalling in the generation of these cells or in the early phase of neuronal development, suggesting that the development of the MTN is regulated in a manner different to dorsal neurons elsewhere in the developing neural tube. Finally, our explant data suggest that the generation of MTN neurons is intrinsic to the dorsal midbrain, starting from relatively early stages following the specification of AP and DV identities, and that neither the isthmus nor the roof plate have any direct role in the emergence of these cells although they do play roles in aspects of their early differentiation.

Earlier studies have implicated isthmic signals as playing a role in directing the early development of the MTN in both chick and zebrafish. We previously demonstrated that FGF signalling has a positive role in promoting MTN production in chick, but the role of WNT signalling was unclear [13]. We show here, however, that inhibition of both FGF and WNT signalling in explants results in a reduction in the number of MTN neurons. This contrasts with a recent study in zebrafish which also found roles for both FGF and WNT isthmic signalling in MTN specification [22]. In this species, loss of FGF signalling results in an increase in the number of MTN neurons while loss of WNT signalling results in a decrease; additionally reduced FGF signalling in

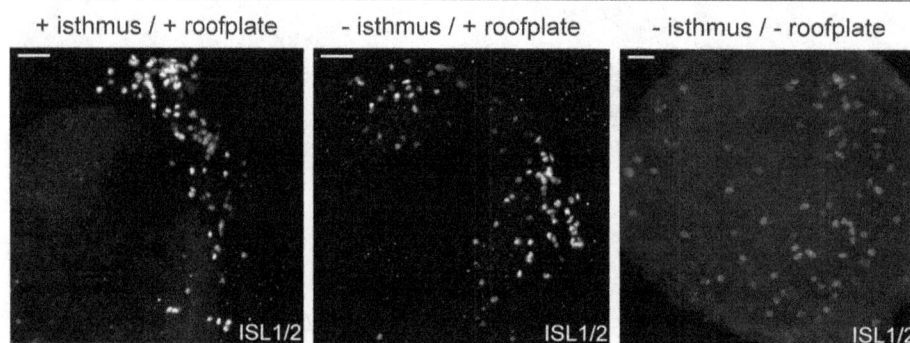

Fig. 8 Cultured explants of midbrain neural tube. Representative wholemount views of midbrain explant cultures. Left, whole midbrain with the isthmus ($n = 6$); middle, midbrain without the isthmus ($n = 22$); right midbrain without the isthmus and roof plate ($n = 38$). Immunostained for ISL1/2. Scale bars. 50 μm

zebrafish results in the differentiation of MTN neurons closer to the isthmus. This suggests that the development of the MTN is differentially controlled by the isthmus in zebrafish versus chick. However, it should be noted that the position of the initial differentiation of MTN neurons differs between these two species. In zebrafish MTN neurons first differentiate in the anterior mesencephalon and not close to isthmus as seen in chick [22]. Studies of MTN development in a number of other species suggest that the situation in zebrafish represents a derived condition while that found in chick is more representative of a plesiomorphic state; in both chondrichthyans (catshark) and mammals (mouse) MTNs also differentiate close to the isthmus [15].

The results presented here show that, while systemic inhibition of FGF or WNT signalling from stages just prior to the onset of neuronal differentiation affects the number of MTN cells being produced, dorsal midbrain cells insensitive to both of these pathways can differentiate as MTN neurons. Thus, both FGF and WNT signalling are likely to affect MTN development via their more general roles in the growth of the midbrain [37], as well as promoting proliferation and cell survival [38–40]. Indeed, if these pathways are inhibited at earlier stages more drastic effects will result in a failure of general midbrain development and, secondarily, in the loss of MTN neurons. However, on a cell intrinsic level these pathways are not immediately required for MTN differentiation. Cells of the dorsal mesencephalon electroporated with inhibitory constructs for FGF and/or WNT signalling will progress to differentiate as MTN neurons. Indeed, we provide direct support for this assertion from our explant studies which show that early dorsal midbrain tissue will go on to generate MTN neurons without isthmic or roof plate cues. This result is in keeping with an earlier analysis of the wnt1 mutant mouse which completely lacks the midbrain and rhombomere 1 but which nonetheless generates dorsal neurons with caudal projections, although the identity of these is ill defined [30].

Yet, our study shows that, while MTN cells are still produced, inhibition of FGF and WNT signalling did affect their development and resulted in a failure to properly establish initial axonal projections. The axons themselves were reduced and rather than projecting towards the presumptive LLF the projections were misdirected. We also found that inhibiting these pathways in vivo resulted in MTN neurons being misplaced apicobasally within the neuroepithelium. Thus, the MTN may represent an example of a post-mitotic neuronal cell type responding to FGF and WNT mediated projection and maturation cues. Notably, the projections of trochlear neurons, which are largely a rhombomere 1 derivative, are also directed by isthmic FGF signalling [41] and

WNT signalling has been implicated in the guidance of a number of different neural populations [42]. While the effects we observed here are most likely cell autonomous, it is possible that electroporated cells could affect their non-electroporated neighbours and this would be worthwhile investigating.

Perhaps the most surprising finding from our study is that BMP signalling has no role in the early development of the MTN. In the spinal cord BMP signalling plays a key role in the generation and patterning of different dorsal interneuron populations [20] suggesting that BMP signalling may also be important for the specification of MTN neurons. These cells are the first born neuronal population of the dorsal mesencephalon, appearing either side of the midline form stage 14 onwards, and at this time the dorsal midline expresses BMPs, in particular GDF7. However, here we show that the generation of MTN neurons occurs independently of such a signal. This suggests that the specification of these neurons takes place outside the framework that underpins the formation of dorsal neuronal cell types in other regions of the developing CNS. Further support for the view that BMP signalling plays little role in early dorsal midbrain patterning arises from the observation that the manipulation of BMPR1B signalling has no effect upon dorsal midbrain specification [43]. In the present study, we further show that the generation of MTN neurons occurs independently of any roof plate influence, even at stages before DV identity in the midbrain is determined. A possible explanation for the absence of a role for the roof plate or BMP signalling in the specification of MTN neurons may lie in the fact that unlike in the spinal cord, there are no cell fate choices to be made in the early midbrain. Thus, while in the dorsal spinal cord BMP signalling specifies the generation of dI1–3 neurons, the only cell type generated in the dorsal midbrain between stages 14 and 23 in the chick are the MTN cells.

Our results therefore suggest that the specification of neurons of the MTN requires only the following three parameters – they are mesencephalic in origin, they are dorsal and they are the first born neurons in this territory. We further find that although the signalling centres of the midbrain, the isthmus and roof plate have no direct inputs into the generation of MTN neurons, they exert profound effects on the MTN, acting to expand this population and to direct their initial axon trajectories.

Finally, the enigmatic location of MTN neurons within the CNS rather than there being a corresponding group of neurons within the trigeminal ganglia is still an unresolved question. There may be two answers to this and both may relate to the evolutionary origins of the MTN. Firstly, the presence of primary sensory neurons within the dorsal CNS is an ancestral feature of chordates: Rohon-Beard cells are present in amphioxus and in larval anamniotes [44] and furthermore, lampreys possess a group of dorsal sensory medullary cells, primary medullary and spinal nucleus of the trigeminal nerve (PMSV) neurons, which display many similarities to Rohon-Beard cells but which persist to adulthood [14]. Thus, we propose that, in the gnathostome lineage, as the jaw apparatus and its associated musculature were assembled, a novel group of sensory neurons emerged in dorsal CNS in proximity to the trigeminal system. The emergence of MTN neurons within dorsal rhombomere 1 may have been precluded by the allocation of this territory to the generation of cerebellar structures and consequently the dorsal midbrain would be the closest CNS area to the trigeminal system with the potential to generate these sensory neurons. Furthermore a midbrain origin would allow MTN neurons to integrate visual information and modulate the position of the jaw in response to that [45]. Secondly, within the cranial sensory ganglia modalities tend to be clearly segregated; for example gustation is associated with the epibranchials, hearing and balance with the vestibuloaccoustic and general somatosensation with the trigeminal placodes [46]. As such the generation of a novel group of proprioceptive neurons within the existing trigeminal ganglia may not have been a possibility and thus dorsal sensory cells of the CNS were co-opted to supply the proprioceptive innervation of the jaw closing muscles.

Conclusions

The mesencephalic trigeminal nucleus (MTN) is an important and enigmatic population forming close to two key signalling centres that impact upon the development of the dorsal midbrain, the isthmus which mediates its effects via FGF and WNT signalling and the roof plate which is a major source of BMP as well as WNT signalling. We show that interfering with either FGF or WNT signalling has pronounced effects on MTN development whilst abrogation of BMP signalling has no effect; inhibition of either FGF or WNT signalling results in the generation of fewer MTN neurons and axonal defects. However, we find cells refractory to either FGF or WNT signalling can differentiate as MTN neurons suggesting that these pathways are not required cell intrinsically for their emergence. We also show that explants of the dorsal mesencephalon lacking the isthmus and roof plate can generate MTN neurons. Our results suggest that the emergence of MTN neurons is an intrinsic property of the dorsal mesencephalon of gnathostomes, and that this population undergoes expansion, and maturation, along with the rest of the dorsal midbrain under the influence of FGF and WNT signalling.

Abbreviations
LLF: Lateral longitudinal fasciculus; MTN or MesV: Mesenecephalic trigeminal nucleus

Acknowledgements
We would like to thank Dr. Suba Poopalasundaram for comments on the manuscript and the BBSRC for funding.

Funding
This work was funded by the BBSRC (UK) – BB/J015261/1.

Authors' contributions
The study was conceived by AG, with ongoing input from ML, TB, AW, and CK. The experimental work was carried out by ML, TB,TL, JL, AW and AG The manuscript was written and revised by AG, ML, CK, TB, TL, JL and AW. All authors read and approved the final manuscript.

Competing interests
The authors declare that they have no competing interests.

Author details
[1]Centre for Developmental Neurobiology, Kings College London, London SE1 1UL, UK. [2]Institute of Clinical Anatomy and Cell Analysis, Department of Anatomy, University of Tübingen, Oesterbergstrasse 3, 72074 Tuebingen, Germany. [3]Universitätsmedizin Berlin, NeuroCure - Institute of Biochemistry, ChariteCrossOver, Virchowweg, 610117 Berlin, Germany. [4]School of Life Sciences, University of Liverpool, Liverpool L69 3BX, UK.

References
1. DAMICOMARTEL A, NODEN D. Contributions of PLACODAL and neural crest cells to avian cranial peripheral ganglia. Am J Anat. 1983;166(4):445–68.
2. Begbie J, Ballivet M, Graham A. Early steps in the production of sensory neurons by the neurogenic placodes. Mol Cell Neurosci. 2002;21(3):502–11.
3. Harlow D, Barlow L. Embryonic origin of gustatory cranial sensory neurons. Dev Biol. 2007;310(2):317–28.
4. O'Neill P, Mak SS, Fritzsch B, Ladher RK, Baker CV. The amniote paratympanic organ develops from a previously undiscovered sensory placode. Nat Commun. 2012;3:1041.
5. Thompson H, Blentic A, Watson S, Begbie J, Graham A. The formation of the superior and jugular ganglia: insights into the generation of sensory neurons by the neural crest. Dev Dyn. 2010;239(2):439–45.
6. COVELL D, NODEN D. Embryonic-development of the chick primary trigeminal sensory-motor complex. J Comp Neurol. 1989;286(4):488–503.
7. CHEDOTAL A, POURQUIE O, SOTELO C. Initial tract formation in the Brain of the chick-embryo - selective expression of the Ben/SC1/dm-grasp cell-adhesion molecule. Eur J Neurosci. 1995;7(2):198–212.
8. Marmigere F, Ernfors P. Specification and connectivity of neuronal subtypes in the sensory lineage. Nat Rev Neurosci. 2007;8(2):114–27.
9. Lallemend F, Ernfors P. Molecular interactions underlying the specification of sensory neurons. Trends Neurosci. 2012;35(6):373–81.
10. Lassiter R, Stark M, Zhao T, Zhou C. Signaling mechanisms controlling cranial placode neurogenesis and delamination. Dev Biol. 2014;389(1):39–49.

11. JERGE C. Organization and function of trigeminal MESENCEPHALIC nucleus. J Neurophysiol. 1963;26(3):379.

12. HISCOCK J, STRAZNICKY C. The formation of axonal projections of the MESENCEPHALIC trigeminal neurons in chick-embryos. J Embryol Exp Morphol. 1986;93:281–90.

13. Hunter E, Begbie J, Mason I, Graham A. Early development of the mesencephalic trigeminal nucleus. Dev Dyn. 2001;222(3):484–93.

14. ANADON R, DEMIGUEL E, GONZALEZFUENTES M, RODICIO C. HRP study of the central components of the trigeminal nerve in the larval sea lamprey - Organization and homology of the primary MEDULLARY and spinal nucleus of the TRIGEMINUS. J Comp Neurol. 1989;283(4):602–10.

15. Ware M, Dupe V, Schubert F. Evolutionary conservation of the early axon scaffold in the vertebrate Brain. Dev Dyn. 2015;244(10):1202–14.

16. Rogers LA, Cowan WM. The development of the mesencephalic nucleus of the trigeminal nerve in the chick. J Comp Neurol. 1973; 147(3):291–320.

17. NARAYANAN C, NARAYANAN Y. Determination of embryonic origin of mesencephalic nucleus of trigeminal nerve in birds. J Embryol Exp Morphol. 1978;43:85–105.

18. Louvi A, Yoshida M, Grove E. The derivatives of the Wnt3a lineage in the central nervous system. J Comp Neurol. 2007;504(5):550–69.

19. Kiecker C, Lumsden A, Hyman S. The role of organizers in patterning the nervous system. Annu Rev Neurosci. 2012;35:347–67.

20. Gouti M, Metzis V, Briscoe J. The route to spinal cord cell types: a tale of signals and switches. Trends Genet. 2015;31(6):282–9.

21. Ulloa F, Briscoe J. Morphogens and the control of cell proliferation and patterning in the spinal cord. Cell Cycle. 2007;6(21):2640–9.

22. Dyer C, Blanc E, Hanisch A, Roehl H, Otto G, Yu T, et al. A bi-modal function of Wnt signalling directs an FGF activity gradient to spatially regulate neuronal differentiation in the midbrain. Development. 2014;141(1):63–72.

23. Li N, Hornbruch A, Klafke R, Katzenberger B, Wizenmann A. Specification of dorsoventral polarity in the embryonic chick mesencephalon and its presumptive role in midbrain morphogenesis. Dev Dyn. 2005;233(3):907–20.

24. HAMBURGER V, HAMILTON H. A series of normal stages in the development of the chick embryo. J Morphol. 1951;88(1):49.

25. Linker C, Stern CD. Neural induction requires BMP inhibition only as a late step, and involves signals other than FGF and Wnt antagonists. Development. 2004;131(22):5671–81.

26. Blentic A, Tandon P, Payton S, Walshe J, Carney T, Kelsh RN, et al. The emergence of ectomesenchyme. Dev Dyn. 2008;237(3):592–601.

27. Robertshaw E, Matsumoto K, Lumsden A, Kiecker C. Irx3 and Pax6 establish differential competence for Shh-mediated induction of GABAergic and glutamatergic neurons of the thalamus. Proc Natl Acad Sci U S A. 2013; 110(41):E3919–26.

28. McMahon AP, Joyner AL, Bradley A, McMahon JA. The midbrain-hindbrain phenotype of Wnt-1–/Wnt-1- mice results from stepwise deletion of engrailed-expressing cells by 9.5 days postcoitum. Cell. 1992;69(4):581–95.

29. Crossley PH, Martinez S, Martin GR. Midbrain development induced by FGF8 in the chick embryo. Nature. 1996;380(6569):66–8.

30. Mastick GS, Fan CM, Tessier-Lavigne M, Serbedzija GN, McMahon AP, Easter SS. Early deletion of neuromeres in Wnt-1–/– mutant mice: evaluation by morphological and molecular markers. J Comp Neurol. 1996;374(2):246–58.

31. Yu PB, Hong CC, Sachidanandan C, Babitt JL, Deng DY, Hoyng SA, et al. Dorsomorphin inhibits BMP signals required for embryogenesis and iron metabolism. Nat Chem Biol. 2008;4(1):33–41.

32. Mohammadi M, McMahon G, Sun L, Tang C, Hirth P, Yeh B, et al. Structures of the tyrosine kinase domain of fibroblast growth factor receptor in complex with inhibitors. Science. 1997;276(5314):955–60.

33. Chen B, Dodge M, Tang W, Lu J, Ma Z, Fan C, et al. Small molecule-mediated disruption of Wnt-dependent signaling in tissue regeneration and cancer. Nat Chem Biol. 2009;5(2):100–7.

34. Hur EM, Zhou FQ. GSK3 signalling in neural development. Nat Rev Neurosci. 2010;11(8):539–51.

35. Dominguez I, Itoh K, Sokol SY. Role of glycogen synthase kinase 3 beta as a negative regulator of dorsoventral axis formation in Xenopus embryos. Proc Natl Acad Sci U S A. 1995;92(18):8498–502.

36. He X, Saint-Jeannet JP, Woodgett JR, Varmus HE, Dawid IB. Glycogen synthase kinase-3 and dorsoventral patterning in Xenopus embryos. Nature. 1995;374(6523):617–22.

37. Liu A, Joyner AL. Early anterior/posterior patterning of the midbrain and cerebellum. Annu Rev Neurosci. 2001;24:869–96.

38. Panhuysen M, Weisenhorn D, Blanquet V, Brodski C, Heinzmann U, Beisker W, et al. Effects of Wnt1 signaling on proliferation in the developing mid–/hindbrain region. Mol Cell Neurosci. 2004;26(1):101–11.

39. Mason I. Initiation to end point: the multiple roles of fibroblast growth factors in neural development. Nat Rev Neurosci. 2007;8(8):583–96.

40. Chi C, Martinez S, Wurst W, Martin G. The isthmic organizer signal FGF8 is required for cell survival in the prospective midbrain and cerebellum. Development. 2003;130(12):2633–44.

41. Irving C, Malhas A, Guthrie S, Mason I. Establishing the trochlear motor axon trajectory: role of the isthmic organiser and Fgf8. Development. 2002; 129(23):5389–98.

42. Yam PT, Charron F. Signaling mechanisms of non-conventional axon guidance cues: the Shh, BMP and Wnt morphogens. Curr Opin Neurobiol. 2013;23(6):965–73.

43. Bobak N, Agoston Z, Schulte D. Evidence against involvement of bmp receptor 1b signaling in fate specification of the chick mesencephalic alar plate at HH16. Neurosci Lett. 2009;461(3):223–8.

44. FRITZSCH B, NORTHCUTT R. Cranial and spinal nerve Organization in amphioxus and lampreys - evidence for an ancestral CRANIATE pattern. Acta Anat. 1993;148(2–3):96–109.

45. Pratt K, Aizenman C. Multisensory integration in Mesencephalic trigeminal neurons in Xenopus tadpoles. J Neurophysiol. 2009;102(1):399–412.

46. Graham A, Begbie J. Neurogenic placodes: a common front. Trends Neurosci. 2000;23(7):313–6.

5

Two Drosophila model neurons can regenerate axons from the stump or from a converted dendrite, with feedback between the two sites

Kavitha S. Rao and Melissa M. Rolls[*] ⓘ

Abstract

Background: After axon severing, neurons recover function by reinitiating axon outgrowth. New outgrowth often originates from the remaining axon stump. However, in many mammalian neurons, new axons initiate from a dendritic site when the axon is injured close to the cell body.

Methods: *Drosophila* sensory neurons are ideal for studying neuronal injury responses because they can be injured reproducibly in a variety of genetic backgrounds. In *Drosophila*, it has been shown that a complex sensory neuron, ddaC, can regenerate an axon from a stump, and a simple sensory neuron, ddaE, can regenerate an axon from a dendrite. To provide a more complete picture of axon regeneration in these cell types, we performed additional injury types.

Results: We found that ddaE neurons can initiate regeneration from an axon stump when a stump remains. We also showed that ddaC neurons regenerate from the dendrite when the axon is severed close to the cell body. We next demonstrated if a stump remains, new axons can originate from this site and a dendrite at the same time. Because cutting the axon close to the cell body results in growth of the new axon from a dendrite, and cutting further out may not, we asked whether the initial response in the cell body was similar after both types of injury. A transcriptional reporter for axon injury signaling, puc-GFP, increased with similar timing and levels after proximal and distal axotomy. However, changes in dendritic microtubule polarity differed in response to the two types of injury, and were influenced by the presence of a scar at the distal axotomy site.

Conclusions: We conclude that both ddaE and ddaC can regenerate axons either from the stump or a dendrite, and that there is some feedback between the two sites that modulates dendritic microtubule polarity.

Keywords: Axon regeneration, Microtubule polarity, Laser surgery

Background

In response to axon severing, many neurons have the capacity to regenerate this part of the cell. Classic axon regeneration involves signaling from the site of injury back to the cell body, followed by initiation of outgrowth from the remaining axon stump [1–3]. In some cases, particularly in the peripheral nervous system, regrowing axons may ultimately reconnect with targets to recover function [3].

Initiation of regeneration from a remaining axon stump has been observed in many types of neurons in vivo, including interneurons in the mouse spinal cord [4], interneurons in snails [5], motor neurons in C.elegans [6] and Drosophila [7] and sensory neurons in C. elegans [8] and Drosophila [9]. It is likely that in all of these scenarios an initial MAP kinase signaling cascade that includes Dual Leucine Zipper Kinase (DLK) is required to initiate regeneration, as it has been shown to be central in all cases where it has been tested [6, 7, 10, 11].

While regeneration from a remaining stump is the most commonly studied type of axon regeneration, in

* Correspondence: mur22@psu.edu
Department of Biochemistry and Molecular Biology, The Pennsylvania State University, University Park, PA 16802, USA

many systems when the axon is severed very close to the cell body (proximal axotomy) a new axonal process arises from the dendrites rather than the cell body or short axon stump. This was first described in reticulospinal neurons of the sea lamprey, a jawless fish, where axon removal resulted in extensive sprouting from dendrites [12], and the ultrastructure of these sprouts resembled that of axons [13]. Similar observations have been made in mammalian neurons. Axon-like processes (ALPs) emerging from distal tips of dendrites after proximal axotomy have been reported in adult feline motoneurons [14–17] and interneurons [18]. Retinal ganglion cells in hamster [19] and spinal neurons in rats [20] also respond to proximal axotomy by sprouting axons from dendrites. Hippocampal neurons in dissociated and slice culture initiate growth of an axon from a dendrite after proximal axotomy, and in this case the new axon was shown to be able to form synapses [21]. More recently, regeneration of an axon from a dendrite was shown to occur after proximal axotomy in Drosophila sensory neurons [22]. This type of regeneration is therefore broadly conserved.

In addition to triggering regeneration from a dendrite, injury of the axon close to the cell body has the potential to induce formation of multiple axons. In feline spinal motoneurons, proximal axotomy often resulted in de novo axon growth from the cell body along with emergence of axons from dendrites [14, 15]. The most detailed description of this phenomenon is in cultured rodent hippocampal neurons, where injuries can be performed at very precise distances from the cell body. When the axon was severed within 35 μm of the cell body, neurons very rarely regrew exclusively from the stump, but fairly frequently initiated stump growth and growth from a dendrite. This "combined response" was only slightly less common than exclusive conversion of a dendrite to a growing axon [21]. When injuries were performed further from the cell body, only the stump regrew [21]. A similar spatial analysis of injury responses was performed in C. elegans DA/DB neurons, and here 30 μm from the cell body was also where the outcome of injury changed. When the stump was 30 μm or longer it was competent for regeneration, and when shorter a new axon emerged from the cell body [23].

We have been using Drosophila sensory neurons as a genetically tractable model system in which to study axon regeneration. However, the basic responses of different sensory neurons to proximal and distal axotomy have not been comprehensively analyzed. Drosophila larval sensory neurons are particularly appealing as a system for studying neuronal injury responses because their cell bodies, dendrites and proximal axon are directly under the cuticle and epidermal cells on the body wall and so are optically accessible in whole animals.

Drosophila dendritic arborization neurons are nonciliated sensory neurons that can be classified into four groups based on complexity of their dendrite arbor [24]. Within these general classes, each neuron can be identified by position in each segment of the animal. Two identified neurons have been used in most of the studies on axon regeneration: ddaE is a Class I (simple) neuron and ddaC is a Class IV (complex) neuron (Fig. 1). The ddaE neuron can regenerate from a dendrite after proximal axotomy [22], but has been reported not to be able to perform classic axon regeneration from the stump after more distal axotomy [25]. In contrast the ddaC neuron regenerates from the axon stump after distal axotomy [9, 25, 26], but has not been tested for regeneration after proximal axotomy. It is also not known whether either of these model cells can generate multiple axons after proximal injury.

In this study we set out to do two things. First, we aimed to complete our basic understanding of the regenerative abilities of the model neurons ddaE and ddaC. Second, we asked whether the remaining axon stump influences the events that convert a dendrite to a new axon. In contrast to a previous study, we show that the Class I ddaE neuron can regenerate an axon from a stump, and therefore has the capacity to do both types

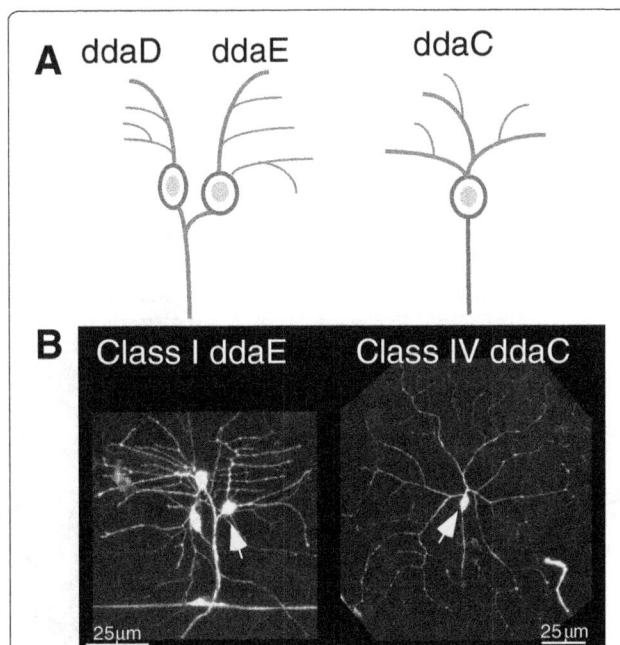

Fig. 1 Neurons used in this study. **a** Schematics of the two larval Class I dendritic arborization neurons in the dorsal cluster are shown on the left, and a similar schematic is shown for the Class IV neuron in the cluster. **b** Confocal images of dorsal Class I and Class IV neurons expressing EB1-GFP are shown. The Gal4-driver used for Class I neurons is 221 and for Class IV is 477. The cell bodies of the ddaE and ddaC neuron are indicated with *arrows*. Ventral is down and posterior is to the right in all images and schematics

of axon regeneration. In addition, we show that the Class IV ddaC neuron can regenerate an axon from a dendrite, and thus also has the complete complement of axon regenerative abilities. We also show that, in Drosophila, as in vertebrates, axons can grow from multiple sites after proximal axotomy. We also identify a novel feedback mechanism between the two regenerating axons, such that when a scar blocks re-growth from the axon stump, the microtubule polarity based changes in the dendrite that converts to an axon become accelerated.

Results

Axons regenerating from dendrites grow along the nerve when they encounter it

Drosophila sensory neurons can be injured precisely using a pulsed UV laser, and regeneration can be tracked in living larvae over several days [22]. Class IV ddaC neurons regenerate robustly from axon stumps after severing at a distance of 20 or more microns from the cell body [9, 25, 26]. In contrast, the Class I ddaE neurons have been reported not to regenerate from axon stumps after similar injury [25]. This result is somewhat confusing as ddaE neurons can convert a dendrite to a regenerating axon and grow on average several hundred microns by 96 h after injury [9, 22, 27], indicating that the cells can activate an axon regeneration program.

One possible explanation for the differential ability of the ddaE cell to regenerate from the stump and from the dendrite is that these types of regeneration are distinct in some way. We previously showed that axons regenerating from dendrites have axonal microtubule polarity and also exclude a dendritic marker [22], however, we were not able to demonstrate that they could follow axonal cues to lead them to their targets in the central nervous system

(CNS) because their point of origination in the dendrite arbor is spatially removed from the nerve and the glial cells that wrap it. Therefore one potential difference between regeneration from the stump and the dendrite is glial vs. non-glial environment. Indeed in mammals, differences in glia are one factor believed to underlie poor regeneration in the CNS compared to the periphery [28].

To test the hypothesis whether contact with glia might influence ddaE regeneration, we collected many examples of axons regenerating from dendrites. After performing hundreds of proximal axotomies on ddaE neurons, we noted rare instances in which the axon growing out of a dendrite randomly encountered the glial wrapping of the nerve. When this happened, the regenerating axon grew along the nerve towards the CNS (Fig. 2). The position of the nerve is indicated by the axon of the other Class I neuron in this region visible with the 221-Gal4 driver. Although not visible, axons from other sensory neurons as well as motor neurons are part of this nerve. This ability to grow along the nerve is similar to that of ddaC neurons regrowing from the axon stump [9]. Thus the ability to use the nerve as a source of guidance cues is another similarity between axons regenerating from the stump and a dendrite. For axons regenerating from the stump the source of guidance cues could either be the other axons or the surrounding glia, while for axons regenerating from a dendrite it would most likely be the glia as the axons would contact the nerve from its outside.

Class I ddaE neurons can regenerate from the axon stump

Because ddaE axons regenerating from a dendrite were not negatively affected by glial contact, we decided to retest the response of ddaE cells to distal axon severing. In the dorsal cluster of neurons that houses the ddaE cell,

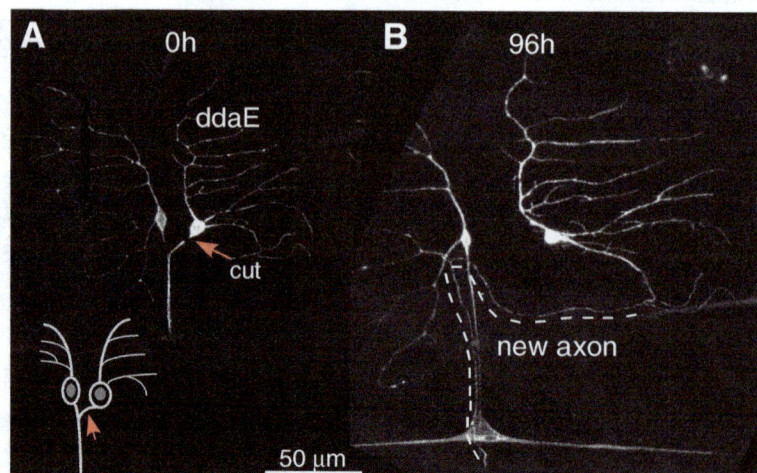

Fig. 2 A new axon emerging from a dendrite can grow along the nerve. **a** The axon of a Class I ddaE neuron was axotomized very close to the cell body. The *orange arrow* shows the cut site, and a schematic is included. **b** The same neuron was imaged 96 h after injury. One of the dendrites converted to an axon and re-joined other axons in the same segment of the larvae. *Dotted line* shows the path of the new axon

there is another Class I neuron, ddaD. All Gal4 drivers that express in ddaE also drive expression in ddaD. Axons from these two cells bundle with one another, and the nerve, 10–20 μm from the cell body. For initial tests on whether the ddaE neuron could regenerate from the stump, we wanted to eliminate the ddaD cell so that we could trace the ddaE axon in isolation. The ddaD neuron was therefore killed by aiming a pulsed UV laser at its nucleus, and the ddaE axon was severed 24 h later (Fig. 3a). In all cases the axon was severed at least 20 μm from the cell body, close to the position of the dorsal bipolar md neuron (dbd). Beyond this cell, the nerve dives below the surface and is more difficult to image at high resolution. We imaged the cell 96 h after severing to determine whether the axon stump had reinitiated growth (Fig. 3b). In 4 out of 10 cells tested, the stump was able to initiate growth indicating these cells are capable of regenerating after distal axotomy (Fig. 3c). Thus ddaE neurons can initiate axon regeneration from a remaining stump, although not in all individual cells. This inability of all cells to initiate regeneration from the stump likely explains the previous lack of regeneration in ddaE compared to ddaC neurons [25].

Class IV ddaC neurons can regenerate from a dendrite after proximal axotomy

To complete our characterization of regeneration capabilities in Class I and Class IV neurons, we wanted to test whether Class IV ddaC neurons can regenerate axons from dendrites after proximal axotomy. Class IV ddaC neurons have been used extensively to study regeneration after distal axotomy [9, 25, 26]. However, it is not known whether the large and highly branched dendrite arbor can support conversion to an axon. We labeled Class IV ddaC neurons by expressing UAS-EB1-GFP under the control of the 477-Gal4 driver. Using a pulsed UV laser, the axon of a single ddaC neuron was severed close to the cell body (Fig. 4a). The same neuron was imaged 4 days post-injury to track regeneration (Fig. 4b). In all cases ($n = 13$), a dendrite converted to an axon and grew extensively (Fig. 4c). In most cases a single dendrite initiated growth, but occasionally more than one changed polarity and grew; no growth was observed from the remaining stump. We conclude that, like ddaE neurons, ddaC neurons can regenerate from either the axon stump or from a dendrite.

New axons can grow from the stump and a dendrite in the same cell

So far we have shown that both Class I and Class IV neurons can regenerate from both the axon stump and dendrite after distal and proximal axotomy respectively. In our studies until this point, we had assayed regeneration either from the stump or the dendrite, but had not tested whether both might occur in the same cell. As injury near the cell body can lead to outgrowth from both sites in mammals, we wished to determine whether *Drosophila* neurons could also support multiple growth sites.

As the experiments in which ddaD is killed to allow imaging of ddaE in isolation (Fig. 3) are somewhat cumbersome, we used an alternative approach to look for multiple sites of outgrowth. To clearly track regeneration from the stump, we severed axons of both ddaD and ddaE at the same point (Fig. 5a). That way, there was a clear gap in the axon bundle to allow tracking of subsequent stump growth. Out of 14 ddaE neurons examined, 4 neurons regenerated by converting a dendrite to an axon, 4 neurons regenerated from the original axon stump and 6 neurons regenerated from both the stump and dendrite (Fig. 5b-c). Axon growth was assessed by acquiring high magnification images of the region where the axons were cut. If the ddaD neuron initiated growth, but the ddaE did not, the blunt stump of ddaE was usually visible. In cases where clear images could not be acquired or there was ambiguity about outgrowth, the cells were not counted.

Similar distal axotomy experiments were conducted in ddaC neurons labeled with EB1-GFP under the control of the 477-Gal4 driver (Fig. 6a). Of the 17 ddaC neurons that were distally axotomized, 9 neurons converted a dendrite to an axon in addition to regeneration from the stump, 4 neurons regenerated only from the stump, and 4 neurons regenerated by dendrite conversion only (Fig.

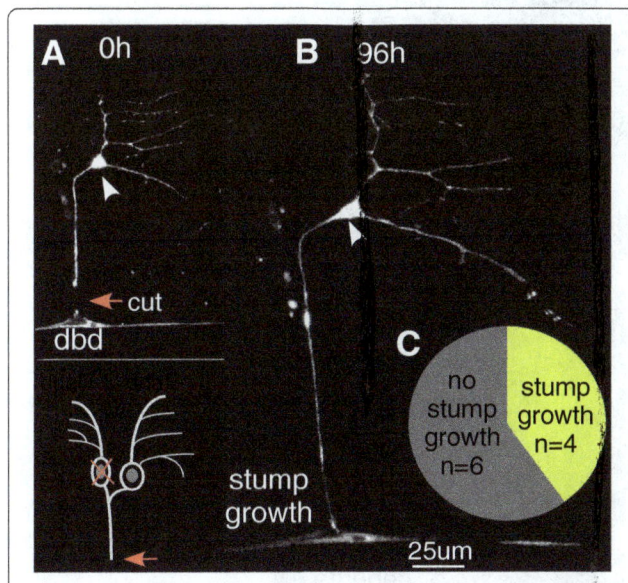

Fig. 3 Class I ddaE neurons can regenerate from the axon stump. **a** An axon of the Class I ddaE neuron (cell body marked with an *arrowhead*) was severed 24 h after laser-mediated ablation of the neighboring Class I ddaD neuron. The site of injury (*orange arrow*) is located near the dorsal bipolar md neuron (dbd). **b** The same neuron was imaged 96 h after injury. Growth from the remaining axon stump was observed. **c** Out of 10 axotomized neurons, 4 neurons showed stump growth and 6 neurons did not grow from the stump

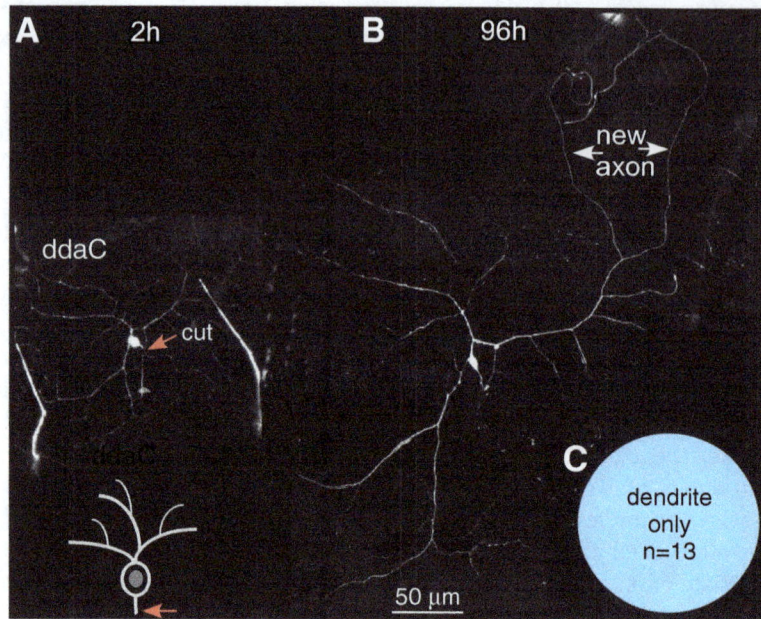

Fig. 4 Proximal axotomy in Class IV ddaC neurons induces regeneration of an axon from a dendrite. **a** An axon of a Class IV ddaC neuron was axotomized very close to the cell body (*orange arrow*) and imaged 2 h after injury. **b** The same neuron was imaged 96 h after injury to track regeneration. *White arrows* indicate a dendrite that has been converted to an axon. The identity of the new axon was confirmed by its plus-end-out microtubule polarity. **c** All 13 axotomized neurons converted a dendrite to an axon following proximal axotomy

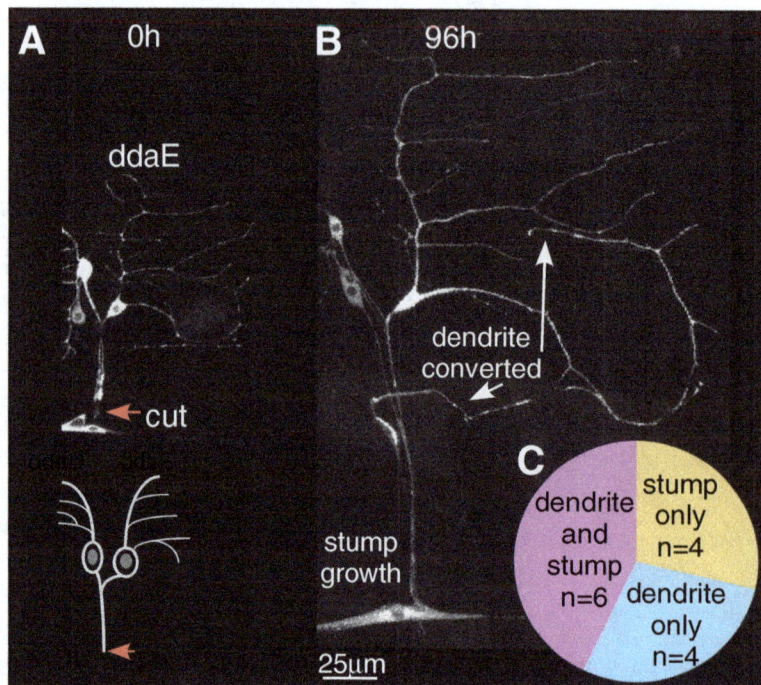

Fig. 5 Distal axotomy often leads to formation of two axons in Class I ddaE neurons. **a** An axon bundle including the ddaE axon was axotomized at least 20 μm from the cell body (*orange arrow*). **b** The same neuron was imaged 96 h after injury. One of the dendrites of the Class I ddaE neuron converted to an axon as indicated by *arrows*, in addition to re-growth from the axon stump. **c** Out of 14 axotomized ddaE neurons, 6 grew from the stump and dendrite, 4 grew from the stump only and 4 grew from the dendrite only

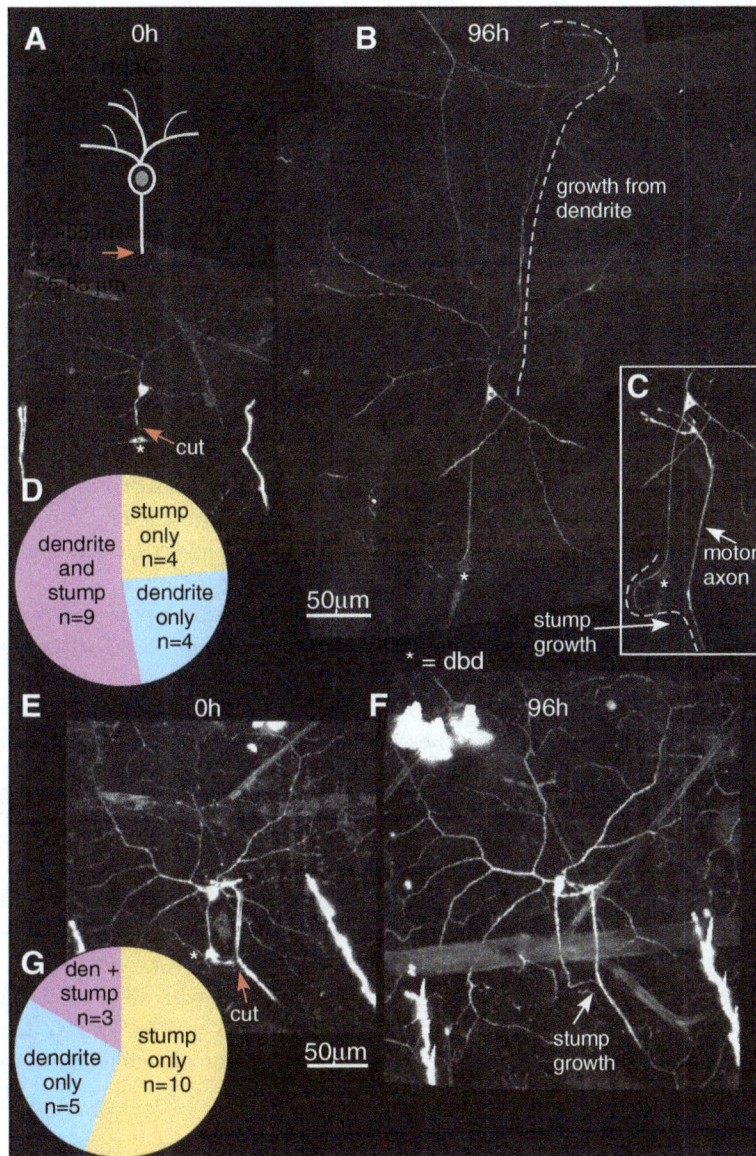

Fig. 6 Distal axotomy often leads to formation of two axons from two locations in Class IV ddaC neurons. **a** An axon of a Class IV ddaC neuron was axotomized (*orange arrow*) more than 30 μm from the cell body. An asterisk indicates the dorsal bipolar md neuron (dbd). **b** The same neuron was imaged 96 h after injury. One of the dendrites converted to an axon as indicated by the *dashed line*. **c** The inset shows the same cell as in A and B, but at a different depth of focus to visualize the re-growing axon joining the nerve. **d** Out of 17 axotomized neurons, 4 neurons regenerated from the axon stump only, 4 neurons regenerated from the dendrite only and 9 neurons regenerated from both locations. **e** An axon of a Class IV ddaC neuron was severed at least 65 μm from the cell body; the cute site is indicated with an *orange arrow*. **f** The same neuron was imaged 96 h after injury. In this example, the remaining axon stump regenerated and joined the motor nerve bundle. **g** Out of 18 injured neurons, 10 neurons regenerated from the stump; 5 neurons regenerated from the dendrite and 3 neurons regenerated from both sites

6b-d); dendrite conversion was assessed using micro-tubule polarity. In earlier studies looking at axon regeneration in ddaC neurons, a plasma membrane marker was used in most cases [9, 25, 26]. The membrane marker labels the entirety of the very complex arbor, including actin-based terminal branches. The marker used here, EB1-GFP, primarily labels regions of the dendrites where microtubules are concentrated. This makes

identifying dendrite tips that have initiated growth more obvious. It is likely that in the previous studies dendrites were also initiating growth, but that it was missed.

In dissociated cultures of rodent hippocampal neurons, the ability to convert a dendrite into a regenerating axon was strongly reduced when axons were injured 35 μm or more from the cell body [21]. We therefore performed an additional set of distal axotomies on ddaC neurons, using the pulsed UV laser to cut 65 μm or more from the cell body (Fig. 6e). As in mammalian neurons, the number of neurons that converted a dendrite to an axon was reduced (although not eliminated) with additional distance from the cell body (Fig. 6f-g).

The transcriptional response to injury is turned on with similar timing after proximal and distal axotomy

Having shown that, like proximal axotomy, distal axotomy can lead to conversion of a dendrite to an axon in both cell types tested, we were interested in determining whether the events that precede regeneration were also similar in these two scenarios. In all model systems where it has been tested, a kinase cascade initiated by DLK is required to initiate the response to axon injury [6, 10, 11, 29]. In Drosophila, this kinase cascade works through the transcription factor fos to activate transcription [7], and one of the genes transcribed is the MAP kinase phosphatase puckered (puc) [7]. A puc-GFP reporter is a good readout of pathway activation [26]. To test whether the timing and approximate level of pathway activation was similar after proximal and distal axotomy, we performed these assays in animals that contained the puc-GFP reporter as well as a membrane marker. The ddaC axon was either severed adjacent to the cell body (proximal) or near the dbd neuron (distal), and images were acquired at 8 h and 24 h after injury (Fig. 7a-b). By 8 h after injury the puc-GFP signal in the nucleus of injured ddaC neurons was about twice as high as in uninjured ddaC neighbors, and by 24 h about five-fold higher (Fig. 7c). Similar increases were seen in cells with proximal and distal axotomy. Thus with this reporter, we did not detect a difference in timing or level of injury-induced transcription after the two types of injury.

Conversion of a dendrite to axonal polarity is faster after proximal axotomy than after distal

Because injury-induced transcription and the ability to regenerate an axon from a dendrite were similar after proximal and distal axotomy, we considered the possibility that the only difference between these two types of injury is the presence of enough of an axon stump to support regeneration. If this were the case, stump regeneration would be entirely independent from regeneration from a dendrite. However, the probability that a dendrite will initiate growth is lower when the axon is cut further from the cell body, so there must be some feedback between the stump and the rest of the cell. The simplest model is that the two potential growth sites compete for resources at the time of outgrowth. To determine whether early feedback might exist, we analyzed microtubule changes required to convert a dendrite to an axon.

Dendrites convert to axons after proximal axotomy by disassembling their minus-end-out microtubule array and rebuilding it into a plus-end-out axonal array [22], so we assayed microtubule polarity after injury to probe early stages of the decision to convert a dendrite to an axon. Microtubule polarity was analyzed in Class IV ddaC neurons expressing EB1-GFP. EB1-GFP labels the plus-ends of growing microtubules, and so the movement of EB1-GFP comets denotes the orientation of microtubules [30]. Either proximal or distal axotomy was performed in the ddaC neuron, and EB1-GFP comets were analyzed in all dendrites at 8 h and 24 h post-axotomy (see methods). Injured ddaC neurons were then binned into one of three categories: 1) neurons with at least one plus-end-out neurite, 2) neurons with all minus-end-out neurites or 3) neurons with one or more mixed neurites (Fig. 8). At the 8 h time-point, in proximally axotomized neurons, 4 out of 7

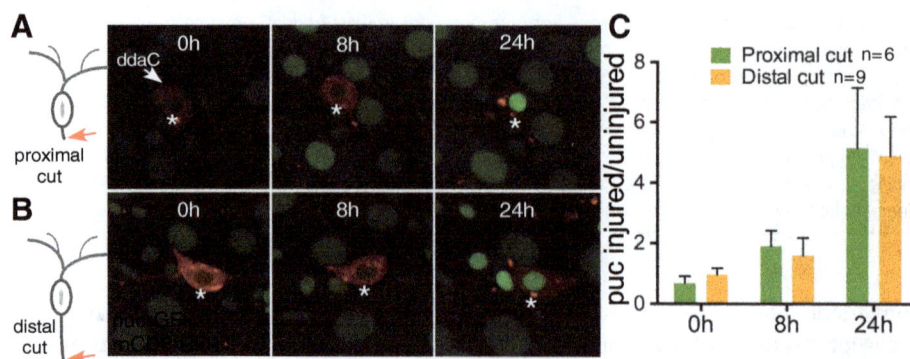

Fig. 7 The post-injury JNK signaling pathway is turned on after proximal and distal axotomies. Class IV ddaC neurons expressing mCD8-RFP and puc-GFP were subjected to either proximal (*top*) or distal axotomy (*bottom*) as shown in the schematic diagrams. **a** Example images of nuclear puc-GFP signal after proximal axotomy are shown at the 0 h, 8 h and 24 h time-points. *Asterisks* indicate nuclei of the injured ddaC neurons. **b** Example images of puc-GFP signal after distal axotomy are shown at the 0 h, 8 h and 24 h time-points. **c** The graph shows the quantification of puc-GFP intensity in the nucleus of the injured ddaC neurons at different time-points, after normalization to the intensity of puc-GFP in the uninjured ddaC neuron in the neighboring segment of the same larva. Average intensities are shown in the bar graph, and error bars are standard deviations

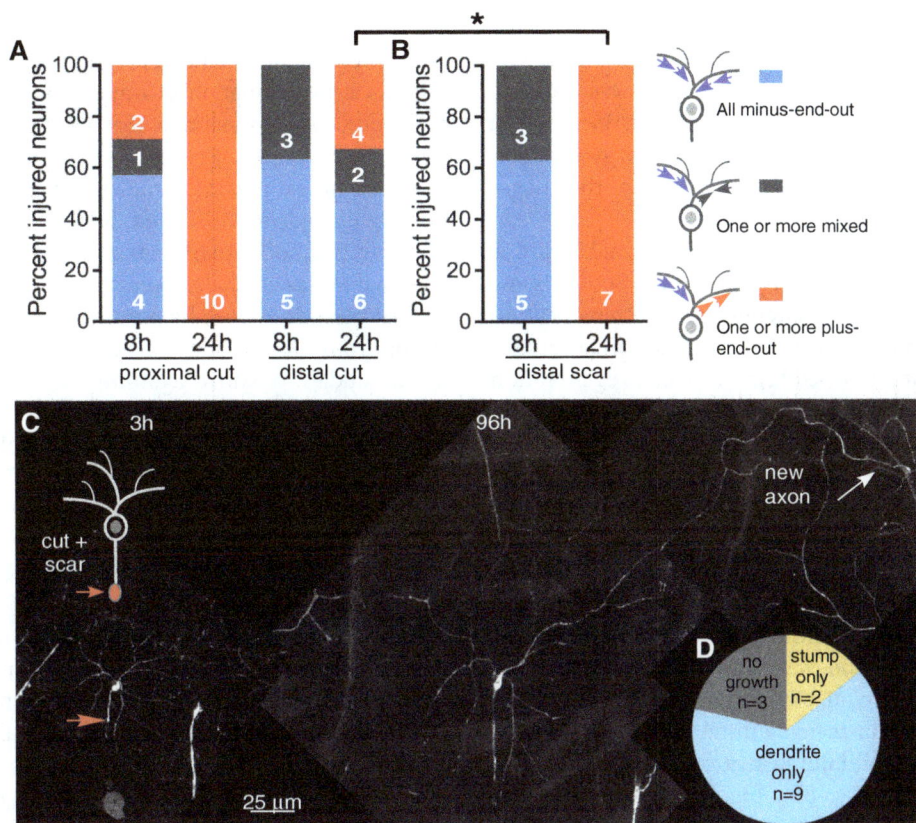

Fig. 8 Conversion of a dendrite to axonal polarity is faster after proximal axotomy than after distal. **a** Class IV ddaC neurons were subjected to proximal or distal axotomy and microtubule polarity in the dendrites was tracked 8 h and 24 h after injury. Neurons with at least one plus-end-out process were placed in the *red* category. Neurons with one or more mixed processes were placed in the *grey* category. Neurons with all minus-end-out processes were placed in the *blue* category. The graph shows percentage of proximally or distally axotomized neurons in each category at 8 h and 24 h after injury. **b** Class IV ddaC neurons were subjected to distal scarring axotomy and microtubule polarity in the dendrites was tracked 8 h and 24 h after injury. Neurons were placed in the same categories shown in **a**. A Fishers Exact test between the red categories in A and B was performed for the 24 h time-points (*$p < 0.05$). **c** Example of a Class IV ddaC neuron subjected to distal scarring axotomy and imaged 3 h after injury. The *orange arrow* shows the cut site. The same neuron was imaged 96 h after injury. The axon stump failed to re-grow. A dendrite converted to an axon and showed extensive growth as indicated by *white arrow*. **d** Out of 14 axotomized neurons, 9 neurons converted a dendrite to an axon, 2 neurons grew from the remaining axon stump and 3 neurons failed to grow from either location

neurons had all minus-end-out neurites, one cell had one or more mixed neurites and two had at least one plus-end-out neurite (Fig. 8a). At 24 h all proximally axotomized neurons had at least one plus-end-out neurite, suggesting that these neurons had completed specification of one of their neurites as an axon (Fig. 8a). In contrast, no distally axotomized ddaC neurons had a plus-end-out process 8 h after injury. Even 24 h post-axotomy, only one third of distally axotomized neurons had a plus-end-out neurite (Fig. 8a). Thus, although the puc-GFP injury reporter was activated with similar timing after proximal and distal axotomy, conversion of a dendrite to axonal polarity was more efficient after proximal axotomy. This difference in early conversion of a dendrite could perhaps account for the later difference in percent of neurons that initiate growth from a dendrite: 100% after proximal axotomy and about 50% after distal axotomy.

Blocking regeneration from the axon stump accelerates microtubule polarity changes in the dendrite after distal axotomy

The difference in early steps in conversion of a dendrite to an axon after proximal and distal axotomy suggests that there is some signal that allows the cell to distinguish between the two injuries. One possibility is that this signal difference is due only to the position of the injury, and another possibility is that the capacity of the stump to regenerate suppresses regeneration from a dendrite. To distinguish between these two possibilities, we tested whether we could block regeneration of the stump after distal axotomy by generating more tissue damage at the injury site than in previous experiments. A scar was created at the injury site by prolonged use of the pulsed UV laser. Typically, the scar appeared as a bright, auto-fluorescent blob at the site of injury (Additional file 1:

Figure S1B). On one occasion, the axon stump immediately retracted from the lesion site (Additional file 1: Figure S1A); in this case it is likely that the entire nerve, including all axons and surrounding glia, was severed. This particular cell did not regenerate, and is included in the results as one of the 3 in the set that did not exhibit regeneration (Fig. 8d). In all other cases the nerve remained connected across the scar.

After distal scarring axotomy 9/14 of injured neurons regenerated via dendrite conversion (Fig. 8c-d). Some neurons (3/14) failed to regenerate from either location and 2/14 of neurons regenerated from the axon stump (Fig 8d). Thus, distal scar axotomy reduced regeneration from the axon stump and frequently led to regeneration via conversion of a dendrite.

Next, we wished to examine whether blocking regeneration from the axon stump would affect microtubule polarity changes in the dendrite. To this end, we performed distal scarring axotomy in ddaC neurons and tracked movement of EB1-GFP comets at 8 h and 24 h post-axotomy. At the 8 h time-point, 5 out of 8 injured neurons had all minus-end-out neurites and the remaining 3 cells had one or more mixed neurites (Fig 8b), very similar to neurons with non-scarring distal injury. However, at the 24 h time-point, all injured neurons had at least one plus-end-out neurite (Fig. 8b), much like neurons after proximal axotomy. This change from initial similarity to distally injured axons to resemblance with proximally injured ones by 24 h implies that a feedback mechanism exists between the two regenerating axons, such that when regeneration from the stump is blocked, polarity reversal in a dendrite occurs more often.

Discussion

Previous studies have shown that many vertebrate neurons have the capacity to regenerate from an axon stump when axons are injured at a distance from the cell body, or from a dendrite when the axon is injured closer to the cell body. Depending on the model, the distances that can be equated with close to the cell body and far vary, but this capacity seems quite general.

In this study, we demonstrate that the highly branched nociceptive ddaC neurons of *Drosophila* larvae respond to proximal axotomy by converting a dendrite to an axon (Fig. 3). This is similar to the response of much simpler ddaE proprioceptive neurons to proximal axotomy [22]. In both cell types the new axon that originates from a dendrite wanders around the body wall, and often grows away from the nerve that leads back to the CNS. There is thus some question about whether these processes are true axons [25]. We were able to reconcile this issue by showing that axons generated by dendrite conversion are able to recognize and grow along the nerve on the rare occasions they encounter it (Fig. 2).

However, it is yet to be demonstrated if this new axon is able to re-innervate targets in the brain.

An interesting outcome of proximal axotomy in vertebrate systems is the formation of multiple axons [14, 15, 21]. In our study, we demonstrate that multiple axons can form after axon loss in the *Drosophila* peripheral nervous system. However, unlike previous studies in vertebrates, two axons were generated in *Drosophila* sensory neurons after distal axotomy but not proximal axotomy. One possible reason for this difference may be the distance of the injury site from the cell body. In mouse hippocampal neurons, a distance of 35 μm from the cell body was considered as proximal [21]. In our studies, proximal axotomy was performed by severing very close to the cell body. Therefore, in most cases, the remaining stump is extremely short, which may make it completely incompetent for growth.

In both ddaC and ddaE neurons, growth from a stump and dendrite at the same time was quite common. It would be very interesting to determine the fate of the two regenerating axons. Since the axon re-growing from the remaining stump seems to retrace its original route towards the ventral nerve cord, it is possible that the axon arising from a dendrite may be eventually pruned or retracted to maintain the 'one-axon' rule that normally governs these cells. With the current larval regeneration assays, the animal pupariates before these observations would be possible, but with long-lived larvae [31] this might be testable in the future. Similarly, while we have now shown that both ddaC and ddaE neurons can be used to study early stages of regeneration from the stump or from a dendrite, long-lived larvae may be necessary to use these model cells to study reinnervation of targets.

Many interesting questions remain about the early stages of axon regeneration that can be investigated in this system. For example, it is not known why severing the axon close to the cell body triggers regeneration from a dendrite, and how a dendrite is converted to a new axon. Moreover, it is not clear how the cell chooses a dendrite to convert to an axon. We did not notice any particular pattern of selection in ddaC neurons, but in ddaE neurons the large dorsal comb-like dendrite is rarely selected [22]. One hypothesis to account for this bias is that the dendrite that is less complex might be easier to convert to opposite polarity. From this study, it is also apparent that the severity of injury can trigger different outcomes: when a scar is generated during injury, conversion of a dendrite to a new axon is much more efficient than injury without a scar. This observation suggests that not only the injury itself is monitored, but perhaps also the type of injury or whether or not an axon growing from a stump encounters an impediment. The nature of the signals that would report to the cell body about type of injury or initial ability of the axon to grow are not known.

Conclusions

Drosophila sensory neurons with simple or complex dendrite arbors have two ways they can regenerate axons: from the remaining stump or by converting a dendrite to a new axon. This suite of responses is similar to those of injured mammalian neurons, meaning that Drosophila is a good model system for understanding conserved repair pathways. The decision to convert a dendrite to an axon is influenced not only by the position of axon injury, but also whether the axon stump encounters a growth obstacle.

Methods

Drosophila stocks

Injury assays in Class IV ddaC neurons were performed by crossing fly lines expressing UAS-EB1-GFP under the control of 447-GAL4, with *yw* flies. Injury assays in Class I ddaE neurons were carried out by crossing fly lines containing 221-Gal4, UAS-EB1-GFP transgenes with *yw* flies. The puc-GFP reporter line was generated as part of a protein trap screen [32].

Live injury assays in *Drosophila* larvae

Adult male and female flies were crossed in bottles capped with 35 mm petri dishes containing standard Drosophila media (food caps) and crosses were maintained at 25 degrees Celsius. Food caps with embryos on them were removed from the cross bottle every day and transferred to 10 cm petri dishes and incubated at 20 degree Celsius. Axotomy assays were performed on 3-day old larvae (3 days of incubation at 20 degrees Celsius) by placing them between a slide and coverslip and secured with tape. A MicroPoint pulsed UV laser system (Andor) was used to sever the axon. For proximal axotomy, the axon was severed very close to the cell body, while being careful to ensure no damage was done to the cell body. For distal axotomy, the axon was severed near the region where the bipolar neuron is situated (20–55 μm from the cell body).

Distal scar axotomy was performed similar to distal axotomy, but a scar was created by prolonged use of the pulsed UV laser. Far distal axotomy was performed by severing the axon 65–85 μm from the cell body. Images were taken immediately after injury (0 h) for proximal axotomy and 2-5 h after distal axotomy to check for complete severing. Regeneration was assessed 96 h after injury. The ddaD neuron was ablated by focusing the pulsed UV laser at the nucleus and the ddaE axon was severed 24 h after elimination. All images were acquired using a Zeiss LSM510 confocal microscope (Carl Zeiss). Z-projections were assembled using ImageJ software. Due to the elaborate branches of Class IV ddaC neurons, images of smaller regions were stitched together using Canvas software (ACD Systems).

Microtubule polarity assay

Microtubule plus-ends were visualized with EB1-GFP in injured neurons at 0 h, 8 h, 24 h or 96 h time-points after axon injury. Time-lapse movies were acquired on the Zeiss LSM510 confocal microscope using a 40× objective at a frame of two images per second. Movement of comets was tracked in all dendrites. Comets were counted manually in ImageJ. Only comets that were in focus for at least three consecutive frames were considered. A neurite was defined as plus-end-out if at least 3 out of 4 comets moved away from the cell body. A neurite was defined as mixed if the number of comets moving towards and away from the cell body was between the thresholds for plus-end-out and minus-end-out. A neurite was defined as minus-end-out if at least 3 out of 4 comets moved toward the cell body. The percentage of neurons with at least one plus-end-out neurite, or mixed or minus-end-out neurites was then plotted using GraphPad Prism 6 software.

puc-GFP reporter assay

Injury-induced activation of the JNK signaling pathway was visualized by crossing flies expressing 477-Gal4, UAS-mCD8-RFP with a puc-GFP protein trap line. Proximal axotomy or distal axotomy of Class IV ddaC neurons were performed and images were acquired immediately after injury (0 h) and 24 h after injury. Nuclear GFP intensity of the injured Class IV ddaC neuron was measured using ImageJ and normalized to nuclear GFP intensity of a neighboring uninjured Class IV ddaC neuron. Average nuclear GFP intensity in the injured/uninjured cells are plotted at each time point using GraphPad Prism 6.

Abbreviations

ALPs: Axon like processes; CNS: Central nervous system; DLK: Dual Leucine Zipper Kinase

Acknowledgements

We are very grateful to the Bloomington Drosophila Stock Center (NIH P40OD018537) for maintaining many of the lines used in this study. We are also grateful to members of the Rolls lab for helpful discussions throughout the project.

Funding

Funding for this work was provided by the National Institutes of Health through grant GM085115 to MMR.

Authors' contributions

MMR oversaw the work and helped with analysis and interpretation. KSR performed the experiments and analyzed the data. MMR and KSR wrote the paper and prepared figures together. Both authors read and approved the final manuscript.

Competing interests
The authors declare they have no competing interests.

References
1. Liu K, Tedeschi A, Park KK, He Z. Neuronal intrinsic mechanisms of axon regeneration. Annu Rev Neurosci. 2011;34:131–52.
2. Rishal I, Fainzilber M. Axon-soma communication in neuronal injury. Nat Rev Neurosci. 2014;15(1):32–42.
3. Navarro X, Vivo M, Valero-Cabre A. Neural plasticity after peripheral nerve injury and regeneration. Prog Neurobiol. 2007;82(4):163–201.
4. Kerschensteiner M, Schwab ME, Lichtman JW, Misgeld T. In vivo imaging of axonal degeneration and regeneration in the injured spinal cord. Nat Med. 2005;11(5):572–7.
5. Murphy AD, Barker DL, Loring JF, Kater SB. Sprouting and functional regeneration of an identified serotonergic neuron following axotomy. J Neurobiol. 1985;16(2):137–51.
6. Hammarlund M, Nix P, Hauth L, Jorgensen EM, Bastiani M. Axon regeneration requires a conserved MAP kinase pathway. Science. 2009; 323(5915):802–6.
7. Xiong X, Wang X, Ewanek R, Bhat P, Diantonio A, Collins CA. Protein turnover of the Wallenda/DLK kinase regulates a retrograde response to axonal injury. J Cell Biol. 2010;191(1):211–23.
8. Wu Z, Ghosh-Roy A, Yanik MF, Zhang JZ, Jin Y, Chisholm AD. Caenorhabditis elegans neuronal regeneration is influenced by life stage, ephrin signaling, and synaptic branching. Proc Natl Acad Sci U S A. 2007;104(38):15132–7.
9. Stone MC, Rao K, Gheres KW, Kim S, Tao J, La Rochelle C, Folker CT, Sherwood NT, Rolls MM. Normal spastin gene dosage is specifically required for axon regeneration. Cell Rep. 2012;2(5):1340–50.
10. Yan D, Wu Z, Chisholm AD, Jin Y. The DLK-1 kinase promotes mRNA stability and local translation in C. elegans synapses and axon regeneration. Cell. 2009;138(5):1005–18.
11. Shin JE, Cho Y, Beirowski B, Milbrandt J, Cavalli V, Diantonio A. Dual leucine zipper kinase is required for retrograde injury signaling and axonal regeneration. Neuron. 2012;74(6):1015–22.
12. Hall GF, Cohen MJ. Extensive dendritic sprouting induced by close axotomy of central neurons in the lamprey. Science. 1983;222(4623):518–21.
13. Hall GF, Poulos A, Cohen MJ. Sprouts emerging from the dendrites of axotomized lamprey central neurons have axonlike ultrastructure. J Neurosci. 1989;9(2):588–99.
14. Linda H, Risling M, Cullheim S. 'Dendraxons' in regenerating motoneurons in the cat: do dendrites generate new axons after central axotomy? Brain Res. 1985;358(1–2):329–33.
15. Linda H, Cullheim S, Risling M. A light and electron microscopic study of intracellularly HRP-labeled lumbar motoneurons after intramedullary axotomy in the adult cat. J Comp Neurol. 1992;318(2):188–208.
16. Rose PK, MacDermid V, Joshi M, Neuber-Hess M. Emergence of axons from distal dendrites of adult mammalian neurons following a permanent axotomy. Eur J Neurosci. 2001;13(6):1166–76.
17. Rose PK, Odlozinski M. Expansion of the dendritic tree of motoneurons innervating neck muscles of the adult cat after permanent axotomy. J Comp Neurol. 1998;390(3):392–411.
18. Fenrich KK, Skelton N, MacDermid VE, Meehan CF, Armstrong S, Neuber-Hess MS, Rose PK. Axonal regeneration and development of de novo axons from distal dendrites of adult feline commissural interneurons after a proximal axotomy. J Comp Neurol. 2007;502(6):1079–97.
19. Cho EY, So KF. Characterization of the sprouting response of axon-like processes from retinal ganglion cells after axotomy in adult hamsters: a model using intravitreal implantation of a peripheral nerve. J Neurocytol. 1992;21(8):589–603.
20. Hoang TX, Nieto JH, Havton LA. Regenerating supernumerary axons are cholinergic and emerge from both autonomic and motor neurons in the rat spinal cord. Neuroscience. 2005;136(2):417–23.
21. Gomis-Ruth S, Wierenga CJ, Bradke F. Plasticity of polarization: changing dendrites into axons in neurons integrated in neuronal circuits. Curr Biol. 2008;18(13):992–1000.
22. Stone MC, Nguyen MM, Tao J, Allender DL, Rolls MM. Global up-regulation of microtubule dynamics and polarity reversal during regeneration of an axon from a dendrite. Mol Biol Cell. 2010;21(5):767–77.
23. Gabel CV, Antoine F, Chuang CF, Samuel AD, Chang C. Distinct cellular and molecular mechanisms mediate initial axon development and adult-stage axon regeneration in C. elegans. Development. 2008;135(6):1129–36.
24. Grueber WB, Jan LY, Jan YN. Tiling of the Drosophila epidermis by multidendritic sensory neurons. Development. 2002;129(12):2867–78.
25. Song Y, Ori-McKenney KM, Zheng Y, Han C, Jan LY, Jan YN. Regeneration of Drosophila sensory neuron axons and dendrites is regulated by the Akt pathway involving Pten and microRNA bantam. Genes Dev. 2012;26(14):1612–25.
26. Stone MC, Albertson RM, Chen L, Rolls MM. Dendrite injury triggers DLK-independent regeneration. Cell Rep. 2014;6(2):247–53.
27. Chen L, Nye DM, Stone MC, Weiner AT, Gheres KW, Xiong X, Collins CA, Rolls MM. Mitochondria and Caspases Tune Nmnat-mediated stabilization to promote axon regeneration. PLoS Genet. 2016;12(12):e1006503.
28. Huebner EA, Strittmatter SM. Axon regeneration in the peripheral and central nervous systems. Results Probl Cell Differ. 2009;48:339–51.
29. Xiong X, Hao Y, Sun K, Li J, Li X, Mishra B, Soppina P, Wu C, Hume RI, Collins CA. The Highwire ubiquitin ligase promotes axonal degeneration by tuning levels of Nmnat protein. PLoS Biol. 2012;10(12):e1001440.
30. Stepanova T, Slemmer J, Hoogenraad CC, Lansbergen G, Dortland B, De Zeeuw CI, Grosveld F, van Cappellen G, Akhmanova A, Galjart N. Visualization of microtubule growth in cultured neurons via the use of EB3-GFP (end-binding protein 3-green fluorescent protein). J Neurosci. 2003;23(7):2655–64.
31. Miller DL, Ballard SL, Ganetzky B. Analysis of synaptic growth and function in Drosophila with an extended larval stage. J Neurosci. 2012;32(40):13776–86.
32. Morin X, Daneman R, Zavortink M, Chia W. A protein trap strategy to detect GFP-tagged proteins expressed from their endogenous loci in Drosophila. Proc Natl Acad Sci U S A. 2001;98(26):15050–5.

6

Evx1 and Evx2 specify excitatory neurotransmitter fates and suppress inhibitory fates through a Pax2-independent mechanism

José L. Juárez-Morales[1], Claus J. Schulte[2], Sofia A. Pezoa[1], Grace K. Vallejo[1], William C. Hilinski[1,3], Samantha J. England[1], Sarah de Jager[2] and Katharine E. Lewis[1*] (iD)

Abstract

Background: For neurons to function correctly in neuronal circuitry they must utilize appropriate neurotransmitters. However, even though neurotransmitter specificity is one of the most important and defining properties of a neuron we still do not fully understand how neurotransmitter fates are specified during development. Most neuronal properties are determined by the transcription factors that neurons express as they start to differentiate. While we know a few transcription factors that specify the neurotransmitter fates of particular neurons, there are still many spinal neurons for which the transcription factors specifying this critical phenotype are unknown. Strikingly, all of the transcription factors that have been identified so far as specifying inhibitory fates in the spinal cord act through Pax2. Even Tlx1 and Tlx3, which specify the excitatory fates of dI3 and dI5 spinal neurons work at least in part by down-regulating Pax2.

Methods: In this paper we use single and double mutant zebrafish embryos to identify the spinal cord functions of Evx1 and Evx2.

Results: We demonstrate that Evx1 and Evx2 are expressed by spinal cord V0v cells and we show that these cells develop into excitatory (glutamatergic) Commissural Ascending (CoSA) interneurons. In the absence of both Evx1 and Evx2, V0v cells still form and develop a CoSA morphology. However, they lose their excitatory fate and instead express markers of a glycinergic fate. Interestingly, they do not express Pax2, suggesting that they are acquiring their inhibitory fate through a novel Pax2-independent mechanism.

Conclusions: Evx1 and Evx2 are required, partially redundantly, for spinal cord V0v cells to become excitatory (glutamatergic) interneurons. These results significantly increase our understanding of the mechanisms of neuronal specification and the genetic networks involved in these processes.

Keywords: Spinal cord, Interneuron, Zebrafish, Evx, Pax2, Glutamatergic, Neurotransmitter, CNS, Transcription factor, V0

Background

Hundreds of millions of people across the world are affected by neurological diseases and injuries. Understanding how functional neuronal circuitry is established in the vertebrate central nervous system (CNS) is essential for developing better treatments for these conditions. How neuronal circuitry develops is also a fundamental question in developmental neuroscience. To answer this question, we need to identify how the functional properties of distinct neurons are specified; since these properties determine which circuits the neurons participate in, the functional roles that the neurons have within those circuits and the resulting outputs of the circuitry. The spinal cord is a powerful system for establishing fundamental principles of neuronal fate specification, function and circuit assembly, as it is relatively simple and experimentally tractable compared to the brain. This has enabled considerable progress in establishing the functions

* Correspondence: kelewi02@syr.edu
[1]Department of Biology, Syracuse University, 107 College Place, Syracuse, NY 13244, USA
Full list of author information is available at the end of the article

of different ventral spinal cord interneurons in loco-motor circuitry (e.g. [1–9]). However, we still know relatively little about how the functional properties of these cells are determined.

For neurons to function correctly they must synthesize and utilize correct neurotransmitters. Within neuronal circuitry, if they inhibit rather than excite their synaptic partners, or vice versa, then the behaviors and functional outputs of those circuits will be dramatically disturbed, and may give rise to pathological conditions. For example, disruptions in the balance of excitatory and inhibitory neurons in the CNS have been implicated in epilepsy, autism, Alzheimer's and many other neurological disorders (e.g. [10–13]). However, even though neurotransmitter specificity is one of the most important and defining properties of a neuron we still do not fully understand how neurotransmitter fates are specified during development.

Many neuronal properties are determined by the transcription factors that cells express as they start to differentiate. We already know a few transcription factors (e.g. Ptf1a, Lhx1, Lhx5, Lbx1, Pax2) that specify the inhibitory (GABAergic and/or glycinergic) fates of several subsets of spinal interneurons [14–18]. Strikingly, most of these transcription factors function in dorsal spinal neurons and all of them act through Pax2 [14–21]. In contrast, we only know two transcription factors, Tlx1 and Tlx3, that are required for the specification of excitatory (glutamatergic) fates and these are only expressed in dorsal dI3, dI5 and DIL$_B$ cells [15, 16, 22]. Interestingly, Tlx1 and Tlx3 determine the glutamatergic fates of dI3 and dI5 cells at least in part by down-regulating Pax2 [15]. These results suggest that Pax2 is a crucial player in neurotransmitter fate specification with its presence being required for inhibitory fates and its absence required for excitatory fates. However, we still do not know which transcription factors regulate the neurotransmitter fates of many excitatory spinal neurons, including those in the ventral spinal cord, whose correct functional specification is essential for locomotion.

In this paper we identify two transcription factors, Evx1 and Evx2, which are required for a subset of excitatory fates in the ventral spinal cord. In mammals, the spinal cord expression of Evx1 and Evx2 is restricted to a population of cells located in an intermediate dorso-ventral position corresponding to V0 cells (e.g. [23–28]). V0 cells are post-mitotic cells that form from the p0 (Dbx1-positive, Nkx6.2-negative) progenitor domain [23, 27–29]. These cells develop into interneurons that are important components of locomotor circuitry and they can be subdivided into an Evx1-positive sub-population called V0$_v$ cells and

an Evx1-negative sub-population called V0$_D$ cells. These names reflect the fact that V0v cells form more ventrally than V0$_D$ cells (e.g. [23–28, 30–34]). Evx2 is expressed in a similar pattern to Evx1 in the mouse CNS, suggesting that it may also be expressed by V0v cells. This is consistent with the observation that Evx2 spinal cord expression is lost in mouse Evx1 mutants [23]. However, co-expression of Evx1 and Evx2 in the mouse spinal cord has not yet been demonstrated [24].

In mammals, both V0v and V0$_D$ interneurons are crucial for correct left-right alternation during locomotion, with V0v cells in particular being required for hindlimb left-right alternation during fast locomotion [9, 34]. While the functions of V0 cells in specific behaviors have so far only been assayed in mouse, these cells have highly conserved commissural axon trajectories in all animals examined so far ([23–28, 32, 33, 35, 36]; this paper), suggesting that their functional properties are likely to be highly conserved across the vertebrate lineage. However, when we started this work the neurotransmitter phenotype of V0v cells had not been identified.

In zebrafish, evx1 and evx2 are expressed in a similar intermediate dorsal-ventral spinal cord position to that observed in other vertebrates [26, 32, 33], although again, co-expression of these two genes has not previously been demonstrated. In this paper, we confirm that evx1 and evx2 are co-expressed by V0v cells and we show that V0v cells are glutamatergic and have a Commissural Ascending (Comissural Secondary Ascending or CoSA) morphology. We also provide the first analysis of evx1;evx2 double mutants in any vertebrate and the first analysis of the spinal cord phenotype of evx2 mutants. Significantly, we demonstrate that Evx1 and Evx2 are required, partially redundantly, to specify the glutamatergic fates of V0v cells. Given that we know so little about how excitatory fates are specified in the spinal cord and particularly the ventral spinal cord, these findings add considerably to our understanding of CNS circuit development.

In the absence of both Evx1 and Evx2, V0v cells lose their glutamatergic fates but other functional characteristics like soma/cell body morphology and axon trajectory are unchanged. In addition, and in contrast to a previously described mouse Evx1 mutant [23], these cells do not express markers of neighboring cell types. This suggests that V0v cells are not transfating into a different class of neuron; they have just changed some of their functional properties. Strikingly, in evx1;evx2 double mutants V0v cells become inhibitory, but they do not express Pax2, suggesting that they are acquiring their inhibitory fates through a novel Pax2-independent mechanism.

Methods

Ethics approval

All zebrafish experiments in this research were approved either by the UK Home Office or by the Syracuse University IACUC committee.

Zebrafish husbandry and fish lines

Zebrafish (Danio rerio) were maintained on a 14 h light/ 10 h dark cycle at 28.5 °C and embryos were obtained from natural, paired and/or grouped spawnings of wild-type (WT) adults (AB, TL or AB/TL hybrids), identified heterozygous or homozygous Tg(slc17a6:EGFP) (used to be called Tg(vGlut2a:EGFP); [36, 37]), Tg(evx1:EGFP)^{SU1} or Tg(evx1:EGFP)^{SU2} adults, double heterozygous evx1^{i232};evx2^{sa140} mutants or double heterozygous evx1^{i232};evx2^{sa140} mutants that also carried one of the Tg(evx1:EGFP) lines (see below). Embryos were reared at 28.5 °C and staged by hours post fertilization (h), days post or prim staging/or prim staging [38].

The evx1^{i232} mutation has been described before [39]. The evx2^{sa140} mutant was received from the Wellcome Trust Sanger Centre, (https://www.sanger.ac.uk/sanger/ Zebrafish_Zmpbrowse). Both mutations produce a single base pair change (a C to a T in the case of evx2^{sa140}) that results in a premature stop codon before the homeobox ([39]; Fig. 1a). Therefore, the truncated proteins, if formed, will lack DNA binding domains. The evx2^{sa140} mutation creates a BfaI recognition site that enables us to genotype individual fish and embryos (see below; Fig. 1b). In this paper we demonstrate that the evx2^{sa140} allele does not make Evx2 protein (Fig. 1c), strongly suggesting that it is a null allele. The evx1^{i232} mutant is also probably a null allele [39]. However, in contrast to the evx1^{i232} mutant which is viable, the evx2^{sa140} mutant is embryonic lethal (see Results and Additional file 1: Results).

Genotyping

Genotyping of mutant alleles was performed on both live adults and fixed embryos using DNA extracted from fin clips and dissected heads respectively. Fin clipping and evx1 genotyping were performed as in [39]. To extract DNA from embryos, heads were removed in 80 % glycerol / 20 % PBS with insect pins. Embryonic trunks were stored in 70 % glycerol / 30 % PBS at 4 °C for later analysis. Heads were incubated in 50 μL of Proteinase K buffer solution (1 M Tris-HCl, pH 8.2; 0.5 M EDTA; 1 M NaCl; 20 % SDS; 10 mg/ml Proteinase K) for 2 h at 55 °C. Proteinase K was heat inactivated at 100 °C for 10 min and tubes were centrifuged for 20 min at 13,000 rpm. DNA was precipitated with 100 % ethanol at -20 °C overnight, centrifuged to pellet the DNA and re-suspended in 20 μL of water. 2 μL of DNA was used for each PCR.

The evx2^{sa140} mutation creates a BfaI recognition site. A genomic region flanking the mutation site was PCR amplified using the following conditions: 94 °C for 60 s, followed by 5 cycles of 92 °C for 30 s, 54 °C for 30 s, 72 °C for 60 s; followed by 40 cycles of 92 °C for 20 s, 52 °C for 30 s, and 72 °C for 60 s, followed by a final extension at 72 °C for 5 min. Forward primer: GTAATGCGATCCCAAAACG. Reverse primer: TTATTTTAGATTTGGCAATGG.

PCR products were digested with BfaI and analysed on a 1 % agarose gel. The WT product is 454 bp, whereas the mutant product is cut into 218 bp and 236 bp fragments. These fragments are close enough in size that they are usually detected as one band on an agarose electrophoresis gel (Fig. 1b).

Creation of Tg(evx1:EGFP) lines

Potential evx1 enhancer regions were identified by multispecies sequence comparisons using the global alignment program Shuffle-LAGAN [40] and visualized using VISTA [41]. Zebrafish (Danio rerio) evx1 genomic sequence (ENSDARG00000099365) and orthologous sequences from human (ENSG00000106038) and mouse (ENSMUSG00000005503) were obtained from Ensembl (http://www.ensembl.org). Zebrafish sequence was used as the baseline and annotated using exon/intron information from Ensembl. The alignment was performed using a 100 bp window and a cutoff score of 70 % identity. A multi-species comparison of approximately 23Kb of Danio rerio genomic DNA sequence containing evx1 and extending 5 Kb into flanking regions revealed high conservation in both coding and non-coding sequences among compared species. We identified three Conserved Non-coding Elements (CNEs) located 5' and 3' to evx1. The first is located 79 bp upstream of zebrafish evx1 coding sequence and extends over 100 bp. The other two are located 3' to evx1. One is 2354 bp downstream of the stop codon and is 184 bp long whereas the other is 2979 bp downstream of the stop codon and extends over 140 bp (Fig. 1d). One amplicon encompassing these two 3' CNEs and the intervening sequence (1.34 Kb) was PCR-amplified from genomic DNA. Forward primer: AAGATTGGAATGGAATGTCT. Reverse primer: GCA TTTTCGCCTTTGCATCA.

The Tg(evx1:EGFP)^{SU1} line was generated by cloning this 3' CNE amplicon into the pDONR^{TM}P4-P1R vector from Invitrogen using Gateway technology [42, 43]. The final construct was assembled using the pENTRbasegfp plasmid and the pCSDest2 vector [44]. This resulted in a vector containing Tol2:1.3Kb 3' zfish evx1:ßcarp minimal promoter:EGFP:Tol2.

The same 3' CNE amplicon was used to generate the Tg(evx1:EGFP)^{SU2} line. In this case, the GAL4VP16;UAS-EGFP cassette was taken from the pBGAL4VP16;UAS-EGFP plasmid [45] and cloned into a middle entry vector

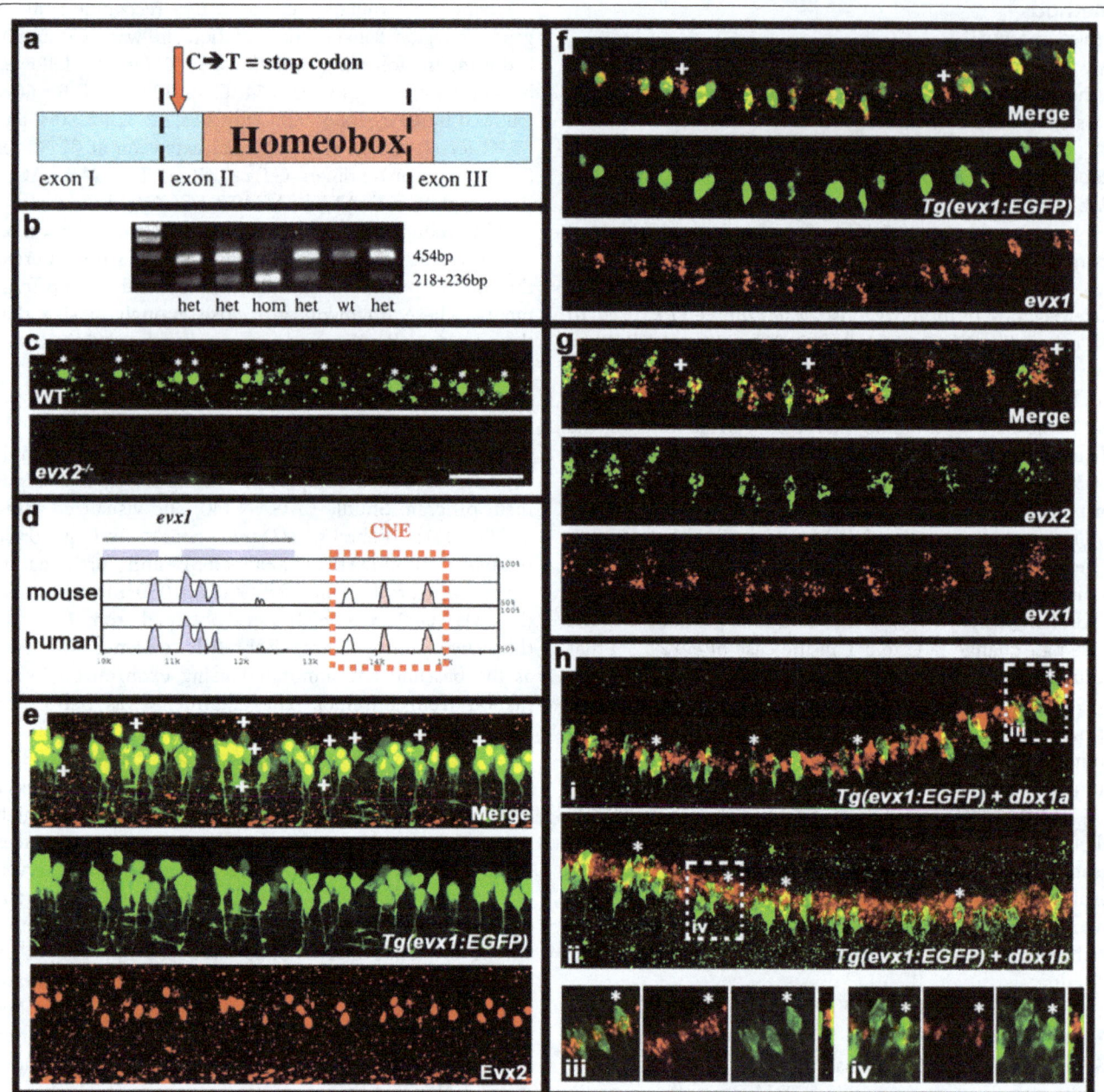

Fig. 1 V0v cells co-express *evx1* and *evx2*. **a** Schematic of Evx2 showing exon boundaries (dotted lines), homeobox-domain (pink) and location of *evx2sa140* mutation (red arrow). **b** Examples of genotyping WT, heterozygous and homozygous *evx2sa140* mutant embryos using gel electrophoresis (see methods). The two fragments from the mutant allele restriction product run at the same position on the gel. **c, e-h** lateral views, dorsal up, anterior left, of spinal cord at 24 h (**f-h**) or 27 h (**c** & **e**). **c** Evx2 immunohistochemistry on WT (*top panel*) and homozygous *evx2sa140* mutant (*bottom panel*) embryos. Stars indicate Evx2-expressing cells. Mutant embryos have no Evx2 expression. **d** Schematic showing Shuffle-LAGAN analysis of *evx1* genomic region with zebrafish sequence as baseline compared to orthologous regions in mouse and human genomes. Conserved coding sequences are indicated in blue, arrow indicates 5'-3' orientation. CNEs in 3' region are indicated in pink. The region amplified to create transgenic lines is indicated with red dotted lines. **e-h** Double staining for (**e**) EGFP (green) and Evx2 (red) in *Tg(evx1:EGFP)SU1* embryos, (**f**) EGFP (green) and *evx1* (red) in *Tg(evx1:EGFP)SU1* embryos, (**g**) *evx1* (red) and *evx2* (green) in WT embryos, (**h**) EGFP (green) and *dbx1a* (red) in *Tg(evx1:EGFP)SU1* embryos (i and iii) and EGFP (green) and *dbx1b* (red) in *Tg(evx1:EGFP)SU1* embryos (ii and iv). In **e-g** and **h_iii - h_iv**, merged and single channel views are provided. White crosses indicate cells that only express *evx1*. In (**f**) these probably represent cells that have just started to express *evx1* as there is a delay in expression of EGFP. White stars in **h** indicate double-labelled cells. Three wider panels at bottom of **h** (iii and iv) are magnified single-confocal-plane views of white dotted rectangle regions in panels **h_i** and **h_ii** respectively. Thin panel on RHS in each case shows a cross-section projection (slice) created in Image J confirming that GFP expression is lateral to *dbx* expression. Scale bar: 50 μm (**c** & **e-h**)

from Invitrogen [42, 43]. An oligonucleotide containing the *cfos* minimal promoter sequence [46] plus 17 bp of the 5' arm of *GAL4* was synthesized and used with a RVeGF-PAttb2 primer to PCR amplify the *GAL4VP16;UAS-EGFP* cassette.

FWcfosGAL4VP16 primer: CACTCATTCATAAAC GCTTGTTATAAAAGCAGTGGCTGCGGCGCCTCG TACTCCAACCGCATCTGCAGCGAGCAACTGAGA AGCCAAGACTGAGCCGGCGGCCTTTGTACAAAA AAGCAG

RVeGFPAttb2 primer: GGGGACCACTTTGTACAAG AAAGCTGGGTTTACTTGTACAGCTCGTCCA.

This PCR product was used to generate a second PCR product using the primer FWattB1cfos: GGGGACAAG TTTGTACAAAAAAGCAGGCTCACTCATTCATAAA ATCGCTT and the RVeGFPAttb2 primer.

The final amplicon was cloned into pDONR™221 using gateway technology. This middle entry vector was used to generate a final vector containing *Tol2:1.3Kb 3' zfish evx1:cfos minimal promoter:GAL4VP16;UAS-EGFP:Tol2*.

Each of these plasmids was separately co-injected with transposase mRNA into 1-2 cell embryos as described by [47]. Embryos were raised to adulthood and out-crossed to identify founders. In each case one stable transgenic line was generated. The *Tg(evx1:EGFP)^SU2* or *Tg(1.3 kb evx1:cfos:GAL4-UAS:EGFP)* line has the advantage that it contains a GAL4-UAS cassette to amplify EGFP expression. This facilitates visualization of axons. However, this line has a slightly more variegated expression than the *Tg(evx1:EGFP)^SU1* or *Tg(1.3Kb evx1:ßcarp:EGFP)* line, presumably because of stochastic silencing of the construct due to the GAL4-UAS sequences [48]. In contrast the *Tg(evx1:EGFP)^SU1* line labels all V0v cells more consistently, but the EGFP expression is slightly weaker and we were never able to obtain *evx1^-/-;evx2^-/-* double mutant embryos that contained this transgene, even though we could obtain *evx1^-/-;evx2^+/+* and *evx1^-/-;evx2^+/-* embryos. This suggests that the *Tg(1.3Kb evx1:ßcarp:EGFP)* construct integrated close to the WT *evx2* allele.

Morpholino injection

Approximately 5 nl of a 1:1 combination of two Evx2 ATG Morpholino antisense oligonucleotides (MOs) at 1.25 mg/ml each were injected into 1-2 cell embryos (evx2-1 MO: TTCTTTTCTTATCCTCTCCATCATG; evx2-2 MO: AATCCAAAGTCCCAGGGCTGGTGCT). In all cases, we confirmed that the MOs had completely knocked down Evx2 using immunohistochemistry for zebrafish Evx2.

Expression profiling V0v cells

To determine which neurotransmitters V0v cells express and to identify additional transcription factors

expressed by these cells, different combinations of spinal cord and trunk cells were extracted from live transgenic zebrafish embryos at 27 h using fluorescence activated cell-sorting (FACS). Prior to FACS, embryos were prim-staged, deyolked, dissected and dissociated as in [49, 50]. In all cases, the heads were removed to ensure that only trunk or spinal cord cells were collected. Pure populations of cells were obtained using combinations of the following transgenic lines: *Tg(elav13:EGFP)*, *Tg(evx1:EGFP)^SU1*, *Tg(pax2a:GFP)*, *Tg(Xla.Tubb:DsRed)* (formerly *Tg(NBT:DsRed))*, *Tg(vsx2:DsRed)* and *Tg(gata1:GFP)* [8, 51–54]. Trunk samples correspond to FAC-sorted trunk cells (spinal cord and other tissues). All neuron samples are EGFP-positive cells from *Tg(elav13:EGFP)* trunks. V0v neurons are EGFP-positive cells from *Tg(evx1:EGFP)^SU1* trunks. V1 neurons are double-positive EGFP-positive, DsRed-positive cells from *Tg(pax2-a:GFP);Tg(Xla.Tubb:DsRed)* trunks. V2a neurons are double-positive DsRed-positive, EGFP-positive cells from *Tg(vsx2:DsRed);Tg(elavl3:EGFP)* trunks. V2b + KA neurons are double-positive EGFP-positive, DsRed-positive cells from *Tg(gata1:GFP);Tg(Xla.Tubb:DsRed)* trunks. Total RNA was extracted using an RNeasy Micro Kit (Qiagen, 74004). RNA quality and quantity was assayed on an Agilent 2100 Bioanalyser (RNA 6000 Pico Kit, Agilent, 5067-1513), before converting to fluorescently-labelled cDNA (Ovation Pico WTA System V2, Pico, 3302) and hybridizing to a custom-designed Agilent microarray (EMBL Genomics Core, Heidelberg). Details of this microarray will be described elsewhere, along with the characterization of additional genes identified from these analyses. Data pre-processing and normalization was performed using Bioconductor software (https://www.bioconductor.org/). Two-class eBayes and three-class ANOVA analyses were performed using GEPAS software (Tárraga, (2008)). All reported statistics were corrected for multiple testing (Benjamini and Hochberg (1995)).

in situ hybridization

Embryos were fixed in 4 % paraformaldehyde and single and double *in situ* hybridizations were performed as previously described [55, 56]. RNA probes were prepared using the following templates, *dbx1a* and *dbx1b* [57], *evx1* [58], *evx2* [32], *eve1* [59], *pax2a, pax2b, pax8* [60] and *eng1b* [14]. To determine neurotransmitter phenotypes we used probes for genes that encode proteins that transport or synthesize specific neurotransmitters. A mixture of two probes (*glyt2a* and *glyt2b*) for *slc6a5* (previously called *glyt2*) was used to label glycinergic cells [61, 62]. *slc6a5* encodes for a glycine transporter necessary for glycine reuptake and transport across the plasma membrane. A mixture of two probes to *gad1b* (previously called *gad67*, probes used to be called *gad67a* and *gad67b*) and one probe to *gad2* (previously called *gad65*) was used to label GABAergic cells [61, 62]. *gad1b* and *gad2* encode for glutamic acid decarboxylases, necessary for the synthesis of GABA from glutamate. A mixture of *slc17a6b* (formerly called *vglut2.1*) and *slc17a6a* (formerly called *vglut 2.2*) probes was used to label glutamatergic cells [61, 62]. These genes encode proteins responsible for transporting glutamate to the synapse. In all of these cases, a mix of equal concentrations of the relevant probes was used [61, 62]. We also used *slc32a1* (formerly called *viaat)*, which encodes for a vesicular inhibitory amino acid transporter, to label all inhibitory cells [8].

The DNA template for the *skor2* (ZDB-GENE-060825-57) probe was generated by PCR-amplifying the 3' region of *skor2* from cDNA using a reverse primer containing a T3 promoter sequence at the 5' end (indicated in italics below). Total RNA was extracted by homogenizing 50-100 mg of 27hpf wild-type zebrafish embryos in 1 mL of TRIzol reagent (Ambion, 15596-026). cDNA was synthesized using Bio-Rad iScript Reverse Transcription Supermix kit (Bio-Rad, 170-8891). A 50 μL PCR was assembled containing 5 μL cDNA and 1 unit of Phusion High-Fidelity DNA Polymerase (NEB, M0530L). PCR conditions were: 94 °C for 3 min followed by 35 cycles of 94 °C for 30 s, 56.5 °C for 30 s, 72 °C for 1.5 min and then a final extension step of 72 °C for 10 min. PCR product was purified by phenol:chloroform extraction. Forward primer: CGCAAGACGCTTTTTATCC

Reverse primer: *AATTAACCCTCACTAAAGGGA*AAA TGGAGAGCTGCCTTTCAG.

ZFIN Identification numbers are provided for all genes in Additional file 1: Table S2.

Immunohistochemistry

Primary antibodies used were rabbit anti-Evx2 (a kind gift from Dr Higashijima, described in Satou et al., 2012, raised against the first 168 amino acids of zebrafish Evx2, a region with no significant homology to zebrafish Evx1, 1:300), mouse anti-GFP (Roche Applied Science, 11814460001, 1:500), rabbit anti-GFP (Molecular Probes A6465, 1:500) and mouse anti-Pax2 (Covance PRB-276P 1:300). The Pax2 antibody recognizes both Pax2a and Pax2b in zebrafish [14]. Antibodies used for fluorescent *in situ* hybridization were mouse anti-Dig (Jackson ImmunoResearch 200-002-156, 1:5000) and rabbit anti-Flu (Invitrogen A889, 1:2500). These were detected with Invitrogen Tyramide kits #12 and #5. Secondary antibodies used were Alexa Fluor 568 goat anti-rabbit (Molecular Probes A11036, 1:500), Alexa Fluor 488 goat anti-rabbit (Molecular Probes A11034, 1:500) and Alexa Fluor 488 goat anti-mouse (Molecular Probes A11029, 1:500).

Embryos for immunohistochemistry were treated with acetone for 15 min (24 h embryos) or 20 min (30 h embryos) to permeabilize them, washed for 5 min in distilled water, then washed 2 x 10 min in PBS. Embryos were treated with Image-iT Signal Enhancer (Invitrogen, I36933) for 30 min, then incubated in block solution (2 % goat serum, 1 % BSA, 10 % DMSO and 0.5 % Triton) for 1 h at room temperature followed by incubation in primary antibody in fresh block solution at 4 °C overnight. Embryos were washed with PBT (PBS + 0.1 % Triton) for 2 h at room temperature and incubated with secondary antibody in block solution at 4 °C overnight. Embryos were then washed with PBT for at 2 h at room temperature and stored in 2 % DABCO (Acros Organics, AC11247-1000).

For 3,3'- diaminobenzidine (DAB) staining, after incubation with primary antibody, samples were incubated in fresh blocking solution with goat anti-rabbit IgG (Covance SMI-5030C, 1:200) at 4 °C overnight. Embryos were then washed with PBT for 2 h and incubated with rabbit PAP (Covance SMI-4010 L, 1:200) in block solution at 4 °C overnight. Embryos were then washed in PBT for 2 h. Staining was performed using Sigma Fast 3,3'- diaminobenzidine tablets (Sigma, D4293).

Imaging

Embryos were mounted in 70 % glycerol, 30 % PBS and DIC pictures were taken using an AxioCam MRc5 camera mounted on a Zeiss Axio Imager M1 compound microscope. Fluorescent images were taken on a Zeiss LSM 710 confocal microscope. Images were processed using Adobe Photoshop software (Adobe, Inc) and Image J software (Abramoff et al., 2004). In some cases different focal planes were merged to show labeled cells at different medial lateral positions in the spinal cord.

Cell counts and statistics

In all cases, cells counts are for both sides of a five-somite length of the spinal cord adjacent to somites 6-10. Most values are an average of at least 5 embryos. Exceptions are the *skor2 + Tg(evx1:EGFP)* double-labeling experiments, the *skor2 + Tg(slc17a6:EGFP)* double-labeling experiments and the *pax2a* and *eng1b in situ* hybridization results. In all of these cases 4 embryos were counted. Results were analyzed using the student's *t*-test; Error bars indicate standard deviation.

Results

Zebrafish V0v cells express *evx1* and *evx2*

In mouse, *Evx1* is expressed in V0v cells and while double-labeling experiments have not yet been performed, the data suggest that *Evx2* is probably co-expressed by these same cells [23, 24, 27, 28]. Previous reports described *evx1* and *evx2* expression in a similar region of zebrafish spinal cord [32, 33] but didn't determine whether these genes are co-expressed or the specific cell types that express them.

To address these questions, we performed single and double *in situ* hybridization experiments and found that zebrafish *evx1* and *evx2* are co-expressed in an intermediate region of the dorso-ventral axis of the spinal cord (Figs. 1g and 2a & i). We further confirmed that *evx1* and *evx2* are co-expressed in zebrafish spinal cord using an EGFP line, *Tg(evx1:EGFP)^{SU1}*. We constructed this line using enhancer sequences identified downstream of *evx1* (see methods & Fig. 1d). We confirmed that the stable line recapitulates endogenous *evx1* expression (Fig. 1f) and also shows co-expression of EGFP and Evx2 protein (Fig. 1e). Interestingly, at 27 h, all of the cells that express Evx2 also express EGFP (and hence *evx1*) (Fig. 1e), however, a few cells express EGFP but not Evx2. Similarly, at 24 h, a few cells express *evx1* but not *evx2* (Fig. 1g). This is consistent with earlier reports that suggest that *evx1* may be expressed in the spinal

cord slightly earlier than *evx2* [32, 33], although we cannot rule out the possibility that there is a very small subset of *evx1*-expressing V0v cells that do not express *evx2*.

V0 cells develop from the p0 progenitor domain, which expresses *dbx1* [28, 63]. Therefore, to confirm that *evx1/2*-expressing cells are V0v cells we performed EGFP immunohistochemistry and *in situ* hybridization for *dbx1a* and *dbx1b* in *Tg(evx1:EGFP)^{SU1}* embryos. We found that zebrafish *evx* genes are expressed lateral to cells expressing both of these *dbx1* genes, as would be predicted for cells developing from the p0 domain. In addition, *dbx1a* and *dbx1b* expression persists in some EGFP-positive cells (Fig. 1h), suggesting that these genes continue to be expressed by V0v cells for a short while after they become post-mitotic.

Zebrafish also have a third *evx* gene, called *eve1*, but earlier studies suggested that this gene is not expressed in the spinal cord [26, 32, 59, 64]. We confirmed this by

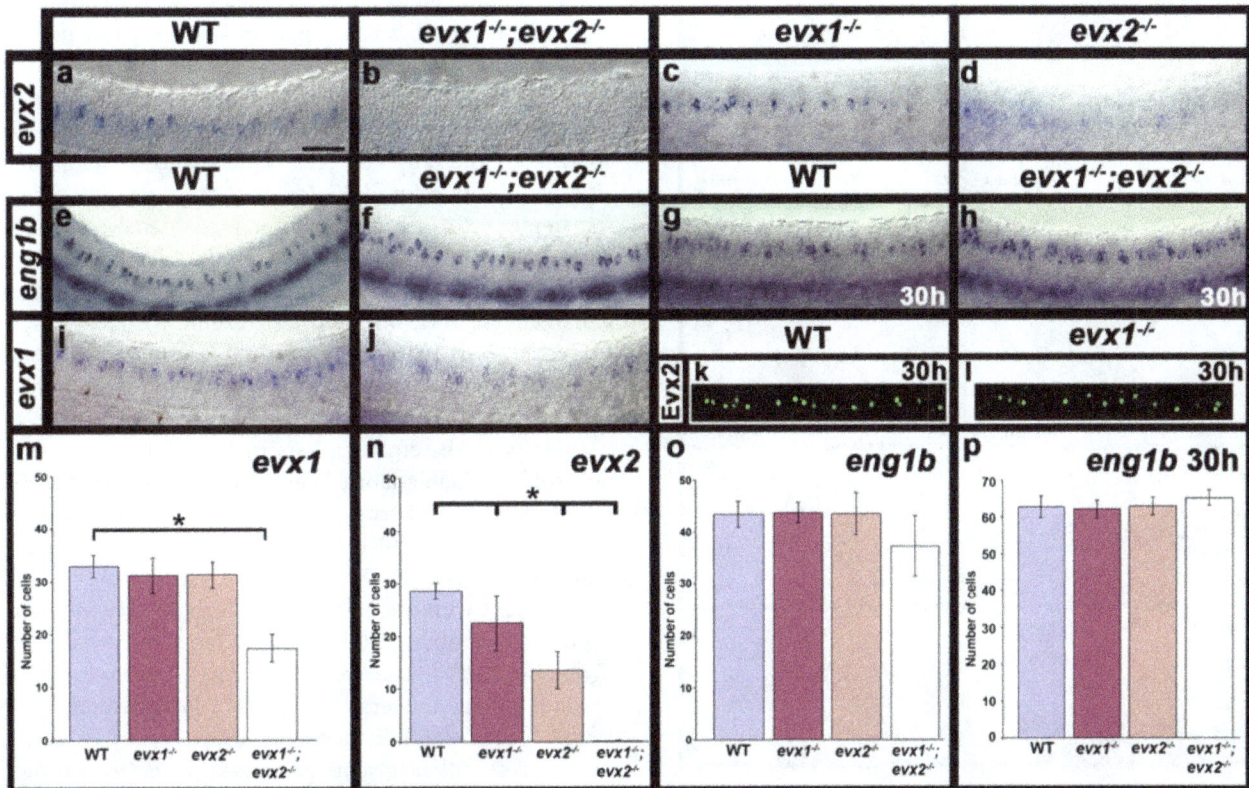

Fig. 2 Expression of *evx* and *eng1b* genes in *evx1;evx2* double mutant embryos. Lateral views of zebrafish spinal cord at 24 h (**a-f, i & j**) or 30 h (**g, h, k & l**). Anterior left, dorsal up. **a-j** *in situ* hybridization for each gene indicated. **e-h** strong ventral expression is in muscle pioneer cells, expression in more individual dorsal cells corresponds to spinal cord V1 cells. **k & l** immunohistochemistry for Evx2. **m-p** Average number of cells (y-axis) expressing indicated marker in spinal cord region adjacent to somites 6-10 in WT embryos and *evx1* and *evx2* single and double mutants (x-axis) at 24 h (**m-o**) or 30 h (**p**). Values are shown as mean +/- standard deviation (values are provided in Table 1). There are no *evx2*-positive cells in the double mutants (**n**). In each case at least 5 embryos were counted, except for *eng1b* where 4 embryos were counted. Statistically significant differences (P < 0.05) from WT values are indicated with brackets and stars. P values for these and other comparisons (e.g differences between single and double mutants) are provided in Table 1. Scale bar: 50 µm (**a-l**)

examining *eve1* expression at multiple stages of spinal cord development (every two somites from 2-somites - 24 h; Fig. 3 and data not shown). In all cases we never saw any spinal cord expression, only expression in the developing tailbud. To check whether *eve1* expression is altered in the absence of Evx1 and/or Evx2 we also examined expression in *evx1;evx2* double mutants. However, we saw no change in *eve1* expression in these double mutants (Fig. 3f). Therefore, this gene is not considered further in this paper. We also confirmed that no additional *evx* genes exist in zebrafish (Additional file 1: Results and Figure S1).

Zebrafish V0v cells develop into commissural ascending interneurons

In mouse, V0v cells develop commissural axons that ascend (grow rostrally) for one to four somite segments [23]. We used both the *Tg(evx1:EGFP)*^{SU1} transgenic line and an additional transgenic line that has stronger expression in

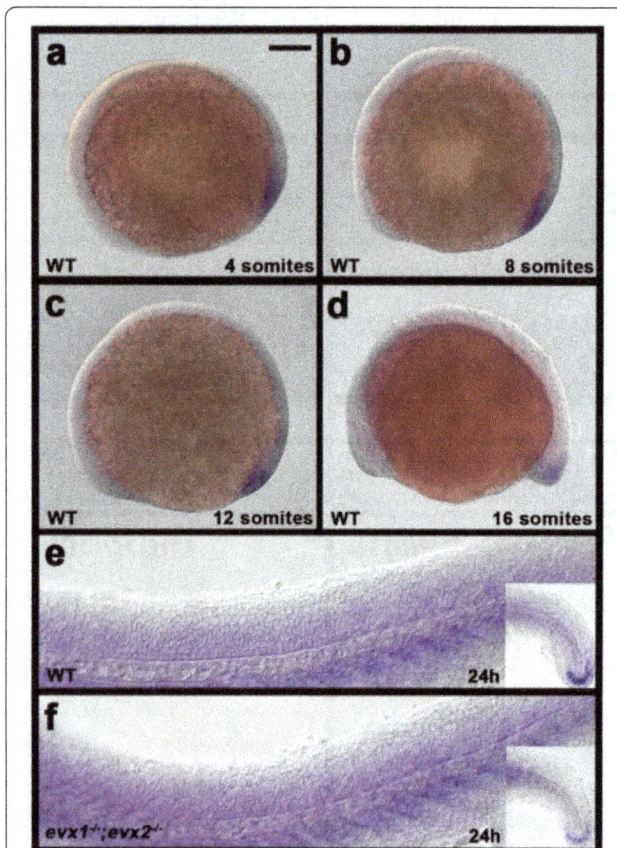

Fig. 3 *eve1* is not expressed in zebrafish spinal cord in WT or *evx1;evx2* double mutant embryos. Lateral views of *in situ* hybridization for *eve1* in 4-somite (**a**), 8-somite (**b**), 12-somite (**c**), 16-somite (**d**) and 24 h (**e & f**) embryos. **a-e** WT; (**f**) *evx1;evx2* double mutant. Anterior is left and dorsal up. Expression is seen in the tail bud region but not the spinal cord. Embryos in (**e & f**) were over-stained to check that there was no weak expression in the spinal cord. The only specific staining seen was at the end of the tail (inset in right bottom corner). The rest is background staining from over-staining. Scale bar: 100 μm

V0v cell axons, *Tg(evx1:EGFP)*^{SU2} (see methods), to examine the morphology of zebrafish V0v cells. We found that by 27-30 h, almost all of the cells have extended their axons ventrally and have at least started to cross the midline to the other side of the spinal cord (Fig 4a & b). By 48 h, most of the cells have reached the other side of the spinal cord and have turned towards the head, giving them a clear commissural ascending, or CoSA [65, 66], morphology (Fig. 4c & f).

V0v cells are glutamatergic

In wild-type mouse spinal cords, V0 cells develop into both inhibitory (glycinergic or GABAergic) and excitatory (glutamatergic) interneurons [27, 28, 36], but when we started this project the neurotransmitter phenotype of V0v cells had not been established. Zebrafish have both excitatory and inhibitory CoSA interneurons [61, 62], so we could not infer the neurotransmitter properties of V0v cells from their morphology alone. Therefore, we performed double-labeling experiments to establish the neurotransmitter fates of these cells. Double immunohistochemistry for Evx2 and EGFP in the *Tg(slc17a6:EGFP)* line which labels glutamatergic interneurons in the zebrafish spinal cord [37, 67] revealed that all of the Evx2-positive cells are glutamatergic (Fig. 5a). As expected, not all of the glutamatergic cells express Evx2, since there are several excitatory cell types in the zebrafish spinal cord and only V0v cells express Evx2. In addition, *in situ* hybridization for *slc17a6 (vglut)* genes, markers of glutamatergic cells (see methods for more details) combined with EGFP immunohistochemistry in *Tg(evx1:EGFP)*^{SU1} embryos also confirmed that *evx1*-expressing cells are glutamatergic (Fig. 5b). We also examined if *evx1* is co-expressed with markers of any other spinal cord neurotransmitter fates. Using double *in situ* hybridization we found no co-expression between *evx1* and markers for glycinergic or GABAergic markers (data not shown). We also observed no double-labeled cells when we performed EGFP immunohistochemistry and *in situ* hybridization for *slc32a1* (formerly called *viaat*) which labels all inhibitory neurons [8, 68, 69] in *Tg(evx1:EGFP)*^{SU2} embryos (Fig. 5c).

Consistent with these analyses, when we FAC-sorted and expression profiled EGFP-labeled V0v cells using the *Tg(evx1:EGFP)*^{SU1} line we found that these cells express markers of glutamatergic fates (*slc17a6a* (formerly called *vglut2.2*) and *slc17a6b* (formerly called *vglut2.1*)) and do not express either glycinergic markers (*slc6a9* (formerly called *glyt1*) or *slc6a5* (formerly called *glyt2*)) or GABAergic markers (*gad1b* or *gad2*) (Fig. 5d & e).

Zebrafish V0v cells do not express Pax2

As discussed above, Pax2 is an important regulator of inhibitory spinal cord fates [14–21]. Given that we had shown that V0v cells are excitatory (glutamatergic) and we had not observed any inhibitory V0v cells

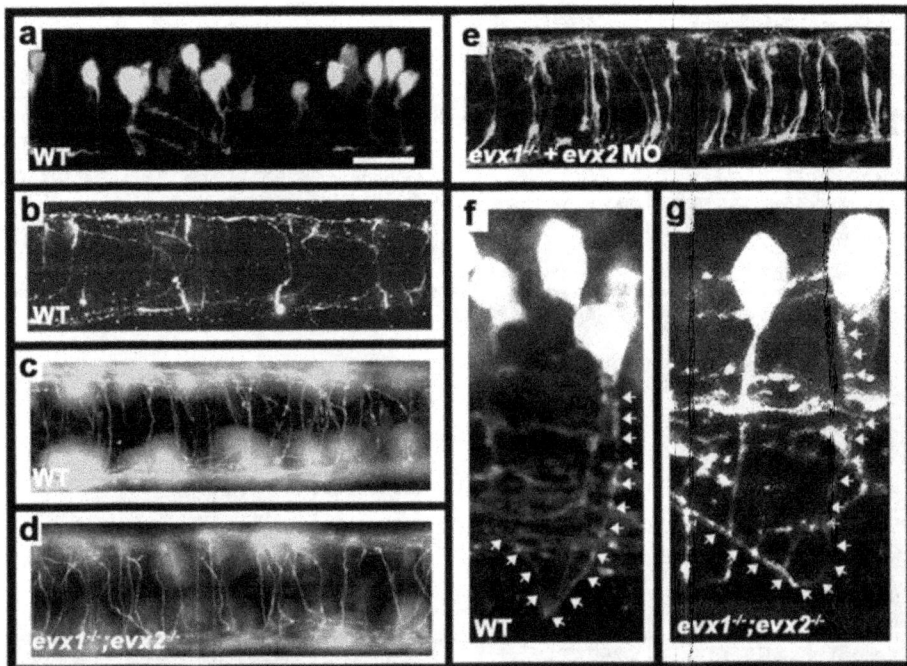

Fig. 4 V0v cells develop into CoSA interneurons. Immunohistochemistry for EGFP in *Tg(evx1:EGFP)^SU1* (**a**, **b** & **e**) or *Tg(evx1:EGFP)^SU2* (**c**, **d**, **f** & **g**) embryos. **a**, **f** & **g** lateral views with dorsal up and anterior left of spinal cord at 27 h (**a**) or 48 h (**f** & **g**). **b-e** dorsal views with anterior left of zebrafish spinal cord at 30 h (**b**) or 48 h (**c**,**e**). **a-c** & **f** WT, (**d** & **g**) *evx1;evx2* double mutant, (**e**) *evx1* mutant injected with *evx2* morpholino. **b** & **c** show increasing number of commissural axons crossing the spinal cord as development proceeds. **d** & **e** demonstrate that V0v axons are still clearly commissural in the absence of Evx1 and Evx2. **f** & **g** show magnified views of commissural ascending V0v axons. White arrows (drawn slightly to the right of the axon so that EGFP expression is still visible) indicate ascending axon trajectories. Scale bar: 50 µm (**a-e**) and 15 µm (**f** & **g**).

(Figs 5a-e), we would not predict that V0v cells would express Pax2. However, the literature contains contradictory evidence as to whether *evx1* and *evx2* are co-expressed with *pax2* in the spinal cord [35, 58, 70, 71]. To resolve this issue, we performed double-labeling experiments for *evx1* and *pax2* using several complementary approaches. These included *in situ* hybridization for *evx1* and immunohistochemistry for Pax2, EGFP immunohistochemistry and *in situ* hybridization for *pax2a*, *pax2b* and *pax8* (three highly-related *pax* genes that are co-expressed in zebrafish spinal cord cells [14]) in *Tg(evx1:EGFP)^SU2* embryos and double immunohistochemistry for EGFP and Pax2 in *Tg(evx1:EGFP)^SU2* embryos. In all cases, we observed no double-labeled cells, suggesting that *evx1* and *evx2* are not co-expressed with *pax2/ pax8* genes in zebrafish spinal cord (Fig. 6g and data not shown). These analyses complement those of Satou and colleagues [36] who recently reported that inhibitory V0 cells, which presumably correspond to V0_D cells, express Pax2, but Evx2-expressing cells do not. Taken together, these data strongly suggest that V0v cells do not express *pax2* genes.

evx2^sa140 is a null allele

To identify the functions of *evx1* and *evx2* in zebrafish V0v cells we used *evx1* and *evx2* mutants (see Methods).

Our previous analyses suggest that *evx1^i232* is a null allele [39]. The *evx2^sa140* mutation introduces a premature stop codon just before the homeodomain, suggesting that if a truncated protein is synthesized it will have no DNA binding activity. However, it is possible that a truncated protein might retain some function in the embryo. To determine if any Evx2 protein is made in mutant embryos, we used an Evx2 antibody that was made against the first 168 amino acids of zebrafish Evx2 (which corresponds exactly to the region upstream of the premature stop codon in the *evx2^sa140* mutant allele). We found that all of the WT (21/51) and heterozygous embryos (20/51) had Evx2 antibody staining but all of the homozygous mutants (10/51) did not (Fig. 1c). This strongly suggests that the *evx2* mutant allele does not produce any protein and is a null allele.

evx2^sa140 homozygous mutants are not viable

Unlike the zebrafish *evx1* mutant, which is homozygous viable [39], we never identified an adult *evx2* homozygous mutant (n = 262 fish from incrosses of heterozygous *evx2* fish, P < 0.0001 using chi-squared test). However, we did obtain fish homozygous for *evx1* and heterozygous for *evx2* (17 fish identified from a total of 191 fish from incrosses of heterozygous double mutants; P = 0.13 using

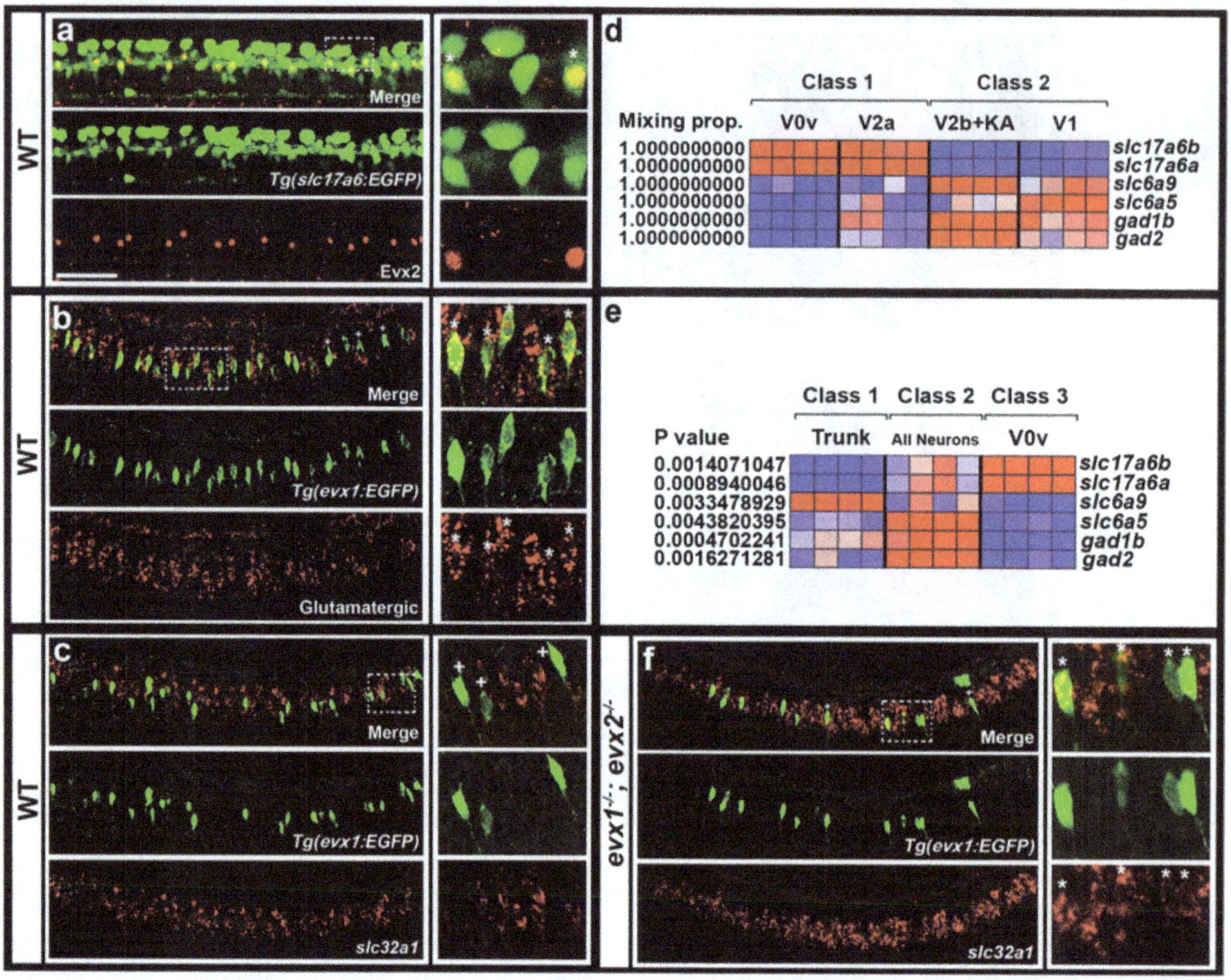

Fig. 5 Neurotransmitter phenotypes of V0v cells. Lateral views of spinal cord at 27 h (**a** & **b**) or 30 h (**c** & **f**). All panels contain merged and single channel views. Smaller images on RHS are single confocal planes of white box regions. Double and single-labeled EGFP-positive cells are indicated in single confocal planes with stars and crosses respectively. **a** EGFP (green) and Evx2 (red) expression in *Tg(slc17a6:EGFP)* embryo. All Evx2-positive cells co-express EGFP. **b** EGFP (green) and glutamatergic marker (*slc17a6b* & *slc17a6a*; red) expression in *Tg(evx1:EGFP)^SU1* embryo. Occasional single-positive cells are indicated with crosses. These may be expressing glutamatergic markers at levels too low to detect (*slc17a6* probes are weak in double-labeling experiments). Remaining cells are double-labeled. **c** & **f** EGFP (green) and *slc32a1* (red) expression in *Tg(evx1:EGFP)^SU2* WT (**c**) and *evx1;evx2* double mutant (**f**) embryos. No V0v cells are inhibitory in WT embryos, but most V0v cells are inhibitory in double mutants (occasional single-labeled cells are indicated with a cross in F). (**d** & **e**) Relative expression profiles of genes (names on right) indicative of neurotransmitter fates at 27 h. Columns represent individual microarray experiments. Rows indicate relative expression levels as normalized data transformed to mean of zero and standard deviation of +1 (highly-expressed, red) to -1 (weakly/not expressed, blue) sigma units. For details of how cells were isolated see methods. **d** Two-class eBayes comparison of excitatory (class 1) versus inhibitory (class 2) cells. Mixing proportion measures posterior probability, or likelihood that genes are differentially expressed (1 = highest probability of differential expression). **e** Three-class ANOVA comparison of V0v cells (class 3) versus trunk cells (class 1) and all post-mitotic neurons (class 2). P values test hypothesis that there is no differential expression between the 3 classes. V0v cells express glutamatergic markers *slc17a6a* and *slc17a6b* and do not express glycinergic or GABAergic markers in both comparisons. Scale bar: 50 μm (**a-c** & **f**)

chi-squared test). Our analyses of incrosses from identified *evx2* heterozygous fish suggest that *evx2* mutant embryos have no obvious morphological defects for the first few days of development but that most of them die by larval stages (see Additional file 1: Results).

V0v cells still form in *evx1;evx2* double mutants

In mouse *Evx1* mutants, expression of Evx2 is lost and there is an increase in the number of cells expressing the V1 marker *En1*. In addition, many of the cells that would normally have expressed *Evx1* develop axon trajectories similar to V1 cells. Most strikingly their axons change from being commissural to ipsilateral [23]. This suggests that in the absence of Evx1, most mouse V0v cells transfate to V1 cells.

In contrast, we found that in zebrafish *evx1* mutants there is only a small reduction in the number of cells expressing *evx2* RNA and Evx2 protein in the spinal cord

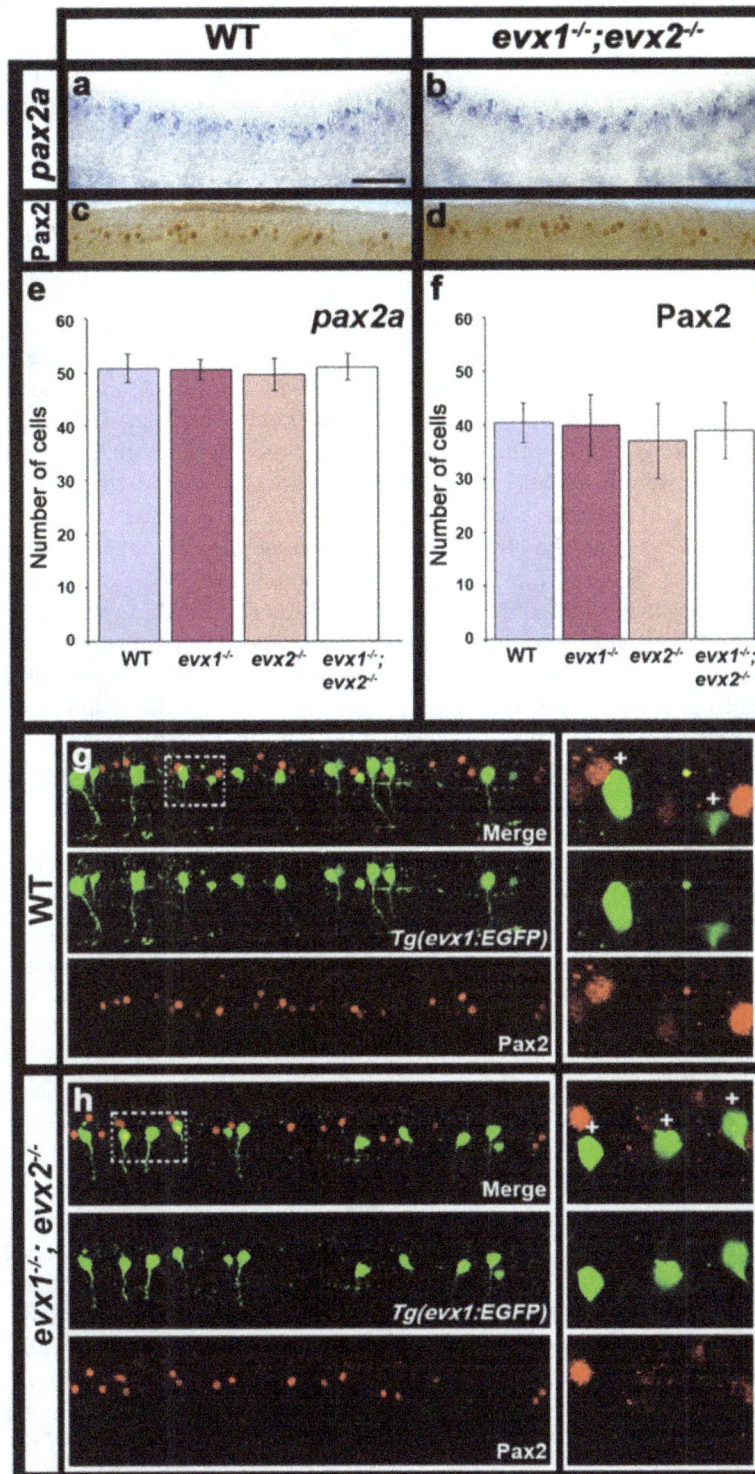

Fig. 6 V0v cells do not express Pax2 in WT or *evx1;evx2* double mutant embryos. Lateral views of zebrafish spinal cord at 24 h (**a-d**) or 30 h (**g** & **h**). Anterior left, dorsal up. **a** & **b** *in situ* hybridization for *pax2a*. **c** & **d** immunohistochemistry for Pax2. The Pax2 antibody recognizes both Pax2a and Pax2b. **e** & **f** Average number of cells (y-axis) expressing these markers (indicated in each case) in spinal cord region adjacent to somites 6-10 in WT embryos and *evx1* and *evx2* single and double mutants (x-axis). Values are shown as mean +/- standard deviation (values are provided in Table 1). In each case at least 5 embryos were counted, except for *pax2a* where 4 embryos were counted. P values for all comparisons are provided in Table 1. **g** & **h** EGFP (green) and Pax2 (red) expression in *Tg(evx1:EGFP)^SU2* WT (**g**) and *evx1;evx2* double mutant (**h**) embryos. No V0v cells express Pax2 in either case. Panels on RHS are magnified single-confocal-plane views of white dotted rectangle regions in panels G and H respectively. White crosses indicate single-positive GFP cells. Scale bar: 50 μm (**a-d**) & 40 μm (**g-h**)

(approximately a 22 % reduction for *evx2* at 24 h and a 32 % reduction for Evx2 at 30 h; Fig. 2c, l & n; Table 1), although expression of *evx2* RNA is lost completely in *evx1;evx2* double mutants (Fig. 2b & n; Table 1). In contrast, there is no difference in *evx1* expression in *evx1* or *evx2* single mutants when compared to WT siblings, although approximately 47 % of V0v cells lose expression of *evx1* in double mutants (Fig. 2j & m; Table 1). Consistent with the down-regulation of *evx1* in double mutants, we observe a 30 % reduction in the number of EGFP-labeled V0v cells in double mutant *Tg(evx1:EGFP)^{SU2}* embryos (22.9 +/- 3.4 cells in WTs; 16.0 +/- 5.5 cells in double mutants). However, strikingly, most V0v cells are still labeled with EGFP and these cells have a normal commissural ascending CoSA morphology (Fig. 4d & g). Unfortunately, we were never able to identify double mutant embryos that carried the *Tg(evx1:EGFP)^{SU1}* transgene, suggesting that this transgene probably integrated in the vicinity of the WT *evx2* allele (see methods). However, consistent with our results using the *Tg(evx1:EGFP)^{SU2}* transgenic line, when we injected *evx2* ATG morpholinos, at a concentration that eliminates Evx2 protein, into *evx1* single mutant *Tg(evx1:EGFP)^{SU1}* embryos, we also observed EGFP-labeled V0v cells with normal CoSA axon trajectories (Fig. 4e).

Consistent with this persistence of V0v cells, we also found no change in the number of *eng1b*-expressing spinal cord cells in *evx1* and *evx2* single or double mutants compared to WT embryos at 24 h. If anything, we observed a slight reduction in the number of *eng1b* cells in the double mutants, although this was not statistically significant (Fig. 2f & o, Table 1). To further confirm that V0v cells were not adopting a V1 fate and turning on *eng1b* expression, we repeated this experiment at 30 h. We still found no change in *eng1b* expression in either single or double mutants when compared to WT embryos (Fig. 2h & p, Table 1).

Taken together, these results suggest that V0v cells are not transfating into V1 cells in zebrafish, even in the absence of both Evx1 and Evx2. Instead at least most of these cells are maintaining their V0v identities. In addition, these data suggest that Evx1 and Evx2 act partially redundantly to maintain each other's expression, although only *evx2* expression requires Evx1/Evx2 activity as more than half of V0v cells still express *evx1* in *evx1;evx2* double mutants.

Evx1 and Evx2 are required for *skor2* expression in V0v cells

To identify additional transcription factors that might be required for specification of V0v functional characteristics, we expression-profiled FAC-sorted V0v cells (see Methods; [50]). From these analyses, we identified *skor2* as a transcription factor gene potentially expressed by V0v neurons.

Our subsequent *in situ* hybridization experiments demonstrated that *skor2* has two clear domains of spinal cord expression, a ventral domain and a more dorsal domain (Fig. 7c). Double labeling experiments show that in the ventral domain, at least most of the *skor2*-expressing cells are V0v cells (Fig. 7a). On average, 97 % of ventral *skor2*-expressing cells co-express EGFP in *Tg(evx1:EGFP)^{SU1}* embryos (73/75 cells counted in 4 embryos). Given this high number of double positive cells and the fact that there is usually a delay in EGFP expression it is possible that all of the ventral *skor2*-expressing cells are V0v cells. Interestingly, double labeling experiments with *skor2* and *Tg(slc17a6:EGFP)* demonstrated that both the ventral and dorsal *skor2*-expressing cells are excitatory cells (Fig. 7b), suggesting that Skor2 may play in role in specifying excitatory fates. As *skor2* is expressed by V0v cells, we tested whether it is regulated by Evx1 and Evx2. We found that the number of cells expressing *skor2* in the ventral spinal cord is reduced in *evx1* and *evx2* single mutants compared to WT embryos. More strikingly, ventral *skor2* expression is completely abolished in double *evx1;evx2* mutants (Figs 7d & e; Table 1), demonstrating that Evx1 and Evx2 are required, partially redundantly for *skor2* expression in V0v cells. In contrast, there was no change in the dorsal expression of *skor2* (Fig. 7d & e; Table 1).

Evx1 and Evx2 are required to specify the glutamatergic fates of V0v cells

Given that V0v cells still form in the absence of Evx1 and Evx2 function and their axon trajectories appear to be unaffected, but expression of a novel excitatory cell marker *skor2* is lost, we decided to test if V0v cell neurotransmitter phenotypes were changed. When we examined the expression of *slc17a6* (*vglut*) genes in embryos from a cross of *evx1;evx2* heterozygous parents, we saw a significant reduction of glutamatergic cells in both of the single mutants when compared to WT embryos and an even more severe reduction in double mutants (Fig. 8a-d & o; Table 1). These data indicate that Evx1 and Evx2 act partially redundantly to specify the glutamatergic phenotype of V0v cells. Strikingly, the number of glutamatergic cells lost in the double mutant (approximately 28 cells in the spinal cord region adjacent to somites 6-10) is equivalent to the number of V0v cells in that region of the spinal cord (approximately 29 cells express *evx2* and 33 cells express *evx1* in this region of the WT spinal cord at this stage; see Table 1), suggesting that probably all of the V0v cells have lost their glutamatergic phenotype.

V0v cells become inhibitory in *evx1;evx* double mutant embryos

Given that V0v cells lose their excitatory phenotype in *evx1;evx2* double mutants, we asked whether they are acquiring an inhibitory neurotransmitter fate instead.

Table 1 Number of cells expressing particular genes and proteins in WT and mutant embryos

Marker	Stage	WT	evx1 mutants	P[a]	evx2 mutants	P[b]	Double mutants	P[c]	P[d]	P[e]
evx1	24 h	33.0 + /-2.0	31.0 + /-3.3	0.32	31.3 + /-2.5	0.56	17.4 + /-2.6	**<0.01**	**<0.01**	**<0.01**
evx2	24 h	28.6 + /-1.6	22.4 + /-50	**0.02**	13.5 + /-3.5	**<0.01**	0.00	**<0.01**	**<0.01**	**<0.01**
Evx2	30 h	33.6 + /-5.2	23.0 + /-4.6	**0.01**	N.D		N.D			
eng1b	24 h	43.3 + /-2.5	43.6 + /-2.0	0.80	43.5 + /-4.0	0.94	37.2 + /-6.0	0.08	0.07	0.10
eng1b	30 h	63.0 + /-3.0	62.0 + /-2.5	0.63	63.0 + /-2.5	0.92	65.2 + /-2.0	0.15	0.06	0.15
slc17a6 (vlgut)	24 h	89.0 + /-10.0	71.3 + /-4.3	**<0.01**	74.6 + /-8.0	**0.01**	60.8 + /-10	**<0.01**	0.08	**0.04**
slc32a1 (viaat)	24 h	157.4 + /-8.0	157.3 + /-10.0	0.75	158.2 + /-4.0	0.86	178.6 + /-7.0	**<0.01**	**<0.01**	**<0.01**
gads (GABAergic)	24 h	50.0 + /-3.0	49.0 + /-4.0	0.59	51.6 + /-2.6	0.31	50.6 + /-2.2	0.66	0.38	0.5
slc6a5 (glyt2a/glyt2b)	24 h	81.0 + /-3.3	93.0 + /-9.0	**<0.01**	87.6 + /-4.5	**0.02**	109 + /-10.0	**<0.01**	**0.02**	**<0.01**
pax2a	24 h	50.6 + /-2.6	50.4 + /-2.0	0.86	49.5 + /-30	0.55	50.8 + /-2.5	0.91	0.75	0.49
Pax2	24 h	40.3 + /-3.8	39.8 + /-5.7	0.83	36.9 + /-6.9	0.23	38.8 + /-5.3	0.41	0.68	0.52
skor2	30 h	24.3 + /-3.0	15.0 + /-5.0	**<0.01**	19.8 + /-4.0	0.07	0.0	**<0.01**	**<0.01**	**<0.01**
skor2 Total cell counts	30 h	46.7 + /-3.7	38.7 + /-3.3	**<0.01**	42.4 + /-1.7	**0.04**	22.6 + /-1.7	**<0.01**	**<0.01**	**<0.01**

Numbers of cells expressing particular markers (first column on left) in spinal cord region adjacent to somites 6-10 and P values of comparisons between embryos with different genotypes. Values are shown as the mean from at least 5 different embryos +/- standard deviation, except for *pax2a* and *eng1b* where 4 embryos were counted. P values are from student's *t*-tests. Statistically significant (P < 0.05) values are indicated in bold. P[a] compares *evx1* single mutants with WT embryos, P[b] compares *evx2* single mutants with WT embryos, P[c], P[d] and P[e] are for comparisons between double mutant embryos and WT (P[c]), *evx1* single mutant (P[d]) and *evx2* single mutant (P[e]) embryos respectively. Mean cell count values are provided to one decimal place and P values to two decimal places. For *skor2*, two sets of values are provided: just the ventral domain of expression and both the ventral and dorsal domains of expression (total cell counts)

When we examined expression of *slc32a1*, which is expressed by all inhibitory neurons [8, 68, 69], there was no significant difference in the number of cells expressing this gene between either of the single mutants and WT embryos (Fig. 8e, g, h & p, Table 1). However, interestingly, there was a significant increase (approximately 21 cells) in the number of *slc32a1*-expressing cells in *evx1;evx2* double mutants (Fig. 8f & p, Table 1). This suggests that Evx1 and Evx2 act redundantly to repress the inhibitory fate in V0v cells.

To further confirm that V0v cells are switching to an inhibitory fate, we performed *in situ* hybridization for *slc32a1* plus immunohistochemistry for EGFP in embryos from a cross of double heterozygous parents that carry the *Tg(evx1:EGFP)^{SU2}* transgene. In WT embryos we see no co-expression of *slc32a1* and EGFP (Fig. 5c). However, in double mutant embryos most V0v cells express *slc32a1* (77 % of EGFP-positive V0v cells (30/39 cells counted in 2 embryos); Fig. 5f).

To determine whether V0v cells are becoming GABAergic and/or glycinergic we examined expression of markers of these two fates. We see no significant difference in the number of cells expressing GABAergic markers in single or double mutant embryos (Fig. 8m, n & r). In contrast, there is an increase in the number of cells expressing glycinergic markers. Interestingly, and in contrast to the *slc32a1* (*viaat*) result, we see a slight increase in both single mutants as well as a more pronounced increase in double mutants (Fig. 8i-l & q, Table 1). The increase in double mutants (approximately 28 cells) suggests that all V0v cells are becoming glycinergic.

V0v cells become glycinergic through a novel Pax2-independent mechanism

All of the transcription factors that have been identified so far as specifying inhibitory spinal fates act through Pax2 [14–21]. In addition, Tlx1 and Tlx3, the only other transcription factors that have been identified as specifying excitatory spinal cord fates [4, 5, 8], work at least in part by down-regulating Pax2 [4]. Therefore, we decided to test if V0v cells turn on Pax2 expression in *evx1;evx2* double mutants. However, when we analyzed *pax2a* expression there was no significant difference in the number of cells expressing this gene in either the single or double mutants compared to WT embryos (Fig. 6b & e; Table 1). To further confirm this result, we performed immunohistochemistry using a Pax2 antibody that recognizes Pax2a and Pax2b [55]. Again, we saw no significant change in the number of cells expressing Pax2 protein in single or double mutants (Fig. 6d & f; Table 1). Finally, we also performed double-labeling experiments for Pax2 and EGFP in WT and mutant embryos that carried the *Tg(evx1:EGFP)^{SU2}* transgene, using either the Pax2 antibody or *in situ* hybridization with a mix of *pax2a*, *pax2b* and *pax8* probes. In each case we examined at least two WT embryos and two double homozygous mutants and we did not observe any double-labeled cells (Fig. 6h and data not shown).

Taken together these results show that V0v cells are becoming glycinergic through a Pax2-independent mechanism. This is the first time that a Pax2-independent mechanism of glycinergic specification has been identified in spinal cord neurons.

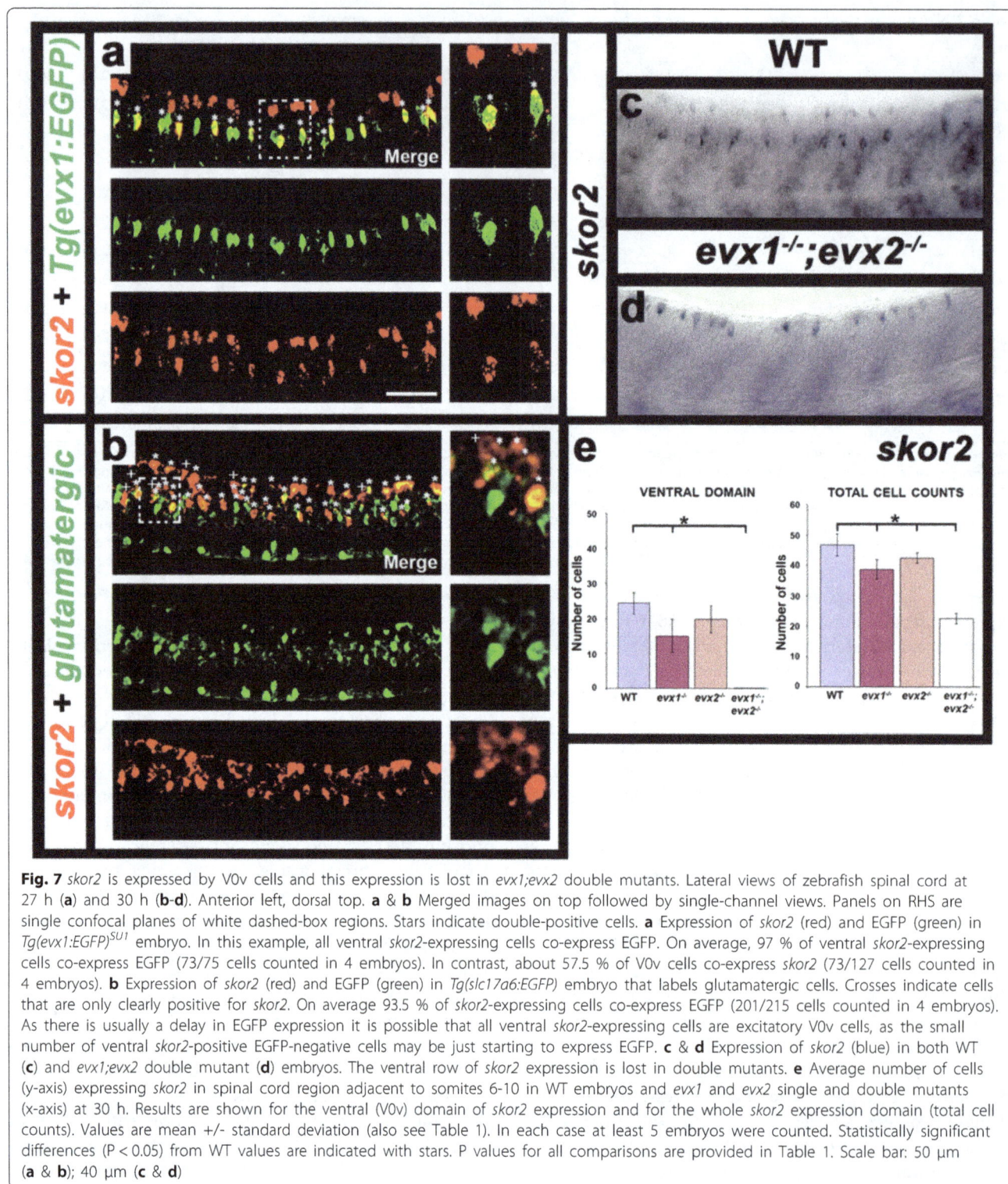

Fig. 7 *skor2* is expressed by V0v cells and this expression is lost in *evx1;evx2* double mutants. Lateral views of zebrafish spinal cord at 27 h (**a**) and 30 h (**b-d**). Anterior left, dorsal top. **a** & **b** Merged images on top followed by single-channel views. Panels on RHS are single confocal planes of white dashed-box regions. Stars indicate double-positive cells. **a** Expression of *skor2* (red) and EGFP (green) in *Tg(evx1:EGFP)^SU1^* embryo. In this example, all ventral *skor2*-expressing cells co-express EGFP. On average, 97 % of ventral *skor2*-expressing cells co-express EGFP (73/75 cells counted in 4 embryos). In contrast, about 57.5 % of V0v cells co-express *skor2* (73/127 cells counted in 4 embryos). **b** Expression of *skor2* (red) and EGFP (green) in *Tg(slc17a6:EGFP)* embryo that labels glutamatergic cells. Crosses indicate cells that are only clearly positive for *skor2*. On average 93.5 % of *skor2*-expressing cells co-express EGFP (201/215 cells counted in 4 embryos). As there is usually a delay in EGFP expression it is possible that all ventral *skor2*-expressing cells are excitatory V0v cells, as the small number of ventral *skor2*-positive EGFP-negative cells may be just starting to express EGFP. **c** & **d** Expression of *skor2* (blue) in both WT (**c**) and *evx1;evx2* double mutant (**d**) embryos. The ventral row of *skor2* expression is lost in double mutants. **e** Average number of cells (y-axis) expressing *skor2* in spinal cord region adjacent to somites 6-10 in WT embryos and *evx1* and *evx2* single and double mutants (x-axis) at 30 h. Results are shown for the ventral (V0v) domain of *skor2* expression and for the whole *skor2* expression domain (total cell counts). Values are mean +/- standard deviation (also see Table 1). In each case at least 5 embryos were counted. Statistically significant differences (P < 0.05) from WT values are indicated with stars. P values for all comparisons are provided in Table 1. Scale bar: 50 μm (**a** & **b**); 40 μm (**c** & **d**)

Discussion

Evx genes are found in a wide range of animals ranging from corals to humans [72]. They encode transcription factors that contain both DNA-binding homeobox and C-terminal repressor domains [73–77]. Amniotes have two *Evx* genes (*Evx1* and *Evx2*) and teleosts, including zebrafish, have three (*evx1*, *evx2* and *eve1*), although only *evx1* and *evx2* are expressed in the spinal cord ([26, 32, 33, 59, 64]; this paper Figs. 2, 3, Additional file 1: Results and Figure S1). Interestingly, the genomic

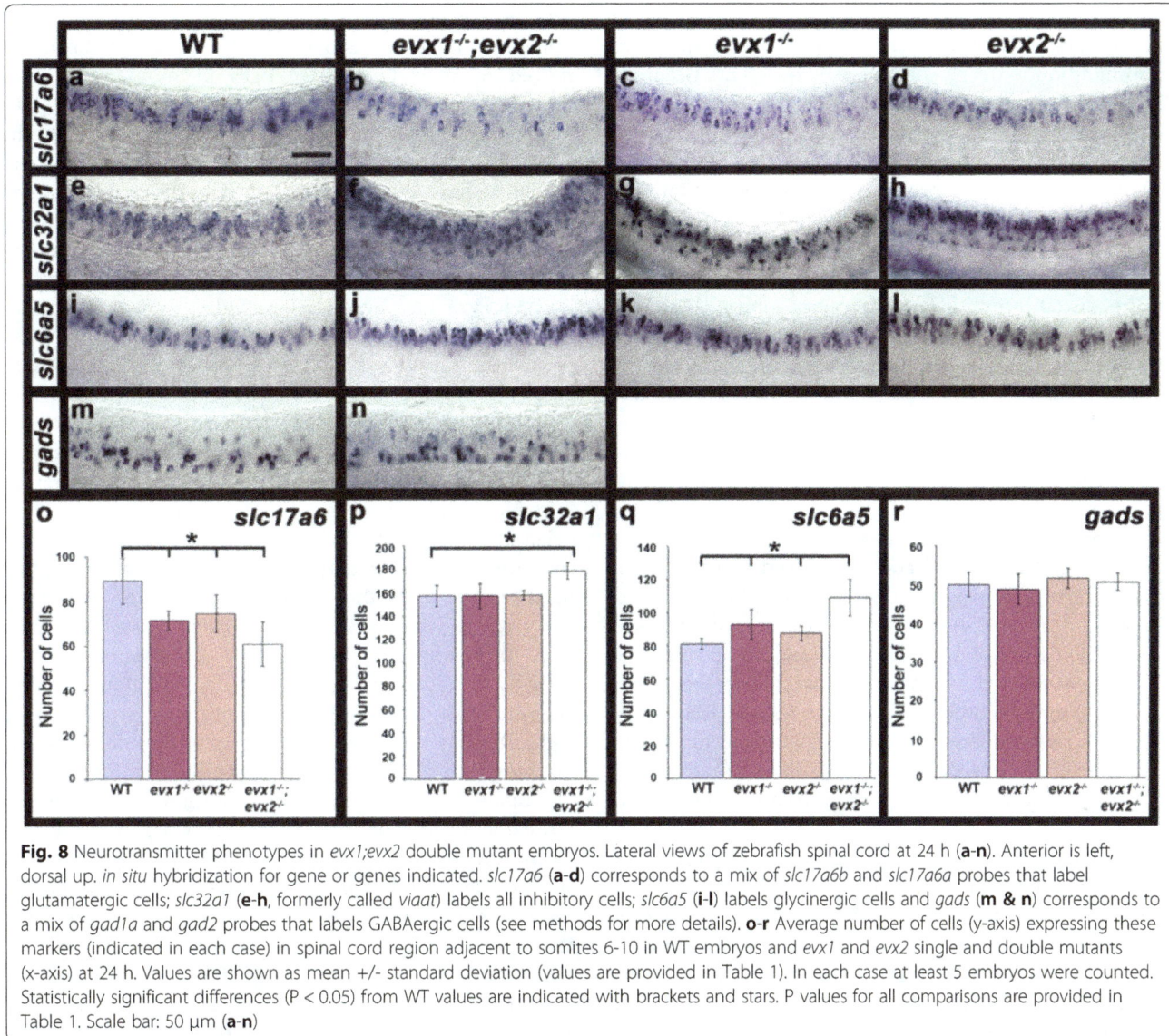

Fig. 8 Neurotransmitter phenotypes in *evx1;evx2* double mutant embryos. Lateral views of zebrafish spinal cord at 24 h (**a-n**). Anterior is left, dorsal up. *in situ* hybridization for gene or genes indicated. *slc17a6* (**a-d**) corresponds to a mix of *slc17a6b* and *slc17a6a* probes that label glutamatergic cells; *slc32a1* (**e-h**, formerly called *viaat*) labels all inhibitory cells; *slc6a5* (**i-l**) labels glycinergic cells and *gads* (**m & n**) corresponds to a mix of *gad1a* and *gad2* probes that labels GABAergic cells (see methods for more details). **o-r** Average number of cells (y-axis) expressing these markers (indicated in each case) in spinal cord region adjacent to somites 6-10 in WT embryos and *evx1* and *evx2* single and double mutants (x-axis) at 24 h. Values are shown as mean +/- standard deviation (values are provided in Table 1). In each case at least 5 embryos were counted. Statistically significant differences (P < 0.05) from WT values are indicated with brackets and stars. P values for all comparisons are provided in Table 1. Scale bar: 50 μm (**a-n**)

positions of these *evx* genes (adjacent to specific *Hox* clusters) along with phylogenetic analyses strongly suggest that the third *evx* gene in teleosts (*eve1*) is not the result of the extra genome duplication in the teleost lineage ([26, 78, 79], Additional file 1). Instead, it is likely that all three of these genes originated from the two rounds of whole genome duplication that occurred early in the vertebrate lineage [80] and *eve1* was later lost in the tetrapod lineage ([26, 78], Additional file 1).

Here we provide the first comprehensive analysis of the functions of Evx1 and Evx2 in spinal cord interneuron development in any vertebrate. We demonstrate that, within the spinal cord, both of these transcription factors are expressed exclusively by V0v cells. We also show that V0v cells are glutamatergic. These findings complement and extend those of Satou and colleagues [36], who reported that Evx2-expressing cells that

develop from the *dbx1b* progenitor domain in zebrafish express the glutamateric maker *slc17a6b* and Talpalar and colleagues [9], who showed that mouse V0v cells express the glutamatergic marker *slc17a6* (*vglut2*). In addition, we confirm and extend previous reports that suggested that V0v neurons extend commissural axons [23, 27, 35, 36] and we identify these neurons as CoSA interneurons. Interestingly, while Satou and colleagues [36] observed similar V0v cell morphologies at the stages that we have examined, at later stages of development they also saw descending and bifurcating commissural excitatory V0 cells, suggesting that V0v cells may diversify morphologically at later developmental stages [36].

In mouse *Evx1* mutants, most V0v cells completely change their fate and acquire characteristics of V1 cells, the cell-type that normally forms ventral to V0v cells. Cells that would have formed V0v interneurons lose expression of Evx1 and Evx2 and instead express the V1 marker Engrailed1 (En1) and develop axon trajectories and migration patterns characteristic of V1 interneurons [23]. Most notably, their axon trajectories change from being contralateral to ipsilateral [23]. In addition, experiments in chick embryos revealed that ectopic Evx is sufficient to suppress Engrailed expression and therefore presumably V1 cell fate [23]. The role of Evx2 in mouse V0v cells is less well understood. Evx2 expression is dependent on Evx1, suggesting that it may be involved in the specification events described above [23], but spinal cord phenotypes of *Evx2* mutants have not been described in mouse and before this study, *Evx1;Evx2* double mutants had not been described in any vertebrate.

These amniote data suggest that Evx1 is required to inhibit the V1 fate in post-mitotic V0v cells. This global cell fate change is unusual for a transcription factor expressed in post-mitotic cells: it is more commonly seen with transcription factors expressed in spinal progenitor domains (e.g. [27–29, 81, 82]). For example, Nkx2.2 is a transcription factor expressed in the p3 progenitor domain and in *Nkx2.2* mutant mice, cells that would have formed V3 interneurons change their fates (transfate) and become motoneurons instead [83]. Similarly, Dbx1 is expressed in the progenitor domain (p0) from which V0 cells develop and in *Dbx1* mutant mice, cells that would have become V0v cells assume the characteristics of V1 cells [27, 28].

Interestingly, our results are different and yield novel insights into Evx1 and Evx2 function in the spinal cord. We see no evidence of V0v cells transfating to V1 cells in zebrafish *evx1* and *evx2* single or double mutants. Notably, there is no increase in the number of cells expressing *eng1b*, which is specifically expressed in V1 cells, or Pax2, which is expressed by V1 and V0$_D$ cells. Instead most V0v cells continue to express *evx1* mRNA and *Tg(evx1:EGFP)* and these EGFP-labelled V0v neurons have what appear to be normal CoSA axon morphologies. These data strongly suggest that V0v cells still form in zebrafish *evx1;evx2* double mutants and that they do not become a different class of neuron. One possible explanation for the differences between our results and the previously reported analyses in mouse might be evolutionary changes in the functions of Evx1 and Evx2. However, it is also possible that the consequences of removing these transcription factors are different in mouse and zebrafish because of variations in the expression of Dbx1 and/or the timing of V0v development. Interestingly, in this paper, we have shown that expression of *dbx1a* and *dbx1b* persists in at least some V0v cells in zebrafish. Therefore, it is possible that in zebrafish *evx1;evx2* mutants, Dbx might be able to inhibit post-mitotic V0v cells from becoming V1 cells

(Fig. 9). Given the speed of zebrafish spinal cord development it is also possible that V0v cells become committed to their fate faster than in mouse and that, therefore, the window of time during which the V1 fate needs to be inhibited in V0v cells is much shorter in zebrafish than in mammals (see [84] for a different example of how the fast speed of zebrafish development can produce changes in spinal cord development). Regardless of how V0v global cell fate specification has evolved, the fact that V0v cells still form in zebrafish lacking Evx1 and Evx2, has provided us with a unique opportunity to identify Evx functions in V0v cells, independent of any role that these transcription factors may also have in repressing the V1 cell fate.

Our results show that in zebrafish, Evx1 and Evx2 act partially redundantly to specify the glutamatergic fate of V0v cells and inhibit an alternative glycinergic fate in these cells. Given that the only spinal cord cells that express *evx1* and *evx2* are V0v cells and that the only other trunk tissue that expresses either of these genes is the posterior gut, which expresses *evx1*, we consider that this requirement for Evx1 and Evx2 function is likely to be cell-autonomous. Interestingly, while there is a reduction of glutamatergic cells in both single and double mutants, expression of the inhibitory marker *slc32a1* is only increased in double mutants, suggesting that the specification of glutamatergic fates and the inhibition of glycinergic fates may be independent processes which require different levels of Evx activity. However, in contrast to *slc32a1*, the number of cells expressing the glycinergic marker *slc6a5* was slightly increased in single mutants, which suggests that the expression of different neurotransmitter transporter proteins is regulated independently and by distinct levels of Evx activity. These results are intriguing as they suggest that the regulation of neurotransmitter transporters and enzymes might be complex, with different components being regulated by distinct mechanisms.

V0v interneurons are a crucial part of locomotor circuitry as they are required for hindlimb left-right alternation during fast locomotion [9, 27, 34]. Therefore, changing the neurotransmitter fate of these cells might be expected to impair fast movements. Unfortunately, as *evx2* mutants die by larval stages, we were not able to assess whether *evx2* single mutants or *evx1;evx2* double mutants have locomotion defects. In addition, *evx1* single mutants lack joints in their fins [39], making it impossible to evaluate if any difference in *evx1* single mutant behavior is due to this fin phenotype or a locomotive defect. Interestingly, we did not observe any obvious changes in V0v cell morphology or axon trajectory in *evx1;evx2* double mutants. Given the changed neurotransmitter

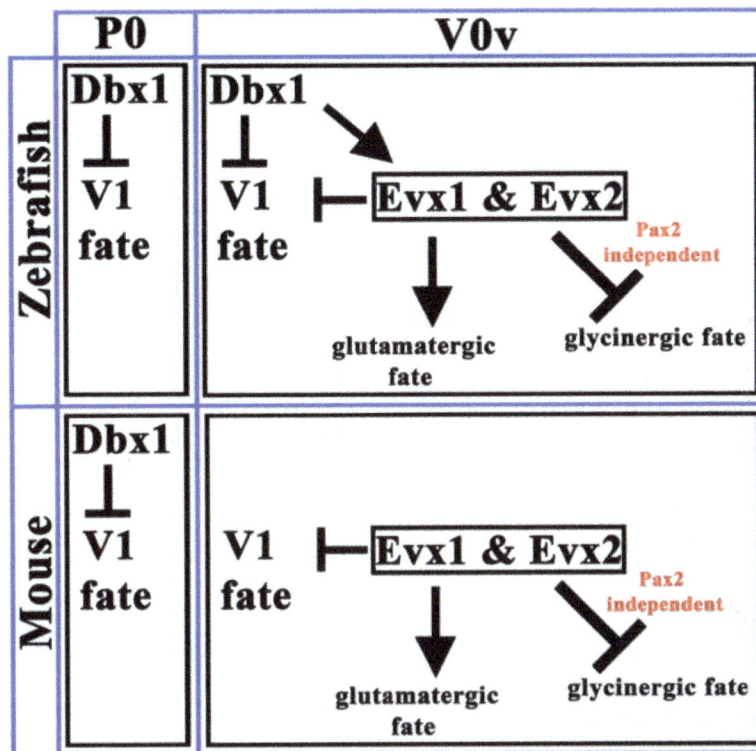

Fig. 9 A Model for Evx Function in V0v cells. A possible model that would reconcile the different phenotypes of mouse and zebrafish *Evx1* mutants. In this model, Dbx1 expression in P0 cells is required for the expression of Evx1 and Evx2 in V0v cells (for simplicity this interaction is not shown) and Dbx1 can also independently repress the V1 fate. In zebrafish, Dbx1 expression persists for a while in newly formed V0v cells. This may be sufficient for the V1 fate to be inhibited in post-mitotic V0v cells, even in the absence of Evx1 and Evx2, thereby revealing other functions of Evx transcription factors. This could explain why V0v cells still form in *evx1;evx2* double mutants, but they express glycinergic rather than gluta-matergic markers. In contrast, in mouse Dbx1 is expressed only in progenitor cells. Therefore, in newly formed V0v cells only Evx1 and Evx2 inhibit the V1 fate and in the absence of these transcription factors V0v cells transfate into V1 cells

phenotype of V0v cells in these animals this might be considered surprising, although it is consistent with our previous analysis of V1 cells, that maintain their ipsilateral axon trajectories even when they lose their inhibitory fates in the absence of Pax2 and Pax8 [14]. It is still possible though that there are subtle changes in V0v cell wiring and/or changes in V0v cell connectivity in *evx1;evx2* double mutants as a result of their change in neurotransmitter fate. As there are fewer GFP-labelled V0v cells in *evx1;evx2* double mutants it is also possible that V0v cells with inappropriate neurotransmitter fates eventually die, although alternatively this reduction in the number of GFP-positive cells may just reflect autoregulation of Evx expression.

In this paper, we also describe the expression of a different transcription factor gene expressed by V0v cells, *skor2*. *Skor2* expression has also been reported in the mouse spinal cord but the cells that express it were not identified [85]. Our results show that *skor2* is expressed by a subset of V0v cells as well as at least one population of more dorsal excitatory spinal cord cells.

We also demonstrate that expression of *skor2* in V0v cells requires Evx1 and Evx2 activity. Given that *skor2* is predominantly expressed by excitatory cells, it is possible that it acts downstream of Evx1 and Evx2 in V0v cells in either the specification of glutamatergic fates and/or the inhibition of glycinergic fates and that it might also have this function in other cells. However it is also possible that Skor2 acts downstream of Evx1 and Evx2 in some other as-yet-unidentified aspect of V0v cell specification. These alternatives can be tested by future loss-of-function analyses of Skor2.

Excitingly, in addition to demonstrating the roles of Evx1 and Evx2 in neurotransmitter specification, our data also show that these transcription factors function independently of Pax2 in specifying glutamatergic fates and inhibiting glycinergic fates. This is the first time that a Pax2-independent mechanism of inhibitory fate specification has been identified in the spinal cord. While several transcription factors have been identified that specify the inhibitory fates of particular spinal cord neurons, so far all of these act upstream of Pax2 [14–18]. In addition, as mentioned before, the only other transcription factors that have been identified as specifying excitatory spinal cord fates, Tlx1 and Tlx3 [4, 5, 8], work at least in part by down-regulating Pax2 [4]. Therefore, our finding that V0v cells become inhibitory in *evx1;evx2* double mutants but do not express Pax2 is a significant one as it demonstrates that there must be an additional Pax2-independent mechanism for specifying inhibitory neurons in the spinal cord.

Conclusions

In conclusion, in this paper we demonstrate that zebrafish V0v cells express *evx1* and *evx2* and develop into excitatory (glutamatergic) CoSA interneurons. We also show that Evx1 and Evx2 are required, partially redundantly for expression of *skor2* and glutamatergic markers and inhibition of glycinergic markers in V0v cells and that in the absence of Evx1 and Evx2 function V0v cells become glycinergic through a novel Pax2-independent mechanism. Taken together, our data significantly increase our understanding of how neurotransmitter fates are specified and the genetic networks involved in these processes.

Abbreviations

CNE: conserved non-coding element; CNS: central nervous system; CoSA: commisural secondary ascending; DAB: 3,3'- diaminobenzidine; dpf: days post fertilization; FACS: fluorescent activated cell sorting; Gads: glutamic acid decarboxylases; h: hours post fertilization; LHS: left hand side; RHS: right hand side; WT: wild type.

Competing interests

The authors have no competing interests.

Authors' contributions

JM created the *Tg(evx:EGFP)* lines and performed most of the experiments in the paper, including most of the single and double labeling experiments in WT, single mutant and double mutant embryos and all of the cell counts except those for the *skor2* double labeling experiments; CS performed initial experiments with the *evx1* mutant and *evx1* and *evx2* morpholinos and helped to formulate many of the hypotheses that this study tests; CS also performed many of the WT expression analyses of *evx1*, *evx2* and *eve1*, including some of the initial double labeling experiments; SE performed the synteny and phylogenetic analyses; SP and GV genotyped embryos and adult fish and helped to establish stable *Tg(evx:EGFP)* WT and mutant lines; SP and GV also examined Evx2 expression in WT and *evx2* single mutant embryos and performed the *evx2* mutant survival experiments; SP also performed the double staining for Evx2 and EGFP in *Tg(slc17a6:EGFP)* embryos; WH performed the initial analysis of *skor2* and the double labeling experiments between *skor2* and other markers; SE and SdJ performed the FACS and expression profiling analyses; KL designed and directed the study; KL and JM wrote most of the paper with input from the other authors.

Acknowledgments

We thank Dr Shinichi Higashijima for kindly providing us with Evx2 antibody, Dr Derek Stemple and everyone working on the zebrafish mutation project at the Wellcome Trust Sanger Centre for the *evx2* mutant allele, ZFIN for providing information on nomenclature and other essential zebrafish resources, Nigel Miller at the Flow Cytometry Facility, Department of Pathology, University of Cambridge, Cambridge, for his expert FAC-sorting, Tomi Ivacevic and Vladimir Benes at the Genomics Core Facility at EMBL, Heidelberg, for RNA amplification, labelling, and hybridization, Uwe Strähle, Olivier Armant and Jasmin Lampert for help with designing microarrays, Nicole Santos for help with genotyping, Henry Putz, Jessica Bouchard, Annika Swanson and several SU undergraduate fish husbandry workers for help with maintaining zebrafish lines and Dr Santanu Banerjee for helpful comments on a previous version of this manuscript.

Funding

This work was supported by NSF IOS-1257583, NIH NINDS R21NS073979, the Spinal Cord Injury Trust Fund through New York State Department of Health Contract #C030177, a Royal Society University Research Fellowship and Syracuse University start-up funds awarded to K.E.L; BBSRC, Cambridge Trust, DAAD and Daimler-Benz-Foundation funding awarded to C.J.S; NSF HRD-0703452 LSAMP and Syracuse University Ruth Meyer funding awarded to S.A.P and NSF HRD-1202480 LSAMP and Syracuse University Ruth Meyer funding awarded to G.K.V.

Author details

[1]Department of Biology, Syracuse University, 107 College Place, Syracuse, NY 13244, USA. [2]Department of Physiology, Development and Neuroscience, University of Cambridge, Downing Street, Cambridge CB2 3DY, UK. [3]Department of Neuroscience and Physiology, SUNY Upstate Medical University, 505 Irving Avenue, Syracuse, NY 13210, USA.

References

1. Goulding M. Circuits controlling vertebrate locomotion: moving in a new direction. Nat Rev Neurosci. 2009;10(7):507–18.
2. Lewis KE. How do genes regulate simple behaviours? Understanding how different neurons in the vertebrate spinal cord are genetically specified. Philos Trans R Soc Lond B Biol Sci. 2006;361(1465):45–66.
3. Gosgnach S, Lanuza GM, Butt SJ, Saueressig H, Zhang Y, Velasquez T, et al. V1 spinal neurons regulate the speed of vertebrate locomotor outputs. Nature. 2006;440(7081):215–9.
4. Li WC, Higashijima S, Parry DM, Roberts A, Soffe SR. Primitive roles for inhibitory interneurons in developing frog spinal cord. J Neurosci. 2004; 24(25):5840–8.
5. Higashijima S, Masino M, Mandel G, Fetcho JR. Engrailed-1 Expression Marks a Primitive Class of Inhibitory Spinal Interneuron. J Neurosci. 2004;24(25): 5827–39.
6. Crone SA, Zhong G, Harris-Warrick R, Sharma K. In mice lacking V2a interneurons, gait depends on speed of locomotion. J Neurosci. 2009;29(21): 7098–109.
7. Crone SA, Quinlan KA, Zagoraiou L, Droho S, Restrepo CE, Lundfald L, et al. Genetic ablation of V2a ipsilateral interneurons disrupts left-right locomotor coordination in mammalian spinal cord. Neuron. 2008;60(1):70–83.
8. Kimura Y, Okamura Y, Higashijima S. alx, a zebrafish homolog of Chx10, marks ipsilateral descending excitatory interneurons that participate in the regulation of spinal locomotor circuits. J Neurosci. 2006;26(21):5684–97.
9. Talpalar AE, Bouvier J, Borgius L, Fortin G, Pierani A, Kiehn O. Dual-mode operation of neuronal networks involved in left-right alternation. Nature. 2013;500(7460):85–8.
10. Xue M, Atallah BV, Scanziani M. Equalizing excitation-inhibition ratios across visual cortical neurons. Nature. 2014;511(7511):596–600.
11. Zadori D, Veres G, Szalardy L, Klivenyi P, Toldi J, Vecsei L. Glutamatergic dysfunctioning in Alzheimer's disease and related therapeutic targets. J Alzheimers Dis. 2014;42 Suppl 3:S177–187.
12. Bateup HS, Johnson CA, Denefrio CL, Saulnier JL, Kornacker K, Sabatini BL. Excitatory/inhibitory synaptic imbalance leads to hippocampal hyperexcitability in mouse models of tuberous sclerosis. Neuron. 2013; 78(3):510–22.
13. Pittenger C, Bloch MH, Williams K. Glutamate abnormalities in obsessive compulsive disorder: neurobiology, pathophysiology, and treatment. Pharmacol Ther. 2011;132(3):314–32.
14. Batista MF, Lewis KE. Pax2/8 act redundantly to specify glycinergic and GABAergic fates of multiple spinal interneurons. Dev Biol. 2008;323(1):88–97.
15. Cheng L, Samad OA, Xu Y, Mizuguchi R, Luo P, Shirasawa S, et al. Lbx1 and Tlx3 are opposing switches in determining GABAergic versus glutamatergic transmitter phenotypes. Nat Neurosci. 2005;8(11):1510–5.

16. Mizuguchi R, Kriks S, Cordes R, Gossler A, Ma Q, Goulding M. Ascl1 and Gsh1/2 control inhibitory and excitatory cell fate in spinal sensory interneurons. Nat Neurosci. 2006;9(6):770–8.

17. Glasgow SM, Henke RM, Macdonald RJ, Wright CV, Johnson JE. Ptf1a determines GABAergic over glutamatergic neuronal cell fate in the spinal cord dorsal horn. Development. 2005;132(24):5461–9.

18. Pillai A, Mansouri A, Behringer R, Westphal H, Goulding M. Lhx1 and Lhx5 maintain the inhibitory-neurotransmitter status of interneurons in the dorsal spinal cord. Development. 2007;134(2):357–66.

19. Guo Z, Zhao C, Huang M, Huang T, Fan M, Xie Z, et al. Tlx1/3 and Ptf1a control the expression of distinct sets of transmitter and peptide receptor genes in the developing dorsal spinal cord. J Neurosci. 2012;32(25):8509–20.

20. Huang M, Huang T, Xiang Y, Xie Z, Chen Y, Yan R, et al. Ptf1a, Lbx1 and Pax2 coordinate glycinergic and peptidergic transmitter phenotypes in dorsal spinal inhibitory neurons. Dev Biol. 2008;322(2):394–405.

21. Hori K, Cholewa-Waclaw J, Nakada Y, Glasgow SM, Masui T, Henke RM, et al. A nonclassical bHLH Rbpj transcription factor complex is required for specification of GABAergic neurons independent of Notch signaling. Gene Dev. 2008;22(2):166–78.

22. Cheng L, Arata A, Mizuguchi R, Qian Y, Karunaratne A, Gray PA, et al. Tlx3 and Tlx1 are post-mitotic selector genes determining glutamatergic over GABAergic cell fates. Nat Neurosci. 2004;7(5):510–7.

23. Moran-Rivard L, Kagawa T, Saueressig H, Gross MK, Burrill J, Goulding M. Evx1 is a postmitotic determinant of V0 interneuron identity in the spinal cord. Neuron. 2001;29(2):385–99.

24. Dolle P, Fraulob V, Duboule D. Developmental expression of the mouse Evx-2 gene: relationship with the evolution of the HOM/Hox complex. Dev Suppl. 1994;143–153.

25. Bastian H, Gruss P. A murine even-skipped homologue, Evx 1, is expressed during early embryogenesis and neurogenesis in a biphasic manner. EMBO J. 1990;9(6):1839–52.

26. Avaron F, Thaeron-Antono C, Beck CW, Borday-Birraux V, Geraudie J, Casane D, et al. Comparison of even-skipped related gene expression pattern in vertebrates shows an association between expression domain loss and modification of selective constraints on sequences. Evol Dev. 2003;5(2):145–56.

27. Lanuza G, Gosgnach S, Pierani A, Jessel T, Goulding M. Genetic Identification of Spinal Interneurons that Coordinate Left-Right Locomotor Activity Necessary for Walking Movements. Neuron. 2004;42:375–86.

28. Pierani A, Moran-Rivard L, Sunshine MJ, Littman DR, Goulding M, Jessell TM. Control of interneuron fate in the developing spinal cord by the progenitor homeodomain protein Dbx1. Neuron. 2001;29(2):367–84.

29. Briscoe J, Pierani A, Jessell TM, Ericson J. A homeodomain protein code specifies progenitor cell identity and neuronal fate in the ventral neural tube. Cell. 2000;101(4):435–45.

30. Ruiz i Altaba A, Melton DA. Bimodal and graded expression of the Xenopus homeobox gene Xhox3 during embryonic development. Development. 1989;106(1):173–83.

31. Ruiz i Altaba A. Neural expression of the Xenopus homeobox gene Xhox3: evidence for a patterning neural signal that spreads through the ectoderm. Development. 1990;108(4):595–604.

32. Sordino P, Duboule D, Kondo T. Zebrafish Hoxa and Evx-2 genes: cloning, developmental expression and implications for the functional evolution of posterior Hox genes. Mech Dev. 1996;59:165–75.

33. Thaeron C, Avaron F, Casane D, Borday V, Thisse B, Thisse C, et al. Zebrafish evx1 is dynamically expressed during embryogenesis in subsets of interneurones, posterior gut and urogenital system. Mech Dev. 2000;99:167–72.

34. Griener A, Zhang W, Kao H, Wagner C, Gosgnach S. Probing diversity within subpopulations of locomotor-related V0 interneurons. Developmental neurobiology. 2015.

35. Suster ML, Kania A, Liao M, Asakawa K, Charron F, Kawakami K, et al. A novel conserved evx1 enhancer links spinal interneuron morphology and cis-regulation from fish to mammals. Dev Biol. 2009;325(2):422–33.

36. Satou C, Kimura Y, Higashijima S. Generation of multiple classes of V0 neurons in zebrafish spinal cord: progenitor heterogeneity and temporal control of neuronal diversity. J Neurosci. 2012;32(5):1771–83.

37. Bae YK, Kani S, Shimizu T, Tanabe K, Nojima H, Kimura Y, et al. Anatomy of zebrafish cerebellum and screen for mutations affecting its development. Dev Biol. 2009;330(2):406–26.

38. Kimmel CB, Ballard WW, Kimmel SR, Ullmann B, Schilling TF. Stages of embryonic development of the zebrafish. Dev Dyn. 1995;203(3):253–310.

39. Schulte CJ, Allen C, England SJ, Juarez-Morales JL, Lewis KE. Evx1 is required for joint formation in zebrafish fin dermoskeleton. Dev Dyn. 2011;240(5):1240–8.

40. Brudno M, Do CB, Cooper GM, Kim MF, Davydov E, Green ED, et al. LAGAN and Multi-LAGAN: efficient tools for large-scale multiple alignment of genomic DNA. Genome Res. 2003;13(4):721–31.

41. Mayor C, Brudno M, Schwartz JR, Poliakov A, Rubin EM, Frazer KA, et al. VISTA : visualizing global DNA sequence alignments of arbitrary length. Bioinformatics. 2000;16(11):1046–7.

42. Sasaki Y, Sone T, Yoshida S, Yahata K, Hotta J, Chesnut JD, et al. Evidence for high specificity and efficiency of multiple recombination signals in mixed DNA cloning by the Multisite Gateway system. J Biotechnol. 2004;107(3):233–43.

43. Suzuki Y, Kagawa N, Fujino T, Sumiya T, Andoh T, Ishikawa K, et al. A novel high-throughput (HTP) cloning strategy for site-directed designed chimerageneis and mutation using the Gateway cloning system. Nucleic Acids Res. 2005;33(12):1–6.

44. Villefranc JA, Amigo J, Lawson ND. Gateway compatible vectors for analysis of gene function in the zebrafish. Dev Dyn. 2007;236(11):3077–87.

45. Köster RW, Fraser SE. Tracing transgene expression in living zebrafish embryos. Dev Biol. 2001;233(2):329–46.

46. Wang Y, Shen J, Arenzana N, Tirasophon W, Kaufman RJ, Prywes R. Activation of ATF6 and an ATF6 DNA binding site by the endoplasmic reticulum stress response. J Biol Chem. 2000;275(35):27013–20.

47. Kawakami K, Takeda H, Kawakami N, Kobayashi M, Matsuda N, Mishina M. A transposon-mediated gene trap approach identifies developmentally regulated genes in zebrafish. Dev Cell. 2004;7(1):133–44.

48. Halpern ME, Rhee J, Goll MG, Akitake CM, Parsons M, Leach SD. Gal4/UAS transgenic tools and their application to zebrafish. Zebrafish. 2008;5(2):97–110.

49. Cerda GA, Hargrave M, Lewis KE. RNA profiling of FAC-sorted neurons from the developing zebrafish spinal cord. Dev Dyn. 2009;238(1):150–61.

50. England S, Hilinski W, de Jager S, Andrzejczuk L, Campbell P, Chowdhury T, Demby C, Fancher W, Gong Y, Lin C et al: Identifying Transcription Factors expressed by Ventral Spinal Cord Interneurons. ZFIN on-line publication 2014, http://zfin.org/ZDB-PUB-140822-10.

51. Park HC, Kim CH, Bae YK, Yeo SY, Kim SH, Hong SK, et al. Analysis of upstream elements in the HuC promoter leads to the establishment of transgenic zebrafish with fluorescent neurons. Dev Biol. 2000;227(2):279–93.

52. Picker A, Scholpp S, Bohli H, Takeda H, Brand M. A novel positive transcriptional feedback loop in midbrain-hindbrain boundary development is revealed through analysis of the zebrafish pax2.1 promoter in transgenic lines. Development. 2002;129:3227–39.

53. Peri F, Nusslein-Volhard C. Live imaging of neuronal degradation by microglia reveals a role for v0-ATPase a1 in phagosomal fusion in vivo. Cell. 2008;133(5):916–27.

54. Kobayashi M, Nishikawa K, Yamamoto M. Hematopoietic regulatory domain of gata1 gene is positively regulated by GATA1 protein in zebrafish embryos. Development. 2001;128(12):2341–50.

55. Batista MF, Jacobstein J, Lewis KE. Zebrafish V2 cells develop into excitatory CiD and Notch signalling dependent inhibitory VeLD interneurons. Dev Biol. 2008;322(2):263–75.

56. Concordet JP, Lewis KE, Moore JW, Goodrich LV, Johnson RL, Scott MP, et al. Spatial regulation of a zebrafish patched homologue reflects the roles of sonic hedgehog and protein kinase A in neural tube and somite patterning. Development. 1996;122(9):2835–46.

57. Gribble SL, Nikolaus OB, Dorsky RI. Regulation and function of Dbx genes in the zebrafish spinal cord. Dev Dyn. 2007;236(12):3472–83.

58. Thaëron C, Avaron F, Casane D, Borday V, Thisse B, Thisse C, et al. Zebrafish evx1 is dynamically expressed during embryogenesis in subsets of interneurones, posterior gut and urogenital system. Mech Dev. 2000;99(1-2):167–72.

59. Joly JS, Joly C, Schulte-Merker S, Boulekbache H, Condamine H. The ventral and posterior expression of the zebrafish homeobox gene eve1 is perturbed in dorsalized and mutant embryos. Development. 1993;119(4):1261–75.

60. Pfeffer PL, Gerster T, Lun K, Brand M, Busslinger M. Characterization of three novel members of the zebrafish Pax2/5/8 family: dependency of Pax5 and Pax8 expression on the Pax2.1 (noi) function. Development. 1998;125(16):3063–74.

61. Higashijima S, Mandel G, Fetcho JR. Distribution of prospective glutamatergic, glycinergic, and GABAergic neurons in embryonic and larval zebrafish. J Comp Neurol. 2004;480(1):1–18.

62. Higashijima S, Schaefer M, Fetcho JR. Neurotransmitter properties of spinal interneurons in embryonic and larval zebrafish. J Comp Neurol. 2004;480(1):19–37.

63. Pierani A, Brenner-Morton S, Chiang C, Jessell TM. A Sonic Hedgehog Independent Retinoid-Activated Pathway of Neurogenesis in the Ventral Spinal Cord. Cell. 1999;97:903–15.
64. Cruz C, Maegawa S, Weinberg ES, Wilson SW, Dawid IB, Kudoh T. Induction and patterning of trunk and tail neural ectoderm by the homeobox gene eve1 in zebrafish embryos. Proc Natl Acad Sci U S A. 2010;107(8):3564–9.
65. Lewis KE, Eisen JS. From cells to circuits: development of the zebrafish spinal cord. Prog Neurobiol. 2003;69(6):419–49.
66. Bernhardt RR, Chitnis AB, Lindamer L, Kuwada JY. Identification of spinal neurons in the embryonic and larval zebrafish. J Comp Neurol. 1990;302:603–16.
67. Satou C, Kimura Y, Hirata H, Suster ML, Kawakami K, Higashijima S. Transgenic tools to characterize neuronal properties of discrete populations of zebrafish neurons. Development. 2013;140(18):3927–31.
68. McIntire SL, Reimer RJ, Schuske K, Edwards RH, Jorgensen EM. Identification and characterization of the vesicular GABA transporter. Nature. 1997;389(6653):870–6.
69. Sagne C, El Mestikawy S, Isambert MF, Hamon M, Henry JP, Giros B, et al. Cloning of a functional vesicular GABA and glycine transporter by screening of genome databases. FEBS letters. 1997;417(2):177–83.
70. Rabe N, Gezelius H, Vallstedt A, Memic F, Kullander K. Netrin-1-dependent spinal interneuron subtypes are required for the formation of left-right alternating locomotor circuitry. J Neurosci. 2009;29(50):15642–9.
71. Burrill JD, Moran L, Goulding MD, Saueressig H. PAX2 is expressed in multiple spinal cord interneurons, including a population of EN1+ interneurons that require PAX6 for their development. Development. 1997;124(22):4493–503.
72. Ahringer J. Posterior patterning by the Caenorhabditis elegans even-skipped homolog vab-7. Gene Dev. 1996;10(9):1120–30.
73. Briata P, Ilengo C, Van DeWerken R, Corte G. Mapping of a potent transcriptional repression region of the human homeodomain protein EVX1. FEBS letters. 1997;402(2-3):131–5.
74. Biggin MD, Tjian R. A purified Drosophila homeodomain protein represses transcription in vitro. Cell. 1989;58(3):433–40.
75. TenHarmsel A, Austin RJ, Savenelli N, Biggin MD. Cooperative binding at a distance by even-skipped protein correlates with repression and suggests a mechanism of silencing. Mol Cell Biol. 1993;13(5):2742–52.
76. Li C, Manley JL. Even-skipped represses transcription by binding TATA binding protein and blocking the TFIID-TA1A box interaction. Mol Cell Biol. 1998;18(7):3771–81.
77. Han K, Manley JL. Functional domains of the Drosophila Engrailed protein. EMBO J. 1993;12:2723–33.
78. Amores A, Force A, Yan YL, Joly L, Amemiya C, Fritz A, et al. Zebrafish hox clusters and vertebrate genome evolution. Science. 1998;282(5394):1711–4.
79. Taylor JS, Braasch I, Frickey T, Meyer A, Van de Peer Y. Genome duplication, a trait shared by 22000 species of ray-finned fish. Genome Res. 2003;13(3):382–90.
80. Holland PW, Garcia-Fernandez J, Williams NA, Sidow A. Gene duplications and the origins of vertebrate development. Dev Suppl. 1994;125–133.
81. Ericson J, Rashbass P, Schedl A, Brenner-Morton S, Kawakami A, van Heyningen V, et al. Pax6 controls progenitor cell identity and neuronal fate in response to graded Shh signaling. Cell. 1997;90:169–80.
82. Sander M, Paydar S, Ericson J, Briscoe J, Berber E, German M, et al. Ventral neural patterning by Nkx homeobox genes: Nkx6.1 controls somatic motor neuron and ventral interneuron fates. Gene Dev. 2000;14(17):2134–9.
83. Briscoe J, Sussel L, Serup P, Hartigan-O'Connor D, Jessell TM, Rubenstein JL, et al. Homeobox gene Nkx2.2 and specification of neuronal identity by graded Sonic hedgehog signalling. Nature. 1999;398(6728):622–7.
84. England S, Batista MF, Mich JK, Chen JK, Lewis KE. Roles of Hedgehog pathway components and retinoic acid signalling in specifying zebrafish ventral spinal cord neurons. Development. 2011;138(23):5121–34.
85. Arndt S, Poser I, Schubert T, Moser M, Bosserhoff AK. Cloning and functional characterization of a new Ski homolog, Fussel-18, specifically expressed in neuronal tissues. Lab Investig. 2005;85(11):1330–41.

7

Mutations in *dock1* disrupt early Schwann cell development

Rebecca L. Cunningham[1], Amy L. Herbert[1], Breanne L. Harty[1,2], Sarah D. Ackerman[1,3] and Kelly R. Monk[1,2*]

Abstract

Background: In the peripheral nervous system (PNS), specialized glial cells called Schwann cells produce myelin, a lipid-rich insulating sheath that surrounds axons and promotes rapid action potential propagation. During development, Schwann cells must undergo extensive cytoskeletal rearrangements in order to become mature, myelinating Schwann cells. The intracellular mechanisms that drive Schwann cell development, myelination, and accompanying cell shape changes are poorly understood.

Methods: Through a forward genetic screen in zebrafish, we identified a mutation in the atypical guanine nucleotide exchange factor, *dock1*, that results in decreased myelination of peripheral axons. Rescue experiments and complementation tests with newly engineered alleles confirmed that mutations in *dock1* cause defects in myelination of the PNS. Whole mount *in situ* hybridization, transmission electron microscopy, and live imaging were used to fully define mutant phenotypes.

Results: We show that Schwann cells in *dock1* mutants can appropriately migrate and are not decreased in number, but exhibit delayed radial sorting and decreased myelination during early stages of development.

Conclusions: Together, our results demonstrate that mutations in *dock1* result in defects in Schwann cell development and myelination. Specifically, loss of *dock1* delays radial sorting and myelination of peripheral axons in zebrafish.

Keywords: *dock1*, Schwann cell development, Myelination, Zebrafish

Background

Myelin, a lipid-rich multi-membrane structure, is an innovation of jawed vertebrates that enables the efficient conduction of action potentials. Schwann cells are the myelinating glia of the peripheral nervous system (PNS), and one Schwann cell myelinates one axonal segment. Schwann cells are derived from the neural crest and undergo a distinct series of developmental stages [1, 2]. These developmental stages of Schwann cells require migration as well as unique and substantial changes in cell shape. Schwann cell precursors (SCPs) migrate great distances longitudinally down peripheral nerves. SCPs develop into immature Schwann cells, which undergo a unique process called radial sorting in which Schwann cells extend processes into axon bundles and select an

axon to myelinate [3]. Prior to myelination, Schwann cells wrap themselves 1–1.5 times around a selected axon segment in what is termed the pro-myelinating state. A mature Schwann cell extends and wraps its membrane to form a myelin sheath around an axonal segment. Cytoskeletal dynamics are needed to facilitate these different stages of Schwann cell development and extensive changes in cell shape, but the intracellular intermediates between extracellular signals and the re-modeling of the Schwann cell cytoskeleton are not well defined.

The Rho-GTPase Rac1 is well known for its role in facilitating cell shape changes through regulating polymerization of the actin cytoskeleton and mediates Schwann cell development [4]. In Schwann cells, differential levels of Rac1 direct when a Schwann cell stops migrating and begins radial sorting and myelination [5]. Schwann cell-specific ablation of Rac1 in a mouse model causes delays in radial sorting and myelination, as well as aberrant Schwann cell process extension [5–7].

* Correspondence: monk@ohsu.edu
[1]Department of Developmental Biology, Washington University School of Medicine, St. Louis, MO 63110, USA
[2]Vollum Institute, Oregon Health and Science University, Portland, OR 97239, USA
Full list of author information is available at the end of the article

Furthermore, Rac1 can function downstream of β1-integrin in Schwann cells performing radial sorting [5]; however, the intracellular mechanisms that influence the temporal and spatial activation of Rac1 following extracellular signaling during Schwann cell development are not well understood.

Guanine nucleotide exchange factors (GEFs) have the ability to temporally and spatially regulate the activation of RhoGTPases, such as Rac1, because many GEFs can regulate the same RhoGTPase [8]. Roles of specific GEFs during distinct stages of Schwann cell development are beginning to be understood and help to broaden our knowledge of how extracellular signals are translated to intracellular signals in order to facilitate alterations in Schwann cell shape and movement [9–12]. In addition to canonical GEFs, atypical GEFs also have the ability to activate RhoGTPases. One such family of atypical GEFs, the Dock1-related GEFs, is composed of 11 family members, including Dock1 (also known as Dock180). Dock1 is highly evolutionarily conserved across species and can specifically bind and activate Rac1 [13–15]. In vitro and in vivo studies in various model organisms have shown that Dock1 influences a variety of cytoskeletal-related cell processes such as phagocytosis and cell migration [16–19]. Thus, Dock1 represents an ideal intracellular candidate to study for a role in cell shape regulation.

Although Dock1 has been studied in several biological contexts and is expressed in Schwann cells [20], a role for Dock1 has not yet been described in Schwann cell myelination. The ability of Dock1 to initiate changes in cell shape to facilitate phagocytosis and cell migration makes Dock1 an attractive candidate to investigate for a role in regulated cell shape changes throughout the development of Schwann cells, particularly during stages of radial sorting and myelination, when Rac1 levels most influence Schwann cell biology [4]. Two other members of the Dock1 family, Dock7, which activates the RhoGT-Pase Cdc42 [20], and Dock8 [21], which can activate Cdc42 and Rac1, have been shown to influence SCP migration through in vitro and in vivo knockdown experiments. Therefore, other members of the Dock1 family may also be key intracellular signals regulating the timing of Schwann cell development.

In this study, we utilized zebrafish to study Schwann cell myelination [22], and we identify and characterize Dock1 as a regulator of early Schwann cell myelination. Although previous morpholino experiments in zebrafish have implicated *dock1* in myoblast development and vasculature morphogenesis [23–25], a role for Dock1 in Schwann cell development has not been examined. In a screen for genetic regulators of myelination, we identified an early stop codon in *dock1* that causes decreased expression of a mature myelin marker, *myelin basic protein* (*mbp*), in the PNS. Transmission electron microscopy (TEM) revealed that fewer axons are myelinated in mutants during early stages of myelin development, while axon number is not affected. We determined that SCP cell number and migration is not affected in *dock1* mutants. Instead, radial sorting is delayed and early markers of myelination are reduced. These data suggest that Dock1 may contribute to the timely process extension of Schwann cells required for radial sorting and myelination.

Methods and materials
Zebrafish lines and rearing conditions
Zebrafish were reared in accordance with the Washington University IRB and animal protocols and were raised in the Washington University Zebrafish Consortium (http://zebrafish.wustl.edu/husbandry.htm). Zebrafish were crossed as either pairs or harems, and embryos were subsequently raised at 28.5 °C in egg water (5 mM NaCl, 0.17 mM KCl, 0.33 mM $CaCl_2$, 0.33 mM $MgSO_4$). Larvae were staged at hours post fertilization (hpf) and days post fertilization (dpf). The following mutant and transgenic strains were utilized in this study: $dock1^{stl145}$, $dock1^{stl365}$, $dock1^{stl366}$, $Tg(sox10(4.9):nls-eos)$ [26], $Tg(foxd3:gfp)$ [27], and $Tg(kdlr:mcherry)$ [28]. Homozygous $dock^{stl145}$ fish are viable as adults, therefore maternal zygotic (MZ) $dock1^{stl145}$ animals were generated by crossing a $dock^{stl145/stl145}$ female with a $dock1^{stl145/+}$ male.

Genotyping
To identify adult and larval zebrafish for either rearing or phenotypic analyses, the following primers were used to amplify a region of interest by PCR: *stl145* F: 5′-CATA GGCGTTCTTCACTGAG-3′ and R: 5′-CGTATTTCC CACTAAACAGC-3′, *stl365* F: 5′-GCAGCCACTTTAAA GCTTCCCG-3′ and R: 5′-GCTGCTTACCTTGCCCT TGTC-3′, and *stl366* F: 5′-CCAGTGCCTCACTTCATAT CTCC-3′ and R: 5′ CTCTTAGTCTCACGCAACACT CATG-3′. After PCR, a restriction enzyme digest assay was performed and the resulting fragments were analyzed on a 3% agarose gel. The *stl145* C-to-T mutation disrupts a BstNI site so that the wild-type PCR product is cleaved into 48 and 527 base pair (bp) products, and the mutant PCR product is 575 bp. The *stl365* allele contains a one bp insertion that disrupts an EcoRV binding site so that the wild-type PCR product is cleaved into 86 and 159 bp products, and the mutant PCR product is 245 bp. The *stl366* allele contains a 13-bp deletion that disrupts a Hpy-CH4III site so that the wild-type PCR product is cleaved into 323 bp and 165 bp products, and the mutant PCR product is 488 bp.

Zebrafish mutant strain generation
$dock1^{stl145}$ was identified in a forward genetic screen described previously in [29, 30]. Phenotypically wild-type and mutant 5 dpf larvae were pooled and extracted DNA was sent for whole genome sequencing at the

Genome Technology Access Center (GTAC) at Washington University. The wild-type to mutant allele ratio was determined using a bioinformatics pipeline generated in-house, and a SNP subtraction analysis suggested that *dock1* was most likely the gene of interest [30]. *dock1* was confirmed as the gene responsible for the *stl145* mutant phenotype through rescue experiments and complementation tests using two other *dock1* mutant alleles, *dock1^{stl365}* and *dock1^{stl366}*, which were generated by TALENs. The TALEN targeter tool (https://tale-nt.cac.cornell.edu/) and GoldyTALEN kit [31] were utilized to build each TALEN in a pCS2+ backbone. The repeat variable domains chosen for each *stl365* TALEN arm and *stl366* TALEN arm were: *stl365* left arm: NN HD NG HD NI HD HD NG NN NI HD NN HD NI NN NI NN NI NN NI; *stl365* right arm: HD NG NG NG NN NI NN NG NG NN NI HD HD HD NG NN NI NN NG; *stl366* left arm: NN NG NG NI NG NI NG NG HD NI NG HD NG NN NI NI NN NN NI NN; *stl366* right arm: NN HD NG NG NI NI NI HD NI NG NI HD NG NN NI HD HD HD NN HD. The TALEN constructs were transcribed with the mMESSAGE mMACHINE SP6 ULTRA Kit (Ambion) and equal concentrations (~ 50 pg) of left and right arm mRNA were injected into 1-cell stage wild-type embryos. Lesions that were successfully transmitted to the F0 germline were identified by restriction enzyme digest analysis as described above. Mutant bands were gel extracted using a QIAquick Gel Extraction kit (Qiagen) and then Sanger sequenced to identify the lesion.

Posterior lateral line nerve (PLLn) dissection and RNA isolation

Posterior lateral line nerves (PLLn) were dissected from 6-month-old adult zebrafish. Animals were euthanized in ice water until gill motion ceased for 5 min, followed by transection of the hindbrain. Using angled forceps, the skin was pulled back from behind the operculum on both sides of the animal to expose the PLLn. Small spring-loaded dissection scissors were used to cut the PLLn near the operculum and then forceps were used to gently remove the nerve by slowly pulling the nerve toward the anterior of the fish. Both nerves were transferred to microcentrifuge tubes sitting on dry ice and then flash frozen in liquid nitrogen and stored at − 80 °C. To isolate RNA, 40 nerves were pooled from 20 different 6-month-old adult zebrafish and total RNA was obtained using standard TRIzol (Life Technologies) RNA extraction, with the exception of the homogenization method. Nerves were pooled into a total of 500 µl TRIzol and then thoroughly homogenized following these steps in succession: vortexing for 30 s, disruption with a plastic-tipped electric homogenizer for 1 min, and passaged through a syringe

and successively smaller needles (22.5 and 27 gauge), 10 times each.

RT-PCR
To make cDNA, 1 µg of total RNA was reverse transcribed using the High Capacity cDNA Reverse Transcription Kit (Applied Biosystems) using random hexamers as per manufacturer instructions. RT-PCR for *dock1* was performed on adult PLLn cDNA. The following primers were used: F: 5'-CGGAGTGGCCGTCTACAACTATG-3' (bordering exons 1 and 2) and R: 5'-CAAGCCGGAAACAC ACCCTTC-3' (bordering exons 3 and 4). Milli-Q water was used as a substrate for a control RT-PCR.

Rescue experiment
Full-length zebrafish *dock1* was cloned into pCS2+ using Gibson Assembly. *dock1* was amplified in two pieces from zebrafish cDNA using a Phusion mastermix (NEB) and the following primers: part 1: F: 5'-TCTTTTTGCAGGAT CCCATAGAGAAGCGAGAAAAAGTGTG-3' and R: 5'-CTCCATGATGATCTGCACGTG-3' and part 2: F: 5'-T CAGCGACATACTGGAGGTGC-3' and R: 5'-TAATA CGACTCACTATAGTTGAGGTGTCAGCTGCTTTTCC G-3'. Gibson Assembly was then performed using an in-house Gibson reaction mixture (gifted by the Solnica-Krezel lab, Washington University in St. Louis). Briefly, the fragments were gel extracted and purified using the QIAquick Gel Purification Kit (Qiagen). 30 ng of pCS2 +, linearized with ClaI and XbaI, were combined with 5-fold excess of the *dock1* PCR fragments and 15 µl of the Gibson Assembly enzyme-reagent mixture. The mixture was incubated at 50 °C for 1 h and then 10 µl were transformed into DH5 alpha cells and plated on ampicillin plates. Subsequent colonies were grown, miniprepped with a Qiagen Kit, and Sanger sequenced. Synthetic mRNA for injection was generated by linearizing *dock1* in pCS2+ with Not1 and then transcribing with the mMESSAGE mMACHINE SP6 ULTRA Kit (Ambion). Approximately 120 pg of *dock1* mRNA in 2 nl was injected into 1-cell stage embryos generated from a *dock1^{stl145}* heterozygous in-cross. In situ hybridization for *mbp* was performed and scoring of expression was performed blinded to genotype.

Whole mount in situ hybridization and qualitative scoring
Whole mount in situ hybridization (WISH) was performed as described [32, 33] on larvae treated with 0.003% phenylthiourea from 24 h post fertilization (hpf) to inhibit pigmentation until fixation in 4% paraformaldehyde. The previously characterized riboprobes used in this study were: *sox10* [34], *krox20* [35], and *mbp* [36]. All phenotypes were scored with the scorer blinded to genotype. The PLLn was scored for strength of staining: "strong" = strong and consistent expression along the entirety of the PLLn; "reduced" = consistent but reduced *mpb* expression along PLLn; and

"strongly reduced" = patches of *mbp* expression or no expression, similar to scoring as performed previously [37]. "Strong" *mbp* expression was assigned a value of 3, "reduced," a value of 2, and "strongly reduced," a value of 1 to code each phenotype as a number for a Chi-squared anaylsis.

Transmission Electron microscopy and quantifications

TEM was performed on 3 dpf, 5 dpf, and 21 dpf cross-sections of the PLLn according to standard protocols [38, 39]. Larvae were cut between body segments 5 and 6 and juvenile 21 dpf fish were cut immediately posterior to the heart. A Jeol JEM-1400 (Jeol USA) electron microscope and AMT V601 digital camera were used to image samples. Quantification of percent myelinated axons, sorted axons, total axon number, and number of Schwann cell nuclei was performed on the entire cross section of the PLLn. The scorer was blinded to genotype, and quantification was performed manually as described previously [37].

Lifeact microinjections and live imaging

One-cell stage zebrafish embryos were injected with ~ 15–20 ng of *sox10:Lifeact-RFP* (a gift from the Lyons lab, University of Edinburgh) and 25 ng of transposase mRNA. 1 dpf larvae were then screened for expression of *sox10:Lifeact-RFP* in Schwann cells at 24 hpf. For live-imaging, larvae were anesthetized in Tricaine and embedded in 0.8% agarose on a 35 mm glass bottom dish filled with 0.2% Tricaine and covered with a 22×22 mm^2 coverslip on top of vacuum grease [40]. The larvae were then imaged with a Zeiss LSM 880 confocal microscope at 20× for 3 h at 3 min intervals. Still images were captured with a Zeiss LSM 880 II Airyscan FAST confocal microscope at 40xW with a 1.8 zoom. To examine blood vesssls, 4 dpf larvae with *Tg(kdlr:mcherry)* were imaged at 13.5× with a Nikon SMZ18 fluorescent dissecting microscope.

Eos Photoconversion and quantification of Schwann cell number

Tg(foxd3:gfp);dock1$^{stl145/+}$ fish were crossed to *Tg(sox10(4.9):nls-eos);dock1$^{stl145/+}$* fish and offspring were screened for both transgenes at 1 dpf. At 2 dpf, larvae were placed in 0.8% low-melt agarose and mounted for imaging as described above. Before counting, larvae were individually exposed to 30 s of UV light using the DAPI filter with the 20× objective of a Zeiss LSM 880 confocal microscope. The number of GFP and RFP positive cells along the PLLn spanning ~ 8 body segments were the counted manually in ImageJ. The observer was blinded to genotype.

Neuromast labeling and quantification

3 dpf larvae derived from a *dock1^{stl145}* heterozygous in-cross were incubated with 50 µl of DASPEI (40 mg/ 100 mL in distilled water) in 4 mL of egg water for 15 min at room temperature. The DASPEI solution was removed and replaced with fresh egg water. The number of neuromasts along the PLLn were counted under a fluorescent dissecting microscope using a GFP filter.

Immunohistochemistry

Immunohistochemistry for acetylated tubulin was performed as described in [32] with mouse anti-acetylated alpha-tubulin used at a dilution of 1:1000 (Sigma). Larvae were fixed at 4 dpf and were derived from a *dock1^{stl145}* heterozygous in-cross. Heavy myosin within somites was detected with chicken MF 20 antibody at a dilution of 1:20 (Developmental Studies Hybridoma Bank). MF 20 was deposited to the DSHB by Fischman, D.A. (DSHB Hybridoma Product MF 20). For MF 20 staining, embryos were fixed at 1 dpf in 4% paraformaldehyde for 1 h and washed twice with 1X PBS for 10 min. Samples were then blocked with 0.05% Triton in PBS and 10% goat serum and then incubated with MF 20 in block overnight at 4 °C. After incubation, larvae were washed twice with PBS and then incubated secondary antibody in PBS for 2 h at room temperature. Primary antibodies were detected IgG2b with secondary antibody conjugated to either Alexa 568 or 488 (Invitrogen) at a 1:2000 dilution. Immunostained larvae were imaged with a Nikon SMZ18 fluorescent dissecting microscope.

Statistical analyses

GraphPad Prism 7 was utilized to perform statistical tests. Unpaired t-tests with Welch's correction were used to test significance of all TEM, neuromast number, and Schwann cell number data. A Chi-squared analysis was utilized to determine significance for all WISH data. Phenotypes of "strong," "reduced," and "strongly reduced" were assigned a number of 3, 2, or 1, respectively, in order to compare phenotypes with a Chi-squared analysis. An unpaired t-test with Welch's correction showed no significant difference between wild-type and heterozygous animals; therefore, for TEM, WISH, neuromast, and Schwann cell number data, wild-type and heterozygous animals were combined as controls.

Results

Mutations in *dock1* result in decreased *myelin basic protein* expression in the peripheral nervous system

An *N*-ethyl-*N*-nitrosourea-based forward genetic screen to identify novel genetic regulators of myelination [29, 30] uncovered a mutant, allele designation *stl145*, that exhibits reduced *mbp* expression in the PNS by whole mount in situ hybridization (WISH). Reduction of *mbp* expression, scored qualitatively in the posterior lateral line nerve (PLLn) (Additional file 1: Figure S1), is most striking at 3 days post fertilization (dpf) (Fig. 1a, b), during early

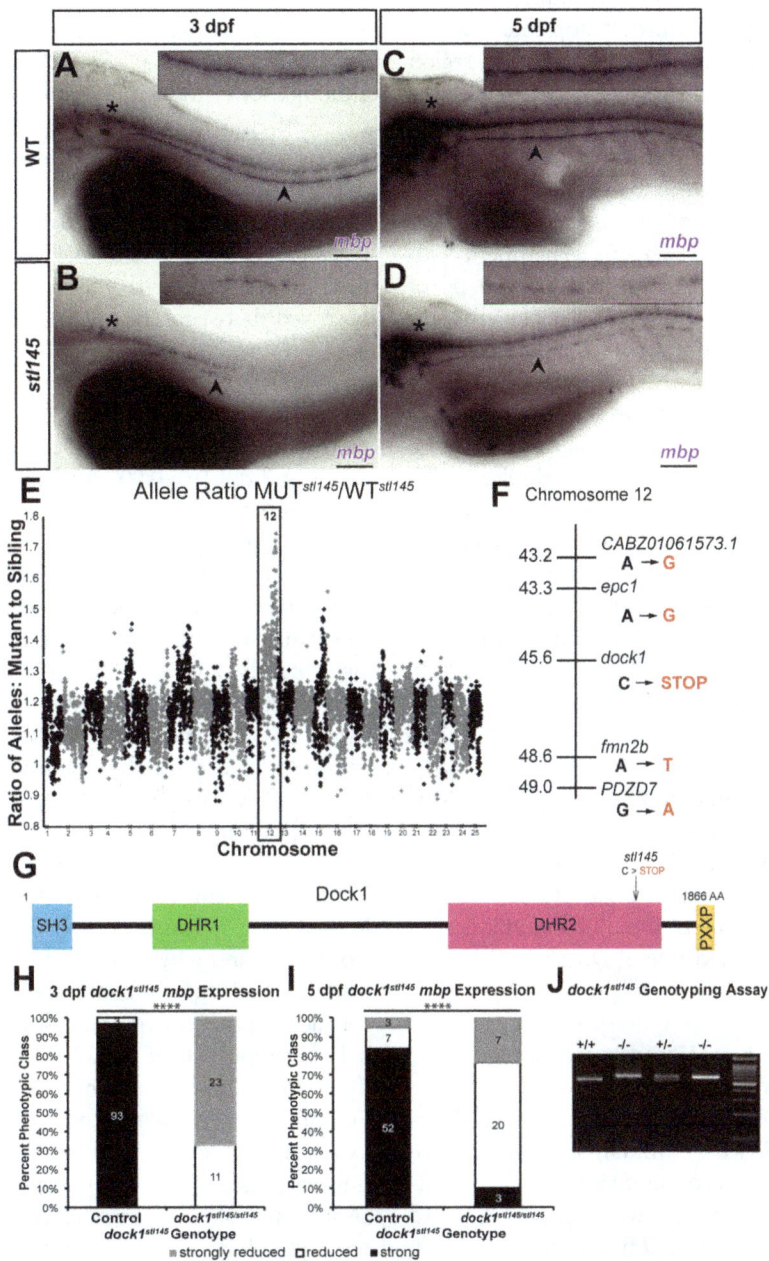

Fig. 1 *stl145* mutants exhibit decreased *mbp* expression in the PNS. **a-d)** Lateral views of *mbp* expression by WISH. Arrowheads indicate the PLLn. Asterisks indicate the central nervous system (CNS). Inset panels show a magnified view of the PLLn. Scale bars = 100 μm. **a)** *mbp* at 3 dpf is strongly expressed in the PLLn of control larva (n = 93/96). **b)** *stl145* mutants at 3dpf exhibit reduced *mbp* expression in the PLLn (n = 34). **c)** *mbp* expression is strongly expressed in the PLLn of control larva at 5 dpf (n = 52/62). **d)** *stl145* mutants at 5 dpf express *mbp*, but at reduced levels compared to control siblings (n = 27/30). **e)** Analysis of whole genome sequencing data showed that chromosome 12 exhibited the highest mutant to wild-type allele ratio. **f)** Within the most highly linked region of chromosome 12, *dock1* was the only gene that contained an early stop codon. **g)** A schematic of the protein structure of Dock1 and the location of the *stl145* lesion. The SH3 and proline rich domains can bind adaptor proteins. The DHR-1 domain interacts with PtdIns(3,4,5)P$_3$ and the DHR-2 domain is the catalytic domain can that catalyzes the exchange of GDP for GTP in Rac1. **h-i)** Quantification of WISH for *mbp* at 3 dpf **(h)** and 5 dpf **(i)**, respectively, based on phenotypic classes and genotypes for the *stl145* lesion. **** p < 0.0001, Chi-squared analysis. **j)** Genotyping assay for the *stl145* lesion. The PCR amplified product is digested with BstN1 and run on a 3% agarose gel

stages of PNS myelination. At 5 dpf, *mbp* expression has increased in the *stl145* mutant PLLn, but is still reduced compared to sibling controls (Fig. 1c, d). To identify the causative mutation, we employed whole genome sequencing

(WGS) of DNA pools from phenotypically mutant and phenotypically wild-type siblings. Analysis of WGS data [30] showed the causative mutation was located on chromosome 12 (Fig. 1e). Within the most highly linked region of chromosome 12, the most likely causative mutation was a C-to-T transition resulting in a premature stop codon within the Rac1 binding domain (DHR2 domain) encoding region of *dock1* (Fig. 1f, g). Genotyping revealed that $dock1^{stl145/stl145}$ homozygous mutations corresponded to decreased levels of *mbp* expression in the PNS at 3 dpf ($p < 0.0001$) and at 5 dpf (p < 0.0001) (Fig. 1h-j). To definitively demonstrate that this premature stop codon was causative for the *stl145* phenotype, we performed a rescue experiment with wild-type *dock1* synthetic mRNA. Injection of 120 pg of full-length synthetic *dock1* mRNA into 1-cell stage embryos derived from an intercross of $dock1^{stl145}$ heterozygotes suppressed the *mbp* phenotype in *stl145* mutants at 3 dpf ($p = 0.0001$) (Fig. 2 a-e). Additionally, we generated two new alleles of *dock1* using TALENs. The *stl365* allele generates a premature stop codon in the DHR2 domain, similar to the *stl145* allele (Fig. 2 f; Additional file 2: Figure S2 A,B). The *stl366* allele causes a premature stop codon generated just after the SH3 domain (Fig. 2 f; Additional file 2: Figure S2 C,D). Both alleles exhibit decreased *mbp* expression in the PNS ($p < 0.0001$) and fail to complement with the *stl145* allele ($dock1^{stl145/stl365} = 4/4$, $dock1^{stl145/stl365} = 6/6$; Fig. 2 g-l). To confirm that *dock1* is expressed in Schwann cells of zebrafish in addition to mammalian Schwann cells [20], RT-PCR for *dock1* was performed on cDNA from adult PLLn, which is enriched in Schwann cell nuclei. This analysis showed that *dock1* is expressed in the PLLn (Additional file 2: Figure S2 E,F). Together, these results confirm that the *stl145* phenotype is the result of the premature stop codon in *dock1*. The phenotype of these new mutants suggests a previously unappreciated role of Dock1 in Schwann cell development.

Schwann cell myelination is significantly reduced in $dock1^{stl145}$ mutants at early stages

We next investigated which stages of Schwann cell development are affected in $dock1^{stl145}$ mutants. To interrogate if the decrease of *mbp* expression in $dock1^{stl145}$ mutants is the result of decreased myelination, we employed TEM to analyze the ultrastructure of the PLLn at 3 dpf and 5 dpf. At 3 dpf, consistent with WISH for *mbp*, the percentage of myelinated axons in the PLLn of $dock1^{stl145}$ mutants is significantly reduced compared to siblings ($p < 0.0001$), while the number of axons is not significantly altered ($p = 0.0983$) (Fig. 3a-d). At 5 dpf, $dock1^{stl145/stl145}$ mutant axon number is similarly unaffected ($p = 0.3031$) while mutants did exhibit a significant decrease in the percentage of myelinated axons compared to controls ($p = 0.0003$), although this phenotype is more variable compared to the mutant phenotype at 3 dpf (Fig. 3 e-h). $dock1^{stl145/+}$ larvae do not exhibit decreased myelination compared to wild-type siblings at 3 dpf ($p = 0.6549$ percent myelinated axons; $p = 0.7258$ total axon number) or 5 dpf ($p = 0.7297$ percent myelinated axons;

$p = 0.6924$ total axon number); thus, wild-type and heterozygous siblings were combined as controls. The presence of myelinated axons at 5 dpf in $dock1^{stl145/stl145}$ larvae, although fewer in number compared to controls, illustrates that Schwann cells do possess the capability to myelinate axons in *dock1* mutants. Maternal zygotic (MZ) $dock1^{stl145}$ mutants at 5 dpf also exhibit a reduction in the number of myelinated axons compared to MZ $dock1^{stl145}$ heterozygotes ($p = 0.0183$) (Additional file 3: Fig. S3 a-d). No significant difference in the percent myelinated axons was observed between zygotic $dock1^{stl145}$ mutants and MZ $dock1^{stl145}$ mutants ($p = 0.8300$). To test if a defect in myelination is consistent between alleles, we performed TEM on $dock1^{stl366}$ mutants and siblings. These mutants also display a significantly decreased percentage of myelinated axons at 3 dpf ($p = 0.0072$) with no significant difference in axon number ($p = 0.3775$) (Additional file 3: Figure S3 E-H). A slight reduction in the percent myelinated axons of the PLLn persists at 21 dpf in MZ $dock1^{stl145}$ mutants ($p = 0.0155$), while axon number ($p = 0.5831$) and Schwann cell nuclei number ($p = 0.1583$) are not significantly altered compared to MZ $dock1^{stl145}$ heterozygous controls (Additional file 4: Figure S4). These results show that *dock1* mutations lead to reductions in the number of myelinated axons, and that these effects are more pronounced at early stages of development.

Neither Schwann cell migration nor number are affected in $dock1^{stl145}$ mutants

To understand why myelination is decreased in $dock1^{stl145}$ mutants at 3 dpf, we examined earlier stages of Schwann cell development, beginning with SCPs. Importantly, global development of $dock1^{stl145}$ mutants is normal and overt PLLn defects are not observed (Additional file 5: Figure S5 A-F). Acetylated tubulin staining shows that axons extend down the trunk of larvae and neuromast number is not significantly altered ($p = 0.7518$), (Additional file 5: Figure S5 G-I). $dock1^{stl145/+}$ larvae and wild-type siblings do not exhibit a significant difference in neuromast number ($p = 0.0727$) and were thus combined as a control. Additionally, blood vessels (*kdlr:mcherry* positive) and somites (MF 20 positive) can develop in zygotic $dock1^{stl145}$ mutants (Additional file 5: Figure S5 J-M). Previous studies have demonstrated that Dock1 can regulate cell migration [41], and two other members of the Dock family of GEFs, Dock7 [20] and Dock8 [21] affect Schwann cell migration. Therefore, we examined if cell migration in $dock1^{stl145}$ mutants is perturbed by performing WISH for *sox10*, which marks all stages of Schwann cell development, including SCPs. At 2 dpf, SCPs have migrated and populated the PLLn in control larvae as evidenced by strong and consistent expression of *sox10* along the entire length of the PLLn (Fig. 4 a). We found that

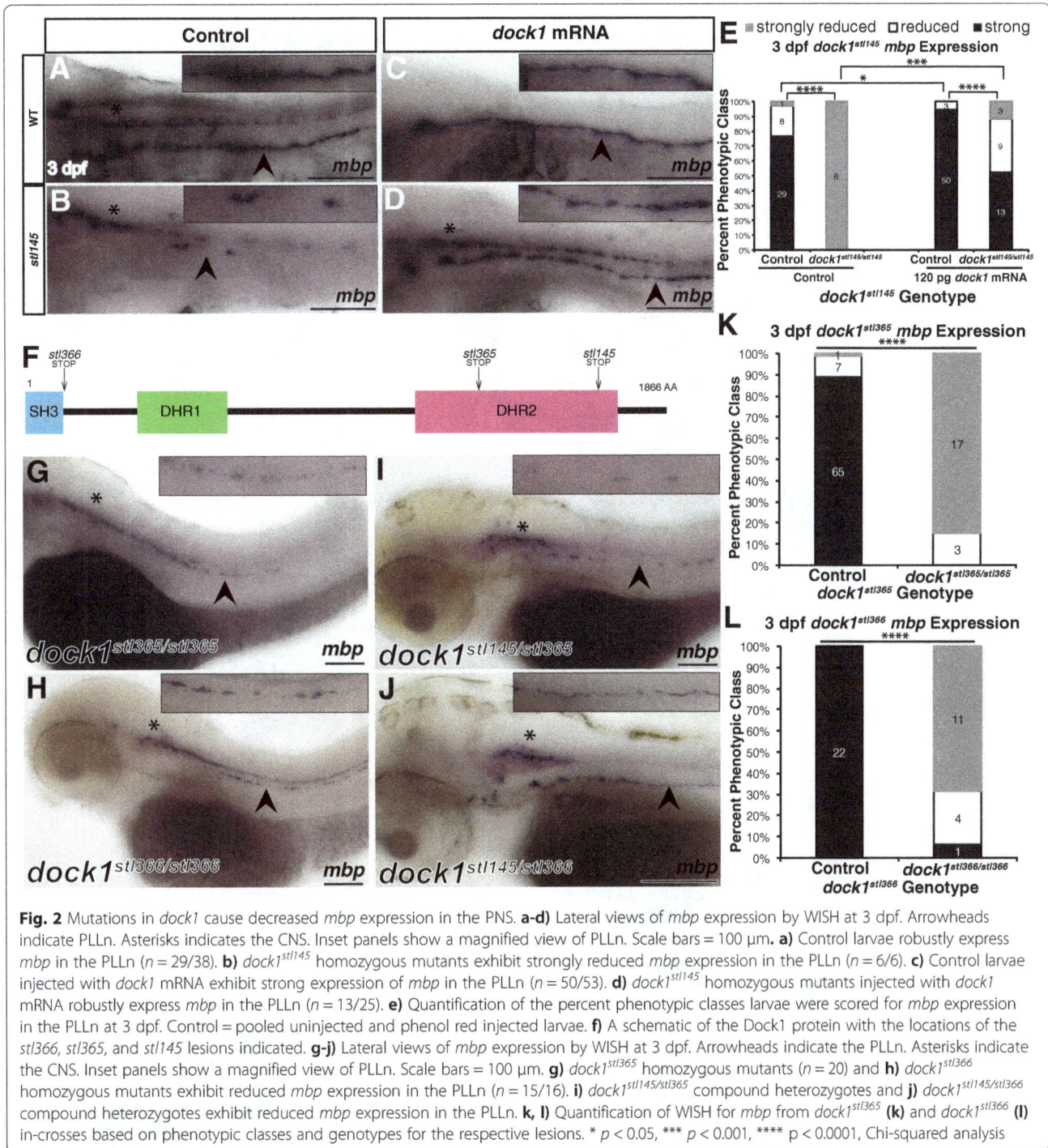

Fig. 2 Mutations in *dock1* cause decreased *mbp* expression in the PNS. **a-d)** Lateral views of *mbp* expression by WISH at 3 dpf. Arrowheads indicate PLLn. Asterisks indicates the CNS. Inset panels show a magnified view of PLLn. Scale bars = 100 µm. **a)** Control larvae robustly express *mbp* in the PLLn (n = 29/38). **b)** *dock1^stl145^* homozygous mutants exhibit strongly reduced *mbp* expression in the PLLn (n = 6/6). **c)** Control larvae injected with *dock1* mRNA exhibit strong expression of *mbp* in the PLLn (n = 50/53). **d)** *dock1^stl145^* homozygous mutants injected with *dock1* mRNA robustly express *mbp* in the PLLn (n = 13/25). **e)** Quantification of the percent phenotypic classes larvae were scored for *mbp* expression in the PLLn at 3 dpf. Control = pooled uninjected and phenol red injected larvae. **f)** A schematic of the Dock1 protein with the locations of the *stl366*, *stl365*, and *stl145* lesions indicated. **g-j)** Lateral views of *mbp* expression by WISH at 3 dpf. Arrowheads indicate the PLLn. Asterisks indicate the CNS. Inset panels show a magnified view of PLLn. Scale bars = 100 µm. **g)** *dock1^stl365^* homozygous mutants (n = 20) and **h)** *dock1^stl366^* homozygous mutants exhibit reduced *mbp* expression in the PLLn (n = 15/16). **i)** *dock1^stl145/stl365^* compound heterozygotes and **j)** *dock1^stl145/stl366^* compound heterozygotes exhibit reduced *mbp* expression in the PLLn. **k, l)** Quantification of WISH for *mbp* from *dock1^stl365^* **(k)** and *dock1^stl366^* **(l)** in-crosses based on phenotypic classes and genotypes for the respective lesions. * p < 0.05, *** p < 0.001, **** p < 0.0001, Chi-squared analysis

*dock1^stl145/stl145^* mutants also exhibit consistent and strong expression of *sox10* along the PLLn (p = 0.3522), demonstrating that SCP migration is not impaired and that Schwann cells populating the PLLn are thus poised to myelinate (Fig. 4b, c). Dock1 has been shown to regulate the actin cytoskeleton in other systems; therefore, we hypothesized that actin cytoskeletal dynamics might be altered during SCP migration in *dock1^stl145^* mutants. We

performed live-imaging of the PLLn in *tg(foxd3:gfp); dock1^stl145^* wild-type, heterozygous, or mutant larvae that also mosaically expressed *sox10:Lifeact-RFP*, which binds and fluorescently labels F-actin in cells expressing *sox10* [42]. Live-imaging from ~ 30–33 hpf did not reveal any overt defects in migration or in actin cytoskeleton localization (Fig. 4d-k; Additional file 6: Movie S1, Additional file 7: Movie S2, Additional file 8: Movie S3

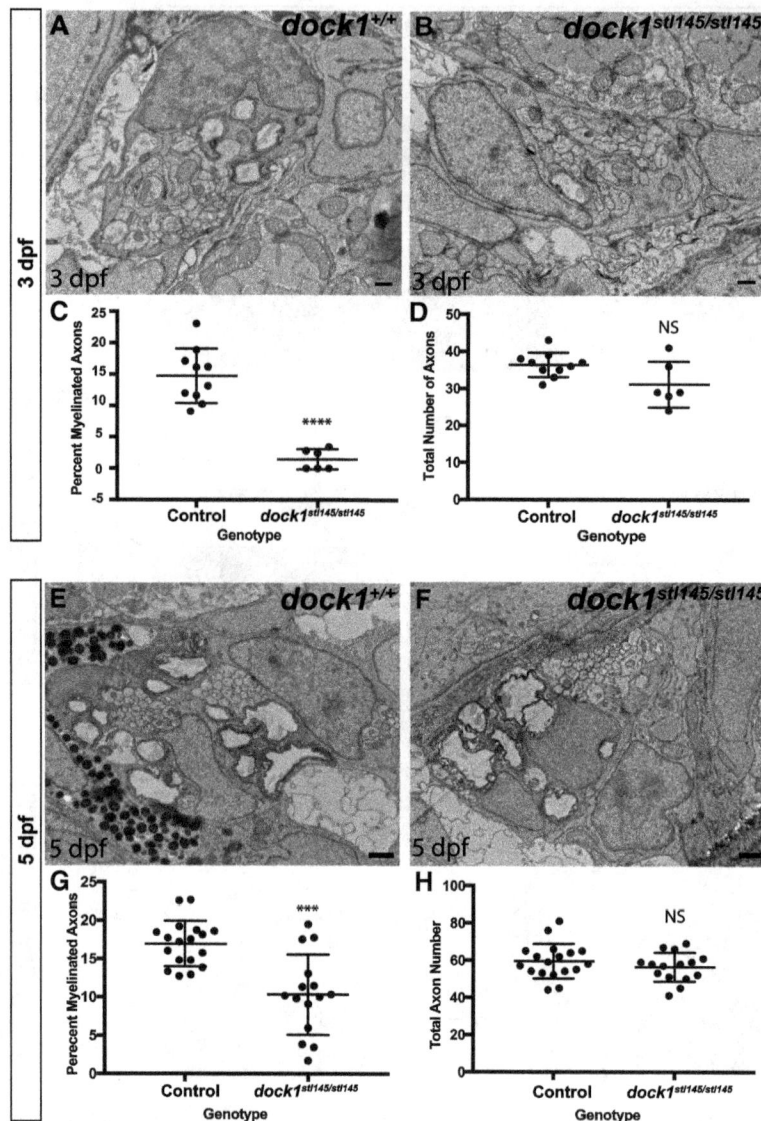

Fig. 3 PNS myelination is significantly reduced in *stl145* mutants. **a, b)** TEM of a cross-section of the PLLn at 3 dpf. Myelinated axons are pseudocolored in green. Scale bars = 500 nm. **a)** Axons in wild-type PLLn begin to be myelinated while **b)** *dock1^{stl145}* homozygous mutant PLLn exhibits fewer myelination of axons. **c)** Quantification of the percent myelinated axons shows a significant difference between control ($n = 6$ animals, 10 nerves) and *dock1^{stl145}* mutants ($n = 4$ animals, 6 nerves). **d)** Quantification of the total number of axons (NS, $p = 0.0983$). **e, f)** Quantification of a cross-section of the PLLn at 5 dpf. Myelinated axons are pseudocolored in green. Scale bars = 500 nm. **e)** The PLLn of a wild-type larva contains numerous myelinated axons whereas **f)** a *dock1^{stl145}* homozygous mutant PLLn contains fewer myelinated axons. **g)** Quantification of the percent myelinated axons shows a significant difference between control ($n = 11$ animals, 18 nerves) and *dock1^{stl145}* mutants ($n = 9$ animals, 15 nerves). **h)** Quantification of the total number of axons (NS, $p = 0.3031$). Bars represent means ± SD. ***$p < 0.001$, ****$p < 0.0001$, unpaired t Test with Welch's correction

and Additional file 9: Movie S4). In both control and *dock1^{stl145}* mutant larvae, F-actin was consistently localized to the back of migrating SCPs. To our knowledge, this is the first time live actin dynamics have been reported in migrating SCPs in vivo. High-resolution still images also show LifeAct distributed throughout the cell with the highest concentration at the back of SCPs (Additional file 10: Figure S6).

Because migration is not affected in *dock1^{stl145}* mutants, we examined whether decreased myelination in *dock1^{stl145}*

mutant nerves was the result of fewer Schwann cells. To do this, we generated and analyzed 2 dpf double transgenic *tg(foxd3:gfp);tg(sox10:nls-eos);dock1^{stl145}* larvae. The *sox10:nls-eos* transgene enabled manual counting of Schwann cell nuclei along the PLLn, while the *foxd3:gfp* transgene provided a co-label to ensure Schwann cell identity. Counting the number of double positive cells at 2 dpf showed that *dock1^{stl145/+}* and wild-type siblings do not exhibit a significant difference in cell number ($p = 0.2218$) and were thus combined as the control group. No

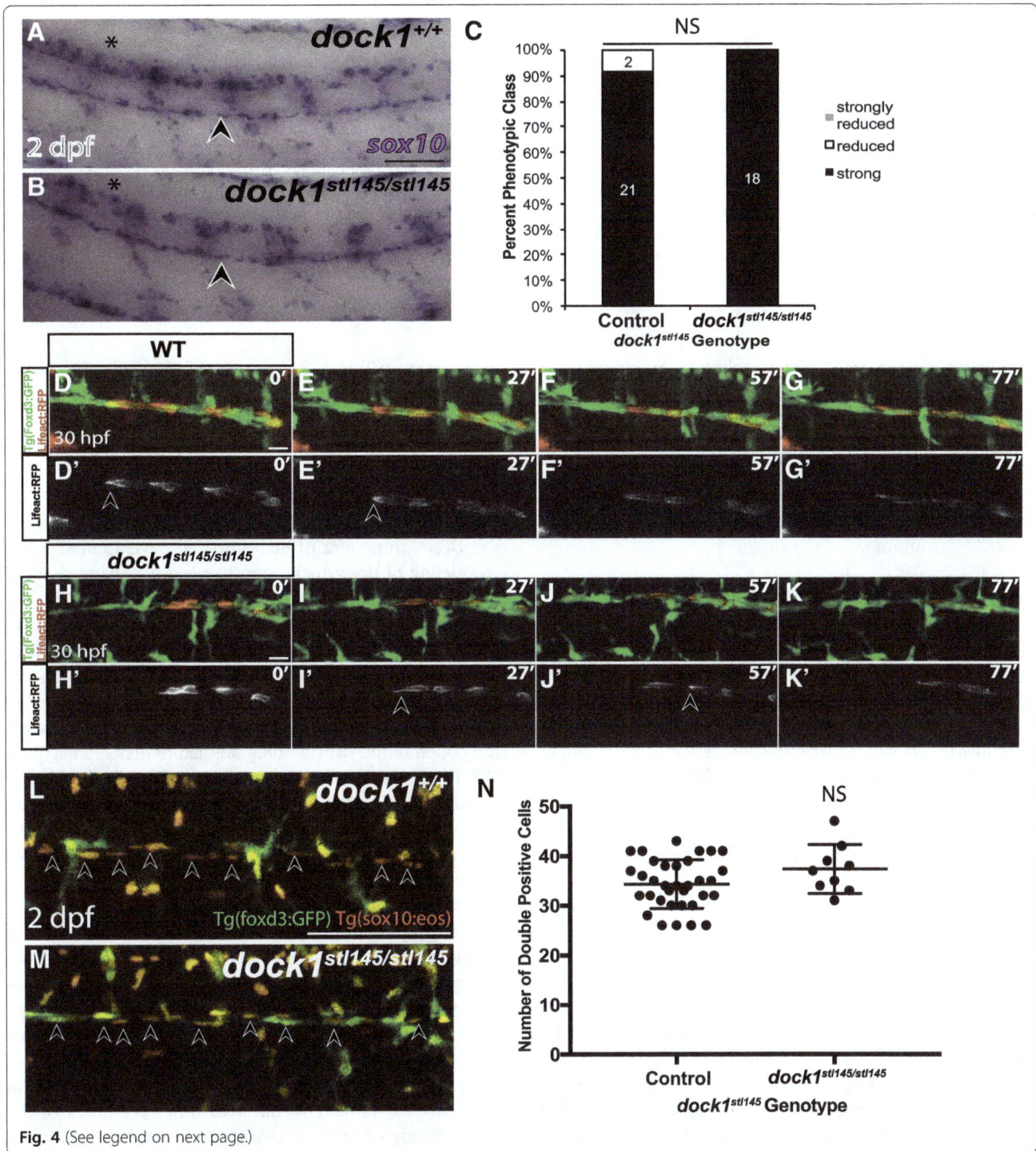

Fig. 4 (See legend on next page.)

Fig. 4 Schwann cell migration and number is not affected in *stl145* mutants. **a, b)** Lateral view of WISH for *sox10* at 2 dpf. Arrowheads indicate the PLLn. Asterisks indicate the CNS. **a)** Strongly expressing *sox10* positive cells are located throughout the PLLn in control larvae ($n = 21/23$), similar to **b)** *dock1*^*stl145* homozygous mutant larva ($n = 18$). **c)** Quantification of WISH for *sox10* at 2 dpf based on phenotypic classes and genotypes for the *stl145* lesion shows no significant difference in expression ($p = 0.3522$, Bars represent means ± SD; Chi-squared analysis). **d, g′)** Still images from time-lapse imaging from 30 to 31.5 hpf in *Tg(foxd3:gfp)* wild-type larvae injected with *sox10:Lifeact-RFP*. Prime panels show Lifeact-RFP strongly localized at the back of migrating Schwann cells (arrowheads). Scale bars = 20 μm. **h-k′)** Still images from time-lapse imaging from 30 to 31.5 hpf in *Tg(foxd3:gfp) dock1*^*stl145/stl145* larvae injected with *sox10:Lifeact-RFP*. Prime panels show Lifeact-RFP strongly localized at the back of migrating Schwann cells (arrowheads). **l, m)** Lateral view of PLLn in 2 dpf larvae containing *Tg(foxd3:gfp)* and *Tg(sox10(4.9):nls-eos)*. Arrows point to examples of double positive Schwann cells. Counting the number of Schwann cells double positive for GFP and RFP in **l)** control ($n = 34$) and **m)** *dock1*^*stl145* homozygous mutants ($n = 9$). Scale bars = 100 μm. **n)** Quantification of the number of Schwann cells within a defined region of the PLLn revealed no significant difference in Schwann cell number (NS, $p = 0.1360$). Bars represent means ± SD; unpaired *t* Test with Welch's correction

significant difference in the number of Schwann cells between mutants and control siblings was observed ($p = 0.1243$), suggesting that a reduction in Schwann cell number is not a contributing factor to decreased myelination of the PNS in *dock1*^*stl145* mutants (Fig. 4 l-n). Overall, these experiments demonstrate that SCP migration and number are not overtly affected in *dock1*^*stl145* mutants.

Defects in Schwann cell development are first observed during radial sorting and myelination initiation

Given that the *dock1*^*stl145* mutation does not alter SCP migration, we next asked if Schwann cell development was affected at the immature and pro-myelinating Schwann cell stages using TEM. At 60 hpf, Schwann cells in MZ *dock1*^*stl145* heterozygous siblings have begun to myelinate axons whereas MZ *dock1*^*stl145* mutants are extending processes into axon bundles and can be found in the promyelinating, but not myelinating state (Fig. 5 a-c′). This phenotype suggests that radial sorting by Schwann cells is delayed in in *dock1*^*stl145* mutants. We then hypothesized that radial sorting delays at 3 dpf in *dock1*^*stl145* mutants might result in higher numbers of Schwann cells associated with axons in a 1:1 ratio at 5 dpf as more Schwann cells have entered the pro-myelinating state. Indeed, compared to 3 dpf, a greater number of Schwann cells are associated in a 1:1 ratio with axons in *dock1*^*stl145* mutants (3 dpf: $p = 0.6068$; 5dpf: $p = 0.0086$) (Fig. 5 d-i). To further test if Schwann cells are developmentally delayed at the pro-myelinating state, we examined expression of *krox20* (*egr2*), a transcription factor that initiates expression of myelin associated genes. By WISH, *krox20* expression is significantly decreased along the PLLn of *dock1*^*stl145/stl145* mutants compared to wild-type and heterozygous control siblings at 3 dpf ($p < 0.0001$), demonstrating that *dock1*^*stl145* mutant Schwann cells are developmentally delayed compared to their siblings (Fig. 5 j-l). This reduction in *krox20* expression is not a result of an absence of Schwann cells because *sox10* positive Schwann cells are present along

the PLLn by WISH at 3 dpf ($p = 0.8141$) (Fig. 5 m-o). Together, these data show that *dock1*^*stl145* mutants exhibit delays in development that begin during radial sorting and extend throughout initial myelination of the PNS in zebrafish.

Discussion

A critical component of Schwann cell development is the remodeling of the cytoskeleton to promote shape changes to facilitate proper myelination of the PNS [3, 43]. Although some of the intracellular components involved in cytoskeletal rearrangements have been identified, such as Rac1, the full complement of proteins involved in this process has not been comprehensively defined. Through a forward genetic screen in zebrafish, we identified an early stop codon in the Rac1 binding domain of *dock1*, an atypical GEF, that causes decreased *mbp* expression in the PNS at 3 dpf and 5 dpf. Rescue experiments and complementation tests with two newly engineered alleles of *dock1* confirmed that mutations in *dock1* result in decreased *mbp* expression.

TEM analysis showed fewer myelinated axons in mutants at 3 dpf, 5 dpf, and 21 dpf, whereas axon number is not significantly affected at any stage assessed. However, we did note that several unmyelinated axons in some mutant nerves were abnormally large in diameter and had many mitochondria (data not shown). We demonstrated that reduced *mbp* expression and the reduction of myelinated axons in mutants is not caused by absence or loss of Schwann cell number. While two other members of the Dock1-family of atypical GEFs, Dock7 and Dock8, affect SCP migration in mammals [20, 21], this does not appear to be the case of Dock1 in zebrafish. This is not entirely unexpected, since loss of Rac1 in mouse Schwann cells did not affect Schwann cell migration [5, 6]. Although overt defects in migration were not detected using live-imaging, these experiments enabled visualization of F-actin localization, which showed that F-actin is localized at the back of migrating Schwann cells. This live-imaging data with Lifeact supports previously reported data from

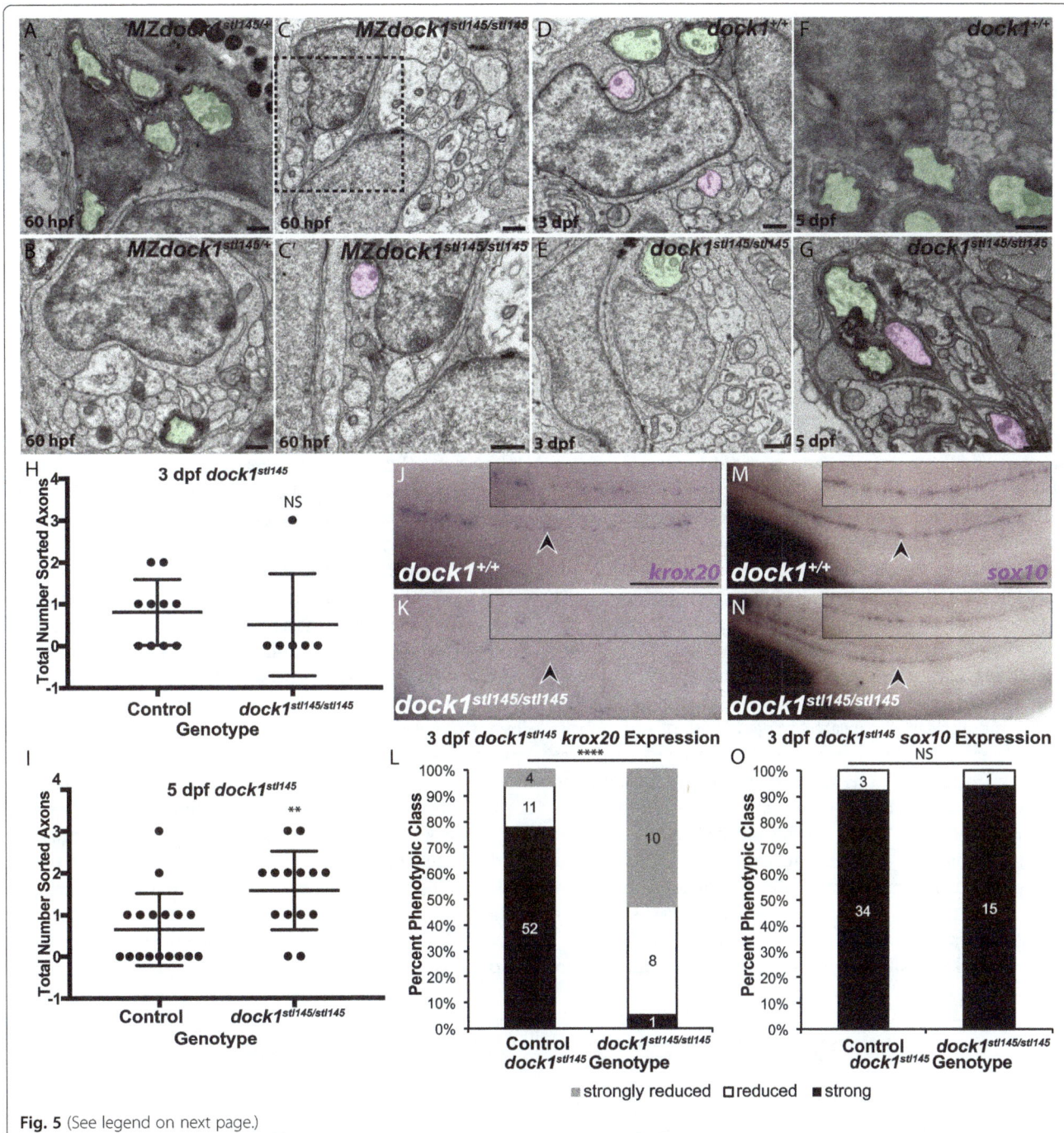

Fig. 5 (See legend on next page.)

(See figure on previous page.)

Fig. 5 *stl145* mutants exhibit delays in radial sorting and decreased expression of *krox20*. **a-g)** TEM of cross-sections of the PLLn. Myelinated axons are pseudocolored in green and axons associated with promyelinating Schwann cells are pseudocolored in purple. Scale bars = 500 nm. **a, b)** Micrographs from the same PLLn within a MZ*dock1*[stl145] heterozygote show Schwann cells myelinating axons at 60 hpf. **C)** An MZ*dock1*[stl145] homozygous larva does not have myelinated axons at 60 hpf, but Schwann cells are extending processes into axon bundles. **C')** Magnification of inset from **C** shows an axon surrounded by a pro-myelinating Schwann cell. **d, e)** Schwann cells can myelinate and sort axons at 3 dpf in wild-type (n = 6 animals, 10 nerves) and mutant larvae (n = 4 animals, 6 nerves). **f, g)** More sorted axons are present in mutants (n = 8 animals, 15 nerves) at 5 dpf compared to controls (n = 11 animals, 17 nerves). Quantification of the number of sorted axons at **h)** 3 dpf and **i)** 5 dpf shows a statistical difference at 5 dpf (unpaired *t* Test with Welch's correction). **j, k)** Lateral view of WISH for *krox20* at 3 dpf. Arrowheads indicate PLLn. Inset panels show a magnified view of the PLLn. Scale bar = 50 μm. **j)** *krox20* is expressed along the PLLn of control larvae (n = 67) whereas **k)** *dock1*[stl145] homozygous mutants express little to no *krox20* along the PLLn (n = 18/19). **l)** Quantification of WISH for *krox20* at 3 dpf based on phenotypic classes and genotypes for the *stl145* lesion (p < 0.0001, Chi-squared analysis). **m, n)** Lateral view of WISH for *sox10* at 3 dpf. Arrowheads indicate the PLLn. Inset panels show a magnified view of the PLLn. Scale bar = 50 μm. **m)** Control larvae exhibit *sox10* positive Schwann cells along the PLLn (n = 37) similar to **N)** *dock1*[stl145] homozygous mutants (n = 16). **o)** Quantification of WISH for *sox10* at 3 dpf based on phenotypic classes and genotypes for the *stl145* lesion (p = 0.8141, Chi-squared analysis). Bars represent means ± SD, **p < 0.001, **** p < 0.0001

3D culture of Schwann cells showing that migrating Schwann cells in vivo move in an amoeboid-like fashion [44], as contractions seem to occur at the back of the cell. In the future, it will be interesting to generate *dock7* and *dock8* zebrafish genetic mutants and observe how migration and F-actin localization is affected in SCPs.

Although a significant reduction in the percent myelinated axons is observed at 5 dpf, Schwann cells in *dock1*[stl145] mutants do have the capability to myelinate axons, suggesting that *dock1* is involved in the timing of myelination onset. It is also possible that other Dock1 family members compensate for *dock1* loss of function in our mutants. Further experiments are needed to determine if Dock1 functions in a Schwann cell-autonomous or non-cell-autonomous manner. Consistent with data showing that *dock1* mutant Schwann cells are delayed in radial sorting and myelination, expression of *krox20*, a transcription factor essential for expression of myelin genes, is decreased in *dock1*[stl145] mutant nerves. Importantly, Schwann cell number is not affected in *dock1*[stl145] mutants and overall PLLn development is not affected in

dock1[stl145] mutants compared to controls, as determined by acetylated tubulin staining and counting neuromast number. Combined, these data demonstrate that Schwann cell radial sorting and myelination are delayed in *dock1* mutants.

How might Dock1 regulate Schwann cell radial sorting and myelination? GEFs are proposed to aid in regulating the spatial and temporal activation of RhoGTPases, such as Rac1 [8]. During the course of development, Schwann cells undergo unique and critical cell shape changes during migration, radial sorting, and myelination. We hypothesize that to regulate the cytoskeletal rearrangements necessary for such functions, Schwann cells utilize a "tool-kit" of GEFs – both canonical and atypical – to activate RhoGTPases, which subsequently remodel the cytoskeleton. For example, Dock7 and Dock8, in addition to canonical GEFs, Dbl's big sister (Dbs) [10] and Tiam1 [9], have already been shown to regulate SCP migration. Dock1 may be activated after Schwann cells have migrated to subsequently promote radial sorting and early myelination. Because few GEFs have been

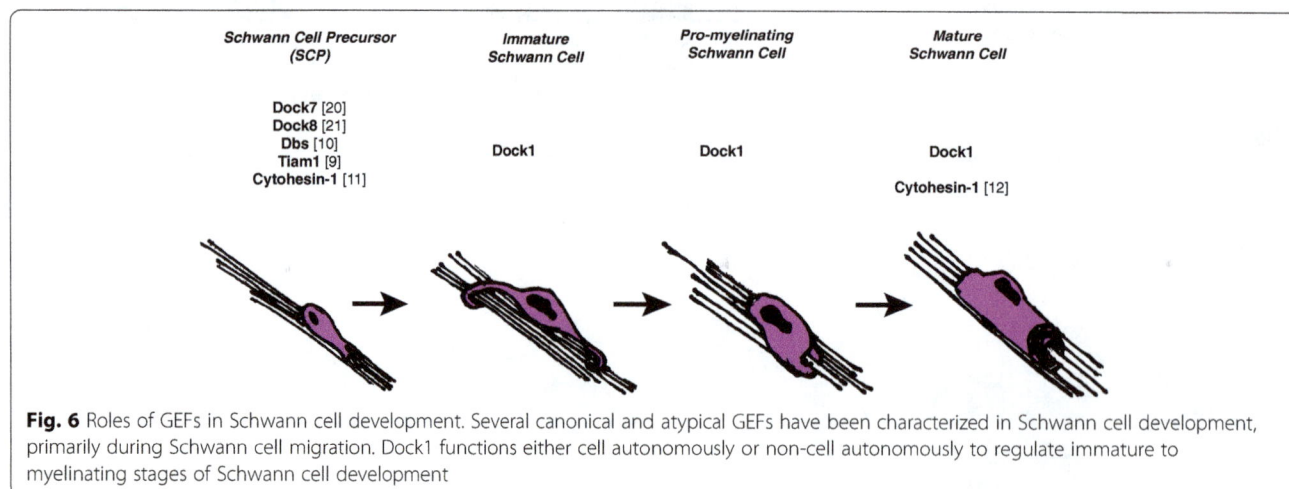

Fig. 6 Roles of GEFs in Schwann cell development. Several canonical and atypical GEFs have been characterized in Schwann cell development, primarily during Schwann cell migration. Dock1 functions either cell autonomously or non-cell autonomously to regulate immature to myelinating stages of Schwann cell development

shown to play a role in Schwann cell development in vivo, important next steps in elucidating the discrete signals necessary for development will be to define the repertoire of active GEFs, particularly after SCP migration (Fig. 6). RhoGTPases, like Rac1, are ubiquitous and important for initiating cytoskeletal rearrangements as well as other cell biological processes; therefore, different GEFs may be utilized to activate RhoGTPases cell-specifically. Previously, it has been shown that Rac1 activation regulates Schwann cell radial sorting and myelination [6] in addition to promoting the transition from Schwann cell migration to radial sorting [5]. Because Dock1 has been shown to specifically bind and activate Rac1 in various biological contexts, we hypothesize that if Dock1 functions cell-autonomously, it may be one of many GEFs that activate Rac1 in Schwann cells. Multiple GEFs working together in concert could increase the total levels of activated Rac1 during a critical period in Schwann cell development to enable the process extensions necessary for radial sorting and myelination. One explanation of our data is that Schwann cell radial sorting and myelination is slower in dock1 mutants because activated Rac1 levels have not reached a critical threshold to promote these processes. In the future, as better in vivo Rac1 sensors are developed, it will be interesting to test this hypothesis. Additionally, Dock1 may function redundantly with other GEFs. As radial sorting and myelination are critical for PNS health, many GEFs may converge on the same pathway such that if only one GEF is dysfunctional, radial sorting and myelination can still proceed, albeit at a slower rate. Alternatively, Dock1 may function in neurons and mutations in dock1 may indirectly affect Schwann cell development.

The cell autonomy of Dock1 function and the upstream signals that trigger Dock1 activation remain to be elucidated. Dock1 has a DHR1 domain that can bind phosphatidylinositols [45] located in the cell membrane, making Dock1 is an attractive candidate to serve as a link between cell surfaces receptor and the cytoskeleton. Additionally, Dock1 could be a representative of a class of drug targets for diseases affecting peripheral myelin, especially because GEFs may contribute to myelination disease states in human patients [4, 46–48]. Although RhoGTPases are critical for cytoskeletal rearrangements, their ubiquity in many cell types limits their ability to serve as useful therapeutic drug targets. Alternatively, GEFs, particularly atypical GEFs like Dock1, could open a door to indirectly affect RhoGTPases in a more cell-specific manner and thus influence the cell shape changes that promote proper Schwann cell development and myelination.

Conclusions
In this study, we demonstrate that mutations in an atypical GEF, dock1, result in defects in Schwann cell radial sorting and myelination. Schwann cells are slower to extend processes into axon bundles and subsequently myelinate fewer axons. Schwann cell number and migration are not affected in these mutants; however, Schwann cells in dock1 mutants fail to robustly express markers such as mbp and krox20 in early development, suggesting that dock1 aids in the temporal regulation of Schwann cell radial sorting and development. Moreover, Dock1 may represent a link between extracellular signals and the intracellular cytoskeletal rearrangements necessary for radial sorting and myelination.

Additional files

Additional file 1: Figure S1. A-C) Lateral view of WISH for mbp. Arrowheads indicate the PLLn. Asterisks indicate the CNS. **A)** Representative image of a PLLn scored as "strong" expression, with mbp strongly and continuously expressed along PLLn **B)** as "reduced" expression, with reduced but consistent mbp expression along PLLn and **C)** as "strongly reduced" with patchy mbp expression along the PLLn.

Additional file 2: Figure S2. A) The stl365 allele was generated by a TALEN that resulted in one base pair insertion causing an early stop. **B)** Genotyping assay for the stl365 lesion. The PCR amplified product is digested with EcoRV and run on a 3% agarose gel. **C)** The stl366 allele was generated by a TALEN that resulted in a 13 base-pair deletion causing an early stop. **D)** Genotyping assay for the stl366 lesion. The PCR amplified product is digested with HpyCH4III and run on a 3% agarose gel. **E)** RT-PCR for dock1 on adult PLLn cDNA shows dock1 is expressed in the PLLn. **F)** Control reaction performed with Milli-q water as a substrate.

Additional file 3: Figure S3. A-B) TEM of a cross-section of the PLLn at 5 dpf in MZ siblings. Myelinated axons are pseudocolored in green. Scale bars = 500 nm. **A)**Axons in MZdock1^stl145 heterozygotes (n = 4 animals, 6 nerves) contain many myelinated axons whereas **B)** MZdock1^stl145 mutants have fewer myelinated axons (n = 5 animals, 8 nerves). **C)** Quantification of the percent myelinated axons. **D)** Quantification of the total number of axons (NS, p = 0.2926). **E-F)** TEM of a cross-section of the PLLn at 3 dpf in dock1^stl366 siblings. Myelinated axons are pseudocolored in green. Scale bars = 500 nm. **E)** Schwann cells in control siblings have myelinated more axons (n = 4 animals, 6 nerves) compared to **F)** dock1^stl366 homozygous mutant nerves (n = 3 animals, 5 nerves). **G)** Quantification of the percent myelinated axons. **H)** Quantification of the total number of axons (NS, p = 0.3775). Bars represent means ± SD. *p < 0.05, **p < 0.01, unpaired t Test with Welch's correction.

Additional file 4: Figure S4. A-B) TEM of a cross-section of the PLLn at 21 dpf in MZ siblings. Scale bars = 10 μm. (**A-B'**) Magnified images. Scale bars = 2 μm. **A-A')** Axons in MZdock1^stl145 heterozygotes (n = 4 animals, 5 nerves) contain many myelinated axons and **B-B')** MZdock1^stl145 mutants have fewer myelinated axons (n = 2 animals, 3 nerves). **C)** Quantification of the percent myelinated axons. **D)** Quantification of the total number of axons (NS, p = 0.5831). **E)** Quantification of the total number of Schwann cell nuclei (NS, p = 0.1583). Bars represent means ± SD. *p < 0.05, unpaired t Test with Welch's correction.

Additional file 5: Figure 5. Gross development is normal at 3 dpf comparing **A)** wild-type, **B)** heterozygous, and **C)** mutant larvae from a dock1^stl145 intercross. Scale bars = 500 μm. **D-F)** Gross development is normal and swim bladders have inflated at 5 dpf comparing **D)** wild-type, **E)** heterozygous, and **F)** mutant from a dock1^stl145 intercross. Scale bars = 500 μm. **G)** Acetylated tubulin shows axons are present and well-fasiculated in both wild-type (n = 3) and **H)** dock1^stl145/stl145 mutant larvae (n = 9) at 4 dpf. **I)** Neuromast number, detected by

DASPEI labeling, did not vary between controls (n = 46) or mutants (n = 16) at 3 dpf (NS, p = 0.7518), indicating that global PLLn development is not affected. Bars represent means ± SD; unpaired t Test with Welch's correction. **J)** Tg(kdlr:mcherry) labeling blood vessels at 4 dpf in wild-type and **K)** dock1^stl14/stl145^ mutants. **L)** MF 20 staining shows defined somite development in wild-type and **M)** dock1^stl14/^~stl145~

mutant larvae at 1 dpf. Scale bars = 100 μm.

Additional file 6: Movie S1. Live-imaging of a Tg(foxd3:gfp) wild-type larva (~ 30–33 hpf) injected with sox10:Lifeact-RFP. The larva was imaged every 3 min for 3 h.

Additional file 7: Movie S2. Grayscale single channel movie of Lifeact as seen in Additional file 6: Movie S1.

Additional file 8: Movie S3. Live-imaging of a Tg(foxd3:gfp) dock1^stl145/^~stl145~ larva (~ 30–33 hpf) injected with sox10:Lifeact-RFP. The larva was imaged every 3 min for 3 h.

Additional file 9: Movie S4. Grayscale single channel movie of Lifeact as seen in Additional file 8: Movie S3.

Additional file 10: Figure S6. A) Zeiss Airyscan image of Tg(foxd3:gfp) wild-type and **B)** Tg(foxd3:gfp) dock1^stl145/+^ larva (~ 30 hpf) injected with sox10:Lifeact-RFP. **A'-B')** Lifeact-RFP localization within Schwann cell precursors. Scale bars = 10 μm.

Abbreviations
bp: Base pair; CNS: Central nervous system; dpf: Days post fertilization; GDP: Guanosine diphosphate; GEF: Guanine nucleotide exchange factor; GTP: Guanosine triphosphate; hpf: Hours post fertilization; mbp: Myelin basic protein; MF 20: Myosin heavy chain antibody; mm: Millimeter; mM: Millimolar; MZ: Maternal zygotic; ng: Nanogram; nl: Nanoliter; PBS: Phosphate buffered saline; PCR: Polymerase chain reaction; pg: Picogram; PLLn: Posterior lateral line nerve; PNS: Peripheral nervous system; PtdIns(3,4,5)P$_3$: Phosphatidylinositol (3,4,5)-trisphosphate; SCP: Schwann cell precursor; SD: Standard deviation; TEM: Transmission electron microscopy; WISH: Whole mount in situ hybridization; WT: Wild-type; μg: Microgram; μm: Micrometer

Acknowledgements
We thank members of the Monk, Solnica-Krezel, and Kaufman laboratories for assistance with the screen and helpful discussions; the Washington University Center for Cellular Imaging; the Washington University Zebrafish Consortium; S. Kucenas (University of Virginia) for the Tg(sox10(4.9):nls-eos) line; D. Lyons for the sox10:lifeact-RFP plasmid; C. Shiau (University of North Carolina) for the Tg(kdlr:mcherry) line; M. Mokallad (Washington University) for the acetylated alpha-tubulin antibody, and the Solnica-Krezel laboratory (Washington University) for the MF 20 antibody.

Author contributions
A.L.H., B.L.H, S.D.A., and K.R.M. performed the genetic screen and identified the stl145 mutant. R.L.C. and K.R.M designed research, and R.L.C. performed research. R.L.C. and K.R.M analyzed data, and R.L.C. and K.R.M. wrote the paper. All authors edited and approved of the manuscript.

Funding
R.L.C. is supported by the National Science Foundation Graduate Research Fellowship (DGE-1745038). This work was also supported by the Philip and Sima Needleman Student Fellowship in Regenerative Medicine (A.L.H.) and by the National Institute of Neurological Disorders and Stroke (NINDS) Grants F31 NS096814 (A.L.H), F31 NS094004 (to B.L.H.), and F31 NS087801 (to S.D.A.), and by a National Institute of Child Health and Human Development Grant R01 HD80601 (to K.R.M.). K.R.M. is a Harry Weaver Neuroscience Scholar of

Competing interests
The authors have no competing interests.

Author details
[1]Department of Developmental Biology, Washington University School of Medicine, St. Louis, MO 63110, USA. [2]Vollum Institute, Oregon Health and Science University, Portland, OR 97239, USA. [3]Institute of Neuroscience, University of Oregon, Eugene, OR 97403, USA.

References
1. Jessen KR, Mirsky R. The origin and development of glial cells in peripheral nerves. Nat Rev Neurosci. 2005;6:671–82.
2. Monk KR, Feltri ML, Taveggia C. New insights on Schwann cell development. Glia. 2015;63:1376–93.
3. Feltri ML, Poitelon Y, Previtali SC. How Schwann cells sort axons: new concepts. Neuroscientist. 2016;22:252–65.
4. Feltri ML, Suter U, Relvas JB. The function of RhoGTPases in axon ensheathment and myelination. Glia. 2008;56:1508–17.
5. Nodari A, Previtali SC, Dati G, Occhi S, Court FA, Colombelli C, et al. Alpha6beta4 integrin and dystroglycan cooperate to stabilize the myelin sheath. J Neurosci. 2008;28:6714–9.
6. Benninger Y, Thurnherr T, Pereira JA, Krause S, Wu X, Chrostek-Grashoff A, et al. Essential and distinct roles for cdc42 and rac1 in the regulation of Schwann cell biology during peripheral nervous system development. J Cell Biol. 2007;177:1051–61.
7. Guo L, Moon C, Niehaus K, Zheng Y, Ratner N. Rac1 controls Schwann cell myelination through cAMP and NF2/merlin. J Neurosci. 2012;32:17251–61.
8. Rossman KL, Der CJ, Sondek J. GEF means go: turning on RHO GTPases with guanine nucleotide-exchange factors. Nat Rev Mol Cell Biol. 2005;6:167–80.
9. Yamauchi J, Miyamoto Y, Tanoue A, Shooter EM, Chan JR. Ras activation of a Rac1 exchange factor, Tiam1, mediates neurotrophin-3-induced Schwann cell migration. Proc Natl Acad Sci U S A. 2005;102:14889–94.
10. Yamauchi J, Chan JR, Miyamoto Y, Tsujimoto G, Shooter EM. The neurotrophin-3 receptor TrkC directly phosphorylates and activates the nucleotide exchange factor Dbs to enhance Schwann cell migration. Proc Natl Acad Sci U S A. 2005;102:5198–203.
11. Miyamoto Y, Torii T, Nakamura K, Takashima S, Sanbe A, Tanoue A, et al. Signaling through Arf6 guanine-nucleotide exchange factor cytohesin-1 regulates migration in Schwann cells. Cell Signal. 2013;25:1379–87.
12. Yamauchi J, Miyamoto Y, Torii T, Takashima S, Kondo K, Kawahara K, et al. Phosphorylation of cytohesin-1 by Fyn is required for initiation of myelination and the extent of myelination during development. Sci Signal. 2012;5 ra69
13. Brugnera E, Haney L, Grimsley C, Lu M, Walk SF, Tosello-Trampont A-C, et al. Unconventional Rac-GEF activity is mediated through the Dock180-ELMO complex. Nat Cell Biol. 2002;4:574–82.
14. Côté J-F, Vuori K. Identification of an evolutionarily conserved superfamily of DOCK180-related proteins with guanine nucleotide exchange activity. J Cell Sci. 2002;115:4901–13.
15. Côté J-F, Vuori K. GEF what? Dock180 and related proteins help Rac to polarize cells in new ways. Trends Cell Biol. 2007;17:383–93.
16. Hasegawa H, Kiyokawa E, Tanaka S, Nagashima K, Gotoh N, Shibuya M, et al. DOCK180, a major CRK-binding protein, alters cell morphology upon translocation to the cell membrane. Mol Cell Biol. 1996;16:1770–6.
17. Reddien PW, Horvitz HR. CED-2/CrkII and CED-10/Rac control phagocytosis and cell migration in Caenorhabditis elegans. Nat Cell Biol. 2000;2:131–6.
18. Ziegenfuss JS, Doherty J, Freeman MR. Distinct molecular pathways mediate glial activation and engulfment of axonal debris after axotomy. Nat Neurosci. 2012;15:979–87.
19. Laurin M, Fradet N, Blangy A, Hall A, Vuori K, Côté J-F. The atypical Rac activator Dock180 (Dock1) regulates myoblast fusion in vivo. Proc Natl Acad Sci U S A. 2008;105:15446–51.
20. Yamauchi J, Miyamoto Y, Chan JR, Tanoue A. ErbB2 directly activates the exchange factor Dock7 to promote Schwann cell migration. J Cell Biol. 2008;181:351–65.
21. Miyamoto Y, Torii T, Kawahara K, Tanoue A, Yamauchi J. Dock8 interacts with Nck1 in mediating Schwann cell precursor migration. Biochem Biophys Rep. 2016;6:113–23.
22. Monk KR, Talbot WS. Genetic dissection of myelinated axons in zebrafish. Curr Opin Neurobiol. 2009;19:486–90.
23. Moore CA, Parkin CA, Bidet Y, Ingham PW. A role for the myoblast city homologues Dock1 and Dock5 and the adaptor proteins Crk and Crk-like in zebrafish myoblast fusion. Development. 2007;134:3145–53.

24. Epting D, Wendik B, Bennewitz K, Dietz CT, Driever W, Kroll J. The Rac1 regulator ELMO1 controls vascular morphogenesis in zebrafish. Circ Res. 2010;107:45–55.

25. Schäker K, Bartsch S, Patry C, Stoll SJ, Hillebrands J-L, Wieland T, et al. The bipartite rac1 guanine nucleotide exchange factor engulfment and cell motility 1/dedicator of cytokinesis 180 (elmo1/dock180) protects endothelial cells from apoptosis in blood vessel development. J Biol Chem. 2015;290:6408–18.

26. McGraw HF, Snelson CD, Prendergast A, Suli A, Raible DW. Postembryonic neuronal addition in zebrafish dorsal root ganglia is regulated by notch signaling. Neural Dev. 2012;7:23.

27. Gilmour DT, Maischein H-M, Nüsslein-Volhard C. Migration and function of a glial subtype in the vertebrate peripheral nervous system. Neuron. 2002;34:577–88.

28. Wang Y, Kaiser MS, Larson JD, Nasevicius A, Clark KJ, Wadman SA, et al. Moesin1 and Ve-cadherin are required in endothelial cells during in vivo tubulogenesis. Development. 2010;137:3119–28.

29. Herbert AL, Fu M-M, Drerup CM, Gray RS, Harty BL, Ackerman SD, et al. Dynein/dynactin is necessary for anterograde transport of Mbp mRNA in oligodendrocytes and for myelination in vivo. Proc Natl Acad Sci U S A. 2017;114:E9153–62.

30. Sanchez NE, Harty BL, O'Reilly-Pol T, Ackerman SD, Herbert AL, Holmgren M, et al. Whole Genome Sequencing-Based Mapping and Candidate Identification of Mutations from Fixed Zebrafish Tissue. G3 (Bethesda). 2017; g3.300212.2017

31. Bedell VM, Wang Y, Campbell JM, Poshusta TL, Starker CG, Ii RGK, et al. *In vivo* genome editing using a high-efficiency TALEN system. Nature. 2012; 491:114–8.

32. Cunningham RL, Monk KR. Whole mount in situ hybridization and immunohistochemistry for zebrafish larvae. Methods Mol Biol. 2018; 1739:371–84.

33. Thisse C, Thisse B. High-resolution in situ hybridization to whole-mount zebrafish embryos. Nat Protoc. 2008;3:59–69.

34. Dutton KA, Pauliny A, Lopes SS, Elworthy S, Carney TJ, Rauch J, et al. Zebrafish colourless encodes sox10 and specifies non-ectomesenchymal neural crest fates. Development. 2001;128:4113–25.

35. Pogoda H-M, Sternheim N, Lyons DA, Diamond B, Hawkins TA, Woods IG, et al. A genetic screen identifies genes essential for development of myelinated axons in zebrafish. Dev Biol. 2006;298:118–31.

36. Lyons DA, Pogoda H-M, Voas MG, Woods IG, Diamond B, Nix R, et al. erbb3 and erbb2 are essential for schwann cell migration and myelination in zebrafish. Curr Biol. 2005;15:513–24.

37. Petersen SC, Luo R, Liebscher I, Giera S, Jeong S-J, Mogha A, et al. The adhesion GPCR GPR126 has distinct, domain-dependent functions in Schwann cell development mediated by interaction with laminin-211. Neuron. 2015;85:755–69.

38. Cunningham RL, Monk KR. Transmission Electron microscopy for zebrafish larvae and adult lateral line nerve. Methods Mol Biol. 2018;1739:385–400.

39. Czopka T, Lyons DA. Dissecting mechanisms of myelinated axon formation using zebrafish. Methods Cell Biol. 2011;105:25–62.

40. Cunningham RL, Monk KR. Live imaging of Schwann cell development in zebrafish. Methods Mol Biol. 2018;1739:401–5.

41. Grimsley CM, Kinchen JM, Tosello-Trampont A-C, Brugnera E, Haney LB, Lu M, et al. Dock180 and ELMO1 proteins cooperate to promote evolutionarily conserved Rac-dependent cell migration. J Biol Chem. 2004;279:6087–97.

42. Riedl J, Crevenna AH, Kessenbrock K, Yu JH, Neukirchen D, Bista M, et al. Lifeact: a versatile marker to visualize F-actin. Nat Methods. 2008;5:605–7.

43. Salzer JL. Schwann cell myelination. Cold Spring Harb Perspect Biol. 2015;7: a020529.

44. Cattin A-L, Burden JJ, Van Emmenis L, Mackenzie FE, Hoving JJA, Garcia Calavia N, et al. Macrophage-induced blood vessels guide Schwann cell-mediated regeneration of peripheral nerves. Cell. 2015;162:1127–39.

45. Côté J-F, Motoyama AB, Bush JA, Vuori K. A novel and evolutionarily conserved PtdIns(3,4,5)P3-binding domain is necessary for DOCK180 signalling. Nat Cell Biol. 2005;7:797–807.

46. Delague V, Jacquier A, Hamadouche T, Poitelon Y, Baudot C, Boccaccio I, et al. Mutations in FGD4 encoding the rho GDP/GTP exchange factor FRABIN cause autosomal recessive Charcot-Marie-tooth type 4H. Am J Hum Genet. 2007;81:1–16.

47. Stendel C, Roos A, Deconinck T, Pereira J, Castagner F, Niemann A, et al. Peripheral nerve demyelination caused by a mutant rho GTPase guanine nucleotide exchange factor, frabin/FGD4. Am J Hum Genet. 2007;81:158–64.

48. Verhoeven K, De Jonghe P, Van de Putte T, Nelis E, Zwijsen A, Verpoorten N, et al. Slowed conduction and thin myelination of peripheral nerves associated with mutant rho guanine-nucleotide exchange factor 10. Am J Hum Genet. 2003;73:926–32.

8

Fate bias during neural regeneration adjusts dynamically without recapitulating developmental fate progression

Jeremy Ng Chi Kei[1], Peter David Currie[1] and Patricia Regina Jusuf[1,2]* iD

Abstract

Background: Regeneration of neurons in the central nervous system is poor in humans. In other vertebrates neural regeneration does occur efficiently and involves reactivation of developmental processes. Within the neural retina of zebrafish, Müller glia are the main stem cell source and are capable of generating progenitors to replace lost neurons after injury. However, it remains largely unknown to what extent Müller glia and neuron differentiation mirror development.

Methods: Following neural ablation in the zebrafish retina, dividing cells were tracked using a prolonged labelling technique. We investigated to what extent extrinsic feedback influences fate choices in two injury models, and whether fate specification follows the histogenic order observed in development.

Results: By comparing two injury paradigms that affect different subpopulations of neurons, we found a dynamic adaptability of fate choices during regeneration. Both injuries followed a similar time course of cell death, and activated Müller glia proliferation. However, these newly generated cells were initially biased towards replacing specifically the ablated cell types, and subsequently generating all cell types as the appropriate neuron proportions became re-established. This dynamic behaviour has implications for shaping regenerative processes and ensuring restoration of appropriate proportions of neuron types regardless of injury or cell type lost.

Conclusions: Our findings suggest that regenerative fate processes are more flexible than development processes. Compared to development fate specification we observed a disruption in stereotypical birth order of neurons during regeneration Understanding such feedback systems can allow us to direct regenerative fate specification in injury and diseases to regenerate specific neuron types in vivo.

Keywords: Neural regeneration, Zebrafish, Fate bias, Retina, Fate specification

Background

All vertebrates show some potential for neural regeneration in the central nervous system, including the retina. In lower vertebrates, such as zebrafish, the adult retina contains multiple neurogenic cell sources including progenitors in the ciliary margin zone, and Müller glia [1–6]. Retinal injuries activate Müller glia to de-differentiate and reactivate neurodevelopmental gene expression cascades in zebrafish [7–13]. Although the regenerative response is more limited in mammals, glia activation and proliferation

has also been observed in rodent [14], and human in vitro studies [15, 16], additional to chick [17] and amphibian (reviewed in [18]). Fate specification during development is controlled primarily by intrinsic gene expression, but also influenced by environmental cues [19–25]. However, little is known about the extent to which regenerating adult progenitors may utilise such cues and whether conserved developmental processes are recapitulated.

Efficient glial driven functional visual recovery [11, 13, 26–30] and regeneration of ablated photoreceptor, ganglion or bipolar cells [26, 31–34] occurs in zebrafish. Proliferative cells show a bias towards generating ablated cell fates, but also generate non-ablated cells [33, 35, 36]. This shows their intrinsic multipotency and may reflect

---

* Correspondence: patricia.jusuf@unimelb.edu.au
[1]Australian Regenerative Medicine Institute, Monash University, Clayton, VIC 3800, Australia
[2]School of Biosciences, University of Melbourne, Parkville, VIC 3010, Australia

recapitulation of intrinsic molecular processes that control temporal cell fate decision as observed in development. Assessing these questions will have profound implications for targeted and efficient regeneration within the tissue to direct regenerative processes including fate choices, differentiation and circuit integration.

Our study has used extended time-course labelling to mark all newly regenerated cells and quantified the proportion of each retinal neuron type regenerated (i.e. ablated vs. non-ablated). Differential neural cell ablation was found to direct fate specification in regenerating progenitors dynamically. In contrast to previous studies, we identify a key early time point at which ablated neurons are almost exclusively regenerated. Subsequently, such cell specific regeneration restores the appropriate neural proportions, and progenitors switch towards an unbiased mode. Unexpectedly and not previously described, our results show a lack of conservation in the developmental histogenic order during regeneration. Thus, regenerating progenitors display a remarkable adaptability by using extrinsic feedback to dynamically adjust fate specification. This correcting of neural composition might aid with appropriate synaptic circuit formation and visual function recovery in vivo.

Methods
Zebrafish husbandry
Zebrafish (*Danio rerio*) of either gender were maintained at FishCore at Monash University or Walter and Eliza Hall Institute of Medical research zebrafish facility in accordance with local animal guidelines. Animals were assigned to the various experimental groups randomly and no animals were excluded from analysis. Fishlines used include TU, Tg(*ptf1a:Gal4*) kindly provided by Prof. Leach [37], Tg(*UAS:nfsb-mCherry*) [38], a gift from Prof. Lieschke, Tg(*gfap:GFP*) generated by Dr. Bernardos and Prof. Raymond [39], Tg(*vsx1:GFP*) provided by Prof. Higashijima [40], Tg(*atoh7:GFP*) generated by Drs Zolessi and Poggi [41]. Lines were crossed to generate double and triple transgenic lines such as Tg(*atoh7:GFP/ptf1a:Gal4/UAS:nfsb-mCherry*) and Tg(*vsx1:GFP/ptf1a:-Gal4/UAS:nfsb-mCherry*). Juveniles were maintained according to standard protocol, staged as previously described [42], and used before and after free feeding stages.

Mechanical ablation (needle stick injury)
One week old zebrafish were anaesthetised in 0.0006% tricaine methanesulfonate and placed on 2% low melt agarose coated petri dishes. Retinal injury was performed using glass needles, pulled from a 1.0 mm O.D × 0.78 mm I.D glass capillary (Harvard Apparatus, Holliston, MA, USA). Injury was conducted at 6 different locations on the eye. The zebrafish were recovered in fresh E3 solution and subsequently monitored for welfare purposes.

Genetic ablation (metronidazole treated nitroreductase injury)
One week old Tg(*ptf1a:Gal4/UAS:nfsb-mCherry*) zebrafish were incubated in 10 mM metronidazole/0.2% DMSO in E3 (NaCl, KCl, $CaCl_2.2H_2O$, $MgCl_2.6H_2O$, methylene blue) solution for 8 h at 28 °C. Zebrafish were rinsed 3 times in fresh E3 media, and monitored for welfare purposes.

5-bromo-2′-deoxyuridine (BrdU) exposure
The proliferative phase and fate tracking of newly generated cells was performed using BrdU incorporation. Larvae were swum in 2 mM BrdU diluted in E3 (pH 7.0). Larvae were swum for 24 h to BrdU at stages 0 to 7 days post injury (dpi). For prolonged BrdU pulse experiments, larvae were swum overnight for 16 h every day from 3 dpi to 7 dpi, and recovered in fresh E3 for 8 h during the day.

Immunohistochemistry
Larvae were fixed in 4% paraformaldehyde (PFA) in phosphate buffered saline (PBS, pH 7.4), cryoprotected in 7.5% gelatine (GL005/500G, Science Supply Australia, Mitcham, Australia) / 15% sucrose in PBS solution, and cryostat sectioned at 14 µm thickness using a Leica CM3050S Cryostat. Antibody staining was performed at room temperature using standard protocols. Sections were blocked in 5% fetal bovine serum (FBS)/0.5% Triton x-100 in PBS, and incubated overnight in primary antibody diluted in the same block solution. Secondary antibodies used (all 1:400 from Thermo Fisher Scientific, Mulgrave, Australia) were anti-mouse Alexa Fluor-488 (cat. number A11001) or Alexa Fluor-546 (cat. number 1256168), anti-rabbit Alexa Fluor-546 (cat. number A11010) and anti-sheep Alexa Fluor-546 (cat. number A21098) diluted in the same block solution. Nuclei were counterstained with 4′,6-diamidino-2-phenylindole (DAPI, cat. number D9542-10MG, Sigma-Aldrich, Castle Hill, Australia) and sections mounted in Mowiol (cat. number 81381-250G, Sigma-Aldrich, Castle Hill, Australia).

Antibodies
Detection of proliferating cells was performed with mouse anti-BrdU (1:500, Sigma Aldrich, cat. number 11170376001, clone BMC9318) [19], which specifically labels BrdU [43].

Characterisation of cell death resulting from each injury paradigm was detected using the terminal deoxynucleotidyl transferase dUTP nick end labeling (TUNEL) with the in situ cell death detection kit, fluorescein including sheep anti-fluorescein Fab fragment antibody (1:500, Sigma Aldrich, cat. number 11684795910, Castle Hill, Australia).

Proliferating cells were detected with rabbit anti-PCNA (proliferating cell nuclear antigen) antibody (1:500, Sigma Aldrich, cat. number SAB2701819), which specifically recognises zebrafish PCNA (manufacturer's information).

Image acquisition

Images of fixed sections were obtained on a Zeiss Z1 (20× objective) using an AxioCam (HRm 13-megapixel, monochrome) with Apotome and Axiovision software. Brightness and contrast were adjusted with Photoshop (Adobe, San Jose, CA, USA).

Analysis

The number of larvae analysed is indicated in the figure legends. Co-labelling quantification was performed only on images taken with the Apotome to provide single optical sections similar to confocal images. For cell death, cell cycle exit, cell fate specification, TUNEL, PCNA, Atoh7:GFP and Vsx1:GFP co-labelled cell were analysed across the central retina, excluding the ciliary margin zone (a region of developmental neurogenesis) and standardized to 400 μm, which represents the width of the layers in an average retinal section. Because the section thickness is the same for all experiments, all quantifications are directly comparable. All results are presented as mean ± SEM. The relative proportion of ablated cell types regenerated at each time point was compared to the control uninjured proportions using student's t-test.

Results

Cell death in distinct neural populations can be efficiently targeted by specificity of injury

In zebrafish, after the initial developmental wave (first 72 h postfertilisation (hpf) [44, 45]), growth via developmental neurogenesis continues in the very peripheral edge in a specialised niche termed the ciliary margin zone (CMZ) [reviewed in 7, 12]. Thus, regenerative neurogenesis can be studied in the spatially separate mature/adult (central) retina, which allowed us to established a nitroreductase-metronidazole induced (genetic) ablation model targeted at ablating inhibitory retinal neurons, namely horizontal and amacrine cells at 7 dpf. The efficacy of this injury model was assessed by characterising and comparing its time course, extent, and specificity to a mechanical injury that targeted all retinal neuron types.

The mechanical needle stick injury is local and we used 6 stabs evenly spaced across the retina to induce wide-spread injury. Immediately after mechanical injury an injury track disrupting all retinal layers was observable (Fig. 1b).

The genetic injury targeted inhibitory neurons using a *ptf1a* promoter [46] to drive the expression of the nitroreductase enzyme, which in turn converts the pro-drug

metronidazole into a cytotoxin. By using a transgenic marker of these inhibitory neurons, Tg(*ptf1a:GFP*), the loss of horizontal cell (HC) and amacrine cell (AC) was observed (Fig. 1d). Cell types could also easily be classified by their laminar location, morphology and co-expression of the m-Cherry tag confined to HCs and ACs. The HCs form a single layer of flattened nuclei in the outermost row of the inner nuclear layer and ACs are weaker DAPI-stained neurons in the inner half of the inner nuclear layer (using Tg(*ptf1a:GFP*) the DAPI label distinctions shows only 4.6% false negative (i.e. GFP labelled amacrine cells erroneously assigned to the brighter DAPI labelling in this layer, n = 995 cells from 7 larvae).The number of inhibitory neurons was reduced by 51% for amacrine cells (41 ± 2 SEM cells/400 μm retinal width untreated vs. 21 ± 1.5 SEM cells/400 μm retinal width post-injury, n = 6 and 7 larvae) and 67% for horizontal cells (9 ± 0.775 SEM cells/400 μm retinal width untreated vs. 3 ± 0.842 SEM cells/400 μm retinal width post-injury, n = 6 or 7 larvae).

Cell death was characterised at 0, 1, 2, 3, 4, 5, 7 and 10 days post injury (dpi) using TUNEL labelling (Fig. 1e-j). After mechanical injury, cell death was observed in 52 ± 25.3 SEM cells/400 μm retinal width and peaked at 1 dpi (56 ± 14.8 SEM cells/400 μm retinal width), being almost completely gone by 3 dpi (2.4 ± 0.89 SEM cells/ 400 μm retinal width) (Fig. 1k). After genetic injury, cell death also peaked at 1 dpi (41 ± 13.8 SEM cells/400 μm retinal width), was reduced by 3 dpi (6.4 ± 0.52 SEM/400 μm retinal width) and almost gone after 5 dpi (Fig. 1l). There was no significant difference between the number of TUNEL labelled cells at any timepoint (student's t-test, p-value range 0.09–0.65) except for 4 dpi (student's t-test, p-value = 0.049), suggesting that cell death after genetic injury may continue a little bit longer. The reduction of TUNEL positive and nitroreductase-mCherry (red) labelled cells as time proceeds is due to the clearing by Müller glia, whose processes can be seen to contain the mCherry transgene at 3 dpi (Fig. 1j). Cell death occurred across the retinal layers after mechanical injury (Fig.1k) and primarily in inhibitory layers 81% ± 3.41 SEM cells/400 μm retinal width after genetic ablation (arrowheads in Fig. 1j) as compared to 34% ± 6.24 SEM cells/400 μm retinal width post mechanical injury. The proportion of inhibitory neurons lost after genetic injury was significantly higher than the proportion of inhibitory neurons lost after mechanical injury at 0–3 dpi (p-value = 0.011 at 0 dpi, 0.0003 at 1 dpi, 0.039 at 2 dpi, 0.004 at 3 dpi) and could not be computed at 4–10 dpi, because there were insufficient TUNEL labelled cells in one or both of the injuries at these timepoints. Consistently, the genetic injury causes a rapid loss of nitroreductase (nfsb) positive cells (Fig. 1l). Thus, differential cell type specific injury with comparable cell death progression was achieved using these two distinct ablation injury models (Fig. 1e-j).

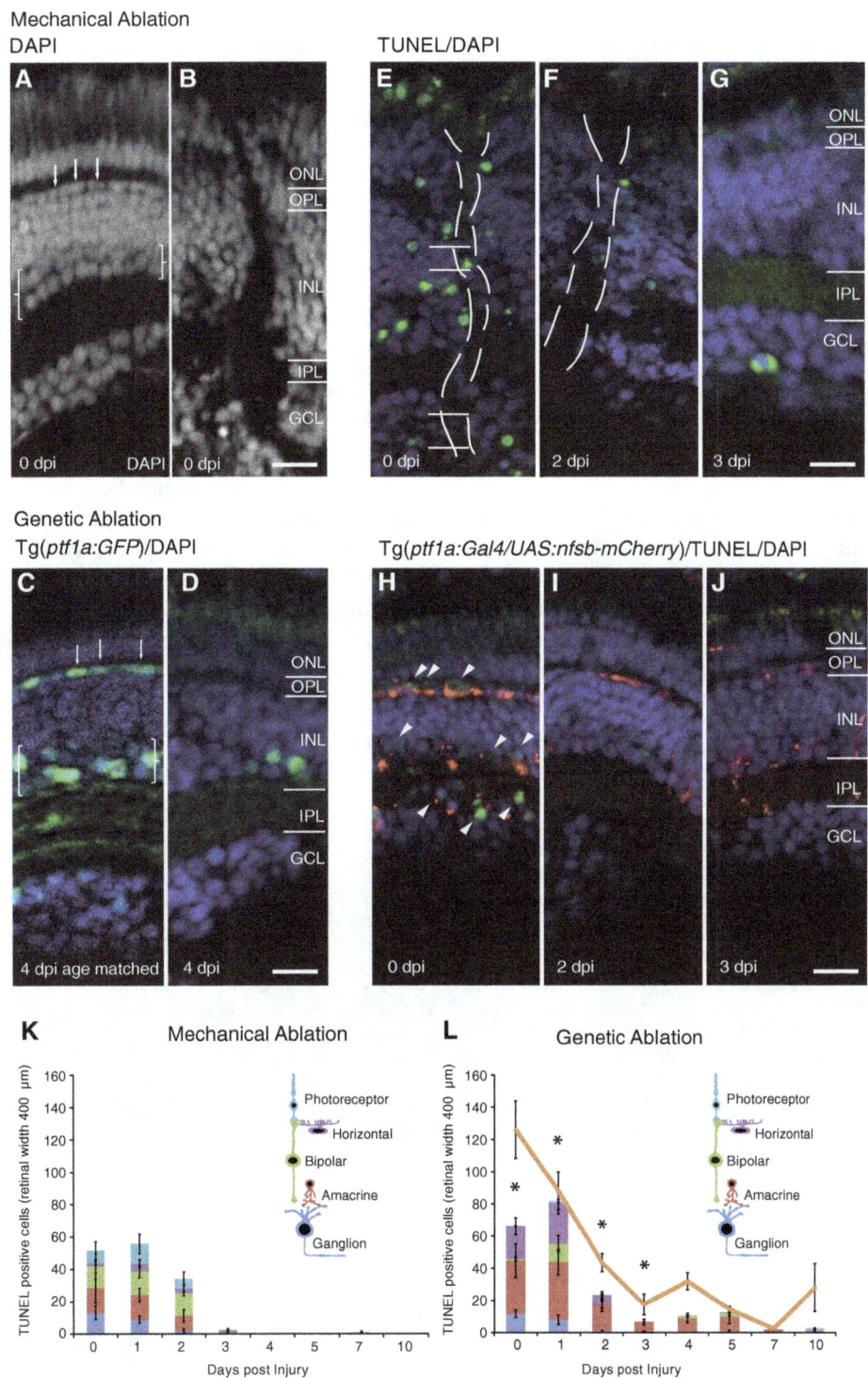

Fig. 1 (See legend on next page.)

(See figure on previous page.)

Fig. 1 Neuron type specific cell death and comparable regenerative time course in two distinct injury models. **a-j** Micrographs of retinal sections after mechanical (**a**, **b**, **e-g**) or metronidazole induced genetic ablation in Tg(*ptf1a:Gal4 / UAS:nfsb-mCherry*) (**c**, **d**, **h-j**, **a**, **c**) Retinal architecture of the uninjured retina at equivalent ages (**b**, **d**). *Brackets* indicate the amacrine neuron layer (weaker DAPI staining in the inner half of the INL) and *arrows* indicate the horizontal neuron layer (first row of flattened nuclei in the inner nuclear layer – INL). **b**, **d** Retinal architecture of injured retina revealed by DAPI staining shows disruption caused by the needle track immediately after ablation injury (0 dpi), affecting neurons types in each retinal layer (**b**), and loss of horizontal cells and amacrine cells (seen by the reduction in Ptf1a:GFP transgene expression, which specifically labels these two cell types) 4 days after injury, which is a timepoint following the main cell death phase (**d**). **e-j** TUNEL labelling at different days post-injury (dpi) in both injury models. TUNEL staining is observed in all retinal layers early after mechanical ablation (**e-g**) and more biased towards horizontal and amacrine cells (*arrowheads* in INL and displaced amacrine cells in GCL) layers among nitroreductase expressing (*red*) cells (**h-j**). **k**, **l** Quantification of TUNEL positive cells in the different retinal layers across days post-injury reveals a peak in cell death in the first two days distributed across all retinal layers in the mechanical ablation (**k**) and primarily confined to inhibitory neurons after genetic ablation (**l**) (*n* = 12 larvae per timepoint). *Asterisks* indicate timepoints at which TUNEL labelling was in a significantly higher proportion of inhibitory neurons in the genetic versus mechanical ablation (*p*-value <0.038). **l** Loss of nitroreductase-mCherry positive cells follows the cell death observed in genetic ablation (orange line, *n* = 12 larvae per timepoint). Results are mean ± SEM. ONL: outer nuclear layer; OPL: outer plexiform layer; IPL: inner plexiform layer; GCL: ganglion cell layer; nfsb: Nitroreductase. Scale bar in D (for **a-d**) = 50 μm, scale bar in J (for **e-j**) = 50 μm

Progenitor proliferation is comparable in mechanical vs. genetic ablation models

The temporal stages of progenitor activation and proliferation were compared using immunohistochemical labelling for proliferating cell nuclear antigen (PCNA), a factor expressed during DNA synthesis. In uninjured age-matched controls of the same transgenic lines, there was little proliferation in this central part of the retina (average 0.25–2 PCNA labelled cells/400 μm retinal width, *n* = 50 retinas). PCNA positive cell clusters suggestive of clones arising from individual cells were observed after mechanical injury (Fig. 2b), with a peak between 4 and 6 dpi (Fig. 2d, 4 dpi: 32.8 ± 8.33 SEM cells/400 μm retinal width; 5 dpi: 16.8 ± 3.82 SEM cells/400 μm retinal width; 6 dpi: 12.8 ± 3.51 SEM cells/400 μm retinal width) and after genetic injury (Fig. 2f), with a peak between 5 and 7 dpi (Fig. 2h; 5 dpi: 19.6 ± 4.34 SEM cells/400 μm retinal width; 6 dpi:

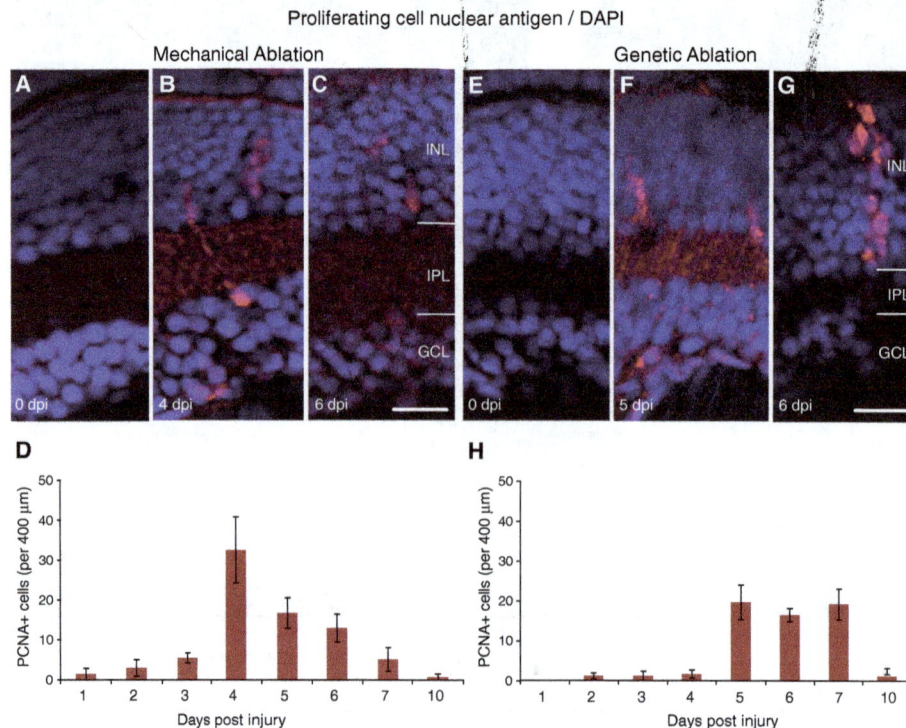

Fig. 2 Timing of PCNA labelled proliferation is comparable between injury models. **a-c**, **e-g** Micrographs of retinal sections after mechanical injury (**a-c**) and genetic ablation injury (**e-g**). Retinal sections stained for PCNA (proliferating cell nuclear antigen, *red*) show cell clusters that span across multiple retinal layers in both injury models (**b**, **f**, **g**). **d**, **h** The graph shows the total number of PCNA cells after mechanical (**d**) and genetic ablation injury (**h**) model, suggesting that broadly, proliferation does not begin until 3–4 dpi and is active for at least three days (*n* = 12 larvae per timepoint per injury model). Results are mean ± SEM. INL: inner nuclear layer; IPL: inner plexiform layer; GCL: ganglion cell layer. Scale bar in G (for **a-c**, **e-g**) = 50 μm

16.4 ± 1.68 SEM cells/400 μm retinal width; 7 dpi: 18.8 ± 3.87 SEM cells/400 μm retinal width). The slightly earlier proliferation after mechanical ablation may be due to the acute cell damage and "death" signal being present immediately, in contrast to the genetic model, which relies on conversion of prodrug, accumulation of toxin, and robust activation of apoptotic pathways. Nonetheless, the period of peak proliferation occurs primarily over a 2-day window at a broadly similar time following either injury.

Regenerating proliferative cells arise from Müller glia

The predominant regenerative cell source after large injuries in the zebrafish retina is the Müller glia [1–3, 11, 14, 32, 47]. A GFP reporter protein was used to label Müller glia Tg(gfap:GFP) in addition to co-labelling with proliferation markers to confirm that progenitors originated from Müller Glia .

Mechanical injury was conducted in Tg(gfap:GFP) and stained for PCNA at 3, 4, 5, 6 & 7 dpi (Fig. 3a-b) confirming previous studies showing that proliferative cells arose from GFAP labelled Müller glia cells. Similarly, genetic injury conducted in Tg(ptf1a:Gal4/UAS:nfsb-mCherry/gfap:GFP) transgenics and stained for PCNA at 1, 2, 3, 4, 5, 6, 7, 8, 9, 10, 11, 12, 14, 21 dpi (Fig. 3c-h) also revealed that Müller glia are the main proliferative cell source following this novel injury paradigm (Fig. 3c-g). At 5 dpi, 97% of all PCNA cells were co-labelled with Gfap:GFP, though most of the co-labelled glia showed a reduction of GFP level as compared to neighbouring non-proliferative glia (Fig. 3a, b). At subsequent days, PCNA labelled cells co-labelled with GFAP:GFP reduced to 57% at 6 dpi and 29% at 7 dpi consistent with de-differentiation (downregulation of GFAP and other glial markers) in these activated cells. This confirms the primary cell source of progenitors in both injury models was the Müller glia cell population.

The environment directs cell type specific regeneration at early stages

In order to determine fate specification during regeneration, we performed prolonged 5-bromo-2′-deoxyuridine (BrdU) labelling across the peak proliferative phase following injury. Because BrdU incorporation and PCNA cell cycle snapshot may differ, we utilised the mechanical injury to compare the proliferative phase identified with PCNA labelling using daily 24 h BrdU pulses . Highest BrdU incorporation occurred at 4 dpi (20.4 ± 0.38 SEM cells/400 μm retinal width) with a reduction by 7 dpi (2 ± 1.07 SEM cells/400 μm retinal width) (Fig. 4a-g), and matched the time course identified by PCNA staining.

Thus, zebrafish were treated after injury with a prolonged BrdU pulse by incubation in BrdU overnight (16 h) and daily from 3 to 7 dpi to encompass the main proliferative stage (Fig. 5a, b). Leaving larvae in BrdU for the entire period unexpectedly resulted in less BrdU labelled cells, and the zebrafish started to show detrimental health, suggesting extensive exposure may have toxic side effects (data not shown). Because BrdU labelled cells can retain the label for additional cell cycles (before being diluted out), this paradigm should label the vast majority, if not all of the newly generated proliferating cells. Control uninjured age-matched tissue labelled only few cells (average 0–0.6 cells/400 μm retinal width, $n = 7$–9 larvae, Fig. 6a, b). The prolonged BrdU pulse labelled 47 cells ±14.88 SEM cells/400 μm retinal width 7 dpi after mechanical injury and 68 cells ±11.66 SEM cells/400 μm retinal width 7 dpi after genetic injury (Fig. 5a, b). Following BrdU exposure withdrawal, the BrdU cell number continued to increase, suggesting that the labelled population may continue dividing.

The proportion of BrdU labelled cells was compared to the normal distribution of retinal neurons in a WT uninjured control, where we quantified 12.5% photoreceptors, 6.4% horizontal cells, 30.4% bipolar cells, 15.5% amacrine cells, 28% displaced amacrine cells and ganglion cells (DAPI labelled Tg(ptf1a:GFP) retinas, $n = 795$ cells from 5 larvae). In particular, we quantified the proportion of BrdU cells that gave rise to the inhibitory neurons that were particularly targeted with the genetic, but not mechanical injury. After mechanical injury (Fig. 5c) BrdU positive cells were found in all retinal layers at all time points. There was no significant difference in the proportion of labelled cells found in inhibitory layer at any of the time points (student's t-test, p-value ranged from 0.10 to 0.74).

After genetic injury (Fig. 5d) at 7 dpi, BrdU positive cells were mainly distributed in the amacrine and horizontal layers (75% ± 4.8% SEM), which was significantly different from the WT distribution of inhibitory cells (student's t-test, p-value = 2.2×10^{-7}). From 10 dpi onwards, proliferating cells were also distributed across other neural layers and showing less pronounced, but still significantly higher representation of inhibitory neurons at 14 dpi (p-value = 0.004), but not 10 dpi (p-value = 0.11) or 17 dpi (p-value = 0.21). By 7 dpi, the retinal laminar architecture started to recover. Quantification of horizontal and amacrine cells following genetic ablation using Tg(ptf1a:GFP) revealed a reduction in GFP positive horizontal and amacrine that was significantly different from 1 dpi (student's t-test, p-values = 0.01 (3 dpi) and 0.01 (4 dpi), and 5 dpi (student's t-test, p-values = 0.018 (3 dpi) and 0.007 (4 dpi). By 5 dpi, there was no significant difference compared to 1 dpi (student's t-test, p-value = 0.50) (Fig. 7), suggesting that the initial wave of biased cell regeneration had re-established cellular proportions. Thus, the bias towards

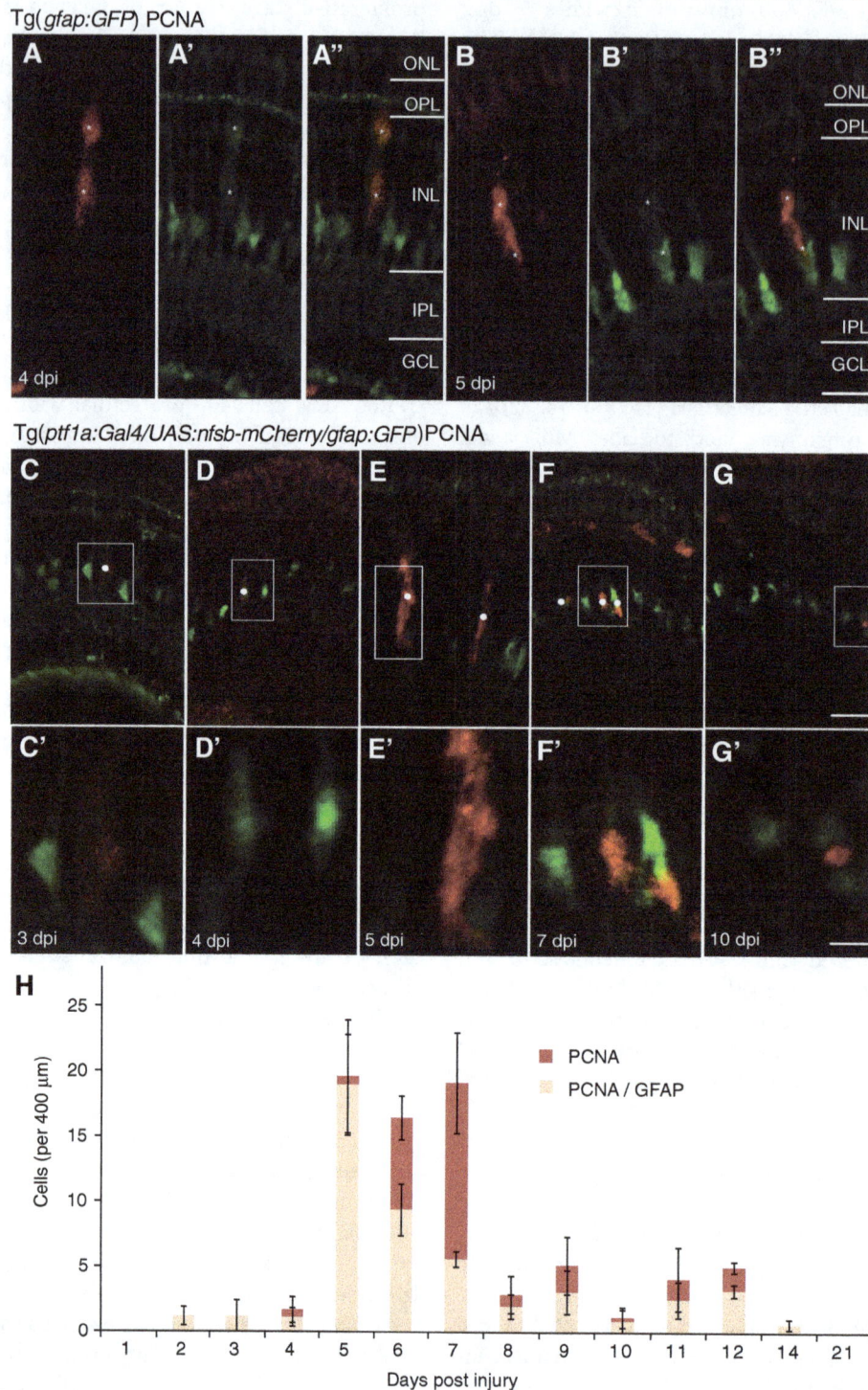

Fig. 3 Progenitors and clones arise from Müller glia. **a-g** Micrographs of retinal sections of Tg(*gfap:GFP*) lines, with Müller glia cells (*green*) stained for PCNA (proliferating cell nuclear antigen red). As previously published, the needle stick injury causes proliferation in Müller glia (**a**). In our newly established genetic injury, PCNA labelled proliferation was also in Müller glia (**b**). **c-h** A detailed time series and quantification (**h**) shows the peak proliferative stage during 5–7 days post-injury (dpi) ($n = 12$ larvae per timepoints 1–10 dpi, $n = 8$ larvae per timepoints 11–14, $n = 6$ larvae at 21 dpi). Proliferative cells in the first 5 dpi also almost exclusively co-labelled with progressively weaker GFAP:GFP, after which time there were also many proliferative cells that no longer expressed detectable GFAP:GFP. White insets (**c'-g'**) show higher power magnification of boxed region indicated in **c-g**. Results are mean ± SEM. ONL: outer nuclear layer; OPL: outer plexiform layer; INL: inner nuclear layer; IPL: inner plexiform layer; GCL: ganglion cell layer. Scale bar B (for **a-b**) = 50 μm, scale bar in G (for **c-g**) = 50 μm, scale bar G' (for **c'-g'**) = 200 μm

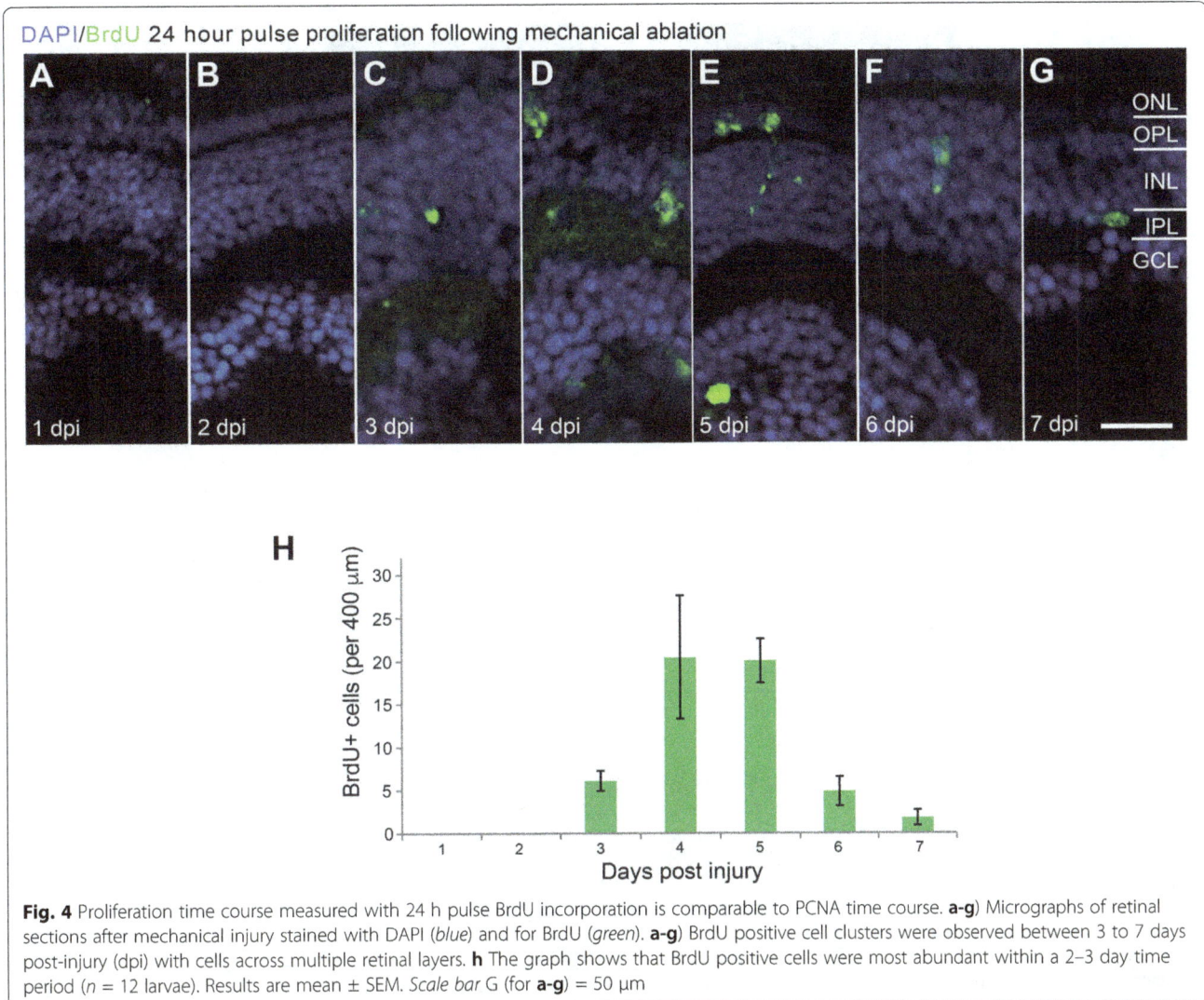

Fig. 4 Proliferation time course measured with 24 h pulse BrdU incorporation is comparable to PCNA time course. **a–g**) Micrographs of retinal sections after mechanical injury stained with DAPI (*blue*) and for BrdU (*green*). **a–g**) BrdU positive cell clusters were observed between 3 to 7 days post-injury (dpi) with cells across multiple retinal layers. **h** The graph shows that BrdU positive cells were most abundant within a 2–3 day time period (*n* = 12 larvae). Results are mean ± SEM. *Scale bar* G (for **a–g**) = 50 µm

specific cell types might remain a dynamic process that continues to adapt to the changing environmental signals as regeneration progresses.

Sequence of fate specification gene expression in proliferative regenerated neurons is distinct from development

During developmental neurogenesis, retinal neuron types are born in a highly conserved histogenic order [48–53]. This process is controlled by the sequential intrinsic expression of fate specification factors. Extrinsic influences can bias or direct fate specification during development at least in part by affecting the timing of such intrinsic fate specification factors [20–25, 54]. Because our injury models result in an initial fate bias, we compared the expression of transcription factors that indicate earliest born (ganglion cell) and latest born (bipolar cell) neurons to assess whether the same sequential gene expression occurs during regeneration.

Both injuries were conducted in transgenic lines Tg(*atoh7:GFP*) (Fig. 6c–e) and Tg(*vsx1:GFP*) (Fig. 6f–h). The bHLH atonal homolog 7 (Atoh7) specifies earliest born ganglion cell fate [20, 55, 56] and the visual homeobox transcription factor 1 (Vsx1) is expressed at medium levels in retinal progenitors and upregulated strongly in differentiating last born bipolar cells [57]. Detection of these transgenes allows us to identify neuron cell specification at an early differentiation stage. Using the prolonged BrdU pulse, we compared the time course of gene expression versus retinal layer distribution of BrdU positive cells at 7, 10, 14 and 17 dpi.

In Tg(*atoh7:GFP*) mechanically injury model, 23% (14.8 ± 8.16 SEM cells/400 µm retinal width) of all BrdU positive cells were located in the ganglion cell layer by 14 dpi, and 75% (11 ± 5.69 SEM cells/400 µm retinal width) of these co-labelled with Atoh7:GFP. Similar results were observed at 17 dpi. Thus, cells within the

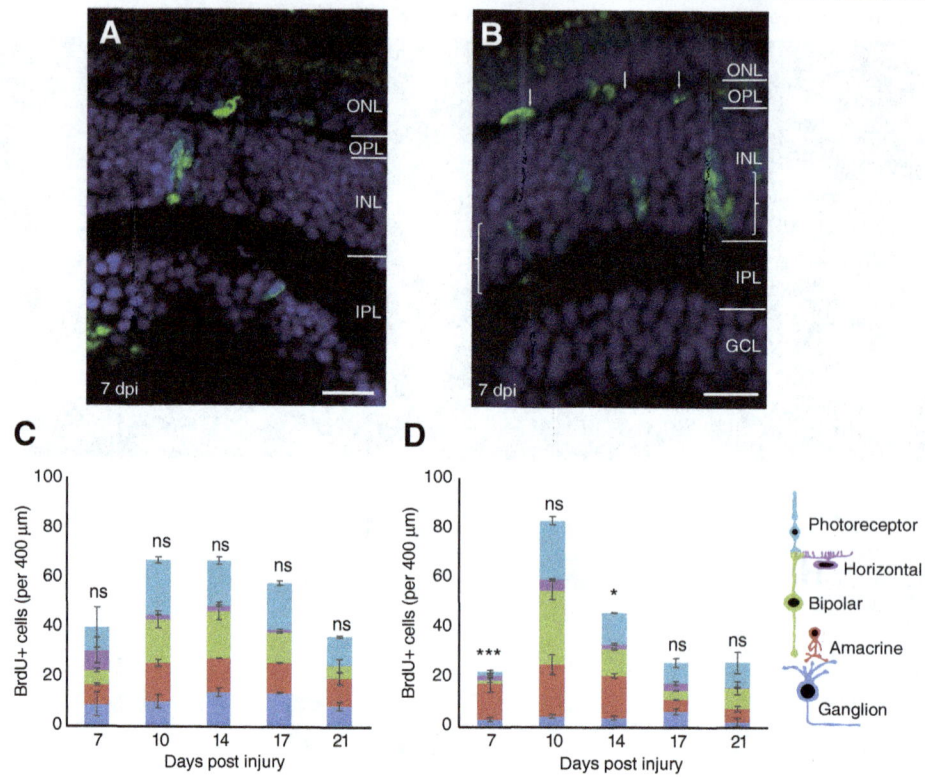

Fig. 5 Prolonged BrdU exposure reveals cell type specific replacement. **a**, **b** Micrographs of mechanical and genetic ablated juveniles in prolonged BrdU exposure between 3 and 7 dpi. Retinal lamination has recovered by this timepoint with horizontal cells (*arrows*) and amacrine cell layer (*brackets*) re-establishing after genetic ablation. **c**, **d** Graphs indicating the total number of BrdU cells in each retinal layer across 5 time points observed in the mechanical (**c**) and genetic (**d**) ablation injury models. Statistics indicate comparison of the proportion of inhibitory neurons compared to age-matched uninjured control composition. After genetic ablation the vast majority of proliferative cells at 7 dpi are confined to the inhibitory layers, most notably the amacrine layer (*** p-value = 2.2×10^{-7} compared to WT proportion). In both injuries, the total number of cells per layer increases after 7 dpi and decreases by 14 dpi (genetic) and 17 dpi (mechanical) (n = 12 larvae at 7 and 10 dpi, 8 larvae at 14 dpi and 6 larvae at 17 and 21 dpi). Ns: not significant (p-value >0.05), * p-value = 0.004. Results are mean ± SEM. ONL: outer nuclear layer; OPL: outer plexiform layer; INL: inner nuclear layer; IPL: inner plexiform layer; GCL: ganglion cell layer; *Scale bars* = 50 μm

ganglion cell layer migrated appropriately and started differentiating at least at 14 dpi. Similarly, 24% of BrdU positive cells were also located in the ganglion cell layer in the genetic ablated Tg(*atoh7:GFP*) cohort by 17 dpi. However, none of these cells expressed Atoh7:GFP at any stage of our analysis, although Atoh7 expression was turned on at 17 dpi in both injuries in BrdU positive cells in the inner half of the inner nuclear layer (20% in mechanical injury; 15% in genetic ablation injury), which is occupied by amacrine cells, a subset of which also arise from this lineage [21, 58]. Thus, after genetic injury, where inhibitory neurons are regenerated first, the generation of ganglion cells and differentiation seems to be delayed relative to the mechanical injury model.

In development, Vsx1 is strongly upregulated in cells as they differentiate into the last born bipolar retinal cell type, which is easily distinguished from the weaker expression in progenitors [57]. In our mechanical injury model, 78% of all BrdU cells in the bipolar layer

(17 ± 8.45 SEM cells/400 μm retinal width) expressed strong Vsx1:GFP signal already at 10 dpi. In the genetic ablation injury model, 73% of all BrdU cells in the bipolar layer (6.8 ± 0.96 SEM BrdU positive cells/400 μm retinal) were co-labelled with Vsx1:GFP at 14 dpi. Vsx1:GFP expression was strongly maintained in all BrdU positive cells in the appropriate retinal bipolar layer at the later stages in mechanical (95%, 14 &17 dpi) and genetic (100%, 17 dpi) ablation models. Thus, as is the case with Atoh7, differentiating Vsx1:GFP expressing bipolar cells are also only generated at a later time point in the genetic ablation model, in which inhibitory neurons are preferentially regenerated first.

These results also indicate that regenerated cells migrate to the their correct laminar location within the retina according to their fate specification. Additionally, after both injuries the timing of expression of Atoh7 (starting 14 dpi in mechanical and 17 dpi in genetic injury) compared to Vsx1 (at 10 dpi in mechanical and

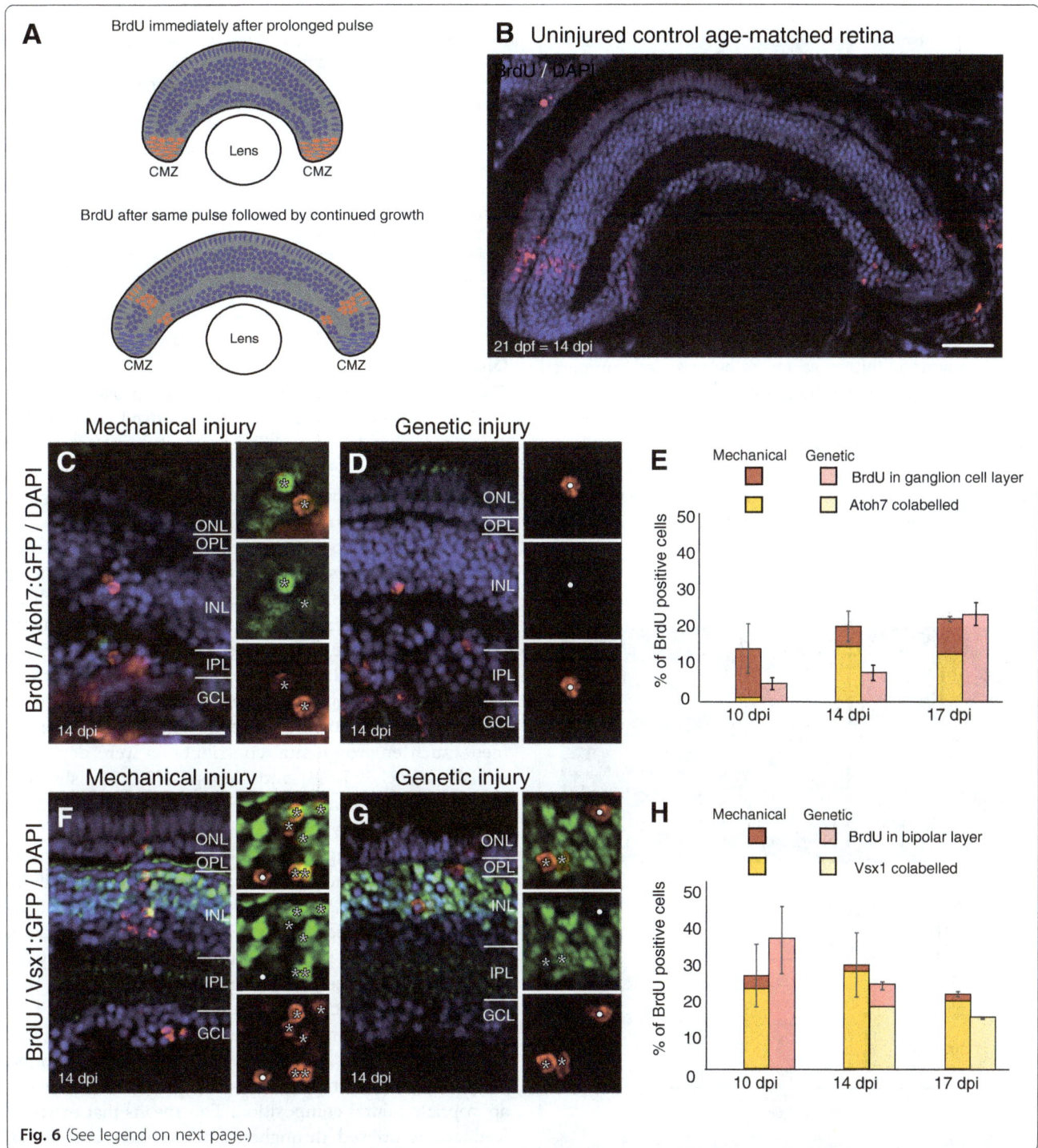

Fig. 6 (See legend on next page.)

Fig. 6 Fate determinant expression during regeneration does not recapitulate developmental sequence after different injuries. **a, b**) In uninjured control, a prolonged BrdU pulse labels neurons in the peripheral ciliary margin zone, which results in a stripe of BrdU positive cells after BrdU withdrawal, as BrdU negative cells continue to be added from the ciliary margin. This BrdU stripe is observed in micrographs from control (**b**). There are no BrdU cells in the mature retina found more centrally. **c-h**) Using prolonged exposure, BrdU labelled cells observed in this central mature retina region reflects regeneration. Micrographs show retinal sections from 14 days post-injury (dpi). The proportion of BrdU positive GCL cells after mechanical injury (n = 17 larvae - 10 dpi, 9 larvae –14 dpi, 12 larvae - 17 dpi) is higher compared to genetic injury (n = 8 larvae - 10 dpi, 15 larvae - 14 dpi, 19 larvae - 17 dpi) at 10 and 14 dpi. The firstborn ganglion cell marker Tg(*atoh7:GFP*) shows more co-labelling after mechanical injury. A large proportion of BrdU positive labelled cells in the bipolar layer (outer half of INL) show high expression of Tg(*vsx1:GFP*) indicative of bipolar differentiation (last born during development) after both injuries, starting earlier after mechanical (n = 13 larvae - 10 dpi, 24 larvae - 14 dpi, 21 larvae - 17 dpi) than genetic (n = 14 larvae - 10 dpi, 21 larvae - 14 dpi, 11 larvae - 17 dpi) injury. For both injuries, strongly labelled Vsx1 cells are observed prior to strongly labelled Atoh7 GCL cells. Results are mean ± SEM ONL: outer nuclear layer; OPL: outer plexiform layer; INL: inner nuclear layer; IPL: inner plexiform layer; GCL: ganglion cell layer. Scale bar B = 100 µm, scale bar C (for **c, d, f, g**) = 50 µm, scale bar in insets C (for *insets* in **c, d, f, g**) = 20 µm

14 dpi in genetic injury) seems to be reversed compared to development. In development Atoh7 is first upregulated at 28 hpf to start generating ganglion cells [20] and Vsx1 is only upregulated at 35 hpf to start generating bipolar cells [57]. Thus, the regeneration of different neuron types may not strictly follow the stereotypical processes observed during development.

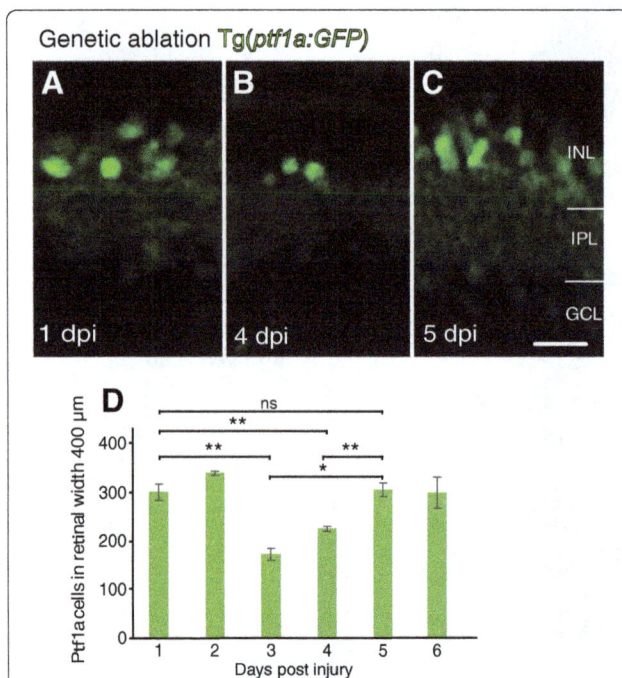

Genetic ablation Tg(*ptf1a:GFP*)

Fig. 7 Following genetic ablation, new horizontal and amacrine cells can be observed prior to the proliferative wave. **a-c**) Micrographs of retinal sections in Tg(*ptf1a:GFP*) larvae at different days post injury (dpi). **d** Quantification shows an initial reduction and subsequent increase in the number of Ptf1a:GFP labelled inhibitory neurons. At 3 and 4 dpi, the number is significantly lower (* p-value = 0.018, ** p-value ≤0.01) compared to 1 dpi (baseline) or 5 dpi (regenerated), which are not significantly different from each other (p-value = 0.50). Ns: not significant (p-value >0.05). Results are mean ± SEM. INL: inner nuclear layer; IPL: inner plexiform layer; GCL: ganglion cell layer. Scale bar C = 50 µm

Discussion

The vertebrate neural retina allows us to assess regenerative processes in a well-characterised and highly organised neural tissue. While signalling pathways involved in retinal regeneration are being identified and expanded, how progenitor cells use these pathways to make fate decisions remains unclear.

Little is known about how pre-programmed versus adjustable fate choices operate in vivo and how the injury environment influences regenerative outcomes, such as determining the fate choice of progenitors to repopulate lost neurons. While the number of each cell type seems to be controlled independently [59] there exists plasticity within the CNS (e.g. neurite arbor size) to compensate by varying in cell type produced [60]. During development, such environmental contributions were described in fish [20, 21, 25, 54] and Xenopus [23, 24], showing that progenitors can be biased towards generating more of the missing subtypes.

There is mounting evidence that regenerating neurons use extrinsic feedback to drive preferential fate specification bias in zebrafish [33, 35, 36]. In our study, we identify a key relative early time point within the first week post injury, where fate specification is biased strongly towards the ablated cell type. Further, our data shows that feedback is dynamic, as progenitors adjust their fate bias as the cell type proportions are restored throughout this regenerative process. Thus, the strong fate bias found early in regeneration reduces as the environment reaches appropriate neural composition. This means that extrinsic feedback is utilised throughout the regenerating period, not only present at the initial stem cell activation phase. Thus, our data supports the hypothesis that intrinsic highly conserved mechanisms such as sequential fate specification factors may be suppressed during regeneration.

Both of our injuries resulted in regenerative responses comparable in timing and extent of cell death and Müller glia driven proliferation. This was important to establish given different paradigms can lead to different regenerative responses [8–10, 47]. Preliminary experiments using 1 or 2 stabs (data not shown) showed a clustered distribution of fewer proliferating cells, consistent with signals triggering regeneration being spatially limited. However, 6 stabs were found to be enough to trigger a proliferative response that was similar in cell number and spatial distribution to that observed in the genetic model. Using prolonged BrdU pulse (3–7 dpi) to label the bulk of regenerating cells, we quantified the differentiation of ablated and non-ablated cell types as regeneration progressed whilst tracking the recovery of retinal architecture and neural proportions. While the prolonged BrdU paradigm consists of 16-h on/8-h off exposure for the benefit of animal health, BrdU can be detected through a few divisions after removal of BrdU. This is consistent with the observation that the number of BrdU cells initially increased beyond 7 dpi (when BrdU exposure was stopped).

At later stages after both injuries, the number of BrdU labelled cells unexpectedly declined and more so after genetic injury. This could be due to newly generated cells undergoing apoptosis, which may be a real biological phenomenon (e.g. cells that do not integrate into circuits) or an artefact of the experimental approach (e.g. cell toxicity due to the prolonged BrdU pulse). Alternatively, proliferation may continue or increase causing a dilution of the BrdU signal.

The mechanical injury resulted in unbiased regeneration of all neuron types. In contrast, genetic ablation resulted in the specific regeneration of the targeted inhibitory neuron types, particularly at early stages of regeneration (7 dpi). Hence, in the genetic ablation model extrinsic fate strongly influenced neural regeneration in line with fate biases and layer selective migration observed in previous zebrafish studies [31–34]. Since our experiments are conducted in young larvae to minimise frequency of metronidazole treatment, the regenerative time course is possibly accelerated compared to adult models [36]. By combining data obtained from labelling different cohorts of proliferative cells [36] with our current work of labelling all cohorts and assessing progression of fate specification throughout the differentiation stages, we propose three key stages of fate determination. Initially, proliferative progenitors may be deployed to all retinal layers in an intrinsic multipotent fashion [36], followed by a second proliferative expansion phase driven by extrinsic feedback to initially replace only the affected neuron types. Finally, at later stages (10 dpi onwards in our genetic injury), proliferative cells also differentiate into non-ablated cell types. Because an initially fate biased regeneration gradually restores normal cell type proportion, the extrinsic feedback will similarly become less fate biased. Thus, the observation that newly generated cells differentiate into all neuron types at later stages suggest progenitors continue to adapt to this new cellular environment to give rise to all retinal cell types. This last phase may still be primarily extrinsically driven rather than requiring a switch back towards an intrinsic pre-programmed mechanism.

The specification of non-ablated neurons at later stages, may indicate an excess number of neurons being regenerated. However, even the peak number of BrdU labelled cells following the prolonged pulse only accounts for half of the number of observed TUNEL positive cells, with TUNEL itself representing only a snapshot of dying cells. Since no striking expansion of layers containing non-ablated cell population was observed, massive overproduction does not seem to be occurring. Nonetheless, it would be an interesting to study newly made non-ablated cell types and assess, how their generation influences overall proportions, neural circuitry and whether appropriate pruning off via cell death occurs.

An intriguing observation following genetic injury is the rapid restoration of retinal inhibitory cells (Fig. 7) by 7 dpi. This occurred despite the number of proliferative cells being too low to account for such extensive regeneration of these ablated neuron types. Therefore, this raises the possibility that restoration of these inhibitory neuron layers may also include non-proliferative contributions from alternate cell sources, which requires further investigation.

Our results show evidence of disruption to the developmental histogenic processes [48, 50, 52, 53, 61]. This was demonstrated by a failure to recapitulate the birth order of last born bipolar cells and first born ganglion cells as both cells expressed transgenes simultaneously. This adds to the evidence of flexibility in cell regeneration processes to shift from the highly co-ordinated gene expression during development towards a more environmental driven process involving more feedback and less rigid intrinsically timed fate progression. A comprehensive fine-scale time course including markers for each fate and clonal analysis would confirm this.

Proliferative cells found in the INL may represent different cell populations. At early regenerative stages, BrdU could be labelling activated Müller glia and early glia derived progenitors, which usually reside in the INL. At intermediate regenerative stages, BrdU labelled cell within the INL could represent progenitor cells undergoing interkinetic nuclear migration (IKNM) cells [62], which occurs during development [63–65], or differentiating cells undergoing their final laminar migration. At late stages, at least after 10 dpi, the co-labelling with the bipolar Vsx1:GFP transgene shows high correlation, suggesting that BrdU labelled cells found in the INL at this stage, are differentiating or mature postmigratory neurons.

Conclusions

We show that the environment after an injury can efficiently and accurately drive neurogenesis, a field that has been previously dominated by contributions of intrinsic gene control. This may be a stronger driver and independent from developmental mechanisms. This data supports alternative approaches to using existing methods that currently direct stem cells in vitro towards a cell specific fate for transplantation therapies. Since visual and other neurodegenerative disorders usually only affect specific neural types, the innate environment may be able to direct the progenitor fate biases. Retinal progenitors introduced early into a host environment may be able to use the extrinsic feedback and existing scaffold to restore correct neuron type proportions. Early integration could also assist other differentiation steps such as migration, pathfinding and re-establishment of neural circuit, that depend on such environmental signals during development. While the processes described during development form an important starting point for our understanding of regeneration, further comparative studies are needed translate such knowledge towards the human clinical setting [16, 66].

Abbreviations

Atoh7: Atonal homolog 7; BrdU: 5-bromo-2'-deoxyuridine; DAPI: 4',6-diamidino-2-phenylindole; dpf: Days postfertilisation; dpi: Days post-injury; hpf: Hours postfertilisation; nfsb: Nitroreductase; PBS: Phosphate buffered saline; PCNA: Proliferating cell nuclear antigen; PFA: Paraformaldehyde; Ptf1a: Pancreas transcription factor 1 a; sem: Standard error of the mean; TUNEL: Terminal deoxynucleotidyl transferase dUTP nick end labelling; UAS: Upstream activating sequence; Vsx1: Visual homeobox transcription factor 1; WT: Wildtype

Acknowledgments

We are grateful for the provisions of transgenic zebrafish from Dr. Zolessi, Dr. Poggi, Prof. Leach, Prof. Lieschke, Prof. Higashijima and Prof. Raymond. We thank Prof. Furness laboratory for microscopy use. We acknowledge FishCore (Monash University) and Walter and Eliza Institute of Medical research zebrafish facility staff for animal maintenance, Ms. Dudczig for technical support and Drs. Brandli, Poggi and Goldshmit for manuscript comments.

Funding

This work was supported by a Faculty of Medicine International Postgraduate Research Scholarship, Monash University to JNCK, and Australian Research Council Discovery Early Career Research Fellowship (DE120101311 to PRJ). The Australian Regenerative Medicine Institute is supported by grants from the State Government of Victoria and the Australian Federal Government.

Authors' contributions

PRJ and JNCK conceived of the study and designed experiments. JNCK carried out the experiments. JNCK, PRJ and PDC, whose laboratory the work was carried out in, wrote the manuscript. All authors read and approved the final manuscript.

Competing interests

The authors declare that they have no competing interests.

References

1. Maier W, Wolburg H. Regeneration of the goldfish retina after exposure to different doses of ouabain. Cell Tissue Res. 1979;202(1):99–118.
2. Hitchcock PF, Raymond PA. Retinal regeneration. Trends Neurosci. 1992; 15(3):103–8.
3. Braisted JE, Essman TF, Raymond PA. Selective regeneration of photoreceptors in goldfish retina. Development. 1994;120(9):2409–19.
4. Fausett BV, Goldman D. A role for alpha1 tubulin-expressing Muller glia in regeneration of the injured zebrafish retina. J Neurosci. 2006;26(23):6303–13.
5. Bernardos RL, et al. Late-stage neuronal progenitors in the retina are radial Muller glia that function as retinal stem cells. J Neurosci. 2007;27(26):7028–40.
6. Goldman D. Muller glial cell reprogramming and retina regeneration. Nat Rev Neurosci. 2014;15(7):431–42.
7. Ng J, Currie PD, Jusuf PR. The regenerative potential of the vertebrate retina: lessons from the Zebrafish. In: Pebay A, editor. Regenerative biology of the eye. New York: Hamana Press Springer Science; 2014. p. 49–82.
8. Vihtelic TS, Hyde DR. Light-induced rod and cone cell death and regeneration in the adult albino zebrafish (Danio rerio) retina. J Neurobiol. 2000;44(3):289–307.
9. Curado S, Stainier DY, Anderson RM. Nitroreductase-mediated cell/tissue ablation in zebrafish: a spatially and temporally controlled ablation method with applications in developmental and regeneration studies. Nat Protoc. 2008;3(6):948–54.
10. Montgomery JE, Parsons MJ, Hyde DR. A novel model of retinal ablation demonstrates that the extent of rod cell death regulates the origin of the regenerated zebrafish rod photoreceptors. J Comp Neurol. 2010;518(6):800–14.
11. Yurco P, Cameron DA. Responses of Muller glia to retinal injury in adult zebrafish. Vis Res. 2005;45(8):991–1002.
12. Raymond PA, et al. Molecular characterization of retinal stem cells and their niches in adult zebrafish. BMC Dev Biol. 2006;6:36.
13. Thummel R, et al. Characterization of Muller glia and neuronal progenitors during adult zebrafish retinal regeneration. Exp Eye Res. 2008;87(5):433–44.
14. Wan J, et al. Preferential regeneration of photoreceptor from Muller glia after retinal degeneration in adult rat. Vis Res. 2008;48(2):223–34.
15. Lawrence JM, et al. MIO-M1 cells and similar muller glial cell lines derived from adult human retina exhibit neural stem cell characteristics. Stem Cells. 2007;25(8):2033–43.
16. Bhatia B, et al. Differences between the neurogenic and proliferative abilities of Muller glia with stem cell characteristics and the ciliary epithelium from the adult human eye. Exp Eye Res. 2011;93(6):852–61.
17. Fischer AJ, Reh TA. Muller glia are a potential source of neural regeneration in the postnatal chicken retina. Nat Neurosci. 2001;4(3):247–52.
18. Hidalgo M, et al. Stem cells and regeneration in the xenopus retina. In: Pebay A, editor. Regenerative biology of the eye. New York: Hamana Press Springer Science; 2014. p. 83–100.
19. Kei JN, et al. Feedback from each retinal neuron population drives expression of subsequent fate determinant genes without influencing the cell cycle exit timing. J Comp Neurol. 2016;524(13):2553–66.
20. Poggi L, et al. Influences on neural lineage and mode of division in the zebrafish retina in vivo. J Cell Biol. 2005;171(6):991–9.
21. Jusuf PR, et al. Origin and determination of inhibitory cell lineages in the vertebrate retina. J Neurosci. 2011;31(7):2549–62.
22. Belliveau MJ, Cepko CL. Extrinsic and intrinsic factors control the genesis of amacrine and cone cells in the rat retina. Development. 1999;126(3):555–66.
23. Reh TA. Cell-specific regulation of neuronal production in the larval frog retina. J Neurosci. 1987;7(10):3317–24.
24. Reh TA, Tully T. Regulation of tyrosine hydroxylase-containing amacrine cell number in larval frog retina. Dev Biol. 1986;114(2):463–9.
25. Tyler MJ, Carney LH, Cameron DA. Control of cellular pattern formation in the vertebrate inner retina by homotypic regulation of cell-fate decisions. J Neurosci. 2005;25(18):4565–76.
26. Fleisch VC, Fraser B, Allison WT. Investigating regeneration and functional integration of CNS neurons: lessons from zebrafish genetics and other fish species. Biochim Biophys Acta. 2011;1812(3):364–80.
27. Fischer AJ, Reh TA. Potential of Muller glia to become neurogenic retinal progenitor cells. Glia. 2003;43(1):70–6.
28. Karl MO, Reh TA. Regenerative medicine for retinal diseases: activating endogenous repair mechanisms. Trends Mol Med. 2010;16(4):193–202.
29. Hitchcock PF, Raymond PA. The teleost retina as a model for developmental and regeneration biology. Zebrafish. 2004;1(3):257–71.
30. Otteson DC, Hitchcock PF. Stem cells in the teleost retina: persistent neurogenesis and injury-induced regeneration. Vis Res. 2003;43(8):927–36.

31. Zhao XF, Ellingsen S, Fjose A. Labelling and targeted ablation of specific bipolar cell types in the zebrafish retina. BMC Neurosci. 2009;10:107.

32. Fimbel SM, et al. Regeneration of inner retinal neurons after intravitreal injection of ouabain in zebrafish. J Neurosci. 2007;27(7):1712–24.

33. Fraser B, et al. Regeneration of cone photoreceptors when cell ablation is primarily restricted to a particular cone subtype. PLoS One. 2013;8(1):e55410.

34. Hochmann S, et al. Fgf signaling is required for photoreceptor maintenance in the adult zebrafish retina. PLoS One. 2012;7(1):e30365.

35. Yoshimatsu T, et al. Presynaptic partner selection during retinal circuit reassembly varies with timing of neuronal regeneration in vivo. Nat Commun. 2016;7:10590.

36. Powell C, et al. Zebrafish Muller glia-derived progenitors are multipotent, exhibit proliferative biases and regenerate excess neurons. Sci Rep. 2016;6:24851.

37. Lin JW, et al. Differential requirement for ptf1a in endocrine and exocrine lineages of developing zebrafish pancreas. Dev Biol. 2004;274(2):491–503.

38. Davison JM, et al. Transactivation from Gal4-VP16 transgenic insertions for tissue-specific cell labeling and ablation in zebrafish. Dev Biol. 2007; 304(2):811–24.

39. Bernardos RL, Raymond PA. GFAP transgenic zebrafish. Gene Expr Patterns. 2006;6(8):1007–13.

40. Kimura Y, Okamura Y, Higashijima S. alx, a zebrafish homolog of Chx10, marks ipsilateral descending excitatory interneurons that participate in the regulation of spinal locomotor circuits. J Neurosci. 2006;26(21):5684–97.

41. Zolessi FR, et al. Polarization and orientation of retinal ganglion cells in vivo. Neural Dev. 2006;1:2.

42. Kimmel CB, et al. Stages of embryonic development of the zebrafish. Dev Dyn. 1995;203(3):253–310.

43. Silvestroff L, et al. Cuprizone-induced demyelination in CNP::GFP transgenic mice. J Comp Neurol. 2010;518(12):2261–83.

44. Easter SS Jr, Nicola GN. The development of vision in the zebrafish (Danio rerio). Dev Biol. 1996;180(2):646–63.

45. Schmitt EA, Dowling JE. Early eye morphogenesis in the zebrafish, Brachydanio rerio. J Comp Neurol. 1994;344(4):532–42.

46. Jusuf PR, Harris WA. Ptf1a is expressed transiently in all types of amacrine cells in the embryonic zebrafish retina. Neural Dev. 2009;4:34.

47. Sherpa T, et al. Ganglion cell regeneration following whole-retina destruction in zebrafish. Dev Neurobiol. 2008;68(2):166–81.

48. La Vail MM, Rapaport DH, Rakic P. Cytogenesis in the monkey retina. J Comp Neurol. 1991;309(1):86–114.

49. Sharma SC, Ungar F. Histogenesis of the goldfish retina. J Comp Neurol. 1980;191(3):373–82.

50. Stiemke MM, Hollyfield JG. Cell birthdays in Xenopus laevis retina. Differentiation. 1995;58(3):189–93.

51. Hollyfield JG. Histogenesis of the retina in the killifish, Fundulus heteroclitus. J Comp Neurol. 1972;144(3):373–80.

52. Fujita S, Horii M. Analysis of cytogenesis in chick retina by tritiated thymidine autoradiography. Arch Histol Jpn. 1963;23:359–66.

53. Rapaport DH, et al. Timing and topography of cell genesis in the rat retina. J Comp Neurol. 2004;474(2):304–24.

54. Ng Chi Kei J, et al. Feedback from retinal neuron population drives expression of subsequent fate determinant genes without influencing the cell cycle exit timing. J Comp Neurol. 2016;524(13):2553-66.

55. Brown NL, et al. Math5 is required for retinal ganglion cell and optic nerve formation. Development. 2001;128(13):2497–508.

56. Ohnuma S, et al. Co-ordinating retinal histogenesis: early cell cycle exit enhances early cell fate determination in the Xenopus retina. Development. 2002;129(10):2435–46.

57. Vitorino M, et al. Vsx2 in the zebrafish retina: restricted lineages through derepression. Neural Dev. 2009;4:14.

58. Jusuf PR, et al. Biasing amacrine subtypes in the Atoh7 lineage through expression of Barhl2. J Neurosci. 2012;32(40):13929–44.

59. Keeley PW, et al. Independent genomic control of neuronal number across retinal cell types. Dev Cell. 2014;30(1):103–9.

60. Reese BE, et al. Developmental plasticity of dendritic morphology and the establishment of coverage and connectivity in the outer retina. Dev Neurobiol. 2011;71(12):1273–85.

61. Nawrocki L, et al. Larval and adult visual pigments of the zebrafish, Brachydanio rerio. Vis Res. 1985;25(11):1569–76.

62. Lahne M, et al. Actin-cytoskeleton- and rock-mediated INM Are Required for Photoreceptor Regeneration in the adult zebrafish retina. J Neurosci. 2015; 35(47):15612–34.

63. Del Bene F, et al. Regulation of neurogenesis by interkinetic nuclear migration through an apical-basal notch gradient. Cell. 2008;134(6):1055–65.

64. Baye LM, Link BA. Interkinetic nuclear migration and the selection of neurogenic cell divisions during vertebrate retinogenesis. J Neurosci. 2007; 27(38):10143–52.

65. Norden C, et al. Actomyosin is the main driver of interkinetic nuclear migration in the retina. Cell. 2009;138(6):1195–208.

66. Giannelli SG, et al. Adult human Muller glia cells are a highly efficient source of rod photoreceptors. Stem Cells. 2011;29(2):344–56.

9

Identification and characterization of mushroom body neurons that regulate fat storage in *Drosophila*

Bader Al-Anzi[1*] and Kai Zinn[2]

Abstract

Background: In an earlier study, we identified two neuronal populations, c673a and Fru-GAL4, that regulate fat storage in fruit flies. Both populations partially overlap with a structure in the insect brain known as the mushroom body (MB), which plays a critical role in memory formation. This overlap prompted us to examine whether the MB is also involved in fat storage homeostasis.

Methods: Using a variety of transgenic agents, we selectively manipulated the neural activity of different portions of the MB and associated neurons to decipher their roles in fat storage regulation.

Results: Our data show that silencing of MB neurons that project into the α'β' lobes decreases de novo fatty acid synthesis and causes leanness, while sustained hyperactivation of the same neurons causes overfeeding and produces obesity. The α'β' neurons oppose and dominate the fat regulating functions of the c673a and Fru-GAL4 neurons. We also show that MB neurons that project into the γ lobe also regulate fat storage, probably because they are a subset of the Fru neurons. We were able to identify input and output neurons whose activity affects fat storage, feeding, and metabolism. The activity of cholinergic output neurons that innervating the β'2 compartment (MBON-β'2mp and MBON-γ5β'2a) regulates food consumption, while glutamatergic output neurons innervating α' compartments (MBON-γ2α'1 and MBON-α'2) control fat metabolism.

Conclusions: We identified a new fat storage regulating center, the α'β' lobes of the MB. We also delineated the neuronal circuits involved in the actions of the α'β' lobes, and showed that food intake and fat metabolism are controlled by separate sets of postsynaptic neurons that are segregated into different output pathways.

Background

Regulation of fat storage and metabolism by the brain requires collaboration among many types of neurons. In mammals, body weight is controlled by specific brain regions, including subdivisions of the hypothalamus [11, 48]. These hypothalamic nuclei contain a variety of neuronal types that can have both behavioral (e.g., feeding and physical activity) and metabolic outputs (e.g., controlling basal metabolic rate, altering rates of de novo fatty acid synthesis) that must be coordinated to ensure that fat content is set at the appropriate levels [11, 12, 53].

In *Drosophila*, genetic screens for alterations in feeding behavior and metabolism have identified many genes.

These include components of the insulin and serotonin pathways, which are known to regulate body weight in mammals [16, 25–27, 36, 39, 44]. *Drosophila* is also an excellent model in which to examine how neuronal activity influences behavior and physiology. This is largely due to the availability of thousands of neuron-specific GAL4 'driver' lines, with which it is possible to turn activity up or down in specific and localized populations of neurons [23, 35].

The mushroom bodies (MBs) are clusters of neurons in the insect brain that project their axons within tracts resembling pairs of mushrooms. The neurons forming this structure are called Kenyon cells (KCs). In fly, there are 2000–2500 KCs per hemisphere [5, 41]. These cells project axons that form the MB lobes. There are two vertical lobes, α and α', and three horizontal lobes, β, β', and γ. αβ KC axons bifurcate and send one branch into

* Correspondence: baderalanzi13@gmail.com
[1]Food & Nutrition Program, Environment & Life Sciences Research Center, Kuwait Institute for Scientific Research, P.O. Box 24885, 13109 Kuwait City, Kuwait

the α lobe and one branch into the β lobe, while α'β' KC axons have one branch in the α' lobe and one branch in the β' lobe. Finally, γ KC axons are unbranched and only project to the γ lobe (see diagram in Fig. 1a, top). A large body of evidence demonstrates that the MB plays critical roles in aversive and appetitive learning, sleep, locomotor activity, and decision making [8, 20, 29, 43].

In an earlier study, we developed a fat-specific thin-layer chromatography (TLC) assay [1, 3], and used it to identify two neuronal populations, defined by the c673a and Fru-GAL4 drivers, that cause obesity when silenced and leanness when hyperactivated. Many of the neurons expressing Fru-GAL4 drivers are γ KCs. In this paper, we describe interactions between specific MB neuron activities that regulate fat content in adult flies. We show that KCs forming the α'β' lobes constitute a new fat regulation center. Perturbation of the activities of KCs that project into the γ lobe produces effects like those previously observed by perturbation of Fru-GAL4 neurons, of which the γ KCs are a subset [3]. We also identified MB input and output neurons that regulate feeding, metabolism, and fat content.

Methods

Drosophila strains

Flies were raised as described in [3]. Males from GAL4 lines obtained from various sources and Split-GAL4 lines from Yoshinori Aso at Janelia Farm Research Campus [5, 7] were crossed with females containing either (UAS-Kir2.1, Tub-Gal80^{ts}), UAS-dTrpA1, UAS-Shi^{ts}, or UAS-NaChBac1. The resulting male progeny were collected for 2 days in groups of 20 individuals. For manipulating neuronal physiology using Kir2.1, dTrpA1, and Shi^{ts}, experimental flies and heterozygote controls were shifted to 30 °C for 7–10 days, while NaChBac1-expressing experimental flies and heterozygote controls were incubated at room temperature for 7–10 days before fat content was analyzed. Wild-type flies were of the Canton-S strain.

It has been reported that feeding habits and metabolic demands of female flies changes with mating [10, 38, 46, 49]. To avoid this additional level of complication, our analysis was restricted to male flies isolated within 24 h after eclosion and aged accordingly on standard media.

Fat level analysis

Stored fats are composed of a glycerol backbone attached to three fatty acids. These fatty acids are typically not uniform in length or saturation levels. This level of chemical heterogeneity necessitates fat measuring methods that are not targeted to specific species of triglyceride fat but have a broad spectrum. We previously developed a fat detecting thin-layer chromatography (TLC) assay that is superior in terms of specificity and accuracy to the frequently used colorimetric assay [1–3]. Fly extracts analyzed using this assay produce four bands. We previously analyzed the composition of these bands by mass spectrometry. Starting from top (near the solvent front) and going through the bands to the bottom (where the samples were pipetted into the TLC plate), the uppermost band has the migration rate and mass spectromeric pattern of waxes and does not exhibit a change in level during starvation. The second band also does not exhibit a change in level during starvation, but due to its low levels we were unable to identify its identity by mass spectrometry. The third band is triglyceride (fat), and three observations confirm its identity: First, the band has the same migration rate as butter, lard, or a triglyceride standard. Second, it gradually disappears with continued starvation, which is expected of stored fat. Third, analysis by mass spectrometry confirms that this band is composed of a mixture of triglycerides. The final bands (near the base of the TLC assay) appear as two concentric circles and hardly migrate on the TLC assay. Mass spectromeric analysis indicates that they are mixtures of mono- and diglycerides, and they do not show any alteration during starvation [1, 3]. The invariant level and migration pattern of the uppermost bands (waxes and other) does not change when the same number of flies are processed with the same volume of solvent, thus making them useful standards to ensure that the same amount of material was loaded in each lane.

Fly fat extraction and TLC analysis was performed as described by [3]. To quantify fat levels, 1 mg/mL lard standard solution dissolved in 2:1 chloroform:methanol solvent was prepared. When test samples were examined, four different lard standard aliquots were pipetted onto the same TLC plate, providing total lard amounts of 0.5, 1, 2, and 4 micrograms. After staining, the TLC plate was scanned and the average pixel density of each standard sample was measured and used to plot a dose-response curve. The test sample pixel densities were then measured and their fat content determined relative to the trend line slope of the standard samples.

To assess the reliability of our data, we compared all pairs of three different genotypes: flies with both driver and transgene lines (test sample), flies with transgene line only (control 1), and flies with driver line only (control 2). Three two-sided independent t-tests were performed: test sample vs. control 1, test sample vs. control 2, and control 1 vs. control 2. Only outcomes in which the mean of the test samples was reliably different from both controls were considered bona fide. Additional file 1: Table S1 presents all comparisons. However, since the controls were all very similar to each other, in the final presentation of the data in the figures we typical show control 1. The exception to this rule was for graphs in which a normal GAL4 and a split-GAL4 line are compared. In these cases (e.g., Fig. 2a), since the GAL4

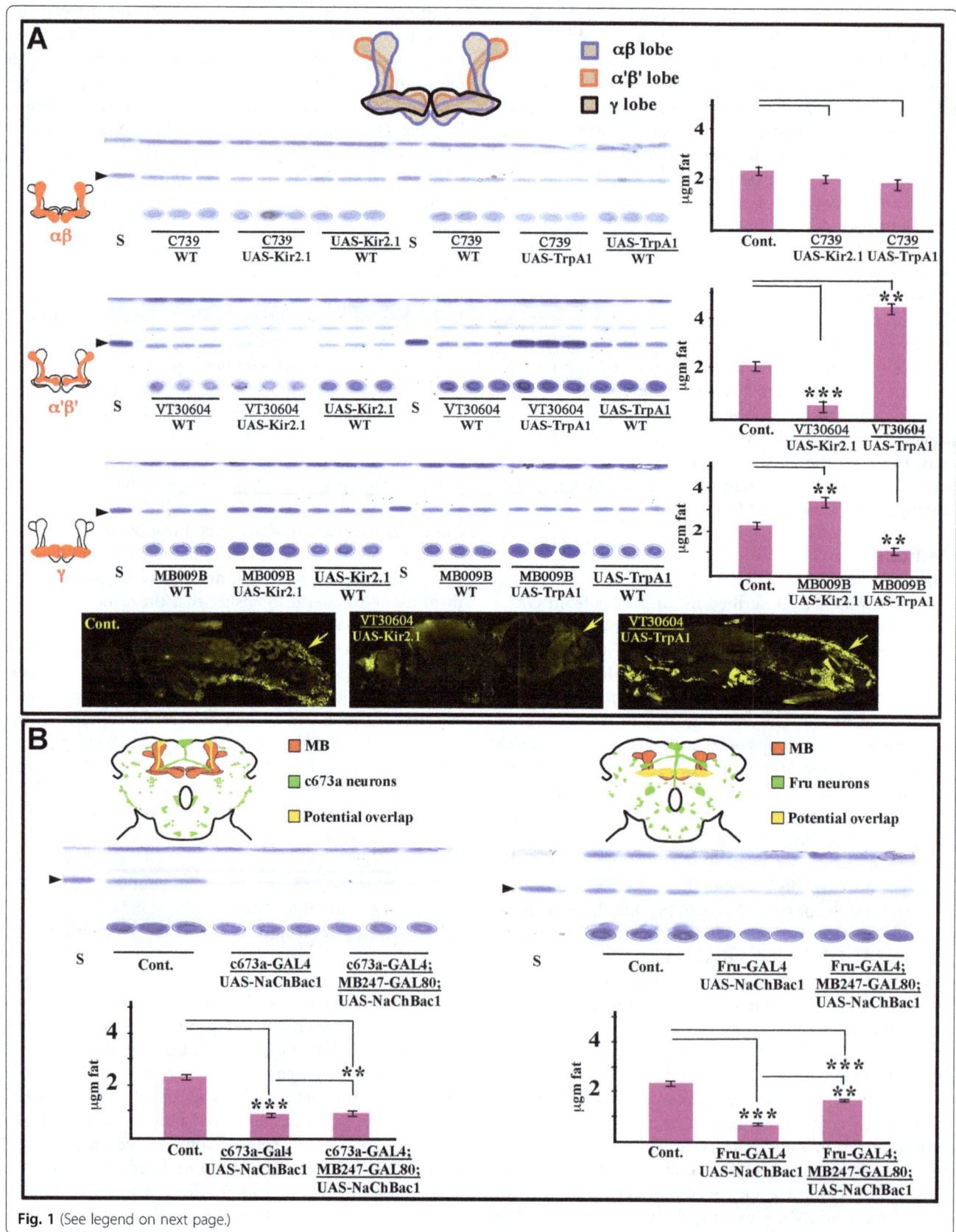

Fig. 1 (See legend on next page.)

heterozygotes would be different, we used UAS-Kir2.1/+ or UAS-dTrpA1/+ for the control bars.

Behavioral and metabolic assays

Nile red histological staining was performed as described by [1, 3]. Behavioral and metabolic analyses were done using UAS-Kir2.1, UAS-dTrpA1, and UAS-Shi[ts] animals and controls 2 days after they were shifted to 30 °C. NaChBac1 animals and their controls were incubated at room temperature for 2 days before being examined. The CAFE feeding assay was performed as described by Ja and others and Al-Anzi and others [4, 22]. The climbing assay was performed as described by Nichols and others [31]. Conversion of consumed radiolabeled amino acids into different metabolites was done as described by [3], except that ^{14}C leucine was replaced by ^{14}C aspartic acid.

Unless stated otherwise, behavioral and metabolic analysis were done on test flies and their controls 2 days after being shifted to 30° C as they were still in the process of either becoming obese or lean.

To assess the reliability of our data, we compared all pairs of three different genotypes: flies with both driver and transgene lines (test sample), flies with driver line only (control 1), and flies with transgene line only (control 2). Three two-sided independent t-tests were performed: test sample vs. control 1, test sample vs. control 2, and control 1 vs. control 2. Only outcomes in which the mean of the test samples was reliably different from both controls were considered bona fide. Additional file 3: Table S3 presents all comparisons. The controls were all very similar to each other, as for the measurement of fat content (see Additional file 1: Table S1). Therefore, in the final presentation of the data, for simplicity we show control 1. The exception to this rule was for graphs in which a normal GAL4 and a split-GAL4 line are compared. In these cases, since the GAL4 heterozygotes would be different, we used UAS-Kir2.1/+ or UAS-dTrpA1/+ for the control bars.

Results

The α'β' and γ lobes of the mushroom body affect fat storage

To determine whether KC activity regulates fat storage, we used MB lobe-specific GAL4 lines to drive the expression of UAS-linked transgenes that cause temperature-dependent conditional neuronal silencing or hyperactivation. To silence neurons, we used an inward rectifier potassium channel, Kir2.1 [9], whose expression is controlled by a ubiquitously expressed temperature-sensitive GAL4 inhibitor, Tub-GAL80[ts] [34]. To hyperactivate neurons, we used a temperature-activated transient receptor potential cation channel, dTrpA1 [17, 33]. We shifted adult flies bearing MB lobe-specific GAL4 drivers and Kir2.1/GAL80[ts] or dTrpA1, respectively, to 30 °C for 7–10 days.

This prolonged incubation, while not physiological with respect to neuronal activation, is necessary to allow for fat accumulation, and was also used in earlier studies [3]. As controls, we subjected lines bearing only the DNA constructs for the GAL4 driver or the UAS effectors to the same temperature shifts. This is the appropriate control, because this is not a conditional experiment with respect to temperature. High temperature is necessary to turn on expression of Kir2.1 (through GAL80[ts] inactivation) and to activate dTrpA1. However, metabolism and fat content change dramatically with temperature, so it would be inappropriate to compare flies at the permissive vs. nonpermissive temperatures. By comparing driver-alone and effector-alone lines to the driver-effector combination at the same temperature, it is possible to accurately assess the effects of the perturbations. In Additional file 1: Table S1, all comparisons to controls are shown. Since the driver-alone and effector-alone lines all have very similar fat contents, in the figures we only show controls 1. Aso and others have generated a large number of split-GAL4 driver lines that label subsets of input mushroom body neurons [7]. The split-GAL4 version they used is based on [35], and is susceptible to GAL80 inhibition.

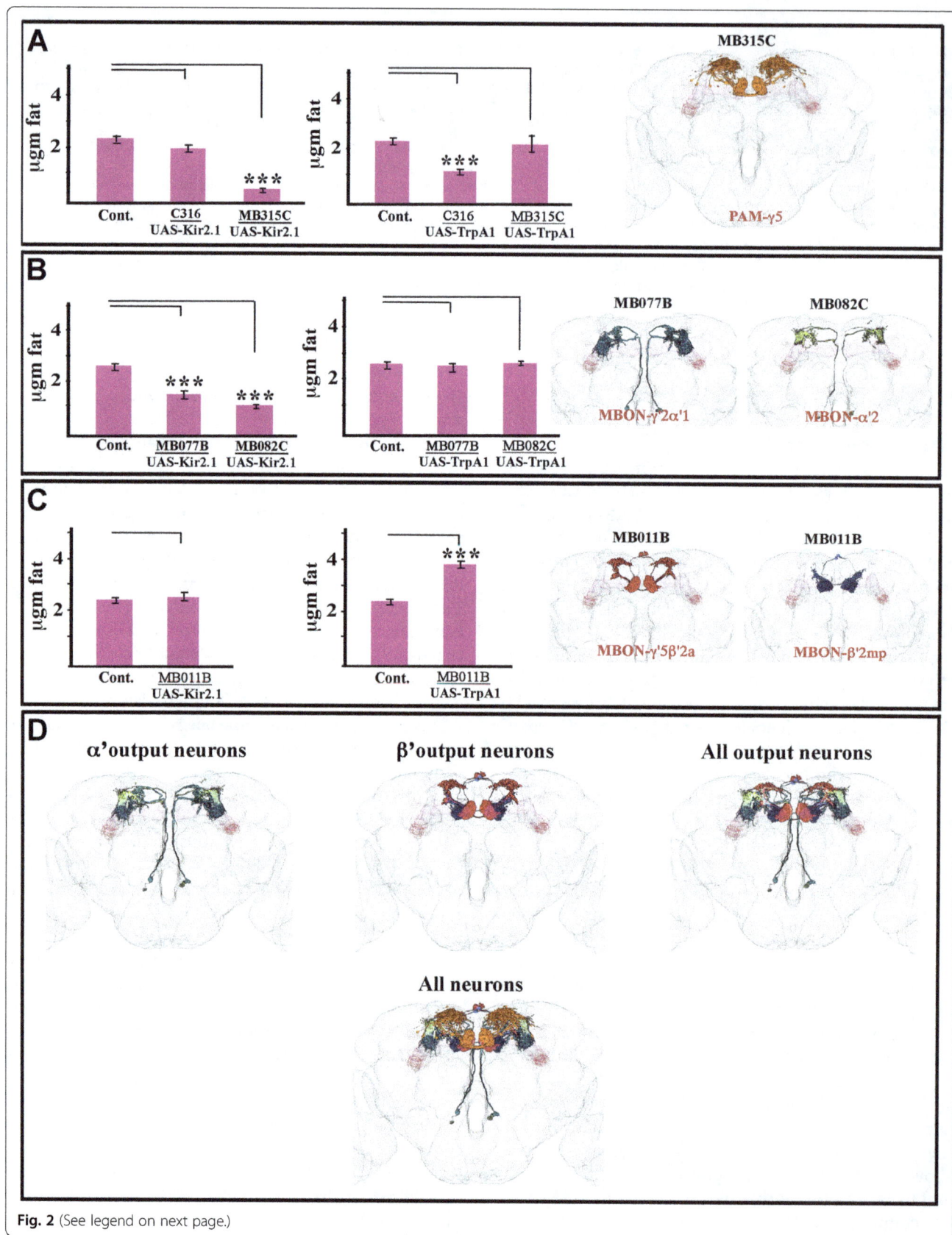

Fig. 2 (See legend on next page.)

Fig. 2 Mushroom body input and output neurons involved in fat storage regulation. **a** Input neurons. Quantitation of fat levels, as measured by TLC, in flies with Kir2.1-mediated silencing (left) or dTrpA1-mediated hyperactivation (right) of DPM neurons using C316-GAL4, or of PAM-γ5 neurons using MB315-GAL4. Far right, Image of PAM-γ5 neurons (orange). In all images in this figure, the brain is a translucent grey skeleton, and the MB lobes are in translucent pink and blue. There are 8–12 PAM-γ5s per brain hemisphere. **b** MBONs innervating α' compartments. Left bar graph shows that Kir2.1-mediated silencing of MBON-γ2α'1 using MB077B-GAL4 and MBON-α'2 using MB082C-GAL4 causes leanness. Right bar graph shows that dTrpA1-mediated hyperactivation of these neurons has no effect. Far right, images of MBON-γ2α'1 (blue-green) and MBON-α'2 (light green). There are 2 MBON-γ2α'1 s and 1 MBON-α'2, per brain hemisphere. **c** MBONs innervating β'2 compartments. Left bar graph shows that Kir2.1-mediated silencing of MBON-γ5β'2a and MBON-β'2mp neurons using MB011B-GAL4 has no effect on fat content. Right bar graph shows that dTrpA1-mediated hyperactivation of the same neurons causes obesity. Far right, images of MBON-γ5β'2a (red) and MBON-β'2mp (blue). There is 1 MBON-γ5β'2a and 1 MBON-β'2mp per brain hemisphere. **d** Combined images at the bottom show superimpositions of all α'-innervating MBONs (left), all β'-innervating MBONs (middle), all MBONs (right), and MBONs plus PAM-γ5s (bottom). Bars indicate means ± SEM, $n = 12$ samples for pooled controls as in Fig. 2 and $n = 4$ for other genotypes, each composed of 10 flies homogenate. Asterisks denote t-test statistical significance: ***, $p < 0.0005$

Silencing or hyperactivation of αβ KCs using C739-GAL4 [5] had no effect on fat content (Fig. 1a, top panels). By contrast, silencing of α'β' KCs using the VT30604-GAL4 driver [50] produced a dramatic decrease (> 5-fold) in the intensities of the triglyceride bands. Conversely, hyperactivation of α'β' KCs increased triglyceride content by more than 2-fold (Fig. 1a, second panel). We confirmed that these changes reflected alterations in the numbers of stored fat droplets by Nile Red staining of cryostat sections (Fig. 1a, bottom panel). Two other α'β' drivers, VT57244-GAL4 [50] and C305a-GAL4 [5], produced similar results (Additional file 1: Table S1). Silencing of γ KCs using the split-GAL4 driver MB009B [7] produced the opposite effect to α'β' silencing, causing a moderate increase in triglyceride content, while hyperactivation produced a decrease in fat (Fig. 1a, third panel).

Transgenic hyperactivation agents such as cation channels can generate sustained neuronal firing rates that are never observed in normal animals, raising the possibility that what is observed when these agents are used may not be relevant to normal physiology, especially when they are kept on for a prolonged period of time as in our experiments. However, in the case of the two groups of MB neurons described above, we demonstrated that silencing of these neurons generates effects opposite to those produced by hyperactivation. This suggests that the activities of these neurons are indeed relevant to fat storage regulation in normal animals.

As stated in the introduction, in our previous work we identified two fat-regulating neuronal populations, defined by their expression of the c673a-GAL4 and Fru-GAL4 drivers. There is little overlap between the two populations, and the overlapping neurons are not responsible for their phenotypes [3]. However, there is some overlap between MB neurons and neurons expressing c673a-GAL4 and Fru-GAL4 (Fig. 1b, top). In particular, most γ KCs express Fru-GAL4 [3, 18], so the effects caused by silencing and hyperactivation of γ KCs might reflect a role of Fru neurons. To test this, we hyperactivated c673a and Fru

neurons with UAS-NaChBac1 (a bacterial cation channel) [32], because dTrpA1-mediated hyperactivation of either of these sets of neurons is lethal. This was done in the presence of a GAL80 repressor element that suppresses GAL4 mediated-expression in the MB. GAL80 expression is driven using a pan-KC promoter element, MB247-GAL80 [42]. MB247-GAL80 had no effect on the leanness phenotype produced by UAS-NaChBac1 hyperactivation of c673a neurons (Fig. 1b, left). However, when we combined Fru-GAL4 and UAS-NaChBac1 with MB247-GAL80, we found that the leanness phenotype was significantly weakened (Fig. 1b, right). This shows that the effect of hyperactivation of Fru neurons on fat content can partially be assigned to γ KCs. However, Fru neurons outside the MB also contribute to fat storage, since flies in which NaChBac1 was shut off in the MB were still significantly leaner than wild-type controls.

Identification of compartment-specific mushroom body input and output neurons that affect fat storage

The MB receives input from many modulatory neurons, including serotonergic/GABAergic Dorsal Median Paired neurons (DPMs)[19, 47] and dopaminergic neurons called DANs [6, 7, 13–15, 24, 37, 40]. It transmits output signals via a small number of mushroom body output neurons, the MBONs [7]. DAN axons and MBON dendrites have spatially restricted innervation patterns that divide the MB into 15 compartments. Various combinations of compartments regulate aspects of mushroom body function such as appetitive learning, aversive learning, and sleep [8].

We screened the Aso collection of split-GAL4 lines expressing in specific MB neuron subtypes by crossing each of the 68 driver lines with UAS-Kir2.1; Tub-GAL80^{ts} or UAS-dTrpA1, respectively, to silence or hyperactivate each DAN and MBON subtype. To identify specific neurons involved in fat storage regulation, we first screened driver lines to identify those that conferred differences in fat levels when crossed with a perturbing agent relative to controls.

Second, driver lines initially scored as hits were verified by retesting for significant differences in fat levels in four independent experiments. Third, in order for us to classify a neuronal type as being involved in fat storage, we required that *all* split-GAL4 driver lines that express in this neuronal type must produce alterations in fat levels. Additional file 2: Table S2 shows results for all split-GAL4 drivers.

The observation that hyperactivation of α'β' KCs causes obesity suggests that α'β' KCs could be postsynaptic to inhibitory neurons that are also involved in fat storage regulation. One potential set of inhibitory neurons are the DPMs. Hyperactivation of DPM neurons with C316-GAL4 causes leanness, while silencing them does not affect fat storage (Fig. 2a). This data suggests that DPM neurons inhibit α'β' KCs and constrain their activity-dependent effect on fat storage.

Of 29 split-GAL4 driver lines specific for input DAN neurons, three lines specific for neurons of the PAM cluster produced significant effects on fat levels when used to drive silencing or hyperactivation agents. For one of these, MB315C-split-GAL4, we identified a small group of DANs, the PAM-γ5 neurons, as responsible for the driver's effect on fat storage (Additional file 2: Table S2). Silencing of these neurons caused leanness, while hyperactivation had no effect (Fig. 2a). For two other two drivers, MB188B-split-GAL4 and MB087C-split-GAL4, we were unable to identify a single neuronal type that was likely to be responsible for their effects (Additional file 2: Table S2).

Among 34 split-GAL4 lines specific for MBON output neurons, we found six that produced significant effects on fat levels when used to drive silencing or hyperactivating agents. For five of these, we were able to assign these effects to specific compartments and MBONs. MB077B and MB077C-split-GAL4s express in only one MBON type (2 cells per brain hemisphere) called MB-γ2α'1, while MB082C-split-GAL4 expresses in MBON-α'2 and MBON-α3. By examining other drivers (Additional file 2: Table S2), we attributed the effects of MB082C-split-GAL4 to MBON-α'2 (1 cell per brain hemisphere). For both MBON-γ2α'1 and MBON-α'2, silencing produced leanness, while hyperactivation had no effect (Fig. 2b).

The effects of MB011B-split-GAL4 and MB074C-split-GAL4 were attributable to output neurons MBON-β'2mp and MBON-γ5β'2a (1 cell each per brain hemisphere) (Additional file 2: Table S2). For these neurons, hyperactivation produced obesity, while silencing had no effect (Fig. 2c). Images of identified fat-regulating neurons are shown in Fig. 2a-d. For the final driver, MB549C-split-GAL4, silencing caused leanness, but we were unable to identify a single neuronal type to which we could attribute its effects (Additional file 1: Table S1 and Additional file 2: Table S2).

Two other split-GAL4 lines are worth mentioning, MB013B and MB022B. The former label the SIFamide neurons, while the latter labels the octopaminergic neurons OA-VPM3 and OA-VPM4. The SIFamide neurons have been implicated in the translation of hunger signals into feeding behavior [28], while OA-VPM3 and OA-VPM4 are known to be involved in appetitive learning [13]. In the TLC assay, hyperactivation of either neuronal type produced a mild increase in fat levels (Additional file 2: Table S2). However, the *p*-values for the significance of this increase as compared to controls are rather modest (0.04 and 0.05, respectively). Thus, we did not examine these drivers further.

Behavioral and metabolic mechanisms involved in control of fat storage by the mushroom body

Fat levels are influenced by a variety of factors, including food intake, the rate of de novo fatty acid synthesis, the rate of fat store utilization, and the animals' physical activity. To evaluate the causes of fat content phenotypes in flies where the activities of specific mushroom body-associated neurons were perturbed, we measured these parameters using behavioral and metabolic assays [3].

Food intake was measured using the capillary feeding assay (CAFE) [4, 22]. The rate of de novo fatty acid synthesis was quantified by feeding flies for 2 days with radioactively labeled amino acids, followed by measuring the amount of radiation incorporated into lipid fractions generated from whole-body extracts [3]. Behavioral activity levels were assessed using a climbing assay [31]. Finally, the rate of fat store utilization was evaluated by measuring the reduction in fat levels due to starvation as described by [3]. Fat was extracted from starved flies in 12 h intervals. The extract was run on the TLC assay, and the fat levels plotted. The slope of the trendline of the fat levels was used to evaluate the rate of fat store depletion as starvation continues. A gentler slope means a slower rate of fat storage depletion.

Hyperactivation of α'β' KCs, which causes obesity, produced a doubling of food intake (Fig. 3a, lower left), but had no effect on de novo fatty acid synthesis (Fig. 3b, lower left). Silencing of the same neurons, which causes leanness, had no effect on food intake (Fig. 3a, top left), but significantly decreased de novo fatty acid synthesis and increased carbohydrate synthesis (Fig. 3b, top left). For γ KCs, the silencing-induced obesity phenotype was associated with a large increase in de novo fatty acid synthesis and increased carbohydrate synthesis, while hyperactivation-induced leanness was associated with a decrease in de novo fatty acid synthesis, but an increase in carbohydrate synthesis (Fig. 3b, left). Food intake was not significantly affected by either hyperactivating or silencing γ KCs. No abnormalities in climbing rate were detected when α'β' or γ KCs were silenced or hyperactivated

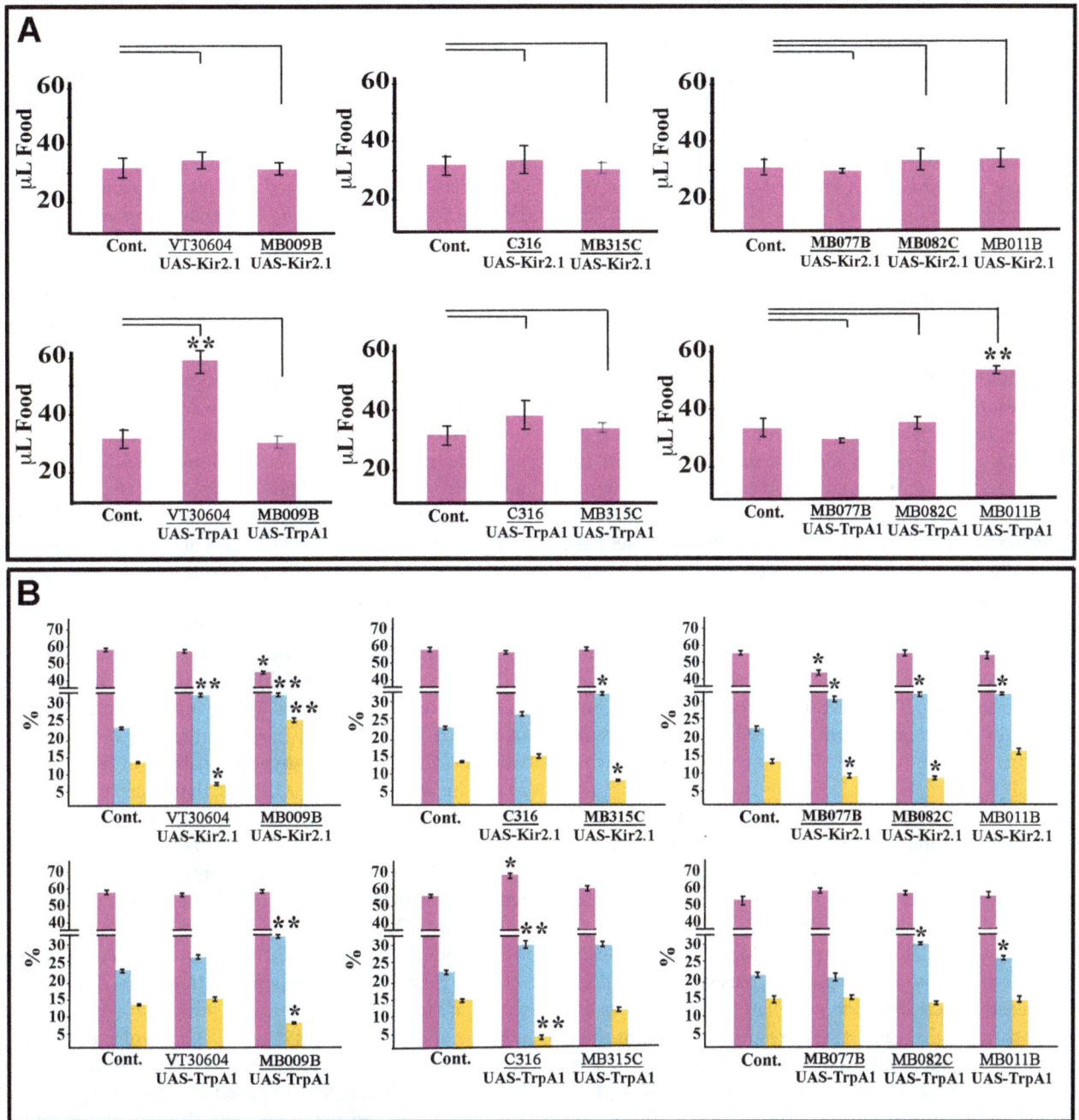

Fig. 3 Behavioral and metabolic phenotypes associated with silenced and hyperactivation of the different mushroom body circuits involved in fat storage regulation. **a** Food intake in flies with silenced or hyperactivated MB. Silencing of any type of mushroom body-associated neuron does not significantly affect food intake (upper row). Hyperactivation of α'β' KCs, using VT30604-GAL4, (lower left) of MBON-γ5β2'a, MBON-β2'mp (MB011B-GAL4 neurons; lower right) cause increases in food intake; all other genotypes are not significantly different from controls. **b** Conversion of ingested ^{14}C aspartic acid to protein (magenta), carbohydrate (light blue), and lipid (yellow) in flies with silenced or hyperactivated MB neurons. Silencing of α'β' KCs (VT30604), MBON-γ2α'1 (MB077B), MBON-α'2 (MB082C), and PAM-γ5 (MB315C) produces decreases in labeled lipids, and silencing γ KCs (MB009B) produces an increase (upper panels). Hyperactivating γ KCs, using MB009-GAL4, and DPM neurons, using C316-GAL4, produces decreases in labeled lipids (lower panels). Bars indicate means ± SEM, $n = 60$ single flies in pooled controls (see Fig. 2) and $n = 20$ for all other genotypes for Café and climbing assay, and $n = 12$ for pooled controls and $n = 4$ for other genotypes for the fat store degradation and ^{14}C incorporation experiments (each sample is a homogenate from 10 flies). Asterisks denote t-test statistical significance: *$p < 0.05$, **$p < 0.005$, ***, $p < 0.0005$

[31]. Additional file 3: Table S3 shows the complete set of comparisons to controls for all of these assays. The results show that the activity of α'β' KCs affects both food intake and metabolism, while γ KC activity affects only metabolism.

We then evaluated the behavioral and metabolic effects caused by silencing or hyperactivating mushroom body input neurons (DPM and PAM-γ5 neurons) or output neurons (MBON-γ2α'1, MBON-α'2, MBON-β'2mp, and MBON-γ5β'2a). Hyperactivation of DPM input neurons, which causes leanness, produced a decrease in de novo fatty acid synthesis. Silencing PAM-γ5 input neurons, which also causes leanness, produced both a decrease in de novo fatty acid synthesis and an increase in carbohydrate synthesis (Fig. 3b). For output neurons, hyperactivation of MBON-β'2mp and MBON-γ5β'2a (with MB011B), like hyperactivation of their corresponding α'β' KC inputs, caused obesity and increased food intake but had no effect on de novo fatty acid synthesis (Fig. 3a, b). Silencing MBON-γ2α'1 and MBON-α'2 (with MB077B and MB082C), like silencing α'β' KCs, caused leanness and produced a decrease in de novo fatty acid synthesis without affecting food intake (Fig. 3a, b). See Additional file 3: Table S3 for the complete dataset.

Hyperactivation and silencing of MBONs involved in fat regulation did not alter climbing rate [31] (Additional file 3: Table S3). These MBONs had previously been assessed for effects on general activity levels, but no major alterations were found when they were silenced or hyperactivated [8, 45].

In summary, we can associate specific MB compartments with behavioral and metabolic effects of perturbation of KCs activity. Increased activity of α'β' KCs causes an increase in food intake and produces obesity, and these responses match the effects produced by hyperactivating the output neurons MBON-β'2mp and MBON-γ5β'2a, which innervate the β'2 compartment. Decreased activity of α'β' KCs causes a decrease in de novo fatty acid synthesis and produces leanness, and these responses match those produced by silencing the output neurons MBON-γ2α'1 and MBON-α'2, which innervate the α'1 and α'2 compartments.

Paired manipulations reveal relationships among fat-regulating neurons and genes

We next examined the functional ordering of pairs of different fat-storage-regulating neurons that (a) either partially or fully overlap with the mushroom body, and (b) have an opposite effect on fat storage when activated. This may provide insights into the functional ordering of these elements. The drivers examined include c673a-GAL4 and Fru-GAL4, which were identified in our earlier study using NaChBac and Shi[ts] [3], and the drivers described in

this paper for α'β' KCs, MBON-β'2mp, MBON-γ5β'2a, and MBON-γ2α'1 (see Fig. 4a for diagram of circuitry).

We first examined interactions between α'β' KCs and the previously identified c673a-GAL4 and Fru-GAL4 neurons [3]; Fru-GAL4 neurons include γ KCs. Hyperactivation with dTrpA1 is lethal with c673a-GAL4 and Fru-GAL4. Since flies can survive without MB (Sweeney et al., 2012), this observed lethality is probably due to Fru-GAL4 and c673a-GAL4 expression in neuronal population outside the MB. In order to examine the combined manipulations of Fru-GAL4 or c673a-GAL4 with different MB drivers, we had to use neuronal hyperactivation mediated by UAS-NaChBac1 that does not cause such lethality (Al-Anzi et al., 2009). However, we observed that UAS-NaChBac1 does not produce effects on fat content when expressed in MB or MB associated neurons (Figure 4), suggesting that the increased activity in these neurons when induced by UAS-NaChBac1 is not sufficient to alter fat storage. However, since we know that these transgenes do cause changes in fat content when used with c673a-GAL4 or Fru-GAL4, we infer that UAS-NaChBac1 is likely to produce an alteration in the activity of MB neurons. In fact, we observed that α'β' KC hyperactivation with UAS-NaChBac1 completely suppressed leanness produced by hyperactivation of c673a or Fru neurons (Fig. 4b, c), confirming that output from α'β' neurons is the most important controller of fat content. In a similar manner, we asked whether the effects of hyperactivation of Fru neurons might be modulated by MBONs that receive input from both α'β' and γ lobes. To do this, we hyperactivated MBON-γ5β'2a and MBON-β'2mp (MB011B neurons), and MBON-γ2α'1 (MB077B) output neurons, together with Fru neurons. We observed that hyperactivation of either MBON-γ5β'2a and MBON-β'2mp, or of MBON-γ2α'1, suppressed the leanness phenotype conferred by Fru neuron hyperactivation (Fig. 4d, e). Note that in all four of these cases the MB driver suppresses the effect of the Fru or c673a driver. We can infer that the Fru and c673a drivers are stronger than the MB drivers since they produce lethality when used to drive dTrpA1, while the MB drivers do not. Thus, the effect of the combined drivers is unlikely to be due to dominance by the stronger GAL4 driver.

Discussion

In this paper, we demonstrate that the mushroom body plays a central role in regulation of fat levels in *Drosophila*. Hyperactivation of α'β' KCs causes obesity, while silencing causing leanness. Hyperactivation and silencing of γ KCs produces the opposite effects (Fig. 1). α'β' KCs are a fat storage regulating center that dominates the fly's physiology, while γ KCs are a subset of the Fru-GAL4 neurons previously implicated in fat store regulation [3]. We also

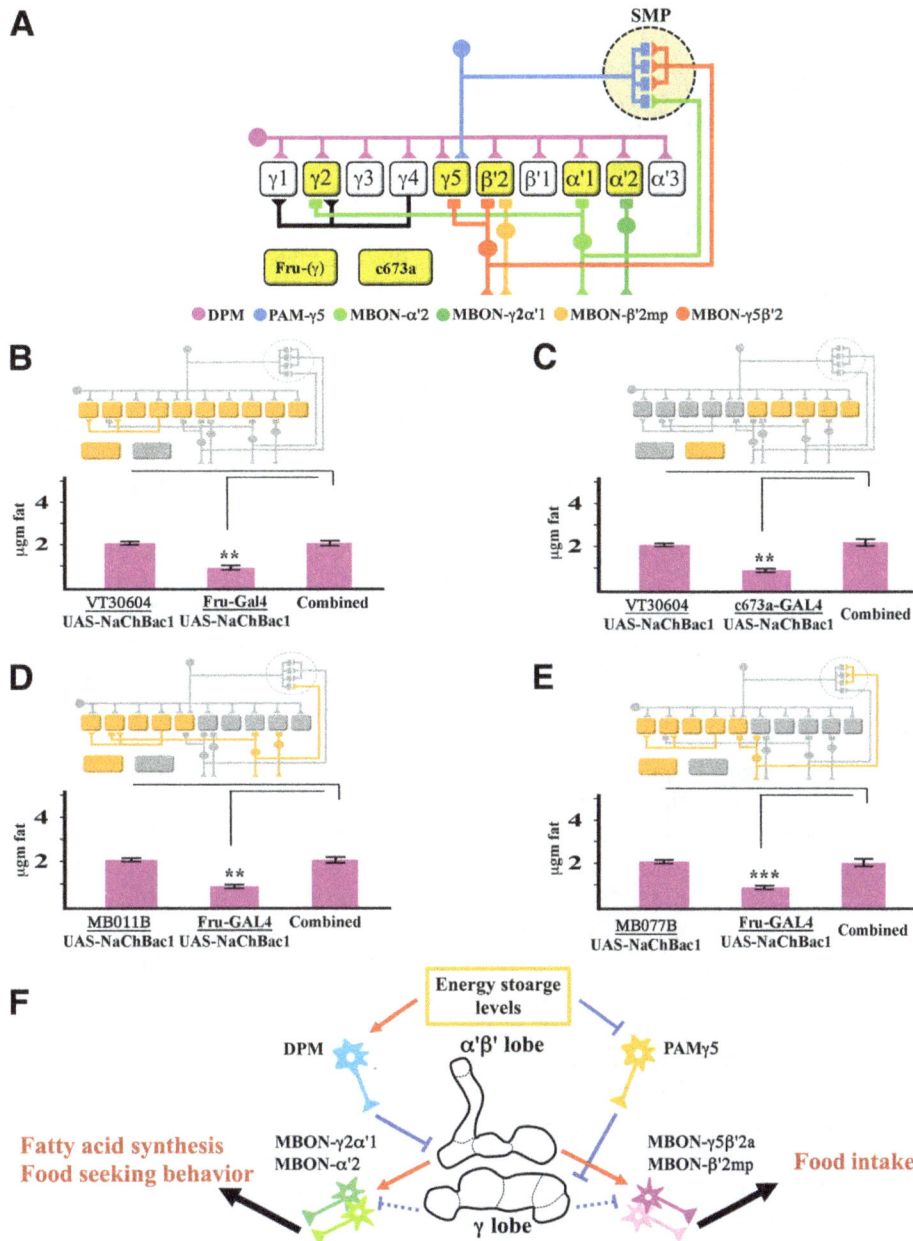

Fig. 4 Paired hyperactivation of neurons with opposing effects on fat storage. **a** Schematic illustration of parts of the MB circuitry, including neurons, examined. Solid rectangles are dendritic arbors, and solid triangles are axon terminals. Selected MB compartments in α'β' and γ lobes are indicated. PAMs and MBONs labeled by the drivers used in this paper are indicated. c673a and non-KC Fru neurons are indicated by unconnected yellow boxes. In the diagrams in the other panels, the method of neural hyperactivation is indicated by red color when dTrpA1 is used and orange color when NaChBac1, highlighted on a grey schematic of the MB circuit. **b** and **c** Combining hyperactivation of α'β' KCs with VT30604-GAL4 with hyperactivation of Fru-GAL4 neurons (**b**) or of c673a-GAL4 neurons (**c**) results in fat levels that are the same as those in flies in which only α'β' KCs are hyperactivated, showing the dominant role of α'β' KC neurons in determining fat content. **d** and **e** Combining hyperactivation of MBON-γ5β'2a and MBON-β'2mp with MB011B (**d**) or of MBON-γ2α'1 with MB077B (**e**) with hyperactivation of Fru-GAL4 neurons results in suppression of the leanness produced by hyperactivation of Fru-GAL4 neurons alone. Bars indicate means ± SEM, $n = 12$ samples for pooled controls and $n = 4$ for other genotypes, as in Fig. 1. Asterisks denote t-test statistical significance: *$p < 0.05$, **$p < 0.005$, ***, $p < 0.0005$. In all experiments, the combined column refers to a single copy of both drivers (GAL4, and split-GAL4) present with a single copy of UAS-NaChBac1 **f**. A model for fat-regulating MB circuitry. α'β' KCs regulate both food consumption (via MBONs innervating β' compartments) and fatty acid synthesis (via MBONs innervating α' compartments). MBON-γ5β'2a and MBON-γ2α'1 also innervate the γ lobes. γ KC activity affects fatty acid synthesis but not food consumption. The phenotypes shown in Fig. 3 and the epistatic relationships shown in Fig. 4 suggest that the output of the γ KCs that is relevant to fat storage is opposite in sign to that of the α'β' KCs. However, we do not know the circuits through which γ KCs regulate fat content, so connections from the γ lobes are shown as dotted lines with inhibition bars

identified MB input and output neurons that mediate these effects.

By combining anatomical analysis and metabolic and behavioral assays, we showed that feeding and fat metabolism are controlled by separate MB output channels (Figs. 2 and 3). Cholinergic MBON-β'2mp and MBON-γ5β'2a (MB011B) output neurons, which innervate the β'2 compartment, regulate food consumption. Glutamatergic MBON-γ2α'1 and MBON-α'2 (MB077B and MB082C) output neurons, which innervate α' compartments, control fat metabolism.

Some of the neurons we found to be involved in fat storage regulation have been previously reported to have functions in food-related behaviors. PAM neurons that innervate the β'2 and γ5 compartments, including PAM-γ5, have been shown to be involved in appetitive learning [21, 51]. DPM neurons are involved in caloric frustration memory, in which flies learn to avoid non-nutritional sweeteners [30]. MBON-γ2α'1, MBON-α'2, MBON-β'2mp, and MBON-γ5β'2a are needed for both visual and odor-associated appetite learning [8]. MBON-γ2α'1 is required for the acquisition, consolidation, and retrieval of appetitive learning [52].

Recently, Tsao and others have shown that inhibiting the activity of KCs increases the time required for hungry flies to find yeast food after starvation. They identified five MBON pathways for which silencing also impairs food-seeking behavior. These included MBON-γ2α'1 and MBON-α'2, which we identified as important for fat regulation in this paper. Silencing of either MBON-γ2α'1 and MBON-α'2 causes leanness (Fig. 2b). They also reported that these neurons exhibited yeast odor-evoked calcium transients that are modulated by starvation [45]. We did not observe that flies in which MBON-γ2α'1 and MBON-α'2 are silenced consumed less food than controls (Fig. 3a). This does not contradict the findings of Tsao et al., however, because the CAFÉ assay we used does not measure food-seeking. In this assay, the flies are continually exposed to food and the amount of food consumed is measured.

It is interesting that both silencing and hyperactivation of α'β' KCs produced changes in fat content, while the MBONs we identified as involved in fat regulation segregated into those for which only silencing affects fat content (MBON-γ2α'1 and MBON-α'2) (MB077B and MB982C) and those for which only hyperactivation affects fat content (MBON-β'2mp and MBON-γ5β'2a) (MB011B). This suggests that outputs from α'β' KCs are compartmentalized, so that the effects of high activity go through a set of cholinergic output MBONs, while the effects of low activity go through a set of glutamatergic MBONs.

Our results, along with previously analyses, are consistent with a model in which the fly uses the activities of α'β' KCs to maintain fat content within normal levels.

A decrease in energy stores might cause a reduction in inhibitory input to α'β' KCs by decreasing GABA release from DPM neurons. As a consequence of reduction in inhibition by DPM neurons, the activity of α'β' KCs would increase, resulting in increased transmitter release from α'1, α'2, and β'2 compartments onto the MBON-γ2α'1, MBON-α'2, MBON-β'2mp, and MBON-γ5β'2a neurons. This will prevent the inhibition of MBON-γ2α'1 and MBON-α'2, leading to an increase in food seeking behavior [45], and may also cause an increase in the activities of MBON-β'2mp and MBON-γ5β'2a. This would in turn increase food consumption, leading to a restoration of energy stores (see diagram in Fig. 4f). Conversely, when energy stores are sufficient, DPM inhibits α'β' activity, resulting in decreased transmitter release from the α'1, α'2, and β'2 compartment onto the above stated MBONs, reducing their activity. This will case a reduction in food seeking behavior and may prevent the release of humoral factors controlling lipid synthesis via MBON-γ2α'1 and MBON-α'2, thus reducing the rate of fat droplet production.

The mechanisms by which the γ KCs influence fat storage are less clear. PAM-γ5 silencing causes leanness and decreased lipid synthesis, like hyperactivation of γ KCs. γ KCs may affect the activities of the MBONs we identified as regulators of lipid synthesis, or act through other MBONs that were not defined by our studies, since the effects of some split-GAL4-mediated perturbations could not be assigned to specific cells (Fig. 4f).

In terms of fat storage regulation, two potential paths of cross-communication between α'β' KCs and γ KCs are histologically feasible. The first one involves the superior medial protocerebrum (SMP), a brain area in which PAM-γ5 input neuron dendrites are contacted by axonal termini of the output neurons identified by our study [7]. The other is the dendritic arbors of MBON-γ2α'1 and MBON-γ5β'2a, which contact both the α'β' and γ lobe, potentially receiving input from both simultaneously [7].

Conclusions

We identified a new fat storage regulating center in the *Drosophila* brain, the α'β' KCs, which project into the α'β' lobes of MB. We identified MB input and output neurons involved in its control of fat content. Our findings show that food intake and fat metabolism are controlled by separate sets of postsynaptic neurons that are segregated into different output pathways.

Additional files

Additional file 1: Table S1. Fat level quantifications for fly strains producing statistically significant effects. These are data that are not included in the main figures. (JPG 785 kb)

Additional file 2: Table S2. Summary of all split-GAL4 line results. GAL4 line numbers are indicated on the left. The top labels indicate MB neurons. The black and grey squares indicate whether the driver is expressed in that neuron, with darker shades representing stronger expression. These data are from Aso and colleagues. The colors represent our analysis, with red rows denoting hits: drivers that produced consistent, statistically significant effects on fat content when used to drive silencing or hyperactivating agents. Yellow rows indicate drivers for which we observed alterations in fat content, but these alterations were small or the effects were not highly reproducible. Blue rows indicate drivers for which no effects on fat content with silencing or hyperactivation were observed. To assign a neuron as relevant for fat storage, we required that all drivers expressed in that neuron have some effect on fat content, and that at least one of these should be classified as red. The nature of the effect produced by the driver is indicated at the right. This table is based on Additional file 1 in Aso and others [8]. (PNG 121 kb)

Additional file 3: Table S3. Summary of CAFÉ assays, climbing assays, fat store degradation, and conversion of ^{14}C-labeled-aspartate to different macro-molecular classes. These are data that are not included in the main figures. (JPG 1336 kb)

Abbreviations
CAFÉ: Capillary assisted feeding assay; DANs: Dopaminergic neurons; DPMs: Dorsal Median Paired neurons; KC: Kenyan cell; Kir2.1: Inward rectifier potassium channel; MB: Mushroom body; MBONs: Mushroom body output neurons; NaChBac: Bacterial cation channel; Shi^{ts}: Temperature sensitive shibire; TLC: Thin-layer chromatography; TrpA1: Temperature-activated transient receptor potential cation channel

Acknowledgements
We thank Yoshinori Aso for generously providing his collection of split-GAL4 lines and for advice on generating images of neurons. We also like to thank Mohammad Khajah for his editorial assistance.

Funding
This work was supported by grants from the NIH (NS083874 and NS28182), and from the Della Martin Foundation to K.Z.

Authors' contributions
BA-A and KZ devised the experimental plan. BA-A conducted all of the analysis of fat content and metabolism. B A-A and KZ, wrote the paper. Both authors read and approved the final manuscript.

Competing interests
The authors declare that they have no competing interests.

Author details
^{1}Food & Nutrition Program, Environment & Life Sciences Research Center, Kuwait Institute for Scientific Research, P.O. Box 24885, 13109 Kuwait City, Kuwait. ^{2}Division of Biology and Biological Engineering, California Institute of Technology, Pasadena, CA 91125, USA.

References
1. Al-Anzi B, Zinn K. Colorimetric measurement of triglycerides cannot provide an accurate measure of stored fat content in Drosophila. PLoS One. 2010;5: e12353.
2. Al-Anzi B, Zinn K. Genetics of fat storage in flies and worms: what went wrong? Front Genet. 2011;2:87.
3. Al-Anzi B, Sapin V, Waters C, Zinn K, Wyman RJ, Benzer S. Obesity-blocking neurons in Drosophila. Neuron. 2009;63:329–41.
4. Al-Anzi B, Armand E, Nagamei P, Olszewski M, Sapin V, Waters C, Zinn K, Wyman RJ, Benzer S. The leucokinin pathway and its neurons regulate meal size in Drosophila. Curr Biol. 2010;20:969–78.
5. Aso Y, Grubel K, Busch S, Friedrich AB, Siwanowicz I, Tanimoto H. The mushroom body of adult Drosophila characterized by GAL4 drivers. J Neurogenet. 2009;23:156–72.
6. Aso Y, Herb A, Ogueta M, Siwanowicz I, Templier T, Friedrich AB, Ito K, Scholz H, Tanimoto H. Three dopamine pathways induce aversive odor memories with different stability. PLoS Genet. 2012;8:e1002768.
7. Aso Y, Hattori D, Yu Y, Johnston RM, Iyer NA, Ngo TT, Dionne H, Abbott LF, Axel R, Tanimoto H, Rubin GM. The neuronal architecture of the mushroom body provides a logic for associative learning. Elife. 2014a;3:e04577.
8. Aso Y, et al. Mushroom body output neurons encode valence and guide memory-based action selection in Drosophila. Elife. 2014b;3:e04580.
9. Baines RA, Uhler JP, Thompson A, Sweeney ST, Bate M. Altered electrical properties in Drosophila neurons developing without synaptic transmission. J Neurosci. 2001;21:1523–31.
10. Barnes AI, Wigby S, Boone JM, Partridge L, Chapman T. Feeding, fecundity and lifespan in female Drosophila melanogaster. Proc Biol Sci. 2008;275:1675–83.
11. Berthoud HR. The neurobiology of food intake in an obesogenic environment. Proc Nutr Soc. 2012;71:478–87.
12. Berthoud HR, Munzberg H. The lateral hypothalamus as integrator of metabolic and environmental needs: from electrical self-stimulation to opto-genetics. Physiol Behav. 2011;104:29–39.
13. Burke CJ, Huetteroth W, Owald D, Perisse E, Krashes MJ, Das G, Gohl D, Silies M, Certel S, Waddell S. Layered reward signalling through octopamine and dopamine in Drosophila. Nature. 2012;492:433–7.
14. Friggi-Grelin F, Iche M, Birman S. Tissue-specific developmental requirements of Drosophila tyrosine hydroxylase isoforms. Genesis. 2003a;35:175–84.
15. Friggi-Grelin F, Coulom H, Meller M, Gomez D, Hirsh J, Birman S. Targeted gene expression in Drosophila dopaminergic cells using regulatory sequences from tyrosine hydroxylase. J Neurobiol. 2003b;54:618–27.
16. Gasque G, Conway S, Huang J, Rao Y, Vosshall LB (2013) Small molecule drug screening in Drosophila identifies the 5HT2A receptor as a feeding modulation target. Sci rep 3:srep02120.
17. Hamada FN, Rosenzweig M, Kang K, Pulver SR, Ghezzi A, Jegla TJ, Garrity PA. An internal thermal sensor controlling temperature preference in Drosophila. Nature. 2008;454:217–20.
18. Hampel S, Chung P, McKellar CE, Hall D, Looger LL, Simpson JH. Drosophila Brainbow: a recombinase-based fluorescence labeling technique to subdivide neural expression patterns. Nat Methods. 2011;8:253–9.
19. Haynes PR, Christmann BL, Griffith LC. A single pair of neurons links sleep to memory consolidation in Drosophila melanogaster. Elife. 2015;4
20. Hige T. What can tiny mushrooms in fruit flies tell us about learning and memory? Neurosci: Res; 2017.
21. Huetteroth W, Perisse E, Lin S, Klappenbach M, Burke C, Waddell S. Sweet taste and nutrient value subdivide rewarding dopaminergic neurons in Drosophila. Curr Biol. 2015;25:751–8.
22. Ja WW, Carvalho GB, Mak EM, de la Rosa NN, Fang AY, Liong JC, Brummel T, Benzer S. Prandiology of Drosophila and the CAFE assay. Proc Natl Acad Sci U S A. 2007;104:8253–6.
23. Jenett A, et al. A GAL4-driver line resource for Drosophila neurobiology. Cell Rep. 2012;2:991–1001.
24. Liu C, Placais PY, Yamagata N, Pfeiffer BD, Aso Y, Friedrich AB, Siwanowicz I, Rubin GM, Preat T, Tanimoto H. A subset of dopamine neurons signals reward for odour memory in Drosophila. Nature. 2012;488:512–6.
25. Liu Y, Luo J, Carlsson MA, Nassel DR. Serotonin and insulin-like peptides modulate leucokinin-producing neurons that affect feeding and water homeostasis in Drosophila. J Comp Neurol. 2015;523:1840–63.

26. Luo J, Becnel J, Nichols CD, Nassel DR. Insulin-producing cells in the brain of adult Drosophila are regulated by the serotonin 5-HT1A receptor. Cell Mol Life Sci. 2012;69:471–84.

27. Luo J, Lushchak OV, Goergen P, Williams MJ, Nassel DR. Drosophila insulin-producing cells are differentially modulated by serotonin and octopamine receptors and affect social behavior. PLoS One. 2014;9:e99732.

28. Martelli C, Pech U, Kobbenbring S, Pauls D, Bahl B, Sommer MV, Pooryasin A, Barth J, Arias CWP, Vassiliou C, Luna AJF, Poppinga H, Richter FG, Wegener C, Fiala A, Riemensperger T. SlFamide translates hunger signals into appetitive and feeding behavior in Drosophila. Cell Rep. 2017;20:464–78.

29. Masek P, Keene AC. Gustatory processing and taste memory in Drosophila. J Neurogenet. 2016;30:112–21.

30. Musso PY, Lampin-Saint-Amaux A, Tchenio P, Preat T. Ingestion of artificial sweeteners leads to caloric frustration memory in Drosophila. Nat Commun. 2017;8:1803.

31. Nichols CD, Becnel J, Pandey UB. Methods to assay Drosophila behavior. J Vis Exp. 2012;

32. Nitabach MN, Wu Y, Sheeba V, Lemon WC, Strumbos J, Zelensky PK, White BH, Holmes TC. Electrical hyperexcitation of lateral ventral pacemaker neurons desynchronizes downstream circadian oscillators in the fly circadian circuit and induces multiple behavioral periods. J Neurosci. 2006;26:479–89.

33. Parisky KM, Agosto J, Pulver SR, Shang Y, Kuklin E, Hodge JJ, Kang K, Liu X, Garrity PA, Rosbash M, Griffith LC. PDF cells are a GABA-responsive wake-promoting component of the Drosophila sleep circuit. Neuron. 2008;60: 672–82.

34. Peabody NC, Diao F, Luan H, Wang H, Dewey EM, Honegger HW, White BH. Bursicon functions within the Drosophila CNS to modulate wing expansion behavior, hormone secretion, and cell death. J Neurosci. 2008;28:14379–91.

35. Pfeiffer BD, Ngo TT, Hibbard KL, Murphy C, Jenett A, Truman JW, Rubin GM. Refinement of tools for targeted gene expression in Drosophila. Genetics. 2010;186:735–55.

36. Pooryasin A, Fiala A. Identified serotonin-releasing neurons induce behavioral quiescence and suppress mating in Drosophila. J Neurosci. 2015;35:12792–812.

37. Powell AM, Davis M, Powell JR. Phenotypic plasticity across 50MY of evolution: drosophila wing size and temperature. J Insect Physiol. 2010;56: 380–2.

38. Ribeiro C, Dickson BJ. Sex peptide receptor and neuronal TOR/S6K signaling modulate nutrient balancing in Drosophila. Curr Biol. 2010;20:1000–5.

39. Smith WW, Thomas J, Liu J, Li T, Moran TH. From fat fruit fly to human obesity. Physiol Behav. 2014;136:15–21.

40. Tanaka NK, Tanimoto H, Ito K. Neuronal assemblies of the Drosophila mushroom body. J Comp Neurol. 2008;508:711–55.

41. Technau GM. Fiber number in the mushroom bodies of adult Drosophila melanogaster depends on age, sex and experience. J Neurogenet. 1984;1: 113–26.

42. Thum AS, Jenett A, Ito K, Heisenberg M, Tanimoto H. Multiple memory traces for olfactory reward learning in Drosophila. J Neurosci. 2007;27: 11132–8.

43. Tomita J, Ban G, Kume K. Genes and neural circuits for sleep of the fruit fly. Neurosci Res. 2017;118:82–91.

44. Trinh I, Boulianne GL. Modeling obesity and its associated disorders in Drosophila. Physiology (Bethesda). 2013;28:117–24.

45. Tsao CH, Chen CC, Lin CH, Yang HY, Lin S. Drosophila mushroom bodies integrate hunger and satiety signals to control innate food-seeking behavior. Elife. 2018;7

46. Vargas MA, Luo N, Yamaguchi A, Kapahi P. A role for S6 kinase and serotonin in postmating dietary switch and balance of nutrients in D. Melanogaster. Curr Biol. 2010;20:1006–11.

47. Waddell S, Armstrong JD, Kitamoto T, Kaiser K, Quinn WG. The amnesiac gene product is expressed in two neurons in the Drosophila brain that are critical for memory. Cell. 2000;103:805–13.

48. Waterson MJ, Horvath TL. Neuronal regulation of energy homeostasis: beyond the hypothalamus and feeding. Cell Metab. 2015;22:962–70.

49. Wong R, Piper MD, Wertheim B, Partridge L. Quantification of food intake in Drosophila. PLoS One. 2009;4:e6063.

50. Wu CL, Shih MF, Lee PT, Chiang AS. An octopamine-mushroom body circuit modulates the formation of anesthesia-resistant memory in Drosophila. Curr Biol. 2013;23:2346–54.

51. Yamagata N, Ichinose T, Aso Y, Placais PY, Friedrich AB, Sima RJ, Preat T, Rubin GM, Tanimoto H. Distinct dopamine neurons mediate reward signals for short- and long-term memories. Proc Natl Acad Sci U S A. 2015;112:578–83.

52. Yamazaki D, Hiroi M, Abe T, Shimizu K, Minami-Ohtsubo M, Maeyama Y, Horiuchi J, Tabata T. Two parallel pathways assign opposing odor valences during Drosophila memory formation. Cell Rep. 2018;22:2346–58.

53. Zeltser LM, Seeley RJ, Tschop MH. Synaptic plasticity in neuronal circuits regulating energy balance. Nat Neurosci. 2012;15:1336–42.

10

Regulation of downstream neuronal genes by proneural transcription factors during initial neurogenesis in the vertebrate brain

Michelle Ware[1,3], Houda Hamdi-Rozé[1,2], Julien Le Friec[1], Véronique David[1,2] and Valérie Dupé[1*]

Abstract

Background: Neurons arise in very specific regions of the neural tube, controlled by components of the Notch signalling pathway, proneural genes, and other bHLH transcription factors. How these specific neuronal areas in the brain are generated during development is just beginning to be elucidated. Notably, the critical role of proneural genes during differentiation of the neuronal populations that give rise to the early axon scaffold in the developing brain is not understood. The regulation of their downstream effectors remains poorly defined.

Results: This study provides the first overview of the spatiotemporal expression of proneural genes in the neuronal populations of the early axon scaffold in both chick and mouse. Overexpression studies and mutant mice have identified a number of specific neuronal genes that are targets of proneural transcription factors in these neuronal populations.

Conclusion: Together, these results improve our understanding of the molecular mechanisms involved in differentiation of the first neuronal populations in the brain.

Keywords: Notch, Embryonic, Early axon scaffold, Neurogenin, Ascl1, Rbpj, Tagln3, Chga

Background

In the embryonic rostral brain, the first neurons differentiate in very specific domains and project axons to give rise to the early axon scaffold. This is an evolutionary conserved structure, formed from longitudinal, transversal and commissural axon tracts that act as a scaffold for the guidance of later axons [12, 55, 57, 59]. Each tract is formed from a small neuronal population, including the nucleus of the medial longitudinal fascicle (nMLF), the nucleus of the tract of the postoptic commissure (nTPOC), the nucleus of the mammillotegmental tract (nMTT), the nucleus of the tract of the posterior commissure (nTPC) and the nucleus of the descending tract of the mesencephalic nucleus of the trigeminal nerve (nmesV) (see Table 1 for abbreviations). Despite the importance of these tracts for ensuring the correct formation of later complex connections, the molecular mechanisms involved in differentiation and specification of the neuronal populations that give rise to the early axon scaffold tracts has largely been ignored.

In all neuronal tissue, expression of specific neuronal transcription factors needs to be tightly controlled to ensure the correct patterning of neuronal populations both temporally and spatially [3]. This patterning is regulated in part by the Notch signalling pathway, which has remained highly conserved throughout vertebrate evolution. Lateral inhibition with feedback regulation allows Notch signalling to maintain the number of neural progenitor cells (NPCs) by controlling the number of neighbouring cells that can exit the cell cycle and subsequently undergo neural differentiation [14]. Cell cycle exit is controlled by a limited number of basic helix-loop-helix (bHLH) proneural genes that are both necessary and sufficient to activate neurogenesis [5, 28]. Loss of function studies indicate that proneural transcription factors direct not only general aspects of neuronal differentiation, but also specific aspects of neuronal identity within NPCs [23, 39, 60]. These proneural transcription factors include ASCL1 and members of the Neurogenin family. In many neuronal tissues these proneural genes are expressed in complementary domains

* Correspondence: valerie.dupe@univ-rennes1.fr
[1]Institut de Génétique et Développement de Rennes, Faculté de Médecine, CNRS UMR6290, Université de Rennes 1, IFR140 GFAS, 2 Avenue du Pr. Léon Bernard, 35043 Rennes Cedex, France
Full list of author information is available at the end of the article

Table 1 Abbreviations used throughout the paper

Cda	Circumferential descending axons
Di	diencephalon
dCortex	dorsal cortex
DMB	diencephalic-mesencephalic boundary
DTmesV	descending tract of the mesencephalic nucleus of the trigeminal nerve
Ep	epiphysis
LC	locus coeruleus
Mes	mesencephalon
MLF	medial longitudinal fascicle
MRB	mesencephalic-rhobencephalic boundary
MTT	mammilotegmental tract
nIII	nucleus of the oculomotor nerve
nIV	nucleus of the trochlear nerve
nmesV	nucleus of the descending tract of the mesencephalic nucleus of the trigeminal nerve
nMLF	nucleus of the medial longitudinal fascicle
nMTT	nucleus of the tract of the mammilotegmental tract
nTPC	nucleus of the tract of the posterior commissure
nTPOC	nucleus of the tract of the postoptic commissure
Os	optic stalk
p1, p2, p3	prosomere 1, prosomere 2, prosomere 3
pros	prosencephalon
Ptec	pretectum
Pth	prethalamus
Rh	rhombencephalon
Tel	telencephalon
TPC	tract of the posterior commissure
TPOC	tract of the postoptic commissure
vCortex	ventral cortex

[5, 13, 32, 37], suggesting that they contribute to the specificity of neuronal populations. In recent years, there has been emphasis on determining their downstream target genes, with proneural transcription factors playing a pivotal role in the transcriptional cascade that specifies neurons by activating general neuronal markers, either directly or indirectly [21]. Global profiling approaches are beginning to identify a large number of target genes that could be directly regulated by ASCL1 [2, 8, 16, 50, 58]. Recently, by inhibiting the Notch signalling pathway with the chemical inhibitor N-[3.5-difluorophenacetyl-L-alanyl)]-S-phenylglycine t-butyl ester (DAPT) during early chick development, new neuronal markers including Transgelin 3 (*Tagln3*), Chromogranin A (*Chga*) and Contactin 2 (*Cntn2*) were identified and introduced to a network of downstream proneural targets genes [43]. Analysis of their expression, as well as the known neuronal markers, *Nhlh1* and Stathmin 2 (*Stmn2*), revealed interesting patterns overlapping with the first neuronal populations of the early axon scaffold in the developing chick brain [44].

Identifying gene regulatory networks are essential for understanding the molecular cascades involved in subtype specification of neurons. Here, we describe the molecular cascade implicating Notch signalling, proneural genes and downstream targets at the level of the first neuronal populations that give rise to the early axon scaffold in both chick and mouse embryos. We identified several target genes that are known neuronal markers (*Nhlh1*, *Tagln3*, *Chga*, *Cntn2* and *Stmn2*), which are likely to play an essential role in the differentiation of these neuronal populations.

Methods

Chick embryos

Fertilised chicken (*Gallus gallus*) eggs were obtained from E.A.R.L. Les Bruyères (France). Eggs were incubated in a humidified incubator at 38 °C until the required developmental stages described according to Hamburger and Hamilton [19].

Generation and genotyping of mutant mouse embryos

To generate conditional RBPj knock-out mice, RBPJ$^{f/f}$ [20] mice were crossed with R26R^{creERT2} [3] mice. To activate cre recombinase, tamoxifen (Sigma) was dissolved in sunflower oil at a concentration of 10 mg/ml. 5 mg of tamoxifen was injected by intraperitoneal (IP) injection at embryonic day (E) 7.5 and embryos were harvested at E9.5. Heterozygous Ascl1 delta null mutant mice were used in this study [18]. Genotyping of RBPj mutant embryos and Ascl1 delta null mutant embryos was performed as previously described [7, 20]. Animal experimentation protocols were reviewed and approved by the Direction Départementale des Services Vétérinaires and are conformed to the European Union guidelines (RL2010/63/EU).

In ovo electroporation

The pCAGGS-IRES-nuclearGFP (pCIG) plasmid was used for control experiments. The overexpression constructs for rat *Ascl1* and mouse *Neurog2* were previously cloned into the pCIG plasmid [9]. The expression constructs were used at a concentration of 1 µg/µL^{-1}, with Fast Green (Sigma) added at 0.2% to facilitate visualisation of the DNA solution. The DNA solution was injected into the rostral neural tube of chick embryos at Hamburger and Hamilton stage (HH) 10-11, using a nanoinjector (Drummond Scientific). Electrodes were placed either side of the neural tube, targeting the mesencephalon. Five pulses of 15 V/50 ms were applied, using a square wave pulse electroporator (CUY21SC; Nepa Gene Co., Ltd). After electroporation, the eggs were sealed and incubated for a further 24 h.

In situ hybridisation and immunohistochemistry

All embryos were fixed in 4% PFA/PBS at 4 °C overnight, rinsed and processed for whole-mount RNA *in situ* hybridisation or immunohistochemistry. Anti-sense probes were generated either from plasmids cloned as previously described [43] or plasmids provided as a gift. The protocol for single and double *in situ* hybridisation has been previously described [43]. For double labelling, Digoxigenin and Fluorescein labelled probes were incubated together. The Digoxigenin antibody (Roche) was added first, followed by the NBT/BCIP reaction. After inactivation of the colour reaction, the embryos were fixed with 4% PFA overnight, then the Fluorescein antibody (Roche) was added, followed by fast red reaction (VectorRed). The immunohistochemistry protocol with anti-HuC/D (1:500; molecular probes; A21271) and anti-

neurofilament (1:1000; Invitrogen; 13–0700) has previously been described [30].

Results

Expression of neuronal markers during early development of the mouse brain

Recently, a number of neuronal markers, described as part of the Notch/proneural network, were shown to be specifically expressed in the early neuronal populations of the chick brain [44]. To investigate the role of this network during formation of these neuronal populations in the developing mouse brain, the expression patterns of those markers, *Nhlh1*, *Tagln3*, *Chga*, *Cntn2* and *Stmn2* were analysed between E8.5 and E10.5 (Fig. 1). The conservation of gene expression was analysed by comparison with chick data (Table 2). Similar to the expression

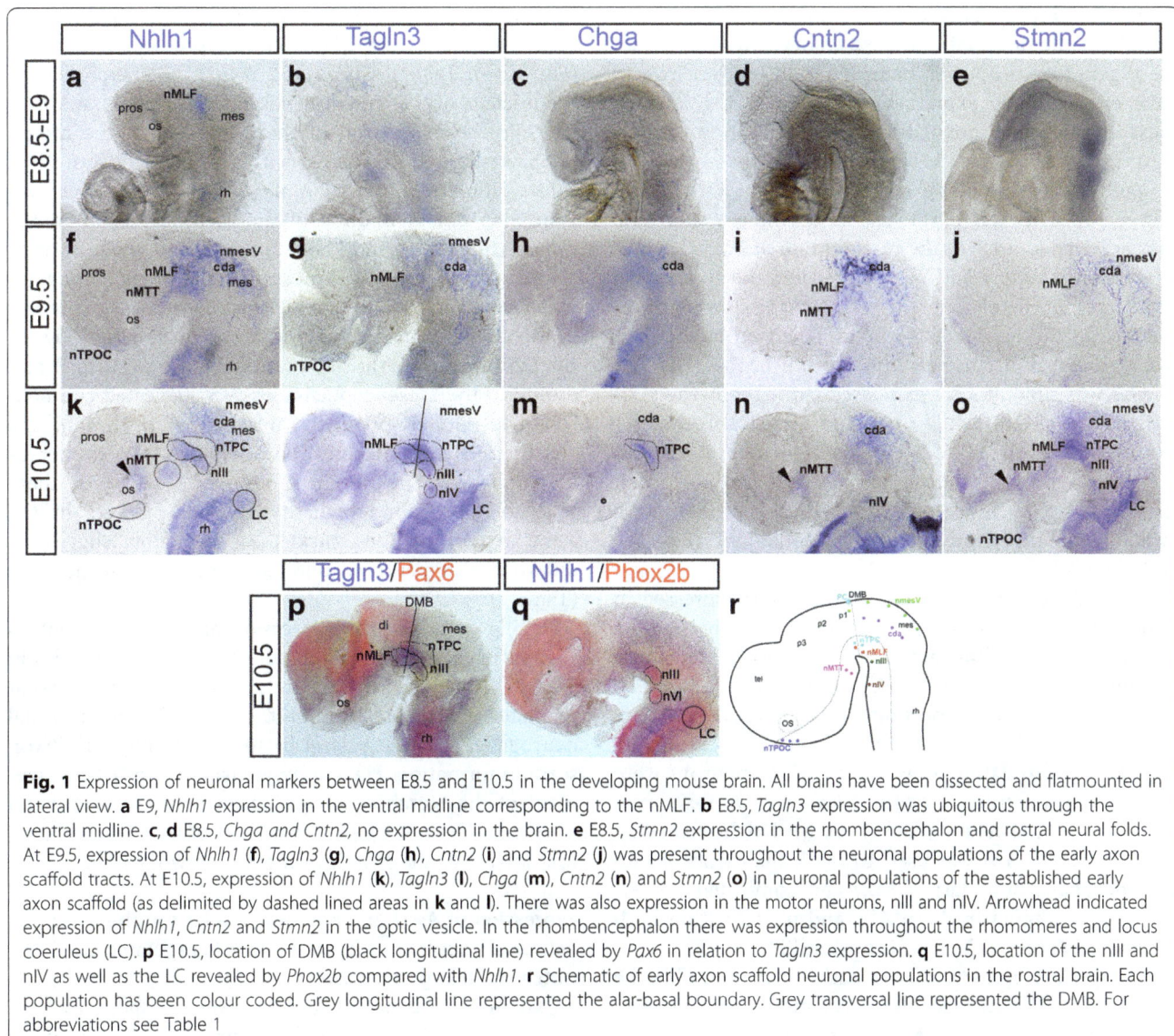

Fig. 1 Expression of neuronal markers between E8.5 and E10.5 in the developing mouse brain. All brains have been dissected and flatmounted in lateral view. **a** E9, *Nhlh1* expression in the ventral midline corresponding to the nMLF. **b** E8.5, *Tagln3* expression was ubiquitous through the ventral midline. **c**, **d** E8.5, *Chga and Cntn2*, no expression in the brain. **e** E8.5, *Stmn2* expression in the rhombencephalon and rostral neural folds. At E9.5, expression of *Nhlh1* (**f**), *Tagln3* (**g**), *Chga* (**h**), *Cntn2* (**i**) and *Stmn2* (**j**) was present throughout the neuronal populations of the early axon scaffold tracts. At E10.5, expression of *Nhlh1* (**k**), *Tagln3* (**l**), *Chga* (**m**), *Cntn2* (**n**) and *Stmn2* (**o**) in neuronal populations of the established early axon scaffold (as delimited by dashed lined areas in **k** and **l**). There was also expression in the motor neurons, nIII and nIV. Arrowhead indicated expression of *Nhlh1*, *Cntn2* and *Stmn2* in the optic vesicle. In the rhombencephalon there was expression throughout the rhomomeres and locus coeruleus (LC). **p** E10.5, location of DMB (black longitudinal line) revealed by *Pax6* in relation to *Tagln3* expression. **q** E10.5, location of the nIII and nIV as well as the LC revealed by *Phox2b* compared with *Nhlh1*. **r** Schematic of early axon scaffold neuronal populations in the rostral brain. Each population has been colour coded. Grey longitudinal line represented the alar-basal boundary. Grey transversal line represented the DMB. For abbreviations see Table 1

Table 2 Expression of *Nhlh1*, *Tagln3*, *Chga*, *Cntn2* and *Stmn2* in the developing chick and mouse brains

	Mouse E9.5-E10.5					Chick HH12-HH17				
	Nhlh1	Tagln3	Chga	Cntn2	Stmn2	Nhlh1	Tagln3	Chga	Cntn2	Stmn2
cda	✓	✓	✓	✓	✓	N/A	N/A	N/A	N/A	N/A
nmesV	✓	✓			✓	✓				✓
nMLF	✓	✓		✓	✓	✓	✓			✓
nMTT	✓	✓		✓	✓	✓	✓		✓	✓
nTPC		✓	✓		✓			✓		
nTPOC	✓	✓			✓	✓	✓	✓		✓
nIII	✓	✓			✓	✓	✓		✓	✓
nIV		✓		✓	✓	✓	✓		✓	✓

Ticks indicate where expression was present in the early axon scaffold populations and the motor neurons. Expression in the mouse brain between E9.5 and E10.5, compared in the chick brain between HH12 and HH17 (taken from [44] and Fig. 7)

patterns observed in the chick embryo [44], these neuronal markers were differentially expressed throughout the early neuronal populations in the brain (Fig. 1 and Table 2), cranial ganglia and spinal cord (data not shown) in the developing mouse embryo. We show that these genes were not pan-neuronal markers, but instead have characteristic expression domains at the level of these first neuronal populations developing in the brain.

At E8.5, there was no expression of these markers along the dorsal midline corresponding to the nmesV (Fig. 1a-e). This was surprising as the nmesV were the first neurons to arise in the rostral brain at E8.5 [12] and expression of *Nhlh1* and *Tagln3* predated the appearance of neurons in the chick brain [44]. *Nhlh1* expression was the first of these markers to be switched on in the ventral diencephalon corresponding to the nMLF (Fig. 1a). *Tagln3* was ubiquitously expressed throughout the ventral brain (Fig. 1b), while *Chga* and *Cntn2* were not yet expressed (Fig. 1c, d). *Stmn2* was expressed at E8.5 in the rostral prosencephalon and the rhombencephalon (Fig. 1e). At E9.5, expression of these markers were switched on in various neuronal populations (Fig. 1f-j and Table 2).

By E10.5, *Nhlh1*, *Tagln3* and *Stmn2* were expressed in almost all the neuronal populations of the brain (Fig. 1 k, l, o), while *Chga* and *Cntn2* were expressed more specifically (Fig. 1m, n). There was a clear gap between the circumferential descending axons (cda) and the nMLF where *Nhlh1* and *Cntn2* were not expressed (Fig. 1k, n), correlating to where the nTPC neurons were located. In contract, *Tagln3*, *Chga* and *Stmn2* were expressed in the nTPC (Fig. 1l, m, o). Double labelling with *Pax6* (Fig. 1p) was used to mark the diencephalic-mesencephalic boundary (DMB) and confirmed the expression of *Tagln3* in the nMLF and nTPC within both the diencephalon and mesencephalon [33].

During development of the early axon scaffold, the oculomotor (III) and trochlear (IV) motor neurons also differentiated at the ventral midline. As the nucleus of the oculomotor nerve (nIII) was not easily identifiable from the nMLF and nTPC at E10.5. Therefore, *Phox2b* was used as a specific marker of the motor neurons [40] to distinguish these populations (Fig. 1q). All the neuronal markers except *Chga* were expressed in the nIII (Fig. 1k-o). *Tagln3*, *Cntn2* and *Stmn2* were expressed in the nucleus of the trochlear nerve (nIV) (Fig. 1l, n, o).

While the expression of these markers in the mouse brain was largely conserved with chick, there were some subtle differences. For example, *Chga* was not expressed along the dorsal midline of the mesencephalon in the mouse (Fig. 1h, m and Table 2). Similar to chick, expression of *Cntn2* was not expressed in the nmesV along the mesencephalic roof, but in contract *Cntn2* was expressed in the cda neurons in the mouse mesencephalon (Fig. 1i, n). Expression of the later markers, *Chga*, *Cntn2* and *Stmn2* in the mesencephalon at E9.5 suggested cda neurons were already present at this stage (Fig. 1h, i, j). The cda neurons were likely to be homologous to the tectobulbar neurons in the chick brain [27]. However, there was no expression of these neuronal markers in the same region of the chick mesencephalon suggesting differences in neuronal differentiation of these neurons (Table 2).

Having described the expression of these genes within the early neuronal populations in the mouse brain (Fig. 1r), the goal of this study was to determine what regulated the expression of these genes during initial neurogenesis in the rostral brain and during early axon scaffold formation. Having previously shown the involvement of the Notch signalling pathway in the expression of *Nhlh1*, *Tagln3*, *Chga*, *Cntn2* and *Stmn2* in chick, we first looked at the Notch/proneural network [43].

Expression of *Ascl1* and neuronal markers in the early neuronal populations in the brain was regulated by Notch signalling in mouse

So far, *Ascl1* has been the only proneural gene to have its expression described in detail during formation of the early neuronal populations in the mouse brain. Expression was first detected in the brain at E8.0 in the nmesV before neuronal differentiation [34, 56]. We wanted to determine if the relationship between *Ascl1* and Notch signalling was similar to that already described in other central nervous system regions [47]. RBPj mutant mice have been commonly used to study the role of Notch inhibition [11, 36]. However, as the full RBPj knock-out mouse was embryonic lethal at E9, before the neuronal populations of the early axon scaffold tracts were fully established, we created a conditional mutant mouse by crossing RBPj$^{f/f}$ [20] and R26R^{creERT2} mice [3]. Initially pregnant females were injected with 5 mg of tamoxifen at E6.5, before Notch signalling was active in the brain. However, the embryos displayed a typical Notch deficient phenotype with a strong developmental delay and it was not possible to compare brain development from this stage (results not shown). After injection of 5 mg tamoxifen, one day later at E7.5, we were able to rescue the early lethality and obtained RBPj$^{f/f}$;R26R^{creERT2} embryos with an apparent similar morphology to the control embryos at E9.5. To confirm Notch signalling was knocked down in these embryos, *Hes5* expression was analysed (Fig. 2a, b; $n = 10$). *Hes5* was downregulated, but expression was not completely lost throughout the RBPj mutant brain (Fig. 2b). This result indicated a partial inhibition of Notch was established in these RBPj mutant embryos.

In the control embryos, *Ascl1* was normally expressed throughout the early neuronal populations, including the nTPOC, nmesV and nTPC (Fig. 2c, c'; $n = 10$). There was also expression along the dorsal and ventral rhombencephalon, the locus coeruleus (LC), the pretectum (Ptec) and the prethalamus (Pth) (Fig. 2c). Expression in the control brain was in a salt-and-pepper like pattern (Fig. 2c', arrowhead). When Notch signalling was knocked down, *Ascl1* expression was upregulated throughout the RBPj mutant brain and the salt-and-pepper like pattern was lost (Fig. 2d, d'; $n = 10$). Although *Ascl1* expression was upregulated, the neuronal populations remained identifiable. This showed that Notch signalling negatively regulates neurogenesis and that lateral inhibition involving *Ascl1* was implicated in the differentiation of the neuronal populations of the early axon scaffold tracts in mouse brain.

Compared to control embryos, there was no *Ascl1* expression in some regions of these RBPj mutant brains, such as, the Pth and nTPC. As *Ascl1* should be expressed in these populations already, this suggested there was already a developmental delay in these mutant embryos (Fig. 2d).

Using this RBPj mutant model, we also investigated the expression of the pan-neuronal markers, *Nhlh1* and *Tagln3* (Fig. 2e-h; $n = 5$). Both genes were upregulated

throughout the neuronal populations that give rise to the early axon scaffold tracts, which genetically confirmed expression of these genes was regulated by the Notch pathway (Fig. 2f, h).

Complementary and restricted expression of proneural genes in the developing mouse brain

As proneural genes are essential transcription factors for neurogenesis [5], we wanted to determine whether they played a role in regulating the expression of these neuronal markers. While the expression patterns of proneural genes have been widely described in populations throughout the peripheral and central nervous systems [18, 31, 32, 48], a detailed description during initial neurogenesis in the brain was lacking. Therefore, we first needed to confirm the expression patterns of proneural genes in these early neuronal populations. The expression patterns of *Neurog1* and *Neurog2* were analysed in the developing mouse brain in comparison to *Ascl1* (Fig. 3 and Table 3). Other proneural genes were not described here, such as *Atoh1*, which was not expressed in the ventral brain (data not shown) and *Neurog3* was only expressed in the developing hypothalamus [41, 52].

Ascl1 was first expressed in the brain from E8 along the dorsal midline of the mesencephalon [56]. *Neurog1* was also first expressed along the dorsal midline of the mesencephalon, slightly later at E8.5 (Fig. 3b). This expression of *Ascl1* (Fig. 3a) and *Neurog1* corresponded to the positioning of the nmesV. *Neurog2* was first expressed at E8.5 in the ventral brain, corresponding to the nMLF (Fig. 3c).

By E9.5, while *Ascl1* expression was mostly restricted to the dorsal midline of the mesencephalon (Fig. 3d), *Neurog1* expression expanded throughout the entire mesencephalon (Fig. 3e) and *Neurog2* was not expressed in the dorsal mesencephalon (Fig. 3f). At this stage, *Ascl1* was also expressed in the nTPOC, nTPC and Pth (Fig. 3d), *Neurog1* was expressed in the nMLF (Fig. 3e) and *Neurog2* was expressed in the nMTT, nMLF, the caudal thalamus (Fig. 3f; unfilled arrowhead) and in the dorsal optic vesicle (Fig. 3f; arrowhead).

At E10.5, *Ascl1*, *Neurog1* and *Neurog2* were differentially expressed throughout the early neuronal populations of the developing brain (Fig. 3g, h, i, j and Table 2). For example, both *Neurog1* and *Neurog2* were expressed in the caudal thalamus (Fig. 3h, i, unfilled arrowhead), the nMLF and the nIII (Fig. 3h, i), while *Ascl1* expression was restricted either side of the caudal thalamus in the Pth and in the Ptec (Fig. 3g). By E10.5, the mesencephalon contained both DTmesV neurons along the dorsal midline and cda neurons that were not clearly distinct from each other [33]. Expression of *Neurog1* overlapped with both the cda and nmesV (Fig. 3h), while *Ascl1* expression was more nmesV specific (Fig. 3g).

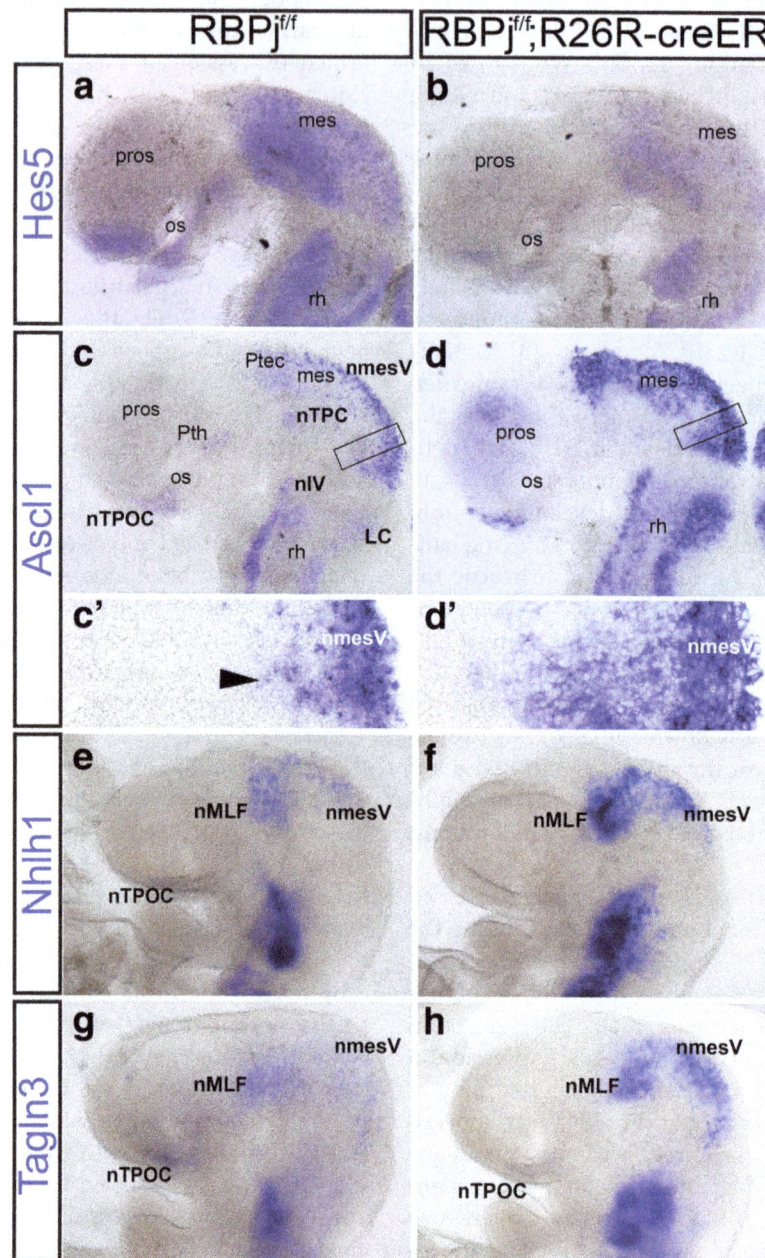

Fig. 2 Loss of Notch signalling affects expression of *Hes5*, *Ascl1*, *Nhlh1* and *Tagln3* in the mouse brain. (**a-d**) All brains have been dissected and flatmounted in lateral view. **e-h** Whole mount embryos. **a**, **b**, *n* = 10 Expression of *Hes5* at E9.5 within the embryonic mouse brain of the control (**a**) and RBPJ mutant (**b**). **c**, *c'*, **d**, *d'*, *n* = 10 *Ascl1* expression in the neuronal populations, which give rise to the early axon scaffold tracts at E9.5 of the control (**c**, *c'*) and RBPj mutant brains (**d**, *d'*). Boxes in **c** and **d** indicate higher magnification in *c'* and *d'* respectively. Arrowhead indicates normal salt-and-pepper like expression of *Ascl1*. Control and mutant embryos were compared from the same littermates. **e**, **f**, *n* = 5 *Nhlh1* expression in control (**e**) and RBPj mutant (**f**). **g**, **h**, *n* = 5 *Tagln3* expression in control (**g**) and RBPj mutant (**h**). Expression of *Nhlh1* and *Tagln3* was upregulated throughout the brain. For abbreviations see Table 1

In the prosencephalon and mesencephalon, there was very little overlap between the expression of *Ascl1* and the two Neurogenin genes. The only exception was at the level of the nmesV (Fig. 3g, h, i; Table 3) where *Ascl1* and *Neurog1* expression overlapped. This mutual exclusivity of proneural gene expression was especially obvious at the level of the nTPC and the cortex (Fig. 3g, h, i). With respect to the neuronal populations of the early axon scaffold tracts, the nTPC and nTPOC were the only populations to express a single proneural gene,

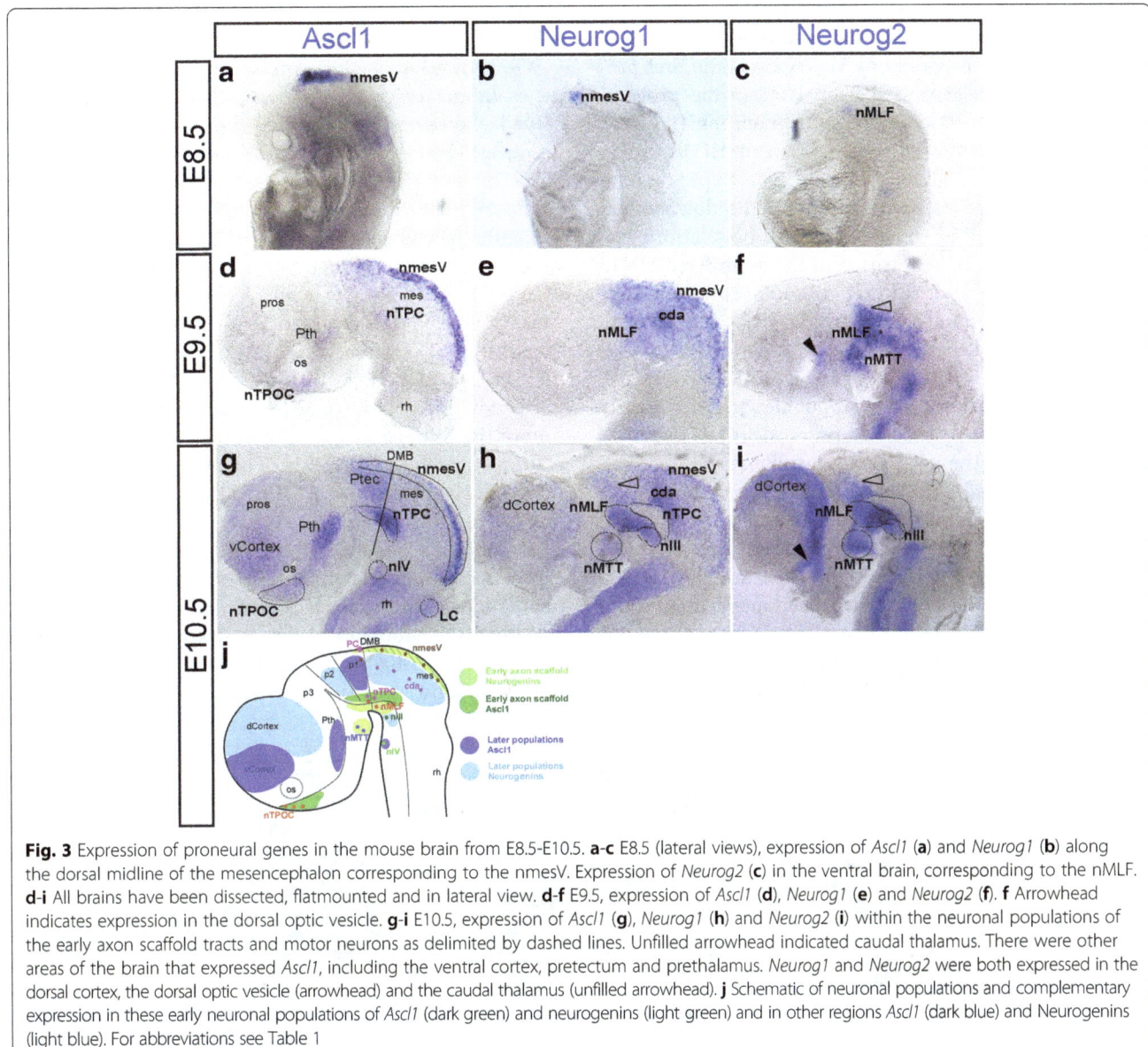

Fig. 3 Expression of proneural genes in the mouse brain from E8.5-E10.5. **a-c** E8.5 (lateral views), expression of *Ascl1* (**a**) and *Neurog1* (**b**) along the dorsal midline of the mesencephalon corresponding to the nmesV. Expression of *Neurog2* (**c**) in the ventral brain, corresponding to the nMLF. **d-i** All brains have been dissected, flatmounted and in lateral view. **d-f** E9.5, expression of *Ascl1* (**d**), *Neurog1* (**e**) and *Neurog2* (**f**). **f** Arrowhead indicates expression in the dorsal optic vesicle. **g-i** E10.5, expression of *Ascl1* (**g**), *Neurog1* (**h**) and *Neurog2* (**i**) within the neuronal populations of the early axon scaffold tracts and motor neurons as delimited by dashed lines. Unfilled arrowhead indicated caudal thalamus. There were other areas of the brain that expressed *Ascl1*, including the ventral cortex, pretectum and prethalamus. *Neurog1* and *Neurog2* were both expressed in the dorsal cortex, the dorsal optic vesicle (arrowhead) and the caudal thalamus (unfilled arrowhead). **j** Schematic of neuronal populations and complementary expression in these early neuronal populations of *Ascl1* (dark green) and neurogenins (light green) and in other regions *Ascl1* (dark blue) and Neurogenins (light blue). For abbreviations see Table 1

Table 3 Comparison of proneural gene expression in the chick and mouse brains

	Ascl1		*Neurog1*		*Neurog2*	
	Chick	Mouse	Chick	Mouse	Chick	Mouse
nmesV	✓	✓	✓	✓	✓	
nMLF			✓	✓	✓	✓
nMTT			✓	✓	✓	✓
nTPC	✓	✓				
nTPOC	✓	✓				
nIII			✓	✓	✓	✓
nIV	✓	✓	✓			

Ticks indicate where expression was located in early axon scaffold neuronal populations and motor neurons at HH18 in chick and E10.5 in mouse

Ascl1 (Fig. 3g). Although the nTPOC only expressed *Ascl1* here, *Neurog3* was also expressed in the hypothalamus, although not in this specific set of the early neurons [52, 53].

These expression studies have revealed a close relationship between proneural and neuronal markers in the developing mouse brain. In order to test whether the neuronal markers described in this study were specific targets of these proneural genes we decided to use the chick model. Therefore, we needed to determine whether expression of the proneural genes was conserved in the early neuronal populations by analysing and comparing the expression patterns of *Ascl1*, *Neurog1* and *Neurog2* in the developing chick brain.

Differential expression of proneural genes was highly conserved between the chick and mouse brains

In the developing chick brain, *Neurog2* was the first proneural gene to be expressed from HH8 in the progenitors that will give rise to the MLF neurons (Fig. 4c). *Ascl1* was first expressed in the brain at HH10 corresponding to the nTPOC (Fig. 4a). The expression of these proneural genes predated any of the downstream target genes and differentiated neuronal populations [44, 57]. *Neurog1* was first expressed in the brain from HH13 within the nmesV and nIII (Fig. 4b). Expression of *Ascl1* expanded to the nmesV from HH11 (data not shown), and then at HH14 the nTPC (Fig. 4d). By HH18, expression of *Ascl1* (Fig. 4g), *Neurog1* (Fig. 4h) and *Neurog2* (Fig. 4i) was in various neuronal populations of the early axon scaffold tracts and the motor neurons. *Neurog2* was expressed in the nMTT and dorsally above the MLF (Fig. 4h, arrowhead). Similar to mouse, the expression of these genes was mostly in complementary populations, expression of all three proneural genes only overlapped in the dorsal mesencephalon within the nmesV (Fig. 4g, h, i). *Neurog1* and *Neurog2* also overlapped in the nIII (Fig. 4h, i). From HH18, proneural genes were expressed in other neuronal populations of the brain. For example, expression of neurogenins dorsal to the MLF in both chick and mouse corresponded to the caudal thalamus (Fig. 4g, h. i, unfilled arrowhead).

We showed that the expression of these proneural genes in the chick and mouse brains was highly conserved, however, there were some slight differences (Table 3). For example, *Neurog2* was expressed in the chick nmesV (Fig. 4i), but not in the mouse (Fig. 3i). Compared with mouse, there was less overlap of all the proneural genes in the chick as *Neurog2* was not as widely expressed throughout the populations in chick (Table 3). Interestingly, while the expression domains were conserved, the timing of expression was not always the same. For example, *Neurog2* expression was switched on first in chick (Fig. 4c), while *Ascl1* expression was switched on first in mouse. This was likely to be a reflection of the difference in timing of the first neuronal populations forming in the brain. The nmesV formed first in mouse [12] and the nMLF formed first in chick [57].

Expression of proneural genes overlapped with the expression of neuronal markers in the early neuronal populations of both the chick and mouse brains

Together, the proneural genes analysed here overlapped with the expression of all the neuronal markers in both the chick and mouse (Figs. 1, 3, 4). However, their

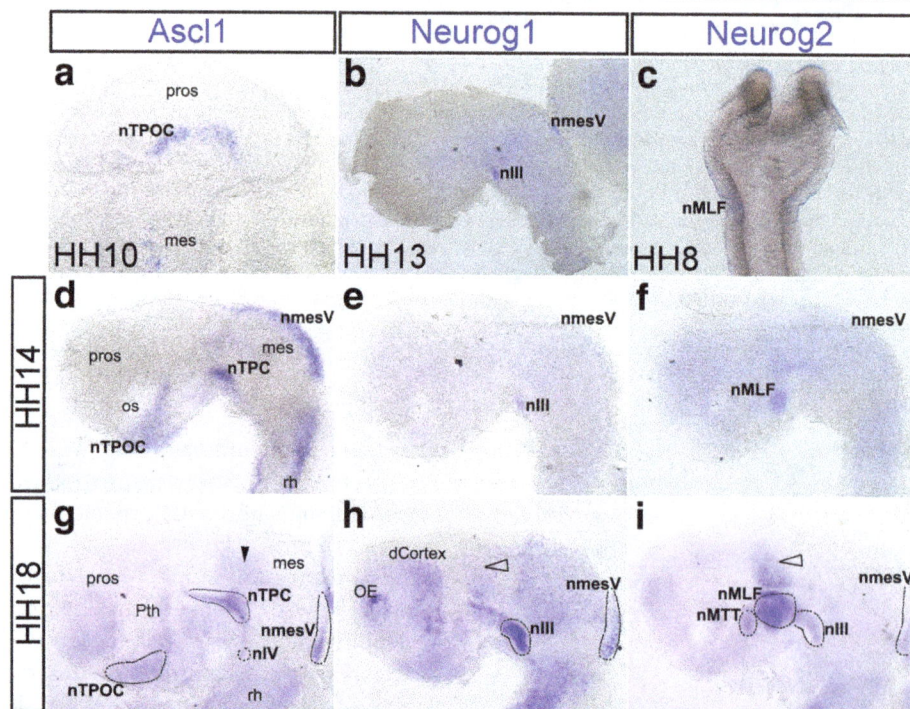

Fig. 4 *Ascl1, Neurog1* and *Neurog2* expression in complementary regions of the chick brain. **a-c** First expression of *Ascl1* (**a**, ventral view) at HH10 in the hypothalamus, *Neurog1* (**b**, dissected, lateral view) at HH13 in the mesencephalon and *Neurog2* (**c**, ventral view) at HH8 in the nMLF. **d-f** HH14 (dissected brain, lateral view). Expression of *Ascl1* (**d**), *Neurog1* (**e**) and *Neurog2* (**f**). **g-i** HH18 (dissected brain lateral view). Expression of *Ascl1* (**g**), *Neurog1* (**h**) and *Neurog2* (**i**). Expression in the pretectum (arrowhead). Expression in the caudal thalamus (unfilled arrowhead). For abbreviations see Table 1

expression did not correlate completely with either the domain of *Ascl1* or the neurogenins. In terms of neuronal marker expression, no single proneural gene completely overlapped with the complete expression of a target gene. *Tagln3* expression, for example, did not completely overlap with *Ascl1* (Figs. 1l and 3g). In chick, *Tagln3* expression was detected in the nMLF and *Neurog2* was the only proneural gene to be expressed in this region, while in mouse both *Neurog1* and *Neurog2* were expressed. This expression analysis suggested that different proneural genes were likely to regulate the same neuronal markers. In contrast to this observation, in both chick and mouse, *Chga* was specifically expressed in the nTPC with *Ascl1* being the only proneural gene in this population (Figs. 1m, 3g, 4g). To test this specificity, we overexpressed *Ascl1* and *Neurog2* in the chick brain.

Ascl1 overexpression induced ectopic neuronal differentiation and misguided axon projection in the developing chick mesencephalon

Previously, upregulation of *Ascl1* in other regions of the embryo led to increased number of neurons [4, 15, 24]. First, the identity of the cells that were electroporated and subsequently overexpressed *Ascl1* was investigated using HuC/D and Neurofilament pan-neuronal antibodies. Embryos were electroporated at HH10, just after neural tube closure, targeting the mesencephalic cells as the proneural and neuronal markers were not widely expressed in this region and there were few post-mitotic neurons (Fig. 5b, d). After 24 h, the number of HuC/D positive post-mitotic neurons increased when *Ascl1* was overexpressed in the chick brain (Fig. 5a, *a'* arrowhead; *n* = 3). These results confirmed that the *Ascl1* construct used here had the ability to induce neurogenesis in cells that were not yet destined to become neurons. Eventually neurons in this region will become tectobular forming the ventral commissure [57]. While HuC/D only showed an increase in the number of neurons, Neurofilament labelled both neurons and their projecting axons (Fig. 5c, d). Interestingly, some of these axons appeared to project along the same path as the DTmesV axons into the rhombencephalon (Fig. 5c, arrow). However, some axons were projecting rostrally back towards the diencephalic-mesencephalic boundary (DMB) (Fig. 5c', unfilled arrowhead), and some axons appeared to be curling back on themselves (Fig. 5c', arrowhead). These results confirmed neurons differentiated from cells that ectopically expressed *Ascl1*, however, their ability to follow the correct path was affected.

Overexpression of *Ascl1* and *Neurog2* caused ectopic expression of the same target genes in the chick brain

To establish a possible specificity of the proneural gene for one of the neuronal markers, we electroporated *Ascl1* and *Neurog2* and analysed the effect on expression of the neuronal markers *Nhlh1*, *Tagln3*, *Chga* and *Stmn2*.

In embryos electroporated with the pCIG control plasmid (n ≥ 3), no ectopic expression of *Nhlh1*, *Tagln3*, *Chga* and *Stmn2* was observed in cells expressing the control plasmid and each gene was normally expressed within the early neuronal populations (Fig. 6a, e, i, m). When either rat *Ascl1* (minimum *n* = 3 for each gene) or mouse *Neurog2* (minimum *n* = 3 for each gene) were overexpressed, cells that ectopically expressed the proneural gene, also expressed the markers *Nhlh1* (Fig. 6b, d), *Tagln3* (Fig. 6f, h), *Chga* (Fig. 6j, l) and *Stmn2* (Fig. 6n, p). As rat and mouse sequences were used, the ectopically expressing cells could be labelled specifically with a rat or mouse RNA riboprobe, therefore highlighting only the cells that were ectopically expressing the gene (Fig. 6; red). As only one half of the brain was electroporated, the other half acted as an internal control (Fig. 6c, g, k, o). The untransfected side of the embryo showed no ectopic expression of the gene and resembled the pCIG embryo. *Pax6* and *Sox10* were tested as negative controls to confirm the specificity of the electroporation, as they were not known to be downstream targets of proneural genes. When *Ascl1* was overexpressed, neither *Pax6* (Additional file 1: Figure S1A, B; *n* = 3) or *Sox10* (data not shown; *n* = 3) were upregulated. Together, these results suggested that both ASCL1 and NEUROG2 were able to regulate the same neuron specific genes tested here.

Loss of *Ascl1* led to discrete loss of *Tagln3* and *Chga* expression in the developing mouse brain

Ascl1 was specifically expressed in some neuronal populations where other proneural gene expression was missing, for example, in the nTPC (Fig. 3g). Therefore, to determine whether *Ascl1* had a specific role in the regulation of the neuronal genes within the early neuronal populations, *Ascl1* null mutant embryos were analysed to investigate the expression of the pan-neuronal gene *Tagln3* (Fig. 7; *n* = 3). Surprisingly, *Ascl1* null mutant embryos still expressed *Tagln3* in all of the neuronal populations at E10 (Fig. 7b), except the LC (Fig. 7b, unfilled arrowhead). The LC was already known to be affected in *Ascl1* mutant mice [22, 37]. We also investigated the expression of *Chga* in *Ascl1* null mutant embryos as its expression was more specific in the early neuronal populations (Fig. 1). Remarkably, in the *Ascl1* mutant embryos, *Chga* expression was specifically lost in the nTPC, while expression in the ganglia was not affected (Fig. 7d, d', filled arrowhead; *n* = 2). *Chga* expression was also downregulated in the cda and in the LC (Fig. 7d, unfilled arrowhead) compared with the control embryos.

Discussion

The organisation of the initial neuronal populations of the brain giving rise to the early axon scaffold has been

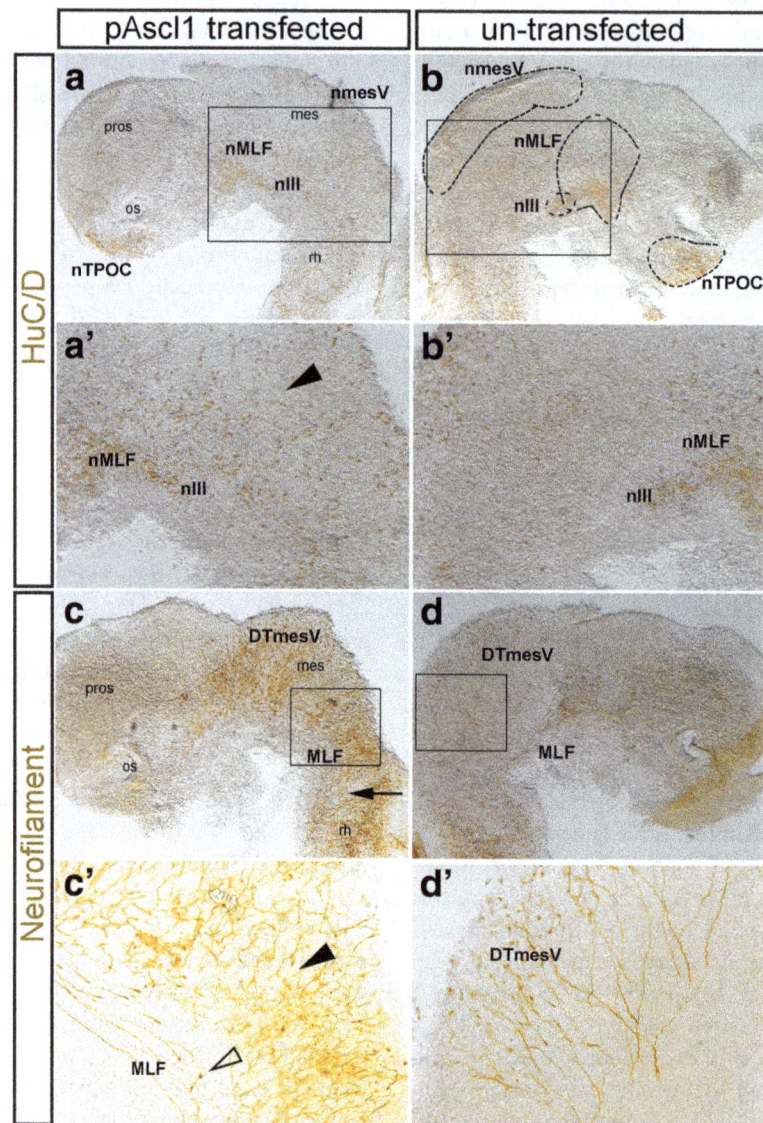

Fig. 5 *Ascl1* overexpression leads to ectopic neuronal differentiation. All brains have been dissected, flatmounted and in lateral view. **a**, **b**, *a'*, *b'*; *n* = 3 The neuronal populations were labelled with HuC/D in the chick brain after electroporation with the pAscl1 plasmids. Box indicates higher magnification image. **a**, *a'* More HuC/D positive cells were visible in the mesencephalon (arrowhead). **b**, *b'* The un-transfected half of the brain showed normal distribution of neurons. **c**, **d**, *c'*, *d'*; *n* = 3 The neuronal populations and their associated axon tracts were labelled with Neurofilament in the chick brain after electroporation with the pAscl1 plasmid. **c** There was an increase in the number of neurons and axons in the mesencephalon. Some of these neurons projected axons into the hindbrain (arrow), not seen in control side (**d**). Box indicates higher magnification image. (*c'*) Some axons did not project correctly. In the ventral brain axons projected rostrally towards the DMB (arrowhead) and other axons within the mesencephalon projected in a curved shape (arrowhead), not directly ventral like the axons in the control (**d**). **d**, *d'* Normal distribution of neurons and axons projected in the correct way. For abbreviations see Table 1

studied in great detail in zebrafish, chick and mouse [33, 57, 59]. However, the molecular mechanisms that underlie the specification of these early differentiating neurons remain undetermined. Our study shows that differentiation of these neurons is tightly regulated by the Notch/proneural network and reveals important new expression descriptions of proneural and neuronal markers in the early axon scaffold in both chick and mouse. This work adds further evidence to suggest evolutionary conservation of the genetic mechanisms that control neuron differentiation between birds and mammals.

Expression of specific neuronal markers reveals genes that potentially play an essential role in the differentiation and specification of the populations that give rise to the early axon scaffold

Very few specific markers are described in the individual neuronal populations of the developing vertebrate brain

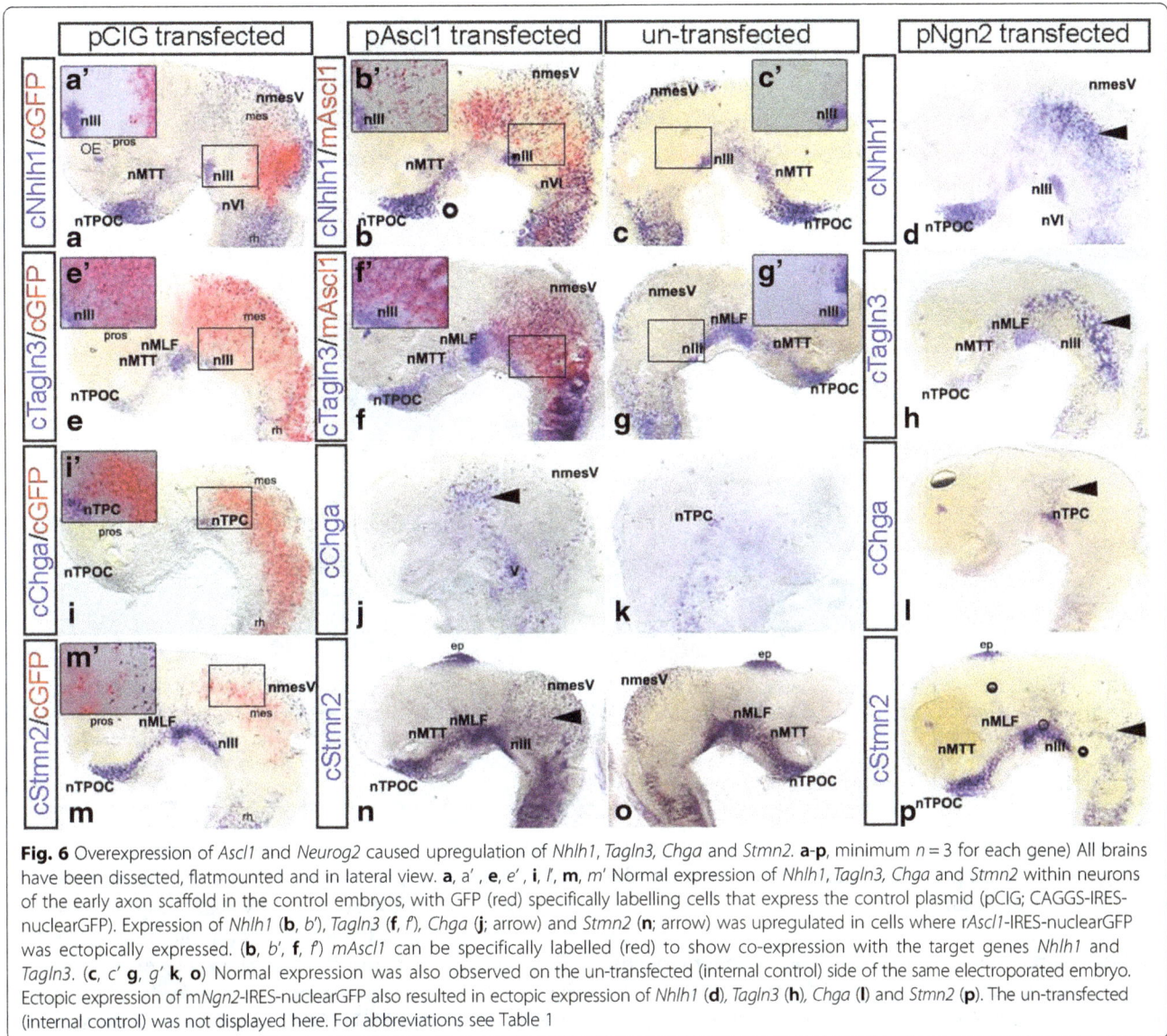

Fig. 6 Overexpression of *Ascl1* and *Neurog2* caused upregulation of *Nhlh1, Tagln3, Chga* and *Stmn2.* **a-p,** minimum *n* = 3 for each gene) All brains have been dissected, flatmounted and in lateral view. **a,** *a'* , **e,** *e'* , **i,** *I'*, **m,** *m'* Normal expression of *Nhlh1, Tagln3, Chga* and *Stmn2* within neurons of the early axon scaffold in the control embryos, with GFP (red) specifically labelling cells that express the control plasmid (pCIG; CAGGS-IRES-nuclearGFP). Expression of *Nhlh1* (**b,** *b'*), *Tagln3* (**f,** *f'*), *Chga* (**j**; arrow) and *Stmn2* (**n**; arrow) was upregulated in cells where r*Ascl1*-IRES-nuclearGFP was ectopically expressed. (**b,** *b'*, **f,** *f'*) m*Ascl1* can be specifically labelled (red) to show co-expression with the target genes *Nhlh1* and *Tagln3*. (**c,** *c'* **g,** *g'* **k, o**) Normal expression was also observed on the un-transfected (internal control) side of the same electroporated embryo. Ectopic expression of m*Ngn2*-IRES-nuclearGFP also resulted in ectopic expression of *Nhlh1* (**d**), *Tagln3* (**h**), *Chga* (**l**) and *Stmn2* (**p**). The un-transfected (internal control) was not displayed here. For abbreviations see Table 1

at early stages during the formation of the early axon scaffold tracts. This study describes 5 genes, *Nhlh1, Tagln3, Chga, Cntn2* and *Stmn2* that are expressed in specific neuronal populations and play a role in the Notch/proneural network. These are all known neuronal markers that mediate critical biological processes required to induce neuronal identity [35, 44]. *Nhlh1* and *Tagln3* are involved in fate determination, whereas *Chga, Cntn2* and *Stmn2* are expressed during terminal differentiation. There is some evidence that these neuronal genes play a specific role in determining the identity or function of these distinct neuronal clusters. For example, *Cntn2* has a role in the guidance of the MLF axons [61], and the specific expression of *Chga* in the nTPC in both the chick and mouse brains, suggests that nTPC may have a neuroendocrine function [49].

Despite the fact that *Nlhh1, Tagln3,* and *Stmn2* are considered pan-neuronal markers they have, to some extent, specific expression at the level of the first neurons establishing the early axon scaffold tracts in the amniote brain [55]. We show that each of these neuronal populations have a specific combination of these neurogenic markers during differentiation (Table 2). This means that very early during development these neurons acquire a specific identity. Most importantly, with a few exceptions, the expression pattern of these neuronal markers is highly conserved between chick and mouse (Table 2). Still, it is surprising to see that *Nhlh1* and *Tagln3* are not expressed in the mouse nmesV until after the first neurons differentiated at E8.5 [55], whereas *Nhlh1* and *Tagln3* are early markers for post-mitotic neurons in the chick [44]. Further analysis will be required to determine

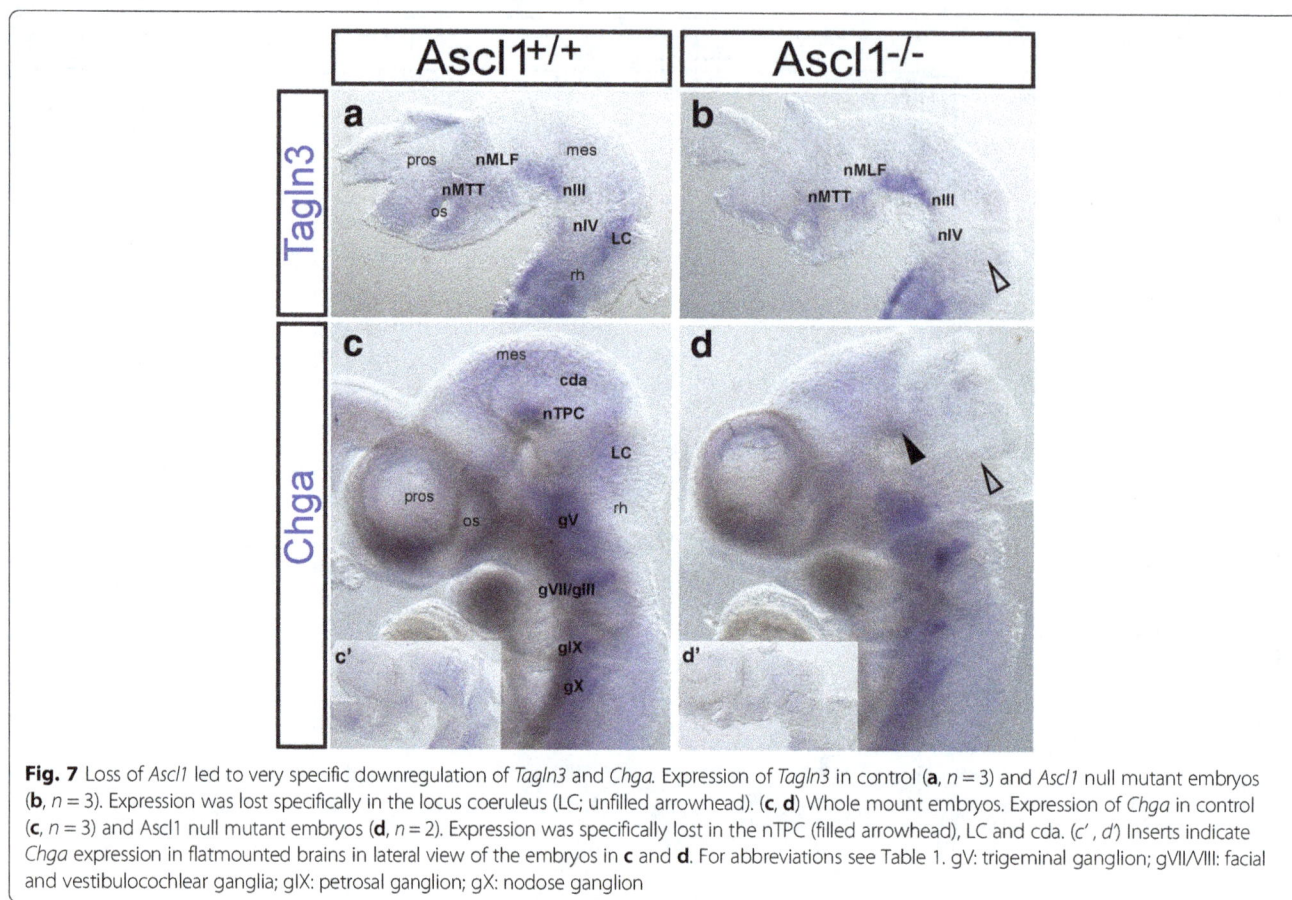

Fig. 7 Loss of *Ascl1* led to very specific downregulation of *Tagln3* and *Chga*. Expression of *Tagln3* in control (**a**, n = 3) and *Ascl1* null mutant embryos (**b**, n = 3). Expression was lost specifically in the locus coeruleus (LC; unfilled arrowhead). (**c, d**) Whole mount embryos. Expression of *Chga* in control (**c**, n = 3) and Ascl1 null mutant embryos (**d**, n = 2). Expression was specifically lost in the nTPC (filled arrowhead), LC and cda. (*c' , d'*) Inserts indicate *Chga* expression in flatmounted brains in lateral view of the embryos in **c** and **d**. For abbreviations see Table 1. gV: trigeminal ganglion; gVII/VIII: facial and vestibulocochlear ganglia; gIX: petrosal ganglion; gX: nodose ganglion

the function of this discrepancy as ultimately these neuronal populations express the same genes in both the chick and mouse brains.

A relationship between Notch signalling, proneural genes and downstream targets is essential for the correct patterning of early neuronal populations in the developing vertebrate brain

Numerous studies support the idea that the Notch signalling pathway and proneural genes act together in a feedback loop to promote initial neurogenesis [5, 10, 29, 43]. However, in the developing brain, this has only been observed in the chick embryo via DAPT treatment [43]. By the inhibition of Notch signalling, this study confirms the role of Notch signalling in the Notch/proneural molecular circuitry that operates within the developing mouse brain similar to the other neural structures to control neurogenesis.

Compensation by proneural genes is not neuronal population specific

We show that a complex pattern of proneural gene expression exists during the generation of the initial neuronal populations in the brain. This seems to be the general situation in most regions of the central nervous

system [32]. Therefore, it is not surprising that *Ascl1* and *Neurog1/2* play a central role in the selection of neuronal progenitor subtypes by regulating downstream target genes [2, 5, 13, 37]. Genomic approaches (CHIP on chip, ChIP-seq and RNA-seq) are powerful tools that have led to the identification of hundreds of targets of ASCL1 [6, 8] and NEUROG2 [28]. However, the relationship between the proneural genes and these target genes, is yet to be functionally shown. In the present study, as the neuronal markers *Nhlh1, Tagln3, Chga, Cntn2* and *Stmn2*, are expressed in very similar expression patterns to the proneural genes, we propose that precise proneural genes regulate expression of specific neuronal genes, including, in specific neuronal populations of the early axon scaffold tracts.

Interestingly, we show that the nTPC has a very specific expression identity. These neurons do not express the pan-neuronal markers *Nhlh1* and *Talgn3*, they are the only neurons to have a strong expression of *Chga*, and *Ascl1* is the exclusively expressed proneural gene. Furthermore, in both the chick and mouse brains, expression of *Chga* is excluded from neuronal populations expressing *Neurog1* and *Neurog2*. This observation strengthens the argument for a specific function of ASCL1 in the development of specific neuroendocrine neurons [34], and this is in accordance with the down-regulation of *Chga* in the *Ascl1* null mutant embryo.

This study shows that regulating expression of the target genes analysed here is not specific to either the over-expression of *Ascl1* or *Neurog2*, suggesting proneural genes are functionally equivalent (at least to induce neuronal identity). Indeed, while proneural genes are expressed in complementary regions, there are numerous studies that show they able to compensate for each other [26, 37, 45]. It has been demonstrated that *Neurog2* has the capacity to rescue the development of *Ascl1*-dependent neurons [34, 37]. It is therefore not surprising that in the *Ascl1* null mutant embryos, the expression of *Tagln3* is not downregulated in neuronal populations expressing more than one proneural gene. This suggests there is compensation of other proneural genes in these populations. However, *Tagln3* expression is not downregulated in the nVI where *Ascl1* is the exclusively expressed proneural gene is unexpected. Other known proneural genes, *Neurog1*, *Neurog2*, *Neurog3* and *Atoh1* seem to be not expressed in the nVI. What is regulating *Tagln3* here is yet to be determined.

The highly conserved expression patterns of the proneural genes in the early ventral forebrain argue against a model of stochastic induction. An important selection pressure may exist to maintain this complementary proneural gene expression within the chick and mouse brains. We still have to determine why these neuronal target genes are expressed in some populations but not others, especially if these genes can be regulated by any proneural gene. It has been demonstrated, that these proneural genes are not always functionally equivalent and this capacity appears to vary in different regions of the nervous system [37]. How the divergent function of the proneural genes is established remain ambiguous. Further analysis of mice containing targeted mutations in both the *Ascl1* and *Neurog2* genes should be informative in answering this question.

The regional cues are likely to be involved in controlling the position of the various neuronal populations that give rise to the early axon scaffold tracts

Questions still remain, including what is controlling the specification of the individual neuronal populations that give rise to the early axon scaffold tracts and other early populations.

If proneural genes can regulate the same target genes, we still need to determine the specific genes or combination of genes (in a cascade) that regulate identity of each individual neuronal population of the early axon scaffold. Although a single proneural gene is sufficient to induce neuronal features, the additional expression of other factors is necessary to generate specific identity, for example, in fibroblasts [51, 54]. Thus, there is another layer of

complexity with other regional cues such as those produced by homeobox genes [17, 42]. Specification of neurons in the neural tube relies on combinations of bHLH and other transcription factors to activate or repress specific neurogenic programs. Homeobox genes, such as, *Sax1* could play a role in specifying the nMLF subtypes [46], as gain of function of *Sax1* results in an enlargement of the nMLF area [1]. However, other homeobox genes need to be found in order to explain the patterning of the neuronal populations of the early axon scaffold tracts.

Initially, a critical step is the establishment of morphogen gradients controlling the distinct sets of transcription factors resulting in the establishment of progenitor domains [25]. Such a mechanism has not yet been described during the establishment of the progenitor domains of the axon scaffold. It may be a different mechanism, as these populations of neurons are not distributed along specific axis. Sonic hedgehog (SHH), one of the main signalling molecules involved in neurogenesis patterning [38] is differentially expressed in the ventral forebrain [56] and mostly likely plays a critical role in the formation of the early axon scaffold tracts [1].

Conclusions

The organisation of the brain is more complex and harbours a greater diversity of neurons compared with the spinal cord. However, to our knowledge, no study investigating the specification of the neuronal populations that give rise to the early axon scaffold in any mutant mouse models has been done. Our present study gives essential tools to explore more accurately the formation of these neuronal populations in mutant models. This will provide a better understanding of how these early neurons differentiate in a specific territory with a specific identity.

Acknowledgements
We would like to thank the members of the David laboratory for suggestions and comments, including Charlotte Mouden for cloning the mouse Neurogenin 2 plasmid. Thank you to for useful discussions throughout the course of this project. Many thanks to Olivier Pourquié (pCIG/pCAGGS-IRES-nuclearGFP), James Briscoe (pAscl1) and François Guillemot (pNgn2) for providing us with plasmids for the overexpression studies. We are grateful to Philippos Mourikis and Shahragim Tajbakhsh for providing the RBPjlox/lox mice and François Guillemot for kindly providing Ascl1 null mutant embryos. We are also grateful to the following people for useful discussion throughout the course of this project and sending plasmids to make RNA probes: Frank Schubert, François Guillemot, Sophie Bel-Vialar, Siew-Lan Ang, Nicholas Greene, Lukas Sommer, Sonia Garel, and Doris Wu. We also thank the animal house platform ARCHE (SFR Biosit, Rennes, France).

Funding
This work was supported by the Agence Nationale de la Recherche (grant no. ANR-12-BSV1-0007-01, Valérie Dupé). Valérie Dupé is supported by the Institut National de la Santé et de la Recherche Médicale (Inserm).

Authors' contributions

M.W. and Va.D. set up and designed the experiments. M.W., H.R. and J.F. performed the experiments. M.W., Ve.D. and Va.D. wrote the manuscript. All authors discussed and edited the manuscript. All authors read and approved the final manuscript.

Competing interests

The authors declare that they have no competing interests.

Author details

[1]Institut de Génétique et Développement de Rennes, Faculté de Médecine, CNRS UMR6290, Université de Rennes 1, IFR140 GFAS, 2 Avenue du Pr. Léon Bernard, 35043 Rennes Cedex, France. [2]Laboratoire de Génétique Moléculaire, CHU Pontchaillou, Rennes Cedex, France. [3]Present address: Department of Physiology, Development and Neuroscience, University of Cambridge, Anatomy Building, Downing Street, CB2 3DY Cambridge, UK.

References

1. Ahsan M, Riley KL, Schubert FR. Molecular mechanisms in the formation of the medial longitudinal fascicle. J Anat. 2007;211:177–87.
2. Augustyn A, Borromeo M, Wang T, Fujimoto J, Shao C, Dospoy PD, Lee V, Tan C, Sullivan JP, Larsen JE, et al. ASCL1 is a lineage oncogene providing therapeutic targets for high-grade neuroendocrine lung cancers. Proc Natl Acad Sci U S A. 2014;111:14788–93.
3. Badea TC, Wang Y, Nathans J. A noninvasive genetic/pharmacologic strategy for visualizing cell morphology and clonal relationships in the mouse. J Neurosci. 2003;23:2314–22.
4. Berninger B, Guillemot F, Gotz M. Directing neurotransmitter identity of neurones derived from expanded adult neural stem cells. Eur J Neurosci. 2007;25:2581–90.
5. Bertrand N, Castro DS, Guillemot F. Proneural genes and the specification of neural cell types. Nat Rev Neurosci. 2002;3:517–30.
6. Borromeo MD, Meredith DM, Castro DS, Chang JC, Tung KC, Guillemot F, Johnson JE. A transcription factor network specifying inhibitory versus excitatory neurons in the dorsal spinal cord. Development. 2014;141:2803–12.
7. Casarosa S, Fode C, Guillemot F. Mash1 regulates neurogenesis in the ventral telencephalon. Development. 1999;126:525–34.
8. Castro DS, Martynoga B, Parras C, Ramesh V, Pacary E, Johnston C, Drechsel D, Lebel-Potter M, Garcia LG, Hunt C, et al. A novel function of the proneural factor Ascl1 in progenitor proliferation identified by genome-wide characterization of its targets. Genes Dev. 2011;25:930–45.
9. Castro DS, Skowronska-Krawczyk D, Armant O, Donaldson IJ, Parras C, Hunt C, Critchley JA, Nguyen L, Gossler A, Gottgens B, et al. Proneural bHLH and Brn proteins coregulate a neurogenic program through cooperative binding to a conserved DNA motif. Dev Cell. 2006;11:831–44.
10. Cau E, Gradwohl G, Fode C, Guillemot F. Mash1 activates a cascade of bHLH regulators in olfactory neuron progenitors. Development. 1997;124:1611–21.
11. de la Pompa JL, Wakeham A, Correia KM, Samper E, Brown S, Aguilera RJ, Nakano T, Honjo T, Mak TW, Rossant J, et al. Conservation of the Notch signalling pathway in mammalian neurogenesis. Development. 1997;124:1139–48.
12. Easter Jr SS, Ross LS, Frankfurter A. Initial tract formation in the mouse brain. J Neurosci. 1993;13:285–99.
13. Fode C, Ma Q, Casarosa S, Ang SL, Anderson DJ, Guillemot F. A role for neural determination genes in specifying the dorsoventral identity of telencephalic neurons. Genes Dev. 2000;14:67–80.
14. Formosa-Jordan P, Ibanes M, Ares S, Frade JM. Lateral inhibition and neurogenesis: novel aspects in motion. Int J Dev Biol. 2013;57:341–50.
15. Geoffroy CG, Critchley JA, Castro DS, Ramelli S, Barraclough C, Descombes P, Guillemot F, Raineteau O. Engineering of dominant active basic helix-loop-helix proteins that are resistant to negative regulation by postnatal central nervous system antineurogenic cues. Stem Cells. 2009;27:847–56.
16. Gohlke JM, Armant O, Parham FM, Smith MV, Zimmer C, Castro DS, Nguyen L, Parker JS, Gradwohl G, Portier CJ, et al. Characterization of the proneural gene regulatory network during mouse telencephalon development. BMC Biol. 2008;6:15.
17. Guillemot F. Spatial and temporal specification of neural fates by transcription factor codes. Development. 2007;134:3771–80.
18. Guillemot F, Joyner AL. Dynamic expression of the murine Achaete-Scute homologue Mash-1 in the developing nervous system. Mech Dev. 1993;42:171–85.
19. Hamburger V, Hamilton HL. A series of normal stages in the development of the chick embryo. J Morphol. 1951;88:49–92.
20. Han H, Tanigaki K, Yamamoto N, Kuroda K, Yoshimoto M, Nakahata T, Ikuta K, Honjo T. Inducible gene knockout of transcription factor recombination signal binding protein-J reveals its essential role in T versus B lineage decision. Int Immunol. 2002;14:637–45.
21. Henke RM, Meredith DM, Borromeo MD, Savage TK, Johnson JE. Ascl1 and Neurog2 form novel complexes and regulate Delta-like3 (Dll3) expression in the neural tube. Dev Biol. 2009;328:529–40.
22. Hirsch MR, Tiveron MC, Guillemot F, Brunet JF, Goridis C. Control of noradrenergic differentiation and Phox2a expression by MASH1 in the central and peripheral nervous system. Development. 1998;125:599–608.
23. Huang HS, Redmond TM, Kubish GM, Gupta S, Thompson RC, Turner DL, Uhler MD. Transcriptional regulatory events initiated by Ascl1 and Neurog2 during neuronal differentiation of P19 embryonic carcinoma cells. J Mol Neurosci. 2015;55:684–705.
24. Jacob J, Kong J, Moore S, Milton C, Sasai N, Gonzalez-Quevedo R, Terriente J, Imayoshi I, Kageyama R, Wilkinson DG, et al. Retinoid acid specifies neuronal identity through graded expression of Ascl1. Curr Biol. 2013;23:412–8.
25. Jessell TM. Neuronal specification in the spinal cord: inductive signals and transcriptional codes. Nat Rev Genet. 2000;1:20–9.
26. Kele J, Simplicio N, Ferri AL, Mira H, Guillemot F, Arenas E, Ang SL. Neurogenin 2 is required for the development of ventral midbrain dopaminergic neurons. Development. 2006;133:495–505.
27. Kroger S, Schwarz U. The avian tectobulbar tract: development, explant culture, and effects of antibodies on the pattern of neurite outgrowth. J Neurosci. 1990;10:3118–34.
28. Lacomme M, Liaubet L, Pituello F, Bel-Vialar S. NEUROG2 drives cell cycle exit of neuronal precursors by specifically repressing a subset of cyclins acting at the G1 and S phases of the cell cycle. Mol Cell Biol. 2012;32:2596–607.
29. Louvi A, Artavanis-Tsakonas S. Notch signalling in vertebrate neural development. Nat Rev Neurosci. 2006;7:93–102.
30. Lumsden A, Keynes R. Segmental patterns of neuronal development in the chick hindbrain. Nature. 1989;337:424–8.
31. Ma Q, Chen Z, del Barco Barrantes I, de la Pompa JL, Anderson DJ. Neurogenin1 is essential for the determination of neuronal precursors for proximal cranial sensory ganglia. Neuron. 1998;20:469–82.
32. Ma Q, Sommer L, Cserjesi P, Anderson DJ. Mash1 and neurogenin1 expression patterns define complementary domains of neuroepithelium in the developing CNS and are correlated with regions expressing notch ligands. J Neurosci. 1997;17:3644–52.
33. Mastick GS, Easter Jr SS. Initial organization of neurons and tracts in the embryonic mouse fore- and midbrain. Dev Biol. 1996;173:79–94.
34. McNay DE, Pelling M, Claxton S, Guillemot F, Ang SL. Mash1 is required for generic and subtype differentiation of hypothalamic neuroendocrine cells. Mol Endocrinol. 2006;20:1623–32.
35. Murdoch JN, Eddleston J, Leblond-Bourget N, Stanier P, Copp AJ. Sequence and expression analysis of Nhlh1: a basic helix-loop-helix gene implicated in neurogenesis. Dev Genet. 1999;24:165–77.
36. Oka C, Nakano T, Wakeham A, de la Pompa JL, Mori C, Sakai T, Okazaki S, Kawaichi M, Shiota K, Mak TW, et al. Disruption of the mouse RBP-J kappa gene results in early embryonic death. Development. 1995;121:3291–301.
37. Parras CM, Schuurmans C, Scardigli R, Kim J, Anderson DJ, Guillemot F. Divergent functions of the proneural genes Mash1 and Ngn2 in the specification of neuronal subtype identity. Genes Dev. 2002;16:324–38.
38. Patten I, Placzek M. The role of Sonic hedgehog in neural tube patterning. Cell Mol Life Sci. 2000;57:1695–708.
39. Pattyn A, Guillemot F, Brunet JF. Delays in neuronal differentiation in Mash1/Ascl1 mutants. Dev Biol. 2006;295:67–75.
40. Pattyn A, Morin X, Cremer H, Goridis C, Brunet JF. Expression and interactions of the two closely related homeobox genes Phox2a and Phox2b during neurogenesis. Development. 1997;124:4065–75.
41. Pelling M, Anthwal N, McNay D, Gradwohl G, Leiter AB, Guillemot F, Ang SL. Differential requirements for neurogenin 3 in the development of POMC and NPY neurons in the hypothalamus. Dev Biol. 2011;349:406–16.

42. Powell LM, Deaton AM, Wear MA, Jarman AP. Specificity of Atonal and Scute bHLH factors: analysis of cognate E box binding sites and the influence of Senseless. Genes Cells. 2008;13:915–29.

43. Ratié L, Ware M, Barloy-Hubler F, Romé H, Gicquel I, Dubourg C, David V, Dupé V. Novel genes upregulated when NOTCH signalling is disrupted during hypothalamic development. Neural Dev. 2013;8:25.

44. Ratié L, Ware M, Jagline H, David V, Dupé V. Dynamic expression of Notch-dependent neurogenic markers in the chick embryonic nervous system. Front Neuroanat. 2014;8:158.

45. Roybon L, Mastracci TL, Ribeiro D, Sussel L, Brundin P, Li JY. GABAergic differentiation induced by Mash1 is compromised by the bHLH proteins Neurogenin2, NeuroD1, and NeuroD2. Cereb Cortex. 2010;20:1234–44.

46. Schubert FR, Lumsden A. Transcriptional control of early tract formation in the embryonic chick midbrain. Development. 2005;132:1785–93.

47. Shi M, Hu ZL, Zheng MH, Song NN, Huang Y, Zhao G, Han H, Ding YQ. Notch-Rbpj signaling is required for the development of noradrenergic neurons in the mouse locus coeruleus. J Cell Sci. 2012;125:4320–32.

48. Sommer L, Ma Q, Anderson DJ. Neurogenins, a novel family of atonal-related bHLH transcription factors, are putative mammalian neuronal determination genes that reveal progenitor cell heterogeneity in the developing CNS and PNS. Mol Cell Neurosci. 1996;8:221–41.

49. Taupenot L, Harper KL, O'Connor DT. The chromogranin-secretogranin family. N Engl J Med. 2003;348:1134–49.

50. Vasconcelos FF, Castro DS. Transcriptional control of vertebrate neurogenesis by the proneural factor Ascl1. Front Cell Neurosci. 2014;8:412.

51. Vierbuchen T, Ostermeier A, Pang ZP, Kokubu Y, Sudhof TC, Wernig M. Direct conversion of fibroblasts to functional neurons by defined factors. Nature. 2010;463:1035–41.

52. Villasenor A, Chong DC, Cleaver O. Biphasic Ngn3 expression in the developing pancreas. Dev Dyn. 2008;237:3270–9.

53. Wang X, Chu LT, He J, Emelyanov A, Korzh V, Gong Z. A novel zebrafish bHLH gene, neurogenin3, is expressed in the hypothalamus. Gene. 2001;275:47–55.

54. Wapinski OL, Vierbuchen T, Qu K, Lee QY, Chanda S, Fuentes DR, Giresi PG, Ng YH, Marro S, Neff NF, et al. Hierarchical mechanisms for direct reprogramming of fibroblasts to neurons. Cell. 2013;155:621–35.

55. Ware M, Dupé V, Schubert FR. Evolutionary conservation of the early axon scaffold in the vertebrate brain. Dev Dyn. 2015;244:1202–14.

56. Ware M, Hamdi-Rozé H, Dupé V. Notch signaling and proneural genes work together to control the neural building blocks for the initial scaffold in the hypothalamus. Front Neuroanat. 2014;8:140.

57. Ware M, Schubert FR. Development of the early axon scaffold in the rostral brain of the chick embryo. J Anat. 2011;219:203–16.

58. Webb AE, Pollina EA, Vierbuchen T, Urban N, Ucar D, Leeman DS, Martynoga B, Sewak M, Rando TA, Guillemot F, et al. FOXO3 shares common targets with ASCL1 genome-wide and inhibits ASCL1-dependent neurogenesis. Cell Rep. 2013;4:477–91.

59. Wilson SW, Ross LS, Parrett T, Easter Jr SS. The development of a simple scaffold of axon tracts in the brain of the embryonic zebrafish, Brachydanio rerio. Development. 1990;108:121–45.

60. Wilson SW, Rubenstein JL. Induction and dorsoventral patterning of the telencephalon. Neuron. 2000;28:641–51.

61. Wolman MA, Sittaramane VK, Essner JJ, Yost HJ, Chandrasekhar A, Halloran MC. Transient axonal glycoprotein-1 (TAG-1) and laminin-alpha1 regulate dynamic growth cone behaviors and initial axon direction in vivo. Neural Dev. 2008;3:6.

11

Charcot-Marie-Tooth 2b associated Rab7 mutations cause axon growth and guidance defects during vertebrate sensory neuron development

Olga Y. Ponomareva[1,2,3,4], Kevin W. Eliceiri[5] and Mary C. Halloran[1,2,3,4]*

Abstract

Background: Charcot-Marie-Tooth2b (CMT2b) is an axonal form of a human neurodegenerative disease that preferentially affects sensory neurons. CMT2b is dominantly inherited and is characterized by unusually early onset, presenting in the second or third decade of life. Five missense mutations in the gene encoding Rab7 GTPase have been identified as causative in human CMT2b disease. Although several studies have modeled CMT2b disease in cultured neurons and in *Drosophila*, the mechanisms by which defective Rab7 leads to disease remain poorly understood.

Results: We used zebrafish to investigate the effects of CMT2b-associated Rab7 mutations in a vertebrate model. We generated transgenic animals expressing the CMT2b-associated mutant forms of Rab7 in sensory neurons, and show that these Rab7 variants cause neurodevelopmental defects, including defects in sensory axon growth, branching and pathfinding at early developmental stages. We also find reduced axon growth and branching in neurons expressing a constitutively active form of Rab7, suggesting these defects may be caused by Rab7 gain-of-function. Further, we use high-speed, high-resolution imaging of endosome transport in vivo and find that CMT2b-associated Rab7 variants cause reduced vesicle speeds, suggesting altered transport may underlie axon development defects.

Conclusions: Our data provide new insight into how disease-associated alterations in Rab7 protein disrupt cellular function in vertebrate sensory neurons. Moreover, our findings suggest that defects in axon development may be a previously unrecognized component of CMT2b disease.

Keywords: CMT2b, Axon guidance, Axon branching, Axon transport, Endosome trafficking, Rab7, Zebrafish, Neurodegeneration

Background

Charcot-Marie-Tooth2b (CMT2b) is an axonal form of peripheral neuropathy characterized by loss of sensation in multiple somatosensory modalities, motor abnormalities, and a very early disease onset in the second or third decade of life [1, 2]. CMT2b is an autosomal dominant disease, caused by five missense mutations in

the Rab7 gene (L129F, K157N, N161I, N161T, V162M) [3–6]. Rab7 is a small GTPase associated with late endosomal membrane compartments that has known roles in conversion of early endosomes to late endosomes, biogenesis of lysosomes, and maturation of autophagosomes [7, 8]. In addition, Rab7 has been shown to regulate retrograde trafficking, signaling and lysosomal degradation of neurotrophin receptors [7–11]. Like other GTPases, Rab7 cycles between a membrane-bound, active, GTP-bound form, and a cytosolic, inactive, GDP-bound form. CMT2b-associated amino acid substitutions occur in the proximity of the GTP-binding pocket and hydrolysis

* Correspondence: mchalloran@wisc.edu
[1]Department of Zoology, University of Wisconsin, 1117 West Johnson St., Madison, WI 53706, USA
[2]Department of Neuroscience, University of Wisconsin, 1111 Highland Ave, Madison, WI 53705, USA
Full list of author information is available at the end of the article

domains, and affect GDP and GTP exchange, increasing both Rab7 activation and hydrolysis-dependent inactivation, resulting in a form of Rab7 that is prone to remain in the active, GTP-bound form [12–14]. This finding, together with the dominant inheritance of the human disease, has led to the hypothesis that the disease is caused by overactivity of Rab7. However, several lines of evidence suggest the mutations do not cause simple gain of Rab7 function, but rather more complex alterations in function. Rab7 proteins containing the CMT2b-associated amino acid substitutions (hereafter referred to as CMT2b Rab7 mutants) show significantly lower affinity for both GDP and GTP [13], suggesting they could have reduced function. Indeed, when CMT2b Rab7 mutants are expressed in *Drosophila* photoreceptors, they are inefficiently recruited to endosomes, consistent with reduced function [15]. In contrast, although the CMT2b Rab7 mutants do cycle between membrane-associated and cytosolic states, they exhibit decreased ability to disassociate from the membrane, which leads to increased activity and augments interaction with several Rab7 effectors [14]. Moreover, the mutations do not interfere with the ability of Rab7 to bind its effector RILP and in some cases CMT2b Rab7 mutants are able to rescue Rab7 loss of function [12, 13, 15], which suggests retention of some wildtype function.

Several studies have investigated mechanisms by which the CMT2b mutations lead to disease by expressing CMT2b Rab7 mutants in cell lines or cultured neurons. CMT2b Rab7 mutants disrupted NGF signaling, NGF-induced neurite outgrowth, and trafficking of TrkA receptors in PC12 cells and DRG neurons [11, 16], suggesting that loss of neurotrophic support may contribute to CMT2B disease. In addition, expression of CMT2b Rab7 mutants in established DRG cultures caused neurite loss, indicating an axon degeneration effect [11]. Expression of CMT2b Rab7 mutants caused decreased neurite outgrowth in neuroblastoma cells, which could be reversed by treatment with valproic acid, an activator of extracellular signal-regulated kinase (ERK) and c-Jun terminal kinase (JNK) signaling pathways, both of the mitogen activated protein kinase (MAPK) superfamily [17, 18], suggesting this signaling pathway plays a role in the disease mechanism. Two recent studies expressed CMT2b Rab7 mutants in *Drosophila* to model the disease [15, 19]. One of these studies found that overexpression of CMT2b Rab7 mutants had no detectable effects on motor neuron or photoreceptor function, and suggested the CMT2b disease effects are due to partial loss of Rab7 function [15]. The second study showed that expression of the L129F CMT2b variant in *Drosophila* sensory neurons causes reduced pain and temperature sensation and is consistent with dominant effects of the mutant variants [19]. However, to date no vertebrate CMT2b models have

been developed for in vivo analysis of the long sensory axons analogous to those affected in human disease.

Analyses of the transport dynamics of vesicles containing the CMT2b Rab7 mutants have also given varied results. CMT2b Rab7 mutants caused increased transport rates of vesicles in DRG neurons, an effect that was mimicked by a constitutively active Rab7, Q67L (CA-Rab7) [11]. Expression of CMT2b Rab7 mutants in *Drosophila* sensory neurons did not alter endosome speed but did result in fewer stationary vesicles [19]. Overall, the diverse and sometimes contradictory findings from studies in different systems and cell types indicate that the CMT2b Rab7 mutants have complex effects on the cell biology of neurons, and highlight the need for additional models for analysis of disease mechanism.

We developed a vertebrate model of CMT2b by expressing CMT2b Rab7 mutants in zebrafish spinal sensory neurons in vivo. The zebrafish model provides a distinct advantage that cellular processes can be analyzed and imaged in vertebrate sensory axons within the intact, living animal. We demonstrate that CMT2b Rab7 mutants cause defects in axon growth, branching and pathfinding in developing sensory neurons. Some of these defects are phenocopied by expression of CA-Rab7, but not by dominant negative Rab7, T22N (DN-Rab7), consistent with a partial gain of function effect of the CMT2b mutants. We also use high speed imaging of vesicle dynamics in developing neurons in vivo and find that CMT2b Rab7 mutants cause reduced vesicle transport speeds, suggesting altered transport may underlie axon development defects. Our data suggest that defects in axon development may be a previously unrecognized component of CMT2b disease.

Results

Peripheral sensory neuron outgrowth and branching are reduced in CMT2b Rab7 mutant expressing neurons

To investigate the effects of CMT2b mutations in a vertebrate model, we used zebrafish Rohon-Beard (RB) spinal sensory neurons. Zebrafish Rab7 shares 97.6 % amino acid identity with the human Rab7 protein, including the amino acid residues that are affected in the human disease, L129F, K157N, N161T, and V162M [3–5] (Fig. 1a), which makes the zebrafish an excellent vertebrate organism in which to model this disease. Using single-site mutagenesis, we generated these CMT2b disease mutations in the zebrafish *rab7* cDNA and expressed these constructs in RB neurons under control of cis-regulatory elements from the *neurogenin1* gene [20] (*-3.1ngn:GFP-Rab7-cmt2b*). In humans CMT2b is autosomal dominant—the presence of only one copy of the mutated gene causes disease. Thus, we modeled the disease by expressing the CMT2b Rab7 mutants in a background containing wildtype Rab7.

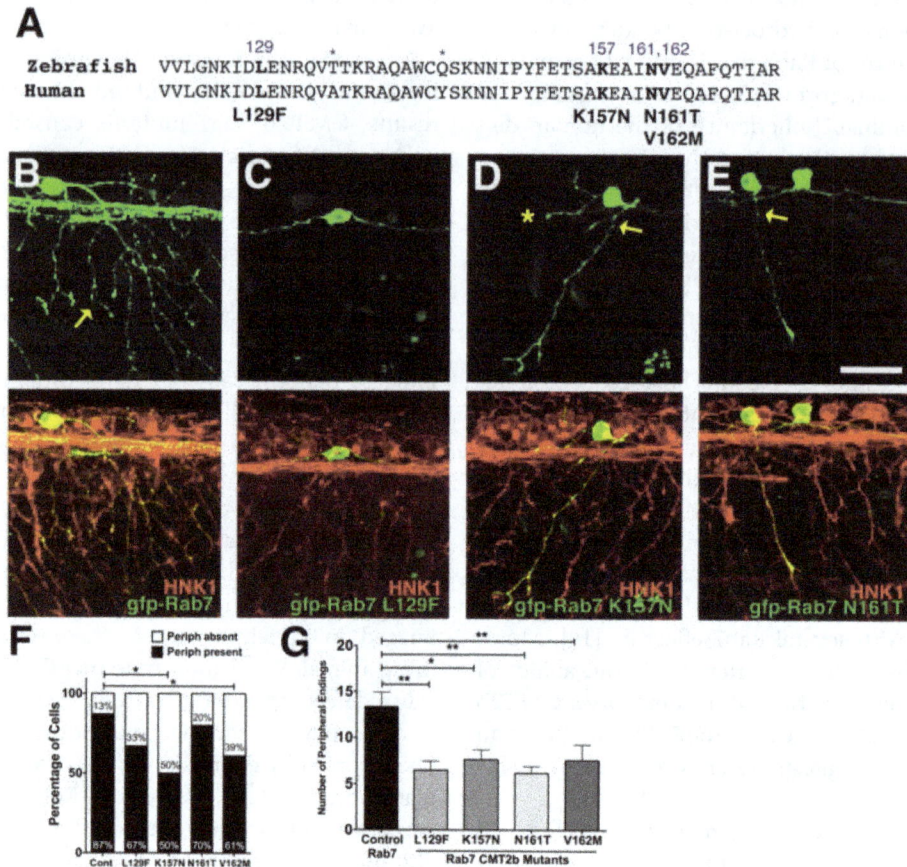

Fig. 1 Decreased peripheral axon branching in sensory neurons expressing CMT2b Rab7 mutants. **a** Comparison of zebrafish and human Rab7 protein sequence in the region of CMT2b mutations. Differences in amino acid sequence indicated by asterisks. Amino acid residues associated with CMT2b are bolded. **b-e** Confocal images of individual RB neurons expressing wildtype GFP-Rab7 (**b**) or CMT2b GFP-Rab7 mutants (**c**) in embryos with all RB neurons labeled with HNK-1 antibody (*red*). Anterior to the left. **b** wildtype Rab7 expressing cell shows wide arborization of peripheral axons (yellow arrow). **c** Lack of peripheral axon outgrowth in Rab7 L129F expressing cell. **d, e** Reduced peripheral branching (yellow arrow) in Rab7 K157N (D) and Rab7 N161T (E) expressing cells. Asterisk = missing central axon. **f** Quantification of number of neurons extending peripheral axons. Cont = wildtype Rab7: $n = 31$ cells in 19 embryos; Rab7 L129F: $n = 33$ cells in 24 embryos, $p = 0.08$; Rab7 K157N: $n = 10$ cells in 10 embryos, $*p = 0.03$; Rab7 N161T: $n = 15$ cells in 14 embryos, $p = 0.6$; Rab7 V162M: $n = 23$ cells in 18 embryos, $*p = 0.05$. Fisher's exact tests. **g** Quantification of peripheral branch endings in CMT2b-associated Rab7 mutations shows a significant decrease in branching. Wildtype Rab7: $n = 20$ cells in 15 embryos; Rab7 L129F: $n = 21$ cells in 18 embryos; Rab7 K157N: $n = 11$ cells in 7 embryos; Rab7 N161T: $n = 12$ cells in 10 embryos; Rab7 V162M: $n = 16$ cells in 14 embryos. $*p = 0.03$, $**p < 0.01$; Unpaired two-tailed t-test. Scale bar = 40 μm

We first expressed the constructs transiently by injecting DNA into 1-cell stage embryos, which results in mosaic labeling of individual sensory neurons, and analyzed the effects on neuronal morphology at 23 hpf, when RB axon arbors are developing. RB neurons have stereotyped morphology; they extend two central axons that ascend and descend ipsilaterally in the spinal cord, and one peripheral axon that extends to the skin where it branches extensively. We first analyzed outgrowth and branching of the peripheral RB axon. Neurons expressing wildtype Rab7 ($n = 31$ cells in 19 embryos) showed normal morphology (Fig. 1b), with most extending a peripheral axon by this stage. Only 13 % of these neurons failed to extend a peripheral axon, which is the same proportion we previously found for wildtype RB

neurons expressing only GFP (4 of 31 cells expressing wildtype Rab7, and 3 of 23 cells expressing GFP alone, failed to extend a peripheral axon, $p = 0.99$, Chi-Square test) [21]. This result suggests that overexpression of wildtype Rab7 in the neuron does not induce axon growth defects. In contrast, expression of CMT2b Rab7 mutants caused defects in outgrowth of the peripheral RB axons (Fig. 1c-f). Overall, 20–50 % of RB neurons expressing CMT2b Rab7 mutants failed to extend a peripheral axon. The effects of the four different mutant variants were variable, and only K157N and V162M showed statistically significant effects on peripheral axon outgrowth (Fig. 1f). In addition, the peripheral axons that did form showed decreased branching. We quantified axon branching by counting the number of peripheral axon endings and found a significant reduction in the number of branches in neurons expressing any of the four CMT2b Rab7 mutants (Fig. 1g). These results suggest that CMT2b Rab7 mutants influence both the ability of the peripheral axon to form and its capacity to extend secondary branches.

Constitutively Active (CA) Rab7 inhibits sensory peripheral axon outgrowth and branching

To ask whether the effect on RB peripheral axon growth and branching is caused by overactive Rab7 or partial loss of Rab7 function, we analyzed the effects of expressing the previously characterized DN-Rab7 (T22N) or CA-Rab7 (Q67L) [22]. We expressed these constructs under control of the -3.1ngn1 sensory neuron promoter. Like the CMT2b Rab7 mutants, expression of CA-Rab7 in wildtype embryos caused defects in RB peripheral axon outgrowth and branching. Significantly fewer RB neurons extended a peripheral axon compared to neurons expressing wildtype Rab7 (Fig. 2a-b, e). Further, the peripheral axons that did grow out had fewer branches (Fig. 2c, f-g). In contrast, DN-Rab7 expression had no significant effect on RB axon development (Fig. 2d, e-g). The similarity in phenotype caused by the CMT2b Rab7 mutants and the CA-Rab7 suggest that CMT2b mutant effects on sensory axon development are caused at least in part by Rab7 gain of function.

CMT2b-associated Rab7 mutants cause central axon guidance defects

We analyzed the RB central axon projections and found that expression of CMT2b Rab7 mutants also caused defects in central axon growth and guidance (Fig. 3). All neurons expressing wildtype Rab7 showed normal central axon growth and trajectories (Fig. 3a), as did all neurons expressing GFP alone analyzed previously [21]. In contrast, a significant percentage of neurons expressing L129F and K157N mutants were lacking a central axon (Fig. 3b, d). Further, we found that expression of the L129F Rab7 mutant caused errors in central axon guidance (Fig. 3c, e). In neurons expressing L129F Rab7, central axons left the dorsal longitudinal fascicle and either extended along the ventral spinal cord, or crossed the midline to join the contralateral fascicle. Misguided central axons were seen in sensory neurons expressing any of the four CMT2b Rab7 mutants, but only at significant numbers for L129F. Interestingly, we did not detect central axon defects in neurons expressing either CA-Rab7 or DN-Rab7 (n = 30 cells expressing CA-Rab7, n = 14 cells expressing DN-Rab7), suggesting this effect is a result of alteration in Rab7 function specifically caused by the disease-related mutation.

Sensory neurons expressing stable CMT2b Rab7 mutant transgenes exhibit central and peripheral axon defects

Transient mosaic expression of plasmid DNA constructs results in variable, and often very high protein expression levels in individual cells. To drive expression at consistent, moderate levels in all RB neurons and thereby more closely model the human disease, we generated stable transgenic lines expressing either GFP-Rab7, GFP-Rab7L129F or GFP-Rab7K157N under control of the -3.1ngn1 promoter, using the Tol2 transposase system, which typically results in integration of single copies of the transgene [23, 24]. We raised F1 carriers of the transgene and examined F2 offspring for expression of the constructs. We found that most or all RB neurons express the GFP-Rab7s and that GFP fluorescence levels appeared lower than in embryos transiently expressing plasmid DNA. We analyzed the whole RB population by labeling Tg(-3.1ngn1:GFP-Rab7-CMT2b) embryos with HNK1 antibody (Fig. 4a-c). We found that similar to cells transiently expressing CMT2b Rab7 mutants, RB neurons in transgenic 23 hpf embryos showed reduced peripheral axon branching compared to those expressing wildtype Rab7. To quantify branching in the population of RB cells, we counted the number of peripheral axon branches that cross the point of the horizontal myoseptum, and found a significant reduction in the embryos expressing the CMT2b Rab7 mutants (Fig. 4g). To analyze individual cell morphology in these embryos, we labeled cells mosaically by injecting -3.1ngn1:TagRFP-CAAX DNA into 1-cell stage transgenic embryos that express the CMT2b Rab7 mutants in all RB neurons. We quantified the number of peripheral axon endings in individually labeled RB neurons, and found a significant reduction in branching of neurons in both the L129F and K157N Rab7 mutant transgenics (Fig. 4h).

To ask whether the reduced branching is due to a failure to initiate peripheral axon branches versus decreased stability or maintenance of branches, we analyzed earlier developmental stages. We again mosaically labeled neurons by injecting -3.1ngn1:TagRFP-CAAX DNA into transgenic embryos that express the CMT2b Rab7 mutants in all RB neurons. We analyzed embryos between 18–21 hpf, stages when peripheral axons are initiating growth. We categorized individually labeled cells into 3 groups: no peripheral axon (example shown in Fig. 4i), a peripheral growth cone just beginning initiation (e.g. Fig. 4j), or a peripheral axon extended out of the spinal cord (e.g. Fig. 4k). We found no significant difference in peripheral axon initiation between wildtype, CMT2b L129F or CMT2b K157N embryos at either 18–19 hpf or 20–21 hpf (Fig. 4l, m). We further measured the number of peripheral branch endings in the cells that had extended peripheral axons, and found no decrease in initial branch formation in the CMT2b Rab7 mutant expressing

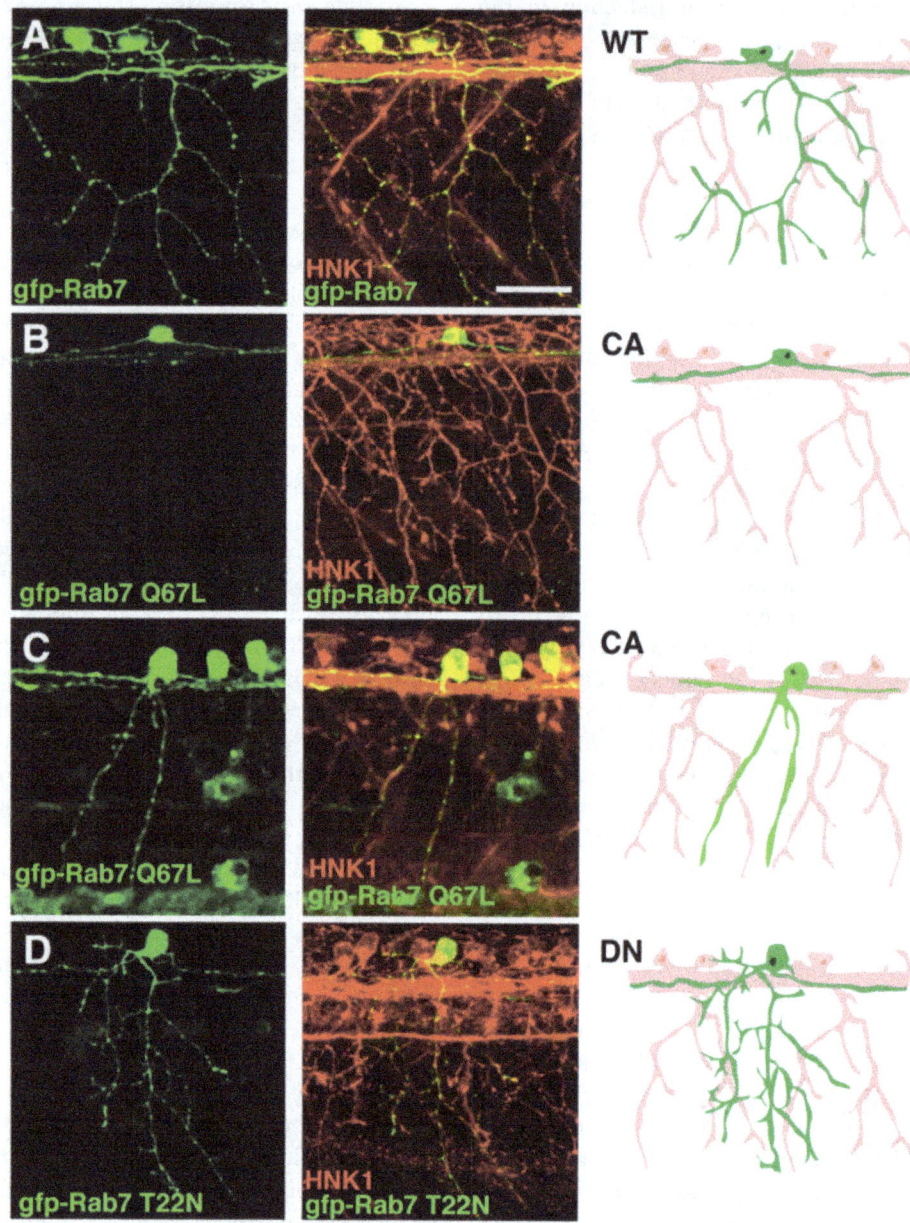

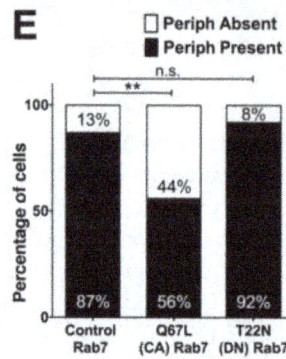

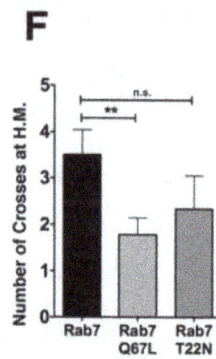

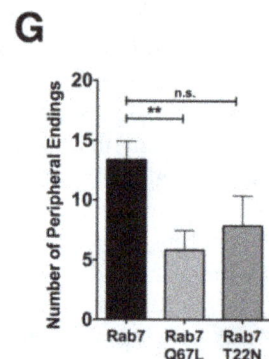

Fig 2 (See legend on next page.)

(See figure on previous page.)

Fig 2 Peripheral axon outgrowth and branching defects in CA-Rab7 expressing neurons. **a-c** Confocal projections of embryos with all RBs labeled with HNK-1 antibody (red) and individual RBs labeled with indicated Rab7 forms (green). Drawings at right highlight morphology of one neuron in green. **a** Individual RB neuron labeled with GFP-Rab7 showing central axons extending anteriorly and posteriorly from the cell body, and peripheral axon branching in the skin. **b** Lack of peripheral axon outgrowth in GFP-Rab7 Q67L (CA) expressing cell. **c** Reduced peripheral branching in GFP-Rab7 Q67L (CA) expressing cell. **d** Normal central outgrowth and peripheral branching in GFP-Rab7 T22N (DN) mutant expressing RB cell. **e** Expression of CA-Rab7, but not DN-Rab7, mutant construct increases percentage of RB neurons that do not extend a peripheral axon. $n = 31$ cells in Rab7 control, 30 cells in CA-Rab7, and 14 cells in DN-Rab7, **$p = 0.006$, Chi-Square test. **f** Number of peripheral axons that cross horizontal myoseptum (H.M.) is reduced in CA-Rab7 expressing cells. CA-Rab7: $n = 9$ cells; wildtype Rab7 control: $n = 12$ cells. **$p = 0.009$, paired t-test. **g** Number of peripheral axon endings in individually labeled neurons **$p = 0.005$, Unpaired two tailed t-test. Wildtype Rab7: 31 cells in 19 embryos; Rab7 Q67L: 30 cells in 15 embryos; Rab7 T22N: 14 cells in 9 embryos. All views anterior to the left. Scale bar = 40 μm

embryos, and in fact a statistically significant increase in the CMT2b K157N embryos (Fig. 4n). These data suggest the earliest stages of outgrowth and branching can occur normally in CMT2b Rab7 mutant expressing neurons, perhaps even to an accelerated degree, but these neurons fail to sustain further growth and branching.

In addition to peripheral axon branching defects, the L129F and K157M transgenic embryos also exhibited central axon guidance defects (Fig. 5), although only in significant numbers for L129F (Fig. 5d). Guidance defects included axons leaving the central axon fascicle (Fig. 5b), and central axons crossing the midline to join the contralateral central axon fascicle (Fig. 5c). Interestingly, some cells had two central axons that correctly entered the ipsilateral fascicle, with an extra axon that crossed the midline to join the contralateral fascicle of central axons. No guidance defects were found in wildtype Rab7 expressing neurons. Together, our data indicate that in addition to known neurodegenerative effects, the CMT2b Rab7 mutants also cause defects in sensory axon guidance and branch formation during development of the sensory circuitry.

CMT2b Rab7 transgenics do not show premature RB cell death

RB neurons normally undergo programmed cell death during larval stages, and their stage of death is regulated in part by neurotrophin signaling [25]. To ask whether the CMT2b Rab7 mutants influence RB cell survival, we analyzed RB cell number at 3 days post fertilization (dpf). We labeled RB cell bodies in 3 dpf embryos with anti-HuC/D, and counted the number of cell bodies in 5 segments beginning at the end of the yolk extension (Fig. 6a, b). We found no reduction in cell number in the CMT2b Rab7 transgenics, and instead found a slight increase in the CMT2b L129F embryos (Fig. 6c). These data suggest that the earlier axon growth defects do not directly inhibit cell survival at later stages.

CMT2b Rab7 mutants disrupt endosome dynamics in vivo

Previous studies of CMT2b Rab7 mutant effects on vesicle transport in cultured cells or in *Drosophila* neurons have given diverse results [11, 19]. To explore the effects of

CMT2b Rab7 mutants on endosome transport in vertebrate embryos, we performed high speed, high resolution in vivo imaging of vesicle movement using swept field confocal microscopy [26], as we have done previously [21]. We transiently expressed either wildtype GFP-Rab7 or the CMT2b Rab7 mutant constructs by DNA injection at the 1-cell stage, and imaged vesicles in neurons at 24 hpf (Fig. 7). To quantify axonal transport rates of labeled endosomes, we generated kymographs and performed several quantifications of endosome dynamics. Because the average speed of vesicle movement is not representative of dynamic, saltatory movement, we first calculated the speed of the fastest run during a 400 s imaging period. We observed a marked decrease in speed of K157N Rab7-containing vesicles (Fig. 7a-d, e). A previous study found that CMT2b L129F Rab7 mutant vesicles pause less often in *Drosophila* sensory neurons [19]. We also quantified the number of stationary versus moving vesicles, and found fewer stationary CMT2b Rab7 mutant containing vesicles, although this result was only significant for the N161T and V162M Rab7 variants (Fig. 7a-d, f). Finally, to ask if the CMT2b mutants affect vesicle directionality, we analyzed the direction of vesicle movement. We found no significant difference in the directionality of CMT2b mutant Rab7 vesicles (73 % of wildtype Rab7 vesicles moved retrogradely, $n = 98$ vesicles in 4 embryos; 83 % of L129F Rab7 vesicles moved retrogradely, $n = 35$ vesicles in 3 embryos, $p = 0.4$; 66 % of N161T Rab7 vesicles moved retrogradely, $n = 76$ vesicles in 7 embryos, $p = 0.3$; 66 % of V162M Rab7 vesicles moved retrogradely, $n = 38$ vesicles in 4 embryos, $p = 0.4$, Fischer's exact test).

Expression of CMT2b Rab7 mutants does not significantly enlarge vesicles in RB sensory neurons

Rab7 is involved in late endosome maturation and formation of lysosomes and autophagosomes [7, 8]. A previous study of cultured cells suggested that CMT2b Rab7 mutants may interfere with Rab7 function in vesicular trafficking and maturation by forming large, vacuolar-like structures, although this effect was seen in PC12 cells, but not in DRG cells [11]. To test the possibility that endosome size is affected by the CMT2b Rab7 mutants in neurons in vivo, we measured the volume of endosomes

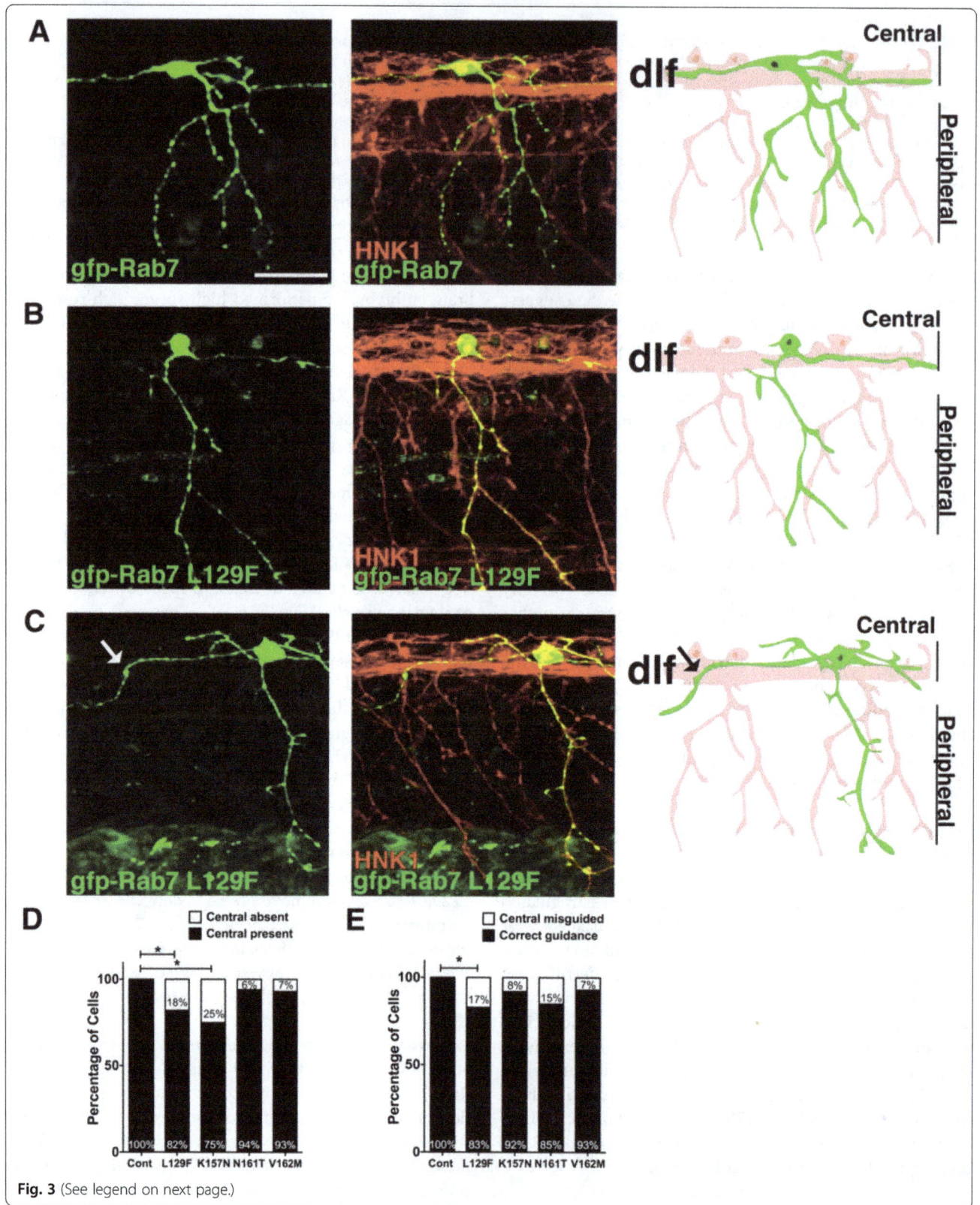

Fig. 3 (See legend on next page.)

Fig. 3 Central axon guidance errors in sensory axons expressing CMT2b Rab7 mutants. **a–c** Confocal projections (lateral views, anterior to the left) of embryos labeled with HNK-1 antibody (*red*) and individual RBs expressing GFP-Rab7 forms (*green*). Drawings at right highlight morphology of one neuron in green. **a** Wildtype GFP-Rab7 expressing neuron with two central axons traveling in the dorsal longitudinal fascicle (DLF), and with one peripheral axon branching in the skin. **b, c** RB neurons expressing GFP-Rab7 L129F show lack of outgrowth of ascending central axon (**b**) or central axon guidance errors (**c**). Central axon leaving DLF indicated by an arrow in (**c**). **d** Quantification of percentage of neurons lacking a central axon. Cont = wildtype Rab7: $n = 30$ cells in 15 embryos; Rab7 L129F: $n = 22$ cells in 20 embryos, *$p = 0.03$; Rab7 K157N: $n = 12$ cells in 8 embryos, *$p = 0.02$; Rab7 N161T: $n = 16$ cells in 11 embryos, $p = 0.3$; Rab7 V162M: $n = 14$ cells in 12 embryos, $p = 0.3$; Fisher's exact tests. **e** Quantification of percentage of cells with central axon guidance errors. Cont = wildtype Rab7: $n = 30$ cells in 15 embryos; Rab7 L129F: $n = 24$ cells in 19 embryos, *$p = 0.03$; Rab7 K157N: $n = 13$ cells in 9 embryos, $p = 0.3$; Rab7 N161T: $n = 13$ cells in 11 embryos, $p = 0.09$; Rab7 V162M: $n = 14$ cells in 12 embryos, $p = 0.3$. Scale bar = 40 μm

in central and peripheral axons and found no significant difference in the vesicular volume between wildtype Rab7 and the CMT2b Rab7 mutants (3.8 ± 0.5 μm³ in wildtype Rab7, $n = 85$ endosomes; 4.1 ± 0.5 μm³ in Rab7 L129F, $p = 0.1$, unpaired, two tailed, *t*-test, $n = 187$ endosomes; 7.0 ± 1.1 μm³ in Rab7 K157N, $p = 0.06$, unpaired, two-tailed *t*-test, $n = 84$ endosomes; 4.7 ± 0.9 μm³ in Rab7 V162M, $p = 0.07$, unpaired two-tailed *t*-test). These results are consistent with a previous finding that CMT2b Rab7 variants did not interfere with endosomal maturation when expressed in *Drosophila* [15].

Discussion

In this study we provide the first vertebrate model to investigate the mechanisms by which CMT2b disease associated mutations affect the cell biology of sensory neurons in vivo. We find that expression of CMT2b Rab7 mutants causes developmental defects in vertebrate sensory neurons, including reduced axon outgrowth, reduced axon branching, as well as axon guidance errors. Furthermore, we use live, high-speed, high-resolution imaging to show that CMT2b Rab7 mutants alter endosome transport during axon development in vivo. Overall, these results suggest there may be a developmental component of CMT2b, and that sensory circuits may not form properly in CMT2b disease.

CMT is an unusual form of a neurodegenerative neuropathy, in that it has an early manifestation during the second or third decade of life. Prior studies have suggested that neurodegeneration of long sensory axons are the primary pathological feature of the disease [2, 15, 27, 28], and have suggested that dysregulated neurotrophin trafficking is one of the main factors influencing early neurodegeneration [11, 16]. Our finding that axon development is affected is consistent with previous studies showing that expression of CMT2b Rab7 mutants can inhibit neurite outgrowth in PC12 and Neuro2A cells in culture [11, 18]. In contrast, recent studies of *Drosophila* sensory neurons showed normal size and complexity of dendritic arbors expressing human L129F Rab7 at larval stages [19], and apparently normal development of photoreceptor neurons [15], suggesting neuronal development was not affected in those models. These contrasting results could be due to

differences in the dependency on subcellular signaling processes between axons and dendrites, or between different cell types. For example, it is possible that photoreceptors are less dependent on neurotrophin signaling, and axons and dendrites likely exhibit differences in their dependencies on neurotrophin signaling. Our vertebrate sensory axon model may be a better representation of the long sensory axons affected in human disease. Developmental effects of CMT2b are perhaps not surprising, as neurotrophin signaling plays multiple important roles in axon growth and branching, as well as in neuronal survival [29–31]. Moreover, the ability to extend an axon during development could affect the neuron's ability to receive trophic support. However, we did not see increased RB cell death at 3 dpf, suggesting neurons are still receiving required trophic support. Our results showing that axons fail to maintain branches during development may partly explain the unusually early onset of CMT2b disease, although we do not know if these axon defects directly participate in later axon degeneration.

The effects we see on vesicle dynamics support the idea that disrupted endosomal transport is a component of the disease mechanism. CMT2b Rab7 mutant effects on transport have been reported in other studies, although there are some differences in findings. An in vitro study of DRG neurons showed that vesicles containing CMT2b Rab7 mutants move faster in the anterograde but not retrograde direction [11]. However, in *Drosophila*, the L129F CMT2b Rab7 mutant did not influence average vesicle speed, but did decrease time spent in the stationary phase [19]. We examined all four CMT2b Rab7 mutants, and found varying effects on vesicle dynamics among the individual mutants. We also saw a significant decrease in the number of stationary vesicles containing N161T Rab7 and V162M Rab7 mutants, but not in cells expressing the other CMT2b mutants. In contrast to the Zhang et al. 2013 [11] study, we found that K157N Rab7, but not the other CMT2b mutants, caused a decrease in vesicle speed. A potential explanation for these differing results may be methodological. We quantified the fastest run speed during a specified time period, whereas Zhang et al. quantified the average vesicle speed. However, there also are substantial differences between in vitro and in vivo

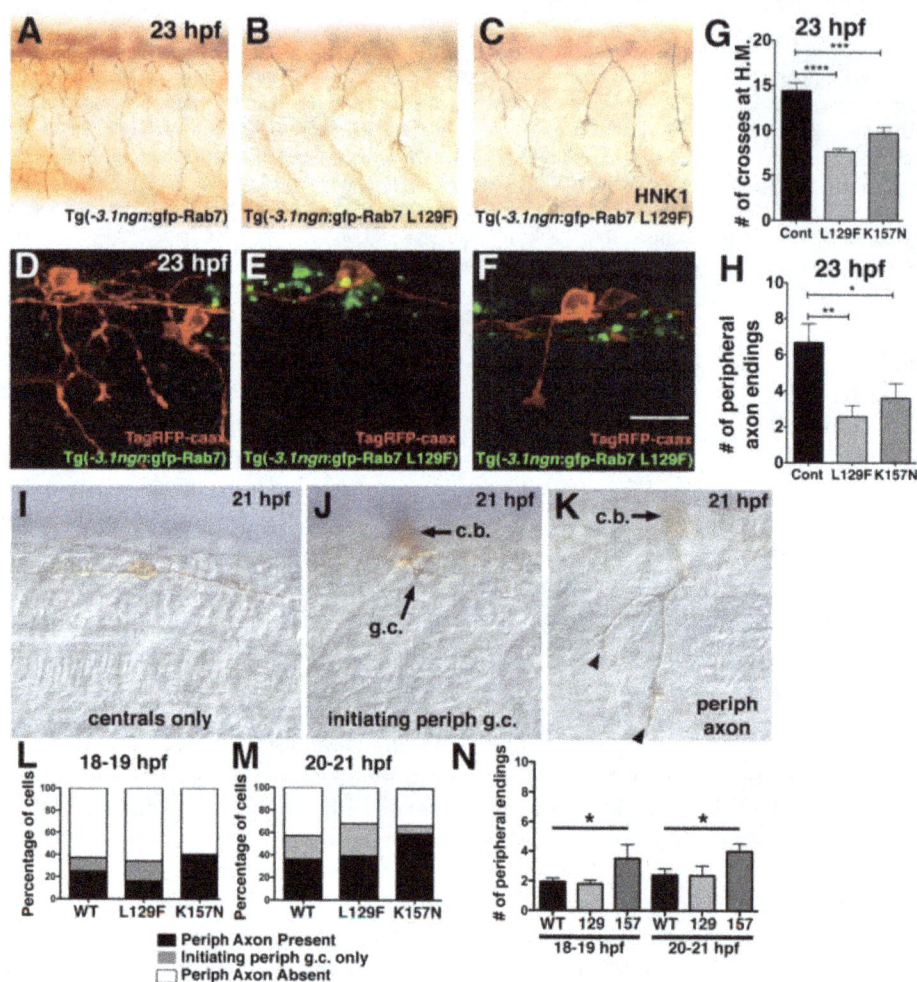

Fig. 4 Decreased peripheral axon branching in transgenics expressing CMT2b Rab7 mutants. **a-c** Lateral views (anterior to the left) of RB neurons labeled with HNK-1 antibody (*brown*) in 23 hpf transgenic embryos expressing wildtype GFP-Rab7 (**a**) or GFP-Rab7 L129F (**b-c**) in all RB neurons, showing decreased branching in Tg(GFP-Rab7L129F) embryos. **d-f** Mosaic labeling of single RB cells with TagRFP-caax membrane label (*red*) in 23 hpf transgenic embryos expressing wildtype GFP-Rab7 (**d**) or GFP-Rab7 L129F (**e, f**) in all RB neurons. **d** Red-labeled RB in wildtype GFP-Rab7 transgenic embryo with widely branched peripheral axon. **e** Red-labeled RB in GFP-Rab7 L129F transgenic embryo does not extend a peripheral axon. **c** Red-labeled RB in GFP-Rab7 L129F transgenic embryo extends a short peripheral axon that does not branch. Scale bar = 20 μm. **g** Quantification of peripheral branches crossing horizontal myoseptum in 23 hpf Tg(-3.1ngn:gfp-Rab7) control (Cont) embryos (n = 14 embryos), Tg(-3.1ngn:gfp-Rab7 L129F) embryos (L129F, n = 63 embryos), and Tg(-3.1ngn:gfp-Rab7 K157N) embryos (K157N, n = 20 embryos). ****$p < 0.0001$, ***$p = 0.0001$. Unpaired, two-tailed t-test. **h** Number of peripheral branch tip endings in 23 hpf Tg(-3.1ngn:gfp-Rab7) control (n = 9 cells in 6 embryos), Tg(-3.1ngn:gfp-Rab7 L129F) (n = 24 cells in 24 embryos), or Tg(-3.1ngn:gfp-Rab7 K157N) (n = 21 cells in 15 embryos) embryos is significantly reduced in embryos expressing CMT2b-associated Rab7 mutants. **$p = 0.002$, *$p = 0.04$. Unpaired, two-tailed t-test. **i-k** Lateral views of 21 hpf embryos injected with *ngn:TagRFP-caax* and labeled with anti-TagRFP antibody. **l**, Example of RB with central axons only and no peripheral axon. **j** Example of RB with a peripheral growth cone (g.c.) just initiating (*arrow*). Cell body (c.b.) is out of focus. **k**, Example of RB with short peripheral (with 2 endings, arrowheads) extended out of the spinal cord. Cell body (c.b.) is out of focus. **l-m** Quantification of percentage neurons with peripheral axons at 18–19 hpf (**l**) and 20–21 hpf (**m**). There are no significant differences between wildtype and CMT2b Rab7 mutants. At 18–19 hpf: wildtype n = 65 neurons, CMT2b L129F n = 61 neurons, CMT2b K157N n = 10 neurons, $p = 0.30$ Chi-Square test. At 20–21 hpf: wildtype n = 75 neurons, CMT2b L129F n = 28 neurons, CMT2b K157N n = 27 neurons, $p = 0.15$ Chi-Square test. **n**, Analysis of peripheral axon branch endings. At 18–19 hpf and 20–21 hpf, wildtype vs. CMT2b K157N, *$p = 0.03$ unpaired student's t-test

systems. Developing neurons in vivo are under the influence of the normal repertoire of extracellular signals and guidance cues, including neurotrophin signaling, which undoubtedly affect intracellular processes such as receptor trafficking. Overall, varied results also may be due to the differences in structural changes in the Rab7 proteins induced by individual CMT2b mutations. The L129F substitution does not map to the nucleotide binding pocket, but is predicted to disrupt the positioning of amino acids adjacent to the binding pocket, thus disrupting GTP-GDP cycling. The K157N and N161T substitutions are predicted to cause a regional loss of secondary

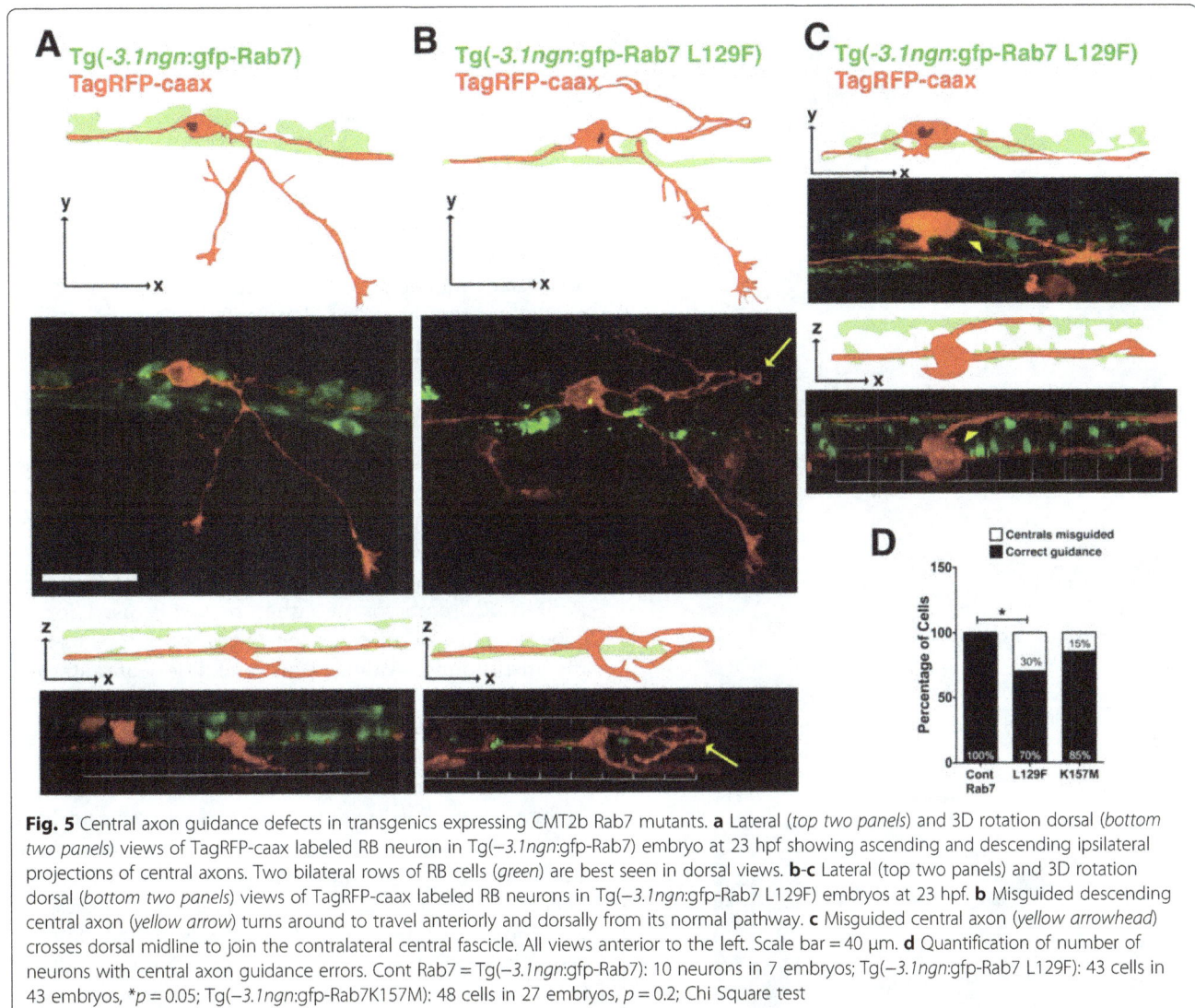

Fig. 5 Central axon guidance defects in transgenics expressing CMT2b Rab7 mutants. **a** Lateral (*top two panels*) and 3D rotation dorsal (*bottom two panels*) views of TagRFP-caax labeled RB neuron in Tg(−3.1ngn:gfp-Rab7) embryo at 23 hpf showing ascending and descending ipsilateral projections of central axons. Two bilateral rows of RB cells (*green*) are best seen in dorsal views. **b-c** Lateral (top two panels) and 3D rotation dorsal (*bottom two panels*) views of TagRFP-caax labeled RB neurons in Tg(−3.1ngn:gfp-Rab7 L129F) embryos at 23 hpf. **b** Misguided descending central axon (*yellow arrow*) turns around to travel anteriorly and dorsally from its normal pathway. **c** Misguided central axon (*yellow arrowhead*) crosses dorsal midline to join the contralateral central fascicle. All views anterior to the left. Scale bar = 40 μm. **d** Quantification of number of neurons with central axon guidance errors. Cont Rab7 = Tg(−3.1ngn:gfp-Rab7): 10 neurons in 7 embryos; Tg(−3.1ngn:gfp-Rab7 L129F): 43 cells in 43 embryos, *p = 0.05; Tg(−3.1ngn:gfp-Rab7K157M): 48 cells in 27 embryos, p = 0.2; Chi Square test

structure around the binding pocket [12, 13]. Thus, specific CMT2b Rab7 mutants may have variable effects on the ability of vesicles to engage with motors and transport along microtubules. Although differences exist in details of study results, it is apparent that CMT2b Rab7 mutants affect endosomal trafficking, potentially in diverse ways.

The question of whether the CMT2b-associated mutations lead to overactive Rab7 versus loss of Rab7 function has been under debate. It appears likely that a more complex alteration of function is involved. CMT2b Rab7 mutants hydrolyze GTP slower than wildtype Rab7 [12, 13], which has led to the hypothesis that disease effects are caused by overactive Rab7. Indeed several previous studies are also consistent with this hypothesis, as the effects they find can be mimicked with CA-Rab7 but not DN-Rab7 [11, 32–34]. The DN-Rab7 T22N variant interferes with GTP binding, and has dominant

negative effects on endosomal trafficking [35]. However, this construct does not have dominant effects in *Drosophila* neurons, suggesting it may not act as a dominant negative under all conditions [15]. CMT2b mutants have reduced binding to both GTP and GDP [12, 13], suggesting these forms may have reduced Rab7 function. In support of this idea, a recent *Drosophila* study showed that CMT2b variants of Rab7 did not have dominant effects and that loss of one *rab7* allele caused defects in photoreceptor synaptic function [15]. These authors conclude that CMT2b disease is in fact caused by reduced Rab7 function. Our results showing decreased peripheral axon branching in both CA-Rab7 and CMT2b Rab7 mutant expressing neurons are consistent with a model in which overactivity of Rab7 contributes to these defects. Interestingly, we found that some aspects of the phenotype caused by CMT2b Rab7 mutant expression in our system, notably, the axon guidance defects, were

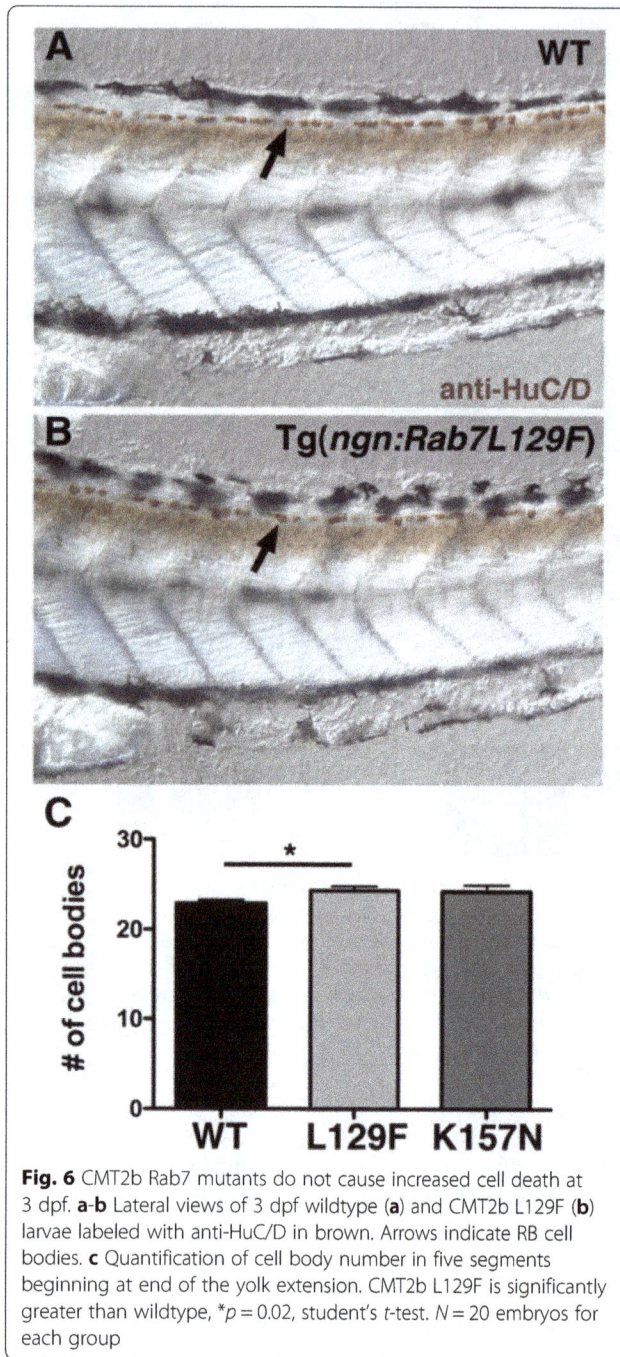

Fig. 6 CMT2b Rab7 mutants do not cause increased cell death at 3 dpf. **a-b** Lateral views of 3 dpf wildtype (**a**) and CMT2b L129F (**b**) larvae labeled with anti-HuC/D in brown. Arrows indicate RB cell bodies. **c** Quantification of cell body number in five segments beginning at end of the yolk extension. CMT2b L129F is significantly greater than wildtype, *$p = 0.02$, student's *t*-test. N = 20 embryos for each group

of multiple in vivo models will be important for unraveling the mechanisms of this complex disease.

Conclusions

In this study, we develop the first vertebrate model to investigate the effects of CMT2b-associated alterations in Rab7 protein on long projection sensory neurons, which are the cells most profoundly affected in human disease. We show previously unrecognized effects of CMT2b-associated mutations on early axon development. These results suggest axon developmental defects may be a component of human CMT2b disease.

Methods
Animals

Adult zebrafish (*Danio rerio*) were kept in a 14/10 h light/dark cycle. Embryos were maintained at 28.5 °C and staged as hours post-fertilization (hpf) as described [36]. Wild type AB strain or transgenic Tg(–3.1ngn1:GFP-Rab7), Tg(–3.1ngn1:GFP-Rab7L129F), Tg(–3.1ngn1:GFP-Rab7K157N) embryos of either sex were used for all experiments. All animal procedures were approved by the Institutional Animal Care and Use Committee at the University of Wisconsin (Animal Welfare Assurance Number A3368-01).

Immunohistochemistry

Embryos were fixed overnight in 4 % paraformaldehyde and labeled with monoclonal anti-HNK1 antibody (ZN-12, 1:250; Zebrafish International Resource Center, Eugene, OR), anti-HuC/D (1:500, Life Technologies), or with mouse or rabbit anti-GFP antibody (1:1000; Invitrogen, Carlsbad, CA) and rabbit anti-TagRFP antibody (1:500, Evitrogen). Antibody detection was performed with a Vectastain IgG ABC detection kit (Vector Laboratories, Burlingame, CA), or for fluorescent labeling, with Alexa-Fluor488 and AlexaFluor568-conjugated secondary anti-mouse or anti-rabbit antibodies (4 µg/mL; Invitrogen, Carlsbad, CA).

Site-directed mutagenesis

The following primers were used to perform PCR-mediated single-site mutagenesis to generate Rab7 L129F, Rab7 K157N, Rab7 N161T, Rab7 V162M, respectively (mutated codon bolded):

(F) 5'-ccttcaagacactggacag**ttc**gagggatgagtttctgatccagg-3'
(R) 5'-cctggatcagaaactcatc**cct**cgaactgtccagtgtcttgaagg-3';
(F) 5'-gagaccagtgcaa**aac**gaggccatcaacgtag-3'
(R) 5'-ctacgttgatggcctc**gtt**tgcactggtctc-3';
(F) 5'-gcaaaggaggccatc**acc**gtagagcaggcattcc-3'
(R) 5'-ggaatgcctgctctac**ggt**gatggcctcctttgc-3':
(F) 5'-ggaggccatcaac**atg**gagcaggcattccag-3'
(R) 5'-ctggaatgcctgctc**cat**gttgatggcctcc-3'

not phenocopied by either CA-Rab7 or DN-Rab7. This result, together with the diversity of findings from all studies of CMT2b mutants, suggests the CMT2b Rab7 mutant proteins affect multiple cellular processes in distinct ways. The specific effects are likely highly context-dependent, and may vary among cell types and processes (e.g. axon growth or neuronal degeneration) depending on how reliant these processes are on particular signals such as neurotrophin signaling. Continued study

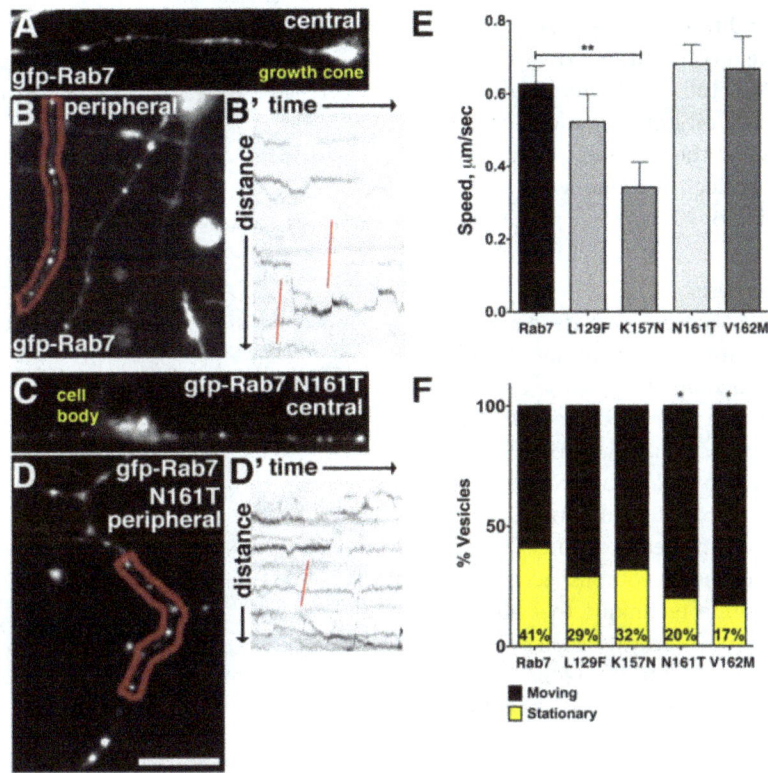

Fig. 7 In vivo imaging of CMT2b Rab7 mutant containing vesicles reveals changes in endosome dynamics. **a-b** Confocal images of neurons with GFP-Rab7 labeled endosomes in central (**a**) and peripheral (**b**) axons. **b'** Kymograph of peripheral RB axon in red region in (**b**). Red lines indicate rapid retrograde vesicle runs. **c-d** Confocal images of neurons with GFP-Rab7 N161T expressing endosomes in central (**c**) and peripheral (**d**) axons. **d'** Kymograph of peripheral axon in red region in (**d**). Red line indicates rapid retrograde vesicle runs. **e** Speeds of vesicles containing Rab7 K157 mutants were significantly reduced in central and peripheral axons. *******p* = 0.009, Unpaired, two-tailed *t*-test. Wildtype Rab7 control: *n* = 97 vesicles in 8 cells in 6 embryos; Rab7 L129F: *n* = 37 vesicles in 6 cells in 4 embryos; Rab7 K157N: *n* = 24 vesicles in 3 cells in 2 embryos; Rab7 N161T *n* = 73 vesicles in 8 cells in 6 embryos; Rab7 V162M *n* = 33 vesicles in 5 cells in 3 embryos. **f** Decreased percentage of stationary vesicles in central and peripheral axons expressing Rab7 N161T and V162M mutants. *p = 0.01, Fisher's exact test. Wildtype Rab7 control: *n* = 39 vesicles in 8 cells in 6 embryos; Rab7 L129F: *n* = 86 vesicles in 6 cells in 4 embryos; Rab7 K157N: *n* = 37 vesicles in 3 cells in 2 embryos; Rab7 N161T *n* = 137 vesicles in 8 cells in 6 embryos; Rab7 V162M *n* = 60 vesicles in 5 cells in 3 embryos

Following PCR-directed mutagenesis, Rab7 constructs were digested with Dpn1 (New England Biolabs) and sequenced.

DNA constructs and injection

DNA expression constructs were made using Multisite Gateway Cloning System (Invitrogen, Carlsbad, CA) into Tol2 vectors [24]. Rab7, Rab7 T22N (DN) and Rab7 Q67L (CA) constructs in Gateway pDONR vectors [22] were obtained from Brian Link (Medical College of Wisconsin), linked with N-terminal GFP, and cloned behind a cis-regulatory element of the *neurogenin1* gene (*-3.1ngn1*) [20] to drive expression in RB neurons as described previously [37]. To mosaically label RB cells, 11 pg of *-3.1ngn1:TagRFP-CAAX* [37], or 25 pg *-3.1ngn1:GFP-Rab7*, *-3.1ngn1:GFP-Rab7L129F*, *-3.1ngn1:GFP-Rab7 K157N*, *-3.1ngn1:GFP-Rab7N161T*, or *-3.1ngn1:GFP-V162M* DNA was injected into one-cell stage embryos.

For transgenesis, AB wildtype embryos at the one-cell stage were co-injected with 25 pg Tol2 transposase mRNA along with 50 pg of either *-3.1ngn1:GFP-Rab7*, *-3.1ngn1:GFP-Rab7L129F* or *-3.1ngn1:GFP-Rab7K157N* DNA. Injected founder embryos were screened for fluorescence and GFP-positive progeny were raised to adulthood.

Brightfield and fluorescent fixed sample imaging

Brightfield images were captured on a Nikon (Tokyo, Japan) TE300 inverted microscope with a Spot RT camera (Diagnostic Instruments, Sterling Heights, MI). Fluorescent images of fixed embryos were captured with an Olympus (Tokyo, Japan) FV1000 laser-scanning confocal microscope with a 40x (UPlan FLN air, NA 0.75) objective.

Time lapse imaging

For live confocal imaging, embryos were anesthetized in 0.02 % tricaine and mounted in 1 % low melting agarose in 10 mM HEPES E3 medium as described [38]. Live high speed imaging of endosomal trafficking was performed on a Bruker Opterra swept field confocal microscope (Bruker Nano Surfaces FM, Middleton, WI) equipped with a Nikon CFI Plan Apo VC 60x oil immersion objective (NA 1.40). Embryos were 23 hpf at the beginning of the experiment, and 1–20 1-μm optical sections were captured every 2 s for a total duration of 400 s.

Quantification and data analysis

Fluorescent images and movies were processed and quantified with Volocity Software (Perkin Elmer, Waltham, MA). For axon growth/branching analysis, the only measurement done in embryos that had all RB neurons labeled with HNK-1 antibody was the counts of axon branches crossing the horizontal myoseptum. Axon crosses over the horizontal myoseptum were counted in somites 8–13 of 23 hpf embryos. All other axon measurements were done on individually labeled neurons (accomplished by mosaic expression of a fluorophore), a technique that allows the entire neuron morphology to be clearly visualized without obstruction from labeled neighboring axons. Neurons were defined as lacking a peripheral axon when the cell body and central axons were visible but no peripheral axon was present. The number of peripheral axon endings were also calculated from individually labeled neurons when the entire arbor including tips of peripheral branches were visible. Axon tips were manually counted from captured images or by examination through the microscope. Axon guidance errors were defined as axons that deviate from the stereotyped pathway and extend into abnormal locations. For cell body number analysis, RB cell bodies labeled with anti-HuC/D were manually counted in a region spanning 5 somite segments, beginning at the end of the yolk extension.

Endosomal trafficking movies were built in Volocity, and corrected for drift in ImageJ [39]. Endosomal speeds were measured in Volocity from kymographs made in ImageJ. Speeds were measured during the fastest run per vesicle in a 400 s imaging period. To determine endosomal direction, we measured the net direction of each individual punctum over 400 s, and categorized vesicle movement as either anterograde (away from the cell body), retrograde (toward the cell body), or no net movement.

All statistical analyses were done using Prism 5.0 (GraphPad Software, Inc.). Errors are reported as standard error of the mean (SEM).

Abbreviations

CA: constitutively active; CMT2b: Charcot-Marie-Tooth 2b; DN: dominant negative; RB: Rohon-Beard.

Competing interests

The authors declare they have no competing interests.

Authors' contributions

OYP conceived of the study, participated in study design, carried out the experiments and data analysis, and co-wrote the manuscript. KWE developed and provided imaging and analytical tools, and helped edit the manuscript. MCH contributed to study conception, experimental design and data interpretation, and co-wrote the manuscript. All authors read and approved the manuscript.

Acknowledgements

This work was supported by National Institutes of Health Grants R56NS086934, R01NS086934, and R01NS042228 to M.C.H., NRSA F31NS074606 to O.Y.P., and R44MH065724 to K.W.E. We thank Julie Last for assistance with swept field confocal microscopy, Jimmy Fong of Bruker Technologies for swept field confocal technical assistance, Brian Link for Rab constructs, Marc Wolman for HuC/D antibody, Aiden Sperry, Jacob Lee and Jacob Miller for technical assistance. We are grateful to Kelsey Baubie, Kassie Ford and Christina Lindop for fish care.

Author details

[1]Department of Zoology, University of Wisconsin, 1117 West Johnson St., Madison, WI 53706, USA. [2]Department of Neuroscience, University of Wisconsin, 1111 Highland Ave, Madison, WI 53705, USA. [3]Neuroscience Training Program, University of Wisconsin, 1111 Highland Ave, Madison, WI 53705, USA. [4]Medical Scientist Training Program, University of Wisconsin, 750 Highland Ave, Madison, WI 53705, USA. [5]Laboratory for Optical and Computational Instrumentation, University of Wisconsin, 1675 Observatory Dr, Madison, WI 53706, USA.

References

1. Barisic N, Claeys KG, Sirotkovic-Skerlev M, Lofgren A, Nelis E, De Jonghe P, et al. Charcot-Marie-Tooth disease: a clinico-genetic confrontation. Ann Hum Genet. 2008;72(Pt 3):416–41. doi:10.1111/j.1469-1809.2007.00412.x.
2. Rotthier A, Baets J, De Vriendt E, Jacobs A, Auer-Grumbach M, Levy N, et al. Genes for hereditary sensory and autonomic neuropathies: a genotype-phenotype correlation. Brain. 2009;132(Pt 10):2699–711. doi:10.1093/brain/awp198.
3. Meggouh F, Bienfait HM, Weterman MA, de Visser M, Baas F. Charcot-Marie-Tooth disease due to a de novo mutation of the RAB7 gene. Neurology. 2006;67(8):1476–8. doi:10.1212/01.wnl.0000240068.21499.f5.
4. Verhoeven K, De Jonghe P, Coen K, Verpoorten N, Auer-Grumbach M, Kwon JM, et al. Mutations in the small GTP-ase late endosomal protein RAB7 cause Charcot-Marie-Tooth type 2B neuropathy. Am J Hum Genet. 2003;72(3):722–7. doi:10.1086/367847.
5. Houlden H, King RH, Muddle JR, Warner TT, Reilly MM, Orrell RW, et al. A novel RAB7 mutation associated with ulcero-mutilating neuropathy. Ann Neurol. 2004;56(4):586–90. doi:10.1002/ana.20281.
6. Wang X, Han C, Liu W, Wang P, Zhang X. A Novel RAB7 Mutation in a Chinese Family with Charcot-Marie-Tooth type 2B disease. Gene. 2013. doi:10.1016/j.gene.2013.10.023.
7. Bucci C, Thomsen P, Nicoziani P, McCarthy J, van Deurs B. Rab7: a key to lysosome biogenesis. Mol Biol Cell. 2000;11(2):467–80.
8. Hyttinen JM, Niittykoski M, Salminen A, Kaarniranta K. Maturation of autophagosomes and endosomes: a key role for Rab7. Biochim Biophys Acta. 2013;1833(3):503–10. doi:10.1016/j.bbamcr.2012.11.018.
9. Saxena S, Bucci C, Weis J, Kruttgen A. The small GTPase Rab7 controls the endosomal trafficking and neuritogenic signaling of the nerve growth factor receptor TrkA. J Neurosci. 2005;25(47):10930–40. doi:10.1523/JNEUROSCI.2029-05.2005.
10. Deinhardt K, Salinas S, Verastegui C, Watson R, Worth D, Hanrahan S, et al. Rab5 and Rab7 control endocytic sorting along the axonal retrograde transport pathway. Neuron. 2006;52(2):293–305. doi:10.1016/j.neuron.2006.08.018.
11. Zhang K, Fishel Ben Kenan R, Osakada Y, Xu W, Sinit RS, Chen L, et al. Defective axonal transport of Rab7 GTPase results in dysregulated trophic signaling. J Neurosci. 2013;33(17):7451–62. doi:10.1523/JNEUROSCI.4322-12.2013.
12. De Luca A, Progida C, Spinosa MR, Alifano P, Bucci C. Characterization of the Rab7K157N mutant protein associated with Charcot-Marie-Tooth type 2B. Biochem Biophys Res Commun. 2008;372(2):283–7. doi:10.1016/j.bbrc.2008.05.060.

13. Spinosa MR, Progida C, De Luca A, Colucci AM, Alifano P, Bucci C. Functional characterization of Rab7 mutant proteins associated with Charcot-Marie-Tooth type 2B disease. J Neurosci. 2008;28(7):1640–8. doi:10.1523/JNEUROSCI.3677-07.200828/7/1640.

14. McCray BA, Skordalakes E, Taylor JP. Disease mutations in Rab7 result in unregulated nucleotide exchange and inappropriate activation. Hum Mol Genet. 2010;19(6):1033–47. doi:10.1093/hmg/ddp567.

15. Cherry S, Jin EJ, Ozel MN, Lu Z, Agi E, Wang D, et al. Charcot-Marie-Tooth 2B mutations in rab7 cause dosage-dependent neurodegeneration due to partial loss of function. Elife. 2013;2:e01064. doi:10.7554/eLife.010642/0/e01064.

16. BasuRay S, Mukherjee S, Romero E, Wilson MC, Wandinger-Ness A. Rab7 mutants associated with Charcot-Marie-Tooth disease exhibit enhanced NGF-stimulated signaling. PLoS One. 2010;5(12):e15351. doi:10.1371/journal.pone.0015351.

17. Yamauchi J, Torii T, Kusakawa S, Sanbe A, Nakamura K, Takashima S, et al. The mood stabilizer valproic acid improves defective neurite formation caused by Charcot-Marie-Tooth disease-associated mutant Rab7 through the JNK signaling pathway. J Neurosci Res. 2010;88(14):3189–97. doi:10.1002/jnr.22460.

18. Cogli L, Progida C, Lecci R, Bramato R, Kruttgen A, Bucci C. CMT2B-associated Rab7 mutants inhibit neurite outgrowth. Acta Neuropathol. 2010;120(4):491–501. doi:10.1007/s00401-010-0696-8.

19. Janssens K, Goethals S, Atkinson D, Ermanoska B, Fransen E, Jordanova A, et al. Human Rab7 mutation mimics features of Charcot-Marie-Tooth neuropathy type 2B in Drosophila. Neurobiol Dis. 2014;65:211–9. doi:10.1016/j.nbd.2014.01.021.

20. Blader P, Plessy C, Strahle U. Multiple regulatory elements with spatially and temporally distinct activities control neurogenin1 expression in primary neurons of the zebrafish embryo. Mech Dev. 2003;120(2):211–8.

21. Ponomareva OY, Holmen IC, Sperry AJ, Eliceiri KW, Halloran MC. Calsyntenin-1 regulates axon branching and endosomal trafficking during sensory neuron development in vivo. J Neurosci. 2014;34(28):9235–48. doi:10.1523/JNEUROSCI.0561-14.201434/28/9235.

22. Clark BS, Winter M, Cohen AR, Link BA. Generation of Rab-based transgenic lines for in vivo studies of endosome biology in zebrafish. Dev Dyn. 2011;240(11):2452–65. doi:10.1002/dvdy.22758.

23. Kawakami K. Tol2: a versatile gene transfer vector in vertebrates. Genome Biol. 2007;8 Suppl 1:S7. doi:10.1186/gb-2007-8-s1-s7.

24. Kwan KM, Fujimoto E, Grabher C, Mangum BD, Hardy ME, Campbell DS, et al. The Tol2kit: a multisite gateway-based construction kit for Tol2 transposon transgenesis constructs. Dev Dyn. 2007;236(11):3088–99. doi:10.1002/dvdy.21343.

25. Williams JA, Barrios A, Gatchalian C, Rubin L, Wilson SW, Holder N. Programmed cell death in zebrafish rohon beard neurons is influenced by TrkC1/NT-3 signaling. Dev Biol. 2000;226(2):220–30. doi:10.1006/dbio.2000.9860.

26. Castellano-Munoz M, Peng AW, Salles FT, Ricci AJ. Swept field laser confocal microscopy for enhanced spatial and temporal resolution in live-cell imaging. Microsc Microanal. 2012;18(4):753–60. doi:10.1017/S1431927612000542.

27. Gemignani F, Marbini A. Charcot-Marie-Tooth disease (CMT): distinctive phenotypic and genotypic features in CMT type 2. J Neurol Sci. 2001;184(1):1–9.

28. Auer-Grumbach M, De Jonghe P, Wagner K, Verhoeven K, Hartung HP, Timmerman V. Phenotype-genotype correlations in a CMT2B family with refined 3q13-q22 locus. Neurology. 2000;55(10):1552–7.

29. Ascano M, Bodmer D, Kuruvilla R. Endocytic trafficking of neurotrophins in neural development. Trends Cell Biol. 2012;22(5):266–73. doi:10.1016/j.tcb.2012.02.005.

30. Aguayo AJ, Clarke DB, Jelsma TN, Kittlerova P, Friedman HC, Bray GM. Effects of neurotrophins on the survival and regrowth of injured retinal neurons. Ciba Found Symp. 1996;196:135–44. discussion 44–8.

31. Gallo G, Letourneau PC. Regulation of growth cone actin filaments by guidance cues. J Neurobiol. 2004;58(1):92–102. doi:10.1002/neu.10282.

32. Taub N, Teis D, Ebner HL, Hess MW, Huber LA. Late endosomal traffic of the epidermal growth factor receptor ensures spatial and temporal fidelity of mitogen-activated protein kinase signaling. Mol Biol Cell. 2007;18(12):4698–710. doi:10.1091/mbc.E07-02-0098.

33. BasuRay S, Mukherjee S, Romero EG, Seaman MN, Wandinger-Ness A. Rab7 mutants associated with Charcot-Marie-Tooth disease cause delayed growth factor receptor transport and altered endosomal and nuclear signaling. J Biol Chem. 2013;288(2):1135–49. doi:10.1074/jbc.M112.417766.

34. Cogli L, Progida C, Thomas CL, Spencer-Dene B, Donno C, Schiavo G, et al. Charcot-Marie-Tooth type 2B disease-causing RAB7A mutant proteins show altered interaction with the neuronal intermediate filament peripherin. Acta Neuropathol. 2013;125(2):257–72. doi:10.1007/s00401-012-1063-8.

35. Feng Y, Press B, Wandinger-Ness A. Rab 7: an important regulator of late endocytic membrane traffic. J Cell Biol. 1995;131(6 Pt 1):1435–52.

36. Kimmel CB, Ballard WW, Kimmel SR, Ullmann B, Schilling TF. Stages of embryonic development of the zebrafish. Dev Dyn. 1995;203(3):253–310.

37. Andersen E, Asuri N, Halloran M. In vivo imaging of cell behaviors and F-actin reveals LIM-HD transcription factor regulation of peripheral versus central sensory axon development. Neural Dev. 2011;6:27.

38. Andersen E, Asuri N, Clay M, Halloran M. Live imaging of cell motility and actin cytoskeleton of individual neurons and neural crest cells in zebrafish embryos. J Vis Exp. 2010;36. http://www.jove.com/video/1726/live-imaging-cell-motility-actinactincytoskeleton-individual-neurons. doi:10.3791/1726.

39. Schneider CA, Rasband WS, Eliceiri KW. NIH Image to ImageJ: 25 years of image analysis. Nat Methods. 2012;9(7):671–5.

12

Genomic analysis of transcriptional networks directing progression of cell states during MGE development

Magnus Sandberg[1]* (ID), Leila Taher[2], Jianxin Hu[3,6], Brian L. Black[3], Alex S. Nord[4,5] and John L. R. Rubenstein[1]*

Abstract

Background: Homeodomain (HD) transcription factor (TF) NKX2–1 critical for the regional specification of the medial ganglionic eminence (MGE) as well as promoting the GABAergic and cholinergic neuron fates via the induction of TFs such as LHX6 and LHX8. NKX2–1 defines MGE regional identity in large part through transcriptional repression, while specification and maturation of GABAergic and cholinergic fates is mediated in part by transcriptional activation via TFs such as LHX6 and LHX8. Here we analyze the signaling and TF pathways, downstream of NKX2–1, required for GABAergic and cholinergic neuron fate maturation.

Methods: Differential ChIP-seq analysis was used to identify regulatory elements (REs) where chromatin state was sensitive to change in the *Nkx2-1*cKO MGE at embryonic day (E) 13.5. TF motifs in the REs were identified using RSAT. CRISPR-mediated genome editing was used to generate enhancer knockouts. Differential gene expression in these knockouts was analyzed through RT-qPCR and in situ hybridization. Functional analysis of motifs within *hs623* was analyzed via site directed mutagenesis and reporter assays in primary MGE cultures.

Results: We identified 4782 activating REs (aREs) and 6391 repressing REs (rREs) in the *Nkx2-1* conditional knockout (*Nkx2-1*cKO) MGE. aREs are associated with basic-Helix-Loop-Helix (bHLH) TFs. Deletion of *hs623*, an intragenic *Tcf12* aRE, caused a reduction of *Tcf12* expression in the sub-ventricular zone (SVZ) and mantle zone (MZ) of the MGE. Mutation of LHX, SOX and octamers, within *hs623*, caused a reduction of *hs623* activity in MGE primary cultures.

Conclusions: *Tcf12* expression in the SVZ of the MGE is mediated through aRE *hs623*. The activity of *hs623* is dependent on LHX6, SOX and octamers. Thus, maintaining the expression of *Tcf12* in the SVZ involves on TF pathways parallel and genetically downstream of NKX2–1.

Keywords: TCF12, SOX, OCT, LHX, MEIS, Medial ganglionic eminence, CRISPR engineering, Transcriptional network, Neurogenesis

Background

Transcription factors (TFs) direct cell fate determination and differentiation through binding to a genomic network consisting of regulatory elements (REs) such as promoters and enhancers. By analyzing epigenetic modifications and transcriptional changes in TF knockouts, we have started to uncover the genomic networks and molecular mechanisms that direct brain development [1]. In-depth understanding of the genetically encoded wiring of the brain is important as perturbation of transcription pathways is implicated in disorders such as autism and intellectual disability [2]. Distantly acting REs have been identified based on conservation and activity [3, 4]. Their spatial activity and dynamic genomic contacts can be predicted using a combination of TF binding profiling, genome-wide 3D chromosome organization mapping and CRISPR/Cas9 editing [5–10].

Mouse genetic experiments have elucidated the functions of many TFs in the development of the subpallial telencephalon [11, 12]. These studies show that the HD protein NKX2–1 is required for regional specification of the MGE by repressing alternative identities, as well as

---
* Correspondence: bmagnussandberg@gmail.com; john.rubenstein@ucsf.edu
[1]Department of Psychiatry, UCSF Weill Institute for Neurosciences, University of California, San Francisco, San Francisco, CA 94143, USA
Full list of author information is available at the end of the article

promoting GABAergic and cholinergic cell fates via the induction of TFs such as LHX6 and LHX8 [13–17]. By integrating genomic data with mouse genetics, we confirmed the repressive function of NKX2–1, however its role in transcriptional activation remains unclear. Moreover, additional data suggests that genes genetically downstream of NKX2–1, such as LHX6 and LHX8, are responsible for the loss of gene expression observed in the $Nkx2–1$cKO [18, 19]. Altogether, the genetic program and molecular mechanisms responsible for promoting GABAergic and cholinergic neuron phenotypes, downstream of NKX2–1 remains largely unexplored.

To investigate the signaling pathways of MGE development downstream of NKX2–1, we extended our earlier analysis of the genomic network directing MGE development that is altered in the $Nkx2–1$ mutant. First we evaluated all loci that showed an epigenetic change, independent of NKX2–1 binding. Via an epigenomic analysis of the NKX2–1 mutant MGE we characterized a large set REs that are implicated in mediating transcriptional repression and activation. Using a combination of genomics, de novo *motif* analysis, CRISPR engineering and primary culture assays we characterize REs and TFs central to patterning of the subpallial telencephalon and promoting MGE characteristics. Gene ontology (GO) analysis showed an enriched association of REs activating transcription (aREs) with E-box binding basic-Helix-Loop-Helix (bHLH) TFs. Using CRISPR engineering we deleted $hs623$, an intronic aRE of the $Tcf12$ gene which encodes a bHLH TF. Deletion of $hs623$ reduced $Tcf12$ expression in the MGE. De novo motif analysis combined with TF motif mutations, showed that OCT/POU and SOX motifs are required for $hs623$'s ability to promote transcription in the MGE.

Methods

Mice
The $Nkx2–1$cKO was earlier described in Sandberg et al. 2016 [18] and generated using mice strains previously reported: $Nkx2–1f/f$ [20], $Olig2-tva$-Cre [21] and $AI14$ Cre-reporter [22]. All experiments with animals complied with federal and institutional guidelines and were reviewed and approved by the UCSF Institutional Animal Care and Use Committee.

Generation of $hs623$ deletion
The $hs623^{Tm1}$ allele was generated by CRISPR-mediated genome editing, using established methods [23]. Guide RNAs sgRNA-$hs623$–1, 5′-GTTTAGTTTTGCTCATAC CA(TGG)-3′ and sgRNA-$hs623$–2, 5′-ATGGTTTCT GTGATCGTAAT(TGG)-3′ (protospacer-adjacent motif [PAM] sequence indicated in parentheses) were transcribed in vitro using the MEGAshortscript T7 kit (Life Technologies, AM1354) and subsequently purified using

the MEGAclear kit (Life Technologies, AM1908). The two guide RNAs were designed to delete a 737 bp intronic region within $Tcf12$ [mm9; chr9:71822812–71823548]. The purified sgRNAs were co-injected into the cytoplasm of fertilized mouse oocytes with in vitro transcribed Cas9 mRNA using standard transgenic procedures as previously described [24]. F0 transgenic founders were identified by PCR screening using $hs623$-KO-F, 5′-GTCATTGTTGCTGTTGGCCT -3′ and $hs623$-KO-R, 5′- CCACCTCACACTAGATTAAGATACA -3′ to identify the $hs623$ null alleles (KO = 250 bp, WT = 1008 bp) and $hs623$-WT-F, 5′-GTGGCTGATGATGTGCTCTGA -3′ and $hs623$-WT-R, 5′-CTCCATCAGGTTCTTGCCC C-3′ to identify the $hs623$-WT allele (462 bp). Four independent F0 founders were each outcrossed to wild type mice, and F1 offspring were used for subsequent $hs623^{Tm1}$ intercrosses to generate $hs623$-null mice. The hs623 mutant strain (CD1-$Tcf12^{em1Jlr}$/Mmucd) is available at MMRC (www.mmrrc.org/) with the number RRID: MMR RC_044027-UCD.

Histology
Immunofluorescence was performed on 16 μm cryosection as previously described [25]. In situ hybridization was performed as previously described [26]. The following primers were used generate the templates used for the in situ probes: Tcf12_F, TCTCGAATGGAAGA CCGC; Tcf12_R, CTCCCTCCTGCCAGGTTT.

Dissection of embryos
RT-qPCR and primary culture experiments were performed on E13.5 micro-dissected MGE. All MGE dissections were performed as follows; the dorsal boundary was defined by the sulcus separating lateral ganglionic eminence (LGE) and MGE. The caudal end of the sulcus defined the caudal boundary. Septum was removed.

Gene expression analysis in $hs623$KO
To assay differential gene expression in the $hs623$KO RNA was purified using RNEasy Mini (Qiagen) and cDNA was generated using Superscript III® First-Strand Synthesis System for RT-PCR (Invitrogen). RT-qPCR analysis was performed on a 7900HT Fast Real-Time PCR System (Applied Biosystems) using SYBR GreenER qPCR SuperMix (Invitrogen, Cat. No. 11760–100). Unpaired t-test was used to test significance in gene expression between $hs623$WT and $hs623$KO using SDHA as internal control [27, 28].

Sequences of RT-qPCR primers used:

SDHA-F, GCTCCTGCCTCTGTGGTTGA
SDHA-R, AGCAACACCGATGAGCCTG
Mns1_ctrl_1F, CTGCTGCTCCGGAAGACG
Mns1_ctrl_1R, TTTTGGTCGCCATCTCGGTT

Myzap_ctrl_2F, TCGAAAGGAAAGATCAGCCTCC
Myzap_ctrl_2R, TCTGATCTTCGCACCACACC
Zfp280d_ctrl_1F, CCCCAGCTCTCATTCAAGAGG
Zfp280d_ctrl_1R, TTCAGGCAGCGTTGACTTGT
TCF12_v1/2-F2, GCTTGTCCCCAACACCTTTC
TCF12_v1/2-R2, TGACAGCCTGAGAGTCCAGA
TCF12_v1/3-F4, TACCAGTCAGTGGCCCAGAG
TCF12_v1/3-R4, AATGCTCGTGAAGTTGCTGC
TCF12_v1/3-F5, TCCCTGGAATGGGCAACAAT
TCF12_v1/3-R5, TCACGGTTGAAATCGTCAGA

Site-directed mutagenesis of TF binding motifs in *hs623*

To study the requirement TF motifs for *hs623* activity LHX6, SOX and octamers were mutated in pCR-Blunt II-TOPO, sequence verified and sub-cloned into a pGL4.23-Luciferase reporter with a minimal β-globin-promoter using BglII and XhoI [18]. Following primers were used to generate the different *hs623* luciferase reporters:

hs623-mut-site#1-R, cgttgctgacaaggctgtttttacagaaattg atgctgagttc
hs623-mut-site#1-F, agccttgtcagcaacgtgattattcaaac
hs623-mut-site#2-F, gatgtgctctgatatgaaaaaagtcattaggt agaatgaatag
hs623-mut-site#3-F, gatgtgctctgatatgtaattagaaaaaaggtag aatgaatag
hs623-mut-site#2 and 3-F, gatgtgctctgatatgaaaaaagaaaa aaggtagaatgaatag
hs623-mut-site#2 and/or 3-R, atatcagagcacatcatcagcca cattc
hs623-mut-site#4-F, gattattcaaacaactctttttttttgttaatgagg
hs623-mut-site#4-R, gagttgtttgaataatcacgttgctgac
hs623-mut-site#5-F, ctcatgcaaatgaaaaagaggccttatttgc
hs623-mut-site#5-R, atttgcatgagttgtttgaataatc
hs623-mut-site#4 and 5-F, caaacaactctttttttttgaaaaaga ggccttatttgc
hs623-mut-site#4 and 5-R, use "*hs623*-mut-site#4-R" for PCR
hs623-mut-site#6-F, gttaatgaggccttaaaaaaatatttattttttcc
hs623-mut-site#6-R, ggcctcattaacatttgcatgagttgtttg
hs623-mut-site#4 and 6-F, caactctttttttttgttaatgaggcctta aaaaaatatttattttttcc
hs623-mut-site#4 and 6-R, cattaacaaaaaaaagagttgtttgaa taatcac
hs623-mut-site#4,5 and 6-F, caactctttttttttgaaaaagaggcc ttaaaaaaatatttattttttcc
hs623-mut-site#4, 5 and 6-R, ggcctcttttttcaaaaaaaaga gttgtttgaataatc
hs623-mut-site#7-F, gcaacgtgattattcccccccctcatgcaaatg
hs623-mut-site#7-R, gaataatcacgttgctgacaagg
hs623-mut-site#4 and 7-F, gtgattattcccccccctcttttttttt gttaatgagg
hs623-mut-site#4 and 7-R, use *hs623*-mut-site#7-R

Analysis of *hs623* activity in MGE primary MGE cultures

MGE tissue was dissected from E13.5 embryos, triturated and plated onto 24-well plates (1 embryo/2wells). Primary cultures were transfected with a total of 500 ng DNA using Lipofectamin 2000 (Thermo Fisher) and cultured in Neurobasal Medium (Thermo Fisher) supplemented with 0.5% Glucose, GlutaMAX (Thermo Fisher Scientific) and B27 (Thermo Fisher Scientific). Luciferase assays were performed 48 h after transfection using Dual Luciferase Reporter Assay System (Promega). Unpaired t-test was used to test significance between the variants of *hs623*.

ChIP-Seq computational analysis

Differential ChIP-seq analysis was performed as described in Sandberg et al. 2016 [18]. After differential H3K4me1, H3K27ac and H3K27me3 analysis we merged overlapping sites. Only merged sites that were enriched in H3K4me1 relative to the input datasets and for which the difference in enrichment between *Nkx2–1* WT and cKO was not significant (for at least one of the sites among the merged sites) were further considered. Of those, merged sites overlapping with blacklisted genomic regions (http://mitra.stanford.edu/kundaje/akundaje/release/black-lists/mm9-mouse/mm9-blacklist.bed.gz) and RepeatMasker annotation (http://hgdownload.cse.ucsc.edu/goldenPath/mm9/database/chr*_rmsk.txt.gz) as well as those exceeding 5000 bp were excluded. We defined aREs based on the following two criteria; 1) more H3K27ac (WT) and no increase in H3K27me3 (WT), H3K27ac (*Nkx2–1*cKO) and H3K4me1 (*Nkx2–1*cKO), 2) more H3K27me3 (*Nkx2–1*cKO) and no increase in H3K27ac (*Nkx2–1*cKO), H3K4me1 (*Nkx2–1*cKO) and H3K27me3 (WT). We defined rREs based on the following two criteria; 1) more H3K27ac (*Nkx2–1*cKO) and no increase in H3K27me3 (*Nkx2–1*cKO), H3K27ac (WT) and H3K4me1 (WT), 2) more H3K27me3 (*WT*) and no increase in H3K27ac (WT), H3K4me1 (*WT*) and H3K27me3 (*Nkx2–1*cKO).

In vivo analysis of aREs and rREs

To assess the in vivo activity of aREs and rREs we used the data published in the VISTA Enhancer Browser (https://enhancer.lbl.gov/) [7]. All aREs and rREs, overlapping with regions tested in the VISTA Enhancer Browser were scored based on their in vivo activity in cortex, MGE and LGE. For the MGE active elements, we also scored their activity in the ventricular zone (VZ), SVZ and MZ.

De novo motif analysis

Motif analysis was performed using RSAT [29], identifying overrepresentation and positional bias of words (6 to 7 nucleotides) in the aREs and rREs using an automated Markov model adapted after the analyzed sequence length. Differential analysis of aREs (rREs as control sequence) and rREs (aREs as control sequence) was also performed to identify overrepresented words in the peak sequence.

Results

Identification of the genomic regulatory network directing MGE identity

We have previously shown that the combined binding of NKX2–1 and LHX6 is a predictive indicator of REs that mediate transcriptional activation in the subventricular (SVZ) and mantle zone (MZ) of the MGE in the developing subpallial telencephalon [18]. There is evidence that NKX2–1 generally acts as a repressor in MGE progenitors (in the ventricular zone [VZ]), whereas LHX6, and potentially other TFs and signaling pathways, some of which are genetically downstream of NKX2–1, are important for activating transcription in the SVZ and MZ of the MGE [18, 30]. By studying aREs, we aimed to further explore the molecular mechanisms underlying the transcriptional network directing differentiation of the secondary progenitors in the SVZ. One important difference between this study and our earlier study [18] is that here we look at all aREs and rREs, independent of NKX2–1 binding.

First we identified aREs and rREs by assessing the genome-wide changes of the two histone marks H3K27ac and H3K27me3 at H3K4me1 positive REs comparing the WT and Nkx2–1cKO MGE [18]. We defined aREs based on the following two criteria; 1) reduced H3K27ac and, 2) increased H3K27me3 in the Nkx2–1cKO. We defined rREs based on the following two criteria; 1) increased H3K27ac and, 2) reduced H3K27me3 in the Nkx2–1cKO (see Methods).

Based on these criteria we identified 4782 aREs and 6391 rREs in the Nkx2–1cKO. See Additional file 1 for a complete list of aREs and rREs. To analyze the in vivo activity patterns of the aREs and rREs we examined transgenic enhancer activity patterns of E11.5 forebrain enhancer activity patterns available in the VISTA database (see VISTA data base; https://enhancer.lbl.gov/) [7]. The activities of rREs were highest in cortex (62% [13 of 21]) and LGE and dorsal MGE (52% [11 of 21]) and lowest in the ventral MGE (24% [5 of 21])(Fig. 1a and b [hs848, hs1172 and hs1187]). In contrast, aREs have the highest activities in the MGE (53% [17 of 32]) when compared to their activities in the LGE (50% [16 of 32]) and cortex (41% [13 of 32]) (Fig. 1a and b [hs676, hs957 and hs1041]). We also found a higher activity of MGE positive aREs in the SVZ (71% [12 of 17]) and MZ (94% [16 of 17]) compared to the VZ (18% [3 of 17]), consistent with our previous results for NKX2–1 bound aREs and rREs (Fig. 1b and c) [18]. See Additional file 1 for a full list of aREs and rREs VISTA transgenics.

To identify TFs motifs enriched in the aRE and rREs we performed a de novo motif discovery using RSAT [29]. This analysis showed a number of motifs enriched in both aREs and rREs such as SOX motifs, homeodomain binding motifs (HOX and POU6f2) and motifs recognized by zinc finger TFs (e.g. SP1 and ZNF384) (Fig. 1d and e). Additional analysis identifying motifs differentially enriched between aREs and rREs showed that aREs have a high frequency of E-boxes (Fig. 1e). Interestingly, we found that rREs are enriched in motifs consistent with the binding site of the TF MEIS2 (Fig. 1d). The Meis2 gene is repressed by NKX2–1, and in turn, its RNA is strongly up-regulated in the MGE of the Nkx2–1cKO [18]. These data suggest that Meis2 is central to activating a genomic network promoting LGE and caudal ganglionic eminence (CGE) characters (through rREs) in the Nkx2–1cKO MGE.

We then examined enrichment of annotation terms among the aREs and rREs candidate target genes using GREAT [31]. Top-ranked GO terms for rREs target genes were associated with WNT signaling (beta-catenin binding and PDZ domain binding), transcriptional regulation (such as RNA polymerase II transcription co-activator activity), and enhancer sequence-specific DNA binding (Fig. 1f). Looking specifically at the associated genes for the rREs containing MEIS2 binding motifs we found several genes (Isl1, Ebf1, Tle4, Zfp503, Efnb1 and Efnb2) with higher expression in the LGE and CGE than the MGE. These findings support the hypothesis that MEIS2 directs LGE and CGE identities. The top-ranked GO terms for aREs target genes were associated with phosphatase activity, E-box binding proteins, L-glutamate transmembrane transporter activity and transmembrane-ephrin receptor activity [31] (Fig. 1f). Two E-box binding TFs, Tcf4 and Tcf12, which are in the region of a large number of aREs, have reduced MGE SVZ and MZ expression in the Nkx2–1cKO [18]. In combination with the high frequency of E-boxes in aREs, our data suggests that Tcf4 and Tcf12 are components of the genomic network regulating gene expression in secondary progenitors of the MGE that are genetically downstream of NKX2–1.

In vivo characterization of hs623 in the MGE of the forebrain

To learn more about the Tcf12 expression and the transcriptional pathways integrated in the aRE network downstream of NKX2–1, we examined aRE hs623, a highly evolutionarily conserved 914 base pair (bp) sequence that is in an intron of the Tcf12 locus (Fig. 2a and b). A previous transgenic study show that hs623 drives LacZ expression at E11.5 [32]. The hs623 transgene is active in the forebrain, hindbrain and the spinal cord (Fig. 2c-e, Additional file 2). A coronal section

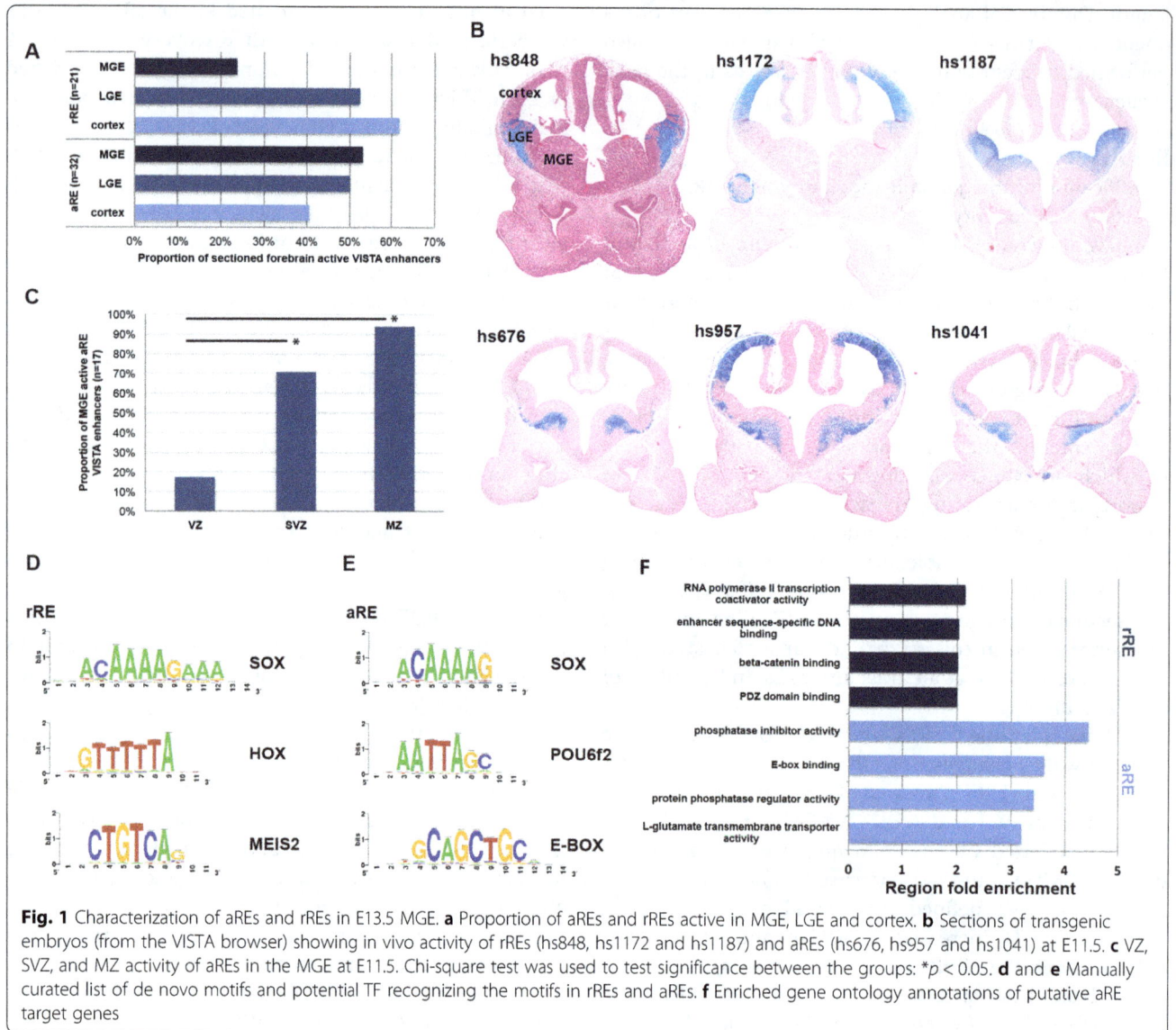

Fig. 1 Characterization of aREs and rREs in E13.5 MGE. **a** Proportion of aREs and rREs active in MGE, LGE and cortex. **b** Sections of transgenic embryos (from the VISTA browser) showing in vivo activity of rREs (hs848, hs1172 and hs1187) and aREs (hs676, hs957 and hs1041) at E11.5. **c** VZ, SVZ, and MZ activity of aREs in the MGE at E11.5. Chi-square test was used to test significance between the groups: *$p < 0.05$. **d** and **e** Manually curated list of de novo motifs and potential TF recognizing the motifs in rREs and aREs. **f** Enriched gene ontology annotations of putative aRE target genes

through the telencephalon shows that *hs623* activity is restricted to the SVZ and MZ of the MGE, and perhaps labels cell tangentially migrating into the LGE (Fig. 2e). This pattern of activity is supported by histone ChIP-seq analysis of the MGE showing that this locus has histone modifications that are characteristic of active enhancer elements (Fig. 2a [H3K4me1+ and H3K27ac+] and 2B). Of note, ChIP-seq analysis of the MGE *Nkx2–1*cKO shows reduced H3K27ac, providing evidence that the activity of the locus is dependent on the activity of the NKX2–1 and/or its target TFs, as reported earlier (Fig. 2b) [18].

Motif logic direct region specific transcriptional activity
Hs623 is flanked by two highly conserved regions and the activity of one of the regions (*hs357)* has been tested in vivo [32]. Similar to *hs623*, *hs357* is active in the

spinal cord, but unlike *hs623* it is active in the pretectum and it lacks activity in the telencephalon, including the MGE (Fig. 2f and g). Therefore, despite the close proximity of *hs623* and *hs357*, they show differences in regional activity, suggesting that their regional activities are more likely due to differences in their primary nucleic acid sequence rather then their genomic location. Consistent with the lack of MGE activity, *hs357* has two NKX2–1 consensus motifs and no LHX6 consensus motifs (Fig. 2b). On the other hand, *hs623* has four LHX6 consensus motifs, which could explain its activity in the MGE (Fig. 2h). Even though *hs623* has NKX2–1 binding, it contains no NKX2–1 consensus motifs. However, the sequences flanking *hs623* do include three NKX2–1 consensus motifs, two within *hs357* (Fig. 2b). In agreement with these observations, we detect NKX2–1 binding covering a wide region that incudes both *hs623* and *hs357*.

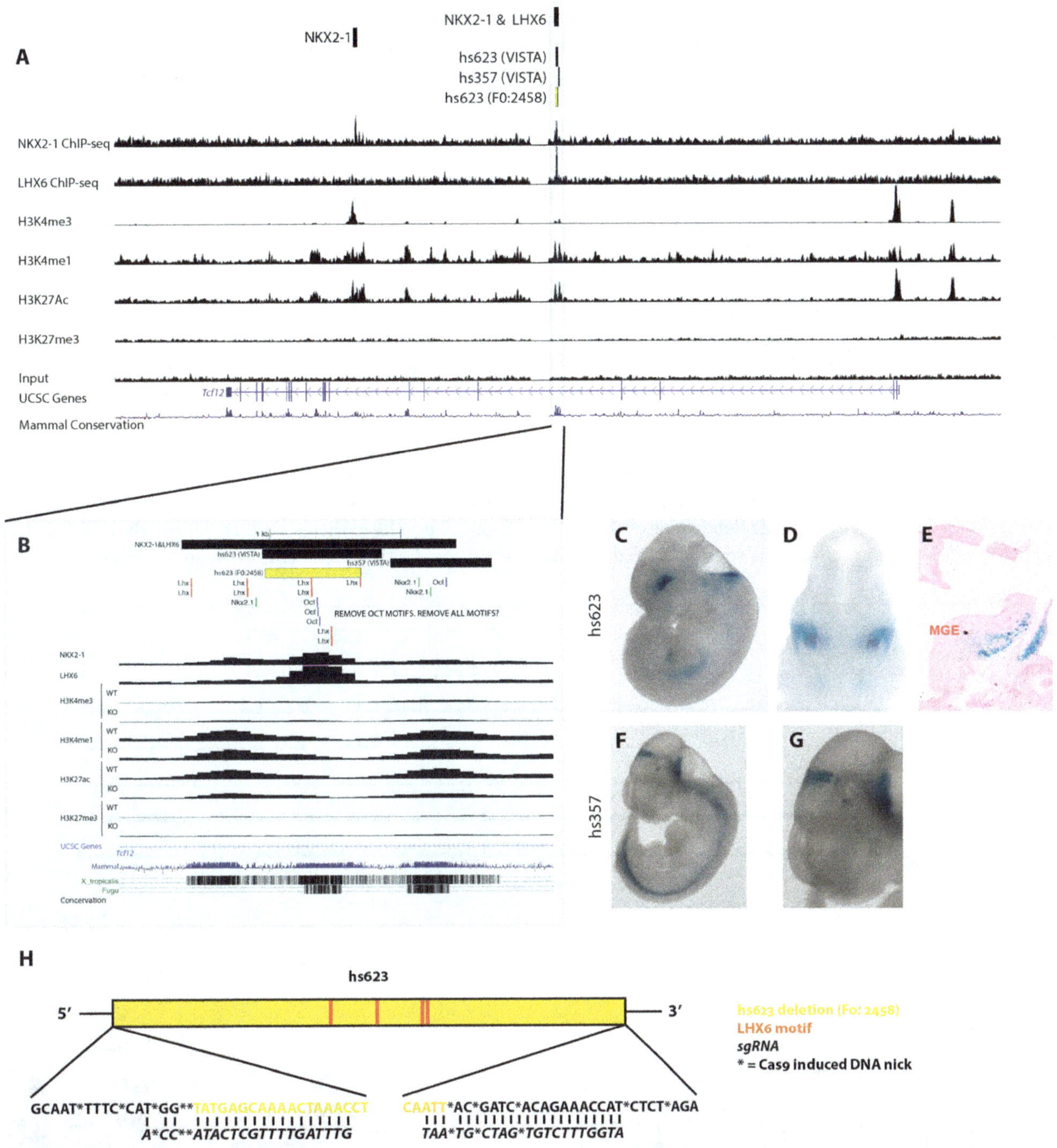

Fig. 2 Deletion of *cis*-regulatory element *hs623* in vivo. **a** Genomic region of the *Tcf12* locus with the ChIP-seq datasets and genomic features shown; NKX2-1 ChIP-seq, LHX6 ChIP-seq, H3K4me3, H3K4me1, H3K27ac, H3K27me3, UCSC genes and mammalian conservation. Histone 3 modifications in MGE at E13.5. *Hs623* region framed and highlighted in blue. **b** Higher resolution view of the *hs623* region with the same ChIP-seq datasets as in Fig. 2a. Called NKX2-1 & LHX6 binding region, VISTA regions, deleted *hs623* region (yellow) and NKX2-1, LHX6 and OCT consensus motifs labeled at the top of the browser. **c-g** VISTA database transgenic embryos showing in vivo activity of *hs623* and *hs357* at E11.5. **h** Schematic description of the generated *hs623* deletions (5 founders). The distribution of LHX6 consensus motifs in *hs623* are indicated. Founder 2458 was used for the analysis presented in this paper

CRISPR/Cas9 mediated deletion of *hs623* in vivo

To functionally test the requirement of *hs623* in vivo, we deleted *hs623* using CRISPR/Cas9 (see VISTA database; http://enhancer.lbl.gov). A pair of sgRNAs was designed to delete the 734 bp core sequence of *hs623*, which has NKX2−1 and LHX6 binding (Fig. 2b and h).

Microinjection of sgRNAs and Cas9 generated a total of 22 pups. 23% (5 of 22) of the pups carried the desired *hs623* deletions and the induced DNA breaks were distributed within 20 bp of the predicted cutting site (5′ and 3′ of *hs623*, Fig. 2h, Additional file 3). To minimize potential off target effects we outcrossed the F0 transgenic founders to wild-type CD1 mice. Four of five founders were fertile and generated a F1 generation; these animals were intercrossed to generate homozygous F2 *hs623KO* animals. *Hs623KOs* in the F2 generation were produced at Mendelian Ratios showing that the enhancer deletion was viable (10[WT]:19[HET]:7[KO], $n = 3$ litters; $\chi^2 = 0.611$; df $= 2$; $p = 0.7367$). Due to the overall similarity of the four fertile founders we decided to focus the following analysis on one of the founders (F0: 2458, Fig. 2h).

Deletion of *hs623* reduces *Tcf12* mRNA levels in the SVZ of MGE

Hs623 is a *Tcf12* intragenic RE that in transgenic assays activates transcription in the SVZ of the MGE (Fig. 2c-e). As noted above, its activity is partly dependent on NKX2–1 activity and *Tcf12* transcription is specifically reduced in

the SVZ of the MGE in the *Nkx2–1cKO* (Fig. 2b) [18]. Together, these data suggest that *hs623* could be a RE activating *Tcf12* transcription in the MGE. To test this hypothesis, we performed RTqPCR on the MGE from *hs623WTs* and *hs623KOs* at E13.5. Primers were designed to target all known mouse protein-coding and non-protein-coding genes in the NCBI RNA reference sequences collection that are found 450 kb up- and downstream of *hs623* (Fig. 3a). From the RTqPCR we found no significant difference in the expression of the following genes in this region: *Myzap*, *Cgln1*, *Zfp280d* and *Mns1* (Fig. 3b). *Tcf12* RNAs include a variety of splice variants. Because of this we designed three separate primer pairs to specifically interrogate the different splice variants of *Tcf12* (Fig. 3a). We found a reduction in the expression of the short isoforms of *Tcf12* isoform 3 and 4 (Fig. 3b, see *Tcf12*_v1/3–4 and *Tcf12*_v1/3–5). Notably, we did not find any difference in the expression levels of the longer isoforms 1 and 2 of *Tcf12* (Fig. 3b, see *Tcf12*_v1/2–2). Together, these results show that *Tcf12* transcription in the MGE is enhanced by *hs623*.

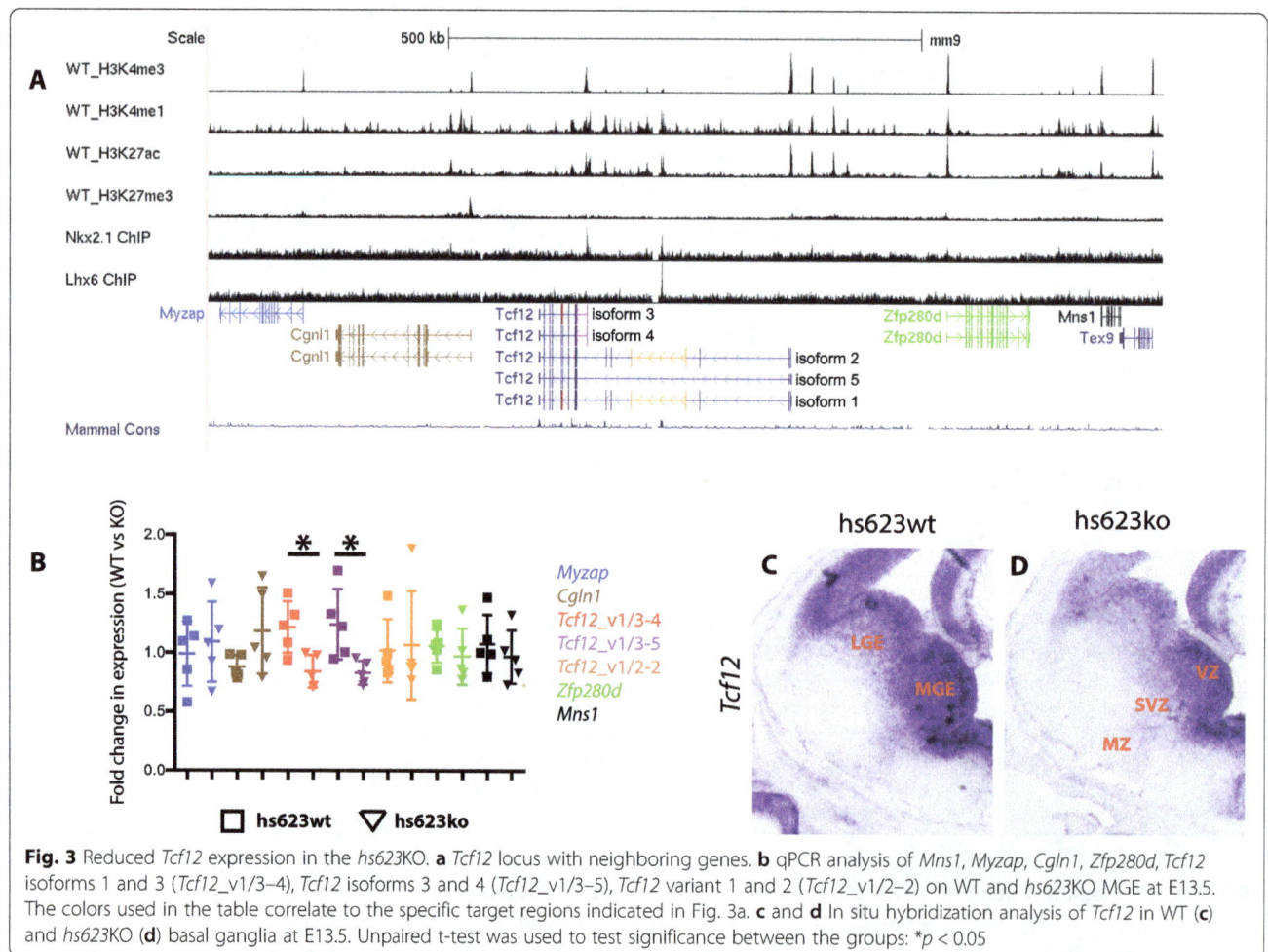

Fig. 3 Reduced *Tcf12* expression in the *hs623*KO. **a** *Tcf12* locus with neighboring genes. **b** qPCR analysis of *Mns1*, *Myzap*, *Cgln1*, *Zfp280d*, *Tcf12* isoforms 1 and 3 (*Tcf12*_v1/3–4), *Tcf12* isoforms 3 and 4 (*Tcf12*_v1/3–5), *Tcf12* variant 1 and 2 (*Tcf12*_v1/2–2) on WT and *hs623*KO MGE at E13.5. The colors used in the table correlate to the specific target regions indicated in Fig. 3a. **c** and **d** In situ hybridization analysis of *Tcf12* in WT (**c**) and *hs623*KO (**d**) basal ganglia at E13.5. Unpaired t-test was used to test significance between the groups: *$p < 0.05$

To obtain spatial information about the reduction of *Tcf12* within the MGE we compared the distribution of *Tcf12* RNA between WT and *hs623KO* telencephalon at E13.5 using in situ RNA hybridization. Normally, *Tcf12* is broadly expressed in the VZ in the pallium and subpallium. In the ganglionic eminences *Tcf12* is also expressed in the SVZ and MZ, with a markedly higher expression in the MGE compared to the LGE. On the other hand, in the *hs623KO* we observed a reduction of *Tcf12* expression that appeared to be specific to the SVZ and MZ of the MGE (Fig. 3c and d). This result is consistent with the spatial activity of *hs623*, which is restricted to the SVZ of the MGE.

Combined activity of POU and SOX TFs are required to maintain gene expression downstream of NKX2–1 in the MGE

To test the functional requirement of the LHX6 motifs in *hs623* we made site directed mutations that removed all four LHX6 motifs (*hs623ΔLHX*). In MGE primary cultures the activity of *hs623ΔLHX* was reduced by half when compared to the non-mutated *hs623* (*hs623*WT, Fig. 4a and b). Together, these experiments provide evidence that *hs623* activity, in part, depends on LHX6 and LHX8 and that there are additional TFs and signaling

pathways required for the activity of *hs623*. Our earlier motif analysis of aREs discovered an enrichment of additional motifs such as HD-binding motifs (POU6f2 and HOX), SOX motifs and E-boxes (Fig. 1e). To identify additional TF pathways responsible for the activity of *hs623* we looked at the other identified de novo motifs within *hs623* (Fig. 1d). Located in the center of *hs623* we found two octamers (bound by POU TFs), of which one is adjacent to a SOX motif. Octamers are known to pair with SOX motifs to form central functional units regulating development in various cell types [33–35]. Initially, we analyzed the activity of the two individual octamers by generating single mutations of the two motifs (Fig. 4a, *hs623ΔOCT1* and *hs623ΔOCT2*). Mutating octamer 1 (*hs623ΔOCT1*) caused a significant reduction of *hs623* activity in MGE primary cultures, whereas mutating octamer 2 (*hs623ΔOCT2*) had no significant effect on *hs623* activity (Fig. 4b). Octamer 2 is located 3 bp from a SOX consensus motif (Fig. 4a). To assess the requirement of this combined motif for *hs623* activity, we generated a compound mutant with a combined mutation of octamer 2 and the paired SOX motif (*hs623ΔOCT2 + SOX*). *Hs623ΔOCT2 + SOX* showed a significantly reduced activity when compared to *hs623*WT as well as, the two individual single mutants, *hs623ΔOCT2* and *hs623ΔSOX* (Fig. 4b).

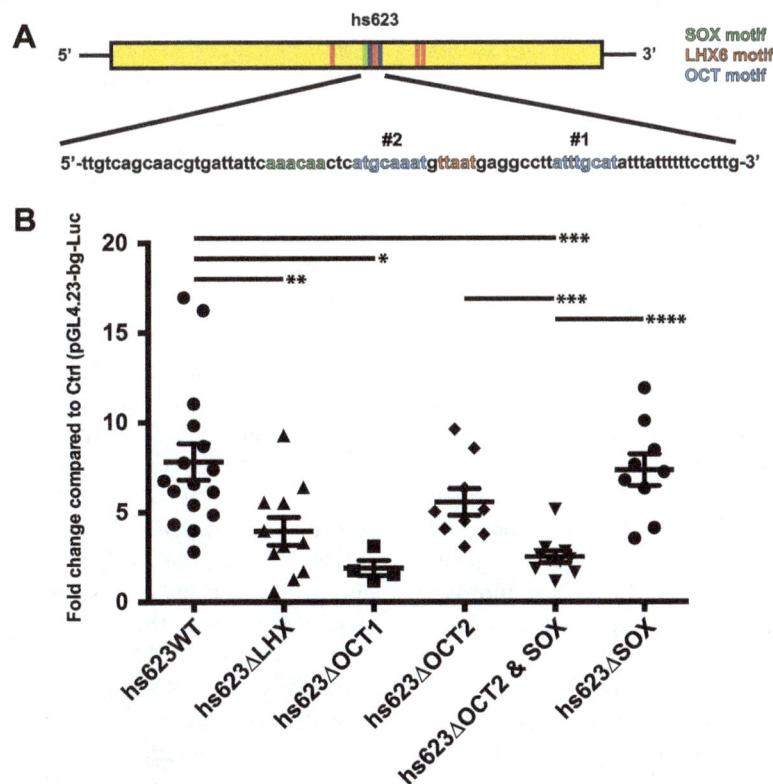

Fig. 4 OCT and SOX motifs required for *hs623* activity in primary MGE cultures. **a** Schematic of *hs623* with LHX6, OCT and SOX motifs. **b** Luciferase reporter assay showing a reduced activity of *hs623* when LHX6, OCT and SOX motifs in *hs623* are mutated. Data are represented as mean ± SEM. Unpaired t-test was used to test significance between the groups: *$p < 0.05$, **$p < 0.01$, ***$p < 0.001$, ****$p < 0.0001$

Altogether, our experiments show that *Tcf12* expression in the SVZ of the MGE is mediated, at least in part, through *hs623*, a RE that is strongly dependent on its OCT and SOX motifs and partially dependent on its LHX6 motifs. We have previously shown that gene expression in the SVZ of the MGE (including *Tcf12*) largely depends on NKX2–1 activity [18]. Existing mechanistic data show that NKX2–1 acts as a transcriptional repressor. Therefore, our findings suggest that the loss of *Tcf12* expression in the SVZ of the MGE *Nkx2–1*cKO is not due to the direct regulation of *Tcf12* by NKX2–1, but is a secondary effect due to changes in expression and activity of LHX6, LHX8, OCT and SOX TFs.

Discussion

Technical advancements in genome wide sequencing, chromosome capture and CRISPR/Cas9 technologies are increasing our understanding of genome organization. These data, combined with data showing RE activities in vivo (https://enhancer.lbl.gov/), TF binding and other epigenetic genomic data, and spatial gene expression data (http://www.brain-map.org/, http://www.eurexpress.org/ee/intro.html), are enabling the field to begin elucidating the genomic networks and the molecular mechanisms that direct brain development. Herein we have used many of these approaches to analyze gene expression in the developing mouse MGE. In the context of the *Nkx2–1*cKO mouse, our analysis of differential (WT vs. cKO) histone ChIP-seq data, and de novo sequence motif analysis, has provided evidence for additional TFs, REs, and signaling pathways that direct MGE development.

In this study, we showed that *Tcf12* expression in the SVZ of the MGE is mediated via *hs623*, an aRE bound by NKX2–1. The activity of *hs623* and the expression of *Tcf12* depend on NKX2–1 activity, suggesting that NKX2–1 promotes *Tcf12* expression in this context. We find no direct evidence showing that NKX2–1 activates *Tcf12* transcription via *hs623*. On the other hand, we show that LHX6, OCT and SOX motives are central to *hs623* activity. In fact, *hs623* lacks NKX2–1 consensus motifs and its interaction with *hs623* can possibly be explained through binding to three flanking regions. Other alternative explanations are that NKX2–1 regulates *hs623* through either uncharacterized NKX2–1 motifs or through indirect binding to transcriptional complexes that bind *hs623*.

We have earlier demonstrated that NKX2–1 represses transcription in the MGE, similar to other NKX HD TFs that specify ventral parts of the developing neural tube [36, 37]. Even at aREs, identified in the *Nkx2–1*cKO MGE, the NKX2–1 motifs mediate transcriptional repression, as exemplified by the intragenic *Tgfb3* RE in Sandberg et al. 2016 [18]. On the other hand, in the case of both the *Tgfb3* RE and *hs623*, LHX6 motifs promote enhancer activity. If NKX2–1 only represses transcription, it is unclear how loci such as LHX6 and LHX8 fail to be activated in the *Nkx2–1* mutants [16–18]. Furthermore it is unclear why NKX2–1 also binds loci that have reduced activity in the *Nkx2–1*cKO. These results suggest that, in some contexts, NKX2–1 may have an activating function. NKX2–1 binding to these loci might be required to keep them poised for subsequent activation by TFs and signaling pathways parallel and genetically downstream of NKX2–1, such as LHX, OCT, SOX and bHLH TFs. A similar model was presented in two studies looking at motor neuron development. In these cells, combinations of NEUROG2 (bHLH TF), LHX3, ISL-1, ONECUT1 and EBF direct the progression of the motor neuron fate through distinct sets of REs [8, 9]. Similar to these models, we find an enrichment of LHX6 binding and e-boxes at aREs, a group of REs with a preferential activity in the SVZ of the MGE. This combination of TF binding and motif enrichment is not seen at NKX2–1 bound rREs, that have a relatively low MGE activity. These data highlight similarities in the molecular mechanisms that direct MGE and motor neuron development over time. In addition to combinatorial activity with other TFs, the activity of NKX2–1 might be affected by changes to chromatin modifications at specific loci over time. Our experimental design lacks the temporal resolution to make these kinds of predictions. For the future, it would be interesting to know; 1) at what time point in the developing MGE (VZ, SVZ or MZ) are the various REs active, 2) and the temporal pattern of TF binding at these REs. This would give us important information that could help elucidate the activating and repressing mechanics through which NKX2–1, LHX6 and other TFs direct MGE development.

The seemingly dual activity of NKX2–1 in the MGE is similar to its double-edged characteristics in regulating cancer development and progression. In this context, NKX2–1 has a role as lineage-survival oncogene in developing lung cancer tumors. On the other hand, NKX2–1 expression is also associated with a favorable prognosis in affected patients, due to its capacity to attenuate the invasive capacity of carcinomas [38]. Interestingly, this has been shown to be mediated through an abrogation of cellular response to TGFβ induced EMT, a signaling pathway that is directly repressed by NKX2–1 in the MGE [18, 39]. By identifying the mechanisms through which NKX2–1 operate in the subpallial telencephalon we might also learn more about its enigmatic role in tumor biology.

The activity of the RE *hs623* depends on two octamers, providing evidence that OCT TFs are central to MGE development. OCT TFs are important regulators of stem cell maintenance and the progression of neurogenesis.

OCT4 is central for propagating undifferentiated embryonic stem cells and has the ability to induce pluripotent stem cells from embryonic and adult fibroblasts [40, 41]. On the contrary, BRN2, together with Ascl1 and Myt1l, can efficiently trans-differentiate embryonic and postnatal fibroblasts into functional neurons [42]. BRN1, BRN2 and OCT6 mutants show defects in layering of the neocortex, due to their role in initiating radial migration of cortical projection neurons, further highlighting their role in promoting neurogenesis [43–45]. Furthermore, we find an enrichment of both octamers and E-boxes in REs promoting gene expression in the MGE, suggesting that the TF machinery directing trans-differentiation of fibroblasts into neurons is similar to the TF machinery inducing neuronal phenotypes in the MGE. Trans-differentiating fibroblast to neurons using Brn2, Ascl1 and Mytl1 generate cells with a mixed neuronal phenotype [42], indicating that these TFs are required for promoting the neuronal fate, without any preference for specific neuronal lineages. Taken together, this suggests a model where neuronal fate and phenotype is directed through separate, although integrated, TF pathways in the MGE.

One of the octamers in *hs623* is paired with a SOX motif. The SOX TF family consists of a large number of genes that direct embryonic development and cell differentiation. They bind loosely to the minor groove of the DNA and their target gene specificity is guided through the interaction with cell type specific partner factors such as OCT TFs. The combined activity of SOX2 and different OCT TFs are important regulators of gene expression in undifferentiated embryonic stem cells (ESCs) and neural progenitor cells (NPCs) [46]. SOX2 and OCT4 (POU5F1) bind REs in ECSs, whereas SOX2 and BRN2 (POU3F2) co-occupy REs in NPCs [34, 46–48]. SOX and OCT motifs have also been shown to direct transcription in both ESCs and NPCs in the forebrain [34, 35]. Today we do not know what specific OCT and SOX TFs that are required to activate transcription in the SVZ of the MGE, via REs like *hs623*, BRN1 (POU3F3), BRN2 (POU3F2), BRN4 (POU3F4), BRN5 (POU6F1) and OCT6 (POU3F1) are all expressed here, but little is know regarding their function in this context. A large number of different SOX TFs are expressed in the MGE and several of them show a reduced expression in the *Nkx2–1*cKO, such as Sox1, Sox2, Sox6, Sox11 and Sox21 constituting possible candidates for promoting *Tcf12* expression via *hs623*. Sox6 is required for patterning of the subpallium and generation on MGE derived interneurons [49, 50], but when looking at *Tcf12* expression in the E13.5 MGE of a conditional *Sox6* mouse [51] with an *Nkx2–1*-Cre line [52], we found no significant change in *Tcf12* expression (Additional file 4). From this we can suggest that SOX6 is not sufficient for promoting *Tcf12* expression. Further studies should be performed

to identify the specific OCT and SOX TFs directing transcriptional activation in the MGE.

Here, in our new analysis of the *Nkx2–1*cKO, we found a large number aREs. Some of these are near the loci of the *Tcf4* and *Tcf12* bHLH TF encoding genes. The *Nkx2–1*cKO shows a near complete loss of *Tcf12* expression in the SVZ and MZ of the MGE. We found an aRE intronic to *Tcf12* (*hs623*) that has activity in the SVZ and MZ of the MGE (Fig. 2e). Deletion of *hs623* leads to a reduced *Tcf12* expression in the VZ and MZ of the MGE. This result suggests that *Tcf12* expression is regulated through several aREs, including *hs623*, and that there is redundancy between these REs. Enhancer redundancy has been demonstrated in the developing telencephalon and limb where REs sharing a similar spatiotemporal activity provides robustness to gene expression [53, 54]. We also find that there are different genetic programs directing *Tcf12* expression in various cell types of the MGE. *Tcf12* expression is initiated in the VZ of the MGE; this expression is largely unaffected in the *Nkx2–1*cKO, indicating that *Tcf12* expression in this region is not mediated through *hs623* and largely NKX2–1 independent.

Altogether, these data provide evidence of transcriptional circuitry that connects the initiation of MGE fate in the VZ by *Nkx2–1* and *Otx2*, to the maturation of cells in the SVZ and MZ by driven through REs such as *hs632*, whose activity integrates signals from LHX, OCT, SOX and bHLH TFs [16, 18, 55]. Future studies will investigate how TFs, chromatin-binding, –reading and -remodeling proteins integrate to direct GABAergic and cholinergic development in the subpallial telencephalon.

Conclusion

In our study we use a combination of genomics, CRISPR/Cas9 engineering and TF motif analysis to investigate the transcriptional networks guiding development of the MGE and its descendants. Whereas NKX2–1 is required for initiating MGE characteristics in the VZ, we provide evidence that a combination of LHX, OCT, SOX and bHLH TFs are central for maintaining gene expression in the SVZ and MZ, genetically down-stream of NKX2–1. Here we generate a mouse mutant in whom we delete a *Tcf12* intragenic RE, showing its requirement for maintaining *Tcf12* transcription in the SVZ and MZ of the MGE. The activity of this *Tcf12* enhancer, in primary cultures of MGE cells, largely depends on an octamer and a combined octamer and SOX motif. Altogether, our study identifies a genomic framework through which a combination of LHX, OCT, SOX and bHLH TFs direct MGE differentiation through the expression terminal effector genes.

Additional files

Additional file 1: aREs and rREs in the Nkx2–1cKO MGE at e13.5. Identified activating (sheet "aRE") and repressing (sheet "rRE") regulatory elements in Nkx2–1cKO MGE at e13.5. In vivo activity of aREs (sheet "VISTA aRE") and rREs (sheet "VISTA rRE") VISTA transgenics at E11.5. (XLSX 696 kb)

Additional file 2: Forebrain activity of hs623. Coronal sections of the hs623 transgene showing its activity in forebrain at E11.5. The sections are arranged rostral (A) to caudal (S). (PDF 135 kb)

Additional file 3: DNA sequences of hs623KO founder mice. DNA sequence of the modified *hs623* locus in the five founder mice carrying the hs623 deletion. (PDF 65 kb)

Additional file 4: Tcf12 expression in Sox6 conditional knockout. In situ analysis of *Tcf12* in WT (A) and *Sox6* conditional knockout (B) forebrain at E13.5. (PDF 4383 kb)

Abbreviations
aREs: activating regulatory element; bHLH: basic-helix-loop-helix; cKO: conditional knockout; E: embryonic day; GO: gene ontology; HD: homeodomain; LGE: lateral ganglionic eminence; MGE: medial ganglionic eminence; MZ: mantle zone; REs: regulatory elements; rREs: repressing regulatory element; SVZ: sub-ventricular zone; TF: transcription factor; VZ: ventricular zone; WT: wild-type

Acknowledgements
We thank members of the Rubenstein, Taher, Black and Nord laboratories for advice and critical evaluation of the data during the course of the study.

Funding
This project was supported by Vetenskapsrådet 2011–38865–83000-30 (M.S.), Svenska Sällskapet för Medicinsk Forskning (M.S.), NIMH R01 MH081880 (J.L.R.R.), NIH R01s HL064658 (B.L.B.) and HL136182 (B.L.B.).

Authors' contributions
MS, JLRR and AN conceived the experiments, interpreted the results, wrote, reviewed and edited the manuscript. MS designed and performed all experiments. JH and BB injected sgRNA and Cas9 to generate *hs623*KO mice. LT performed the differential ChIP-seq enrichment analysis. All authors read and approved the final manuscript.

Competing interests
J.L.R.R. is cofounder, stockholder, and currently on the scientific board of *Neurona*, a company studying the potential therapeutic use of interneuron transplantation.

Author details
[1]Department of Psychiatry, UCSF Weill Institute for Neurosciences, University of California, San Francisco, San Francisco, CA 94143, USA. [2]Division of Bioinformatics, Department of Biology, Friedrich-Alexander Universität Erlangen-Nürnberg, 91054 Erlangen, Germany. [3]Cardiovascular Research Institute, University of California, San Francisco, CA 94143, USA. [4]Department of Psychiatry and Behavioral Sciences, University of California, Davis, Davis, CA 95817, USA. [5]Department of Neurobiology, Physiology, and Behavior, University of California, Davis, Davis, CA 95616, USA. [6]Present address: Biogen, Cambridge 02142, MA, USA.

References
1. Nord AS, Pattabiraman K, Visel A, Rubenstein JLR. Genomic perspectives of transcriptional regulation in forebrain development. Neuron Elsevier Inc. 2015;85:27–47.
2. De Rubeis S, He X, Goldberg AP, Poultney CS, Samocha K, Ercument Cicek A, et al. Synaptic, transcriptional and chromatin genes disrupted in autism. 2014.
3. Pennacchio LA, Ahituv N, Moses AM, Prabhakar S, Nobrega MA, Shoukry M, et al. In vivo enhancer analysis of human conserved non-coding sequences. Nature. Nature Publishing Group. 2006;444:499–502.
4. Visel A, Blow MJ, Li Z, Zhang T, Akiyama JA, Holt A, et al. ChIP-seq accurately predicts tissue-specific activity of enhancers. Nat Publ Group. 2009;457:854–8.
5. Zinzen RP, Girardot C, Gagneur J, Braun M, Furlong EEM. Combinatorial binding predicts spatio-temporal cis-regulatory activity. Nat Publ Group. 2009;462:65–70.
6. Bonev B, Cohen NM, Szabo Q, Fritsch L, Papadopoulos GL, Lubling Y, et al. Multiscale 3D Genome Rewiring during Mouse Neural Development. Cell. Elsevier. 2017;171:557–572.e24.
7. Visel A, Taher L, Girgis H, May D, Golonzhka O, Hoch RV, et al. A high-resolution enhancer atlas of the developing telencephalon. Cell. 2013;152: 895–908.
8. Rhee HS, Closser M, Guo Y, Bashkirova EV, Tan GC, Gifford DK, et al. Expression of terminal effector genes in mammalian neurons is maintained by a dynamic relay of transient enhancers. Neuron. Elsevier. 2016;92:1252–65.
9. Velasco S, Ibrahim MM, Kakumanu A, Garipler G, Aydin B, Al-Sayegh MA, et al. A Multi-step Transcriptional and Chromatin State Cascade Underlies Motor Neuron Programming from Embryonic Stem Cells. Cell Stem Cell. 2016;20:1–13.
10. Lupiáñez DG, Kraft K, Heinrich V, Krawitz P, Brancati F, Klopocki E, et al. Disruptions of topological chromatin domains cause pathogenic rewiring of gene-enhancer interactions. Cell. 2015;161:1012–25.
11. Campbell K. Dorsal-ventral patterning in the mammalian telencephalon. Curr Opin Neurobiol. 2003;13:50–6.
12. Rubenstein JLR, Campbell K. Neurogenesis in the Basal Ganglia. Patterning and Cell Type Specification in the Developing CNS and PNS. Elsevier. 2013: 455–73.
13. Zhao Y, Marin O, Hermesz E, Powell A, Flames N, Palkovits M, et al. The LIM-homeobox gene Lhx8 is required for the development of many cholinergic neurons in the mouse forebrain. Proc Natl Acad Sci U S A. 2011;100:9005–10.
14. Fragkouli A, van Wijk NV, Lopes R, Kessaris N, Pachnis V. LIM homeodomain transcription factor-dependent specification of bipotential MGE progenitors into cholinergic and GABAergic striatal interneurons. Development. 2009; 136:3841–51.
15. Du T, Xu Q, Ocbina PJ, Anderson SA. NKX2.1 specifies cortical interneuron fate by activating Lhx6. Development. 2008;135:1559–67.
16. Sussel L, Marin O, Kimura S, Rubenstein JL. Loss of Nkx2.1 homeobox gene function results in a ventral to dorsal molecular respecification within the basal telencephalon: evidence for a transformation of the pallidum into the striatum. Development. 1999;
17. Butt SJB, Sousa VH, Fuccillo MV, Hjerling-Leffler J, Miyoshi G, Kimura S, et al. The requirement of Nkx2-1 in the temporal specification of cortical interneuron subtypes. Neuron. 2008;59:722–32.
18. Sandberg M, Flandin P, Silberberg S, Su-Feher L, Price JD, Hu JS, et al. Transcriptional networks controlled by NKX2-1 in the development of forebrain GABAergic neurons. Neuron. 2016;91:1260–75.
19. Vogt D, Hunt RF, Mandal S, Sandberg M, Silberberg SN, Nagasawa T, et al. Lhx6 directly regulates Arx and CXCR7 to determine cortical interneuron fate and laminar position. Neuron. 2014;82:350–64.

20. Kusakabe T, Kawaguchi A, Hoshi N, Kawaguchi R, Hoshi S, Kimura S. Thyroid-specific enhancer-binding protein/NKX2.1 is required for the maintenance of ordered architecture and function of the differentiated thyroid. Mol Endocrinol. 2006;20:1796–809.

21. Schüller U, Heine VM, Mao J, Kho AT, Dillon AK, Han Y-G, et al. Acquisition of Granule Neuron Precursor Identity is a critical determinant of progenitor cell competence to form Shh-induced Medulloblastoma. Cancer Cell. 2008; 14:123–34.

22. Madisen L, Zwingman TA, Sunkin SM, Oh SW, Zariwala HA, Gu H, et al. A robust and high-throughput Cre reporting and characterization system for the whole mouse brain. Nat Neurosci Nature Publishing Group. 2010;13:133–40.

23. Wang H, Yang H, Shivalila CS, Dawlaty MM, Cheng AW, Zhang F, et al. One-step generation of mice carrying mutations in multiple genes by CRISPR/ Cas-mediated genome engineering. Cell. 2013;153:910–8.

24. De Val S, Anderson JP, Heidt AB, Khiem D, Xu S-M, Black BL. Mef2c is activated directly by Ets transcription factors through an evolutionarily conserved endothelial cell-specific enhancer. Dev Biol. 2004;275:424–34.

25. Zhao Y, Flandin P, Long JE, Cuesta MD, Westphal H, Rubenstein JLR. Distinct molecular pathways for development of telencephalic interneuron subtypes revealed through analysis of Lhx6 mutants. J Comp Neurol. 2008;510:79–99.

26. Schaeren-Wiemers N, Gerfin-Moser A. A single protocol to detect transcripts of various types and expression levels in neural tissue and cultured cells: in situ hybridization using digoxigenin-labelled cRNA probes. Histochemistry Springer-Verlag. 1993;100:431–40.

27. Schmittgen TD, Livak KJ. Analyzing real-time PCR data by the comparative CT method. Nat Protoc. 2008;3:1101–8.

28. Livak KJ, Schmittgen TD. Analysis of relative gene expression data using real-time quantitative PCR and the 2(−Delta Delta C(T)) method. Methods Academic Press. 2001;25:402–8.

29. Thomas-Chollier M, Darbo E, Herrmann C, Defrance M, Thieffry D, van Helden J. A complete workflow for the analysis of full-size ChIP-seq (and similar) data sets using peak-motifs. Nat Protoc. 2012;7:1551–68.

30. Silberberg SN, Taher L, Lindtner S, Sandberg M, Nord AS, Vogt D, et al. Subpallial enhancer transgenic lines: a data and tool resource to study transcriptional regulation of GABAergic cell fate. Neuron Elsevier. 2016;92:59–74.

31. McLean CY, Bristor D, Hiller M, Clarke SL, Schaar BT, Lowe CB, et al. GREAT improves functional interpretation of cis-regulatory regions. Nat Biotechnol. 2010;28:495–501.

32. Visel A, Minovitsky S, Dubchak I, Pennacchio LA. VISTA enhancer browser--a database of tissue-specific human enhancers. Nucleic Acids Res. 2007;35: D88–92.

33. Kamachi Y, Uchikawa M, Kondoh H. Pairing SOX off: with partners in the regulation of embryonic development. Trends Genet. 2000;16:182–7.

34. Josephson R, Muller T, Pickel J, Okabe S, Reynolds K, Turner PA, et al. POU transcription factors control expression of CNS stem cell-specific genes. Development. 1998;125:3087–100.

35. Bery A, Martynoga B, Guillemot F, Joly J-S, Rétaux S. Characterization of enhancers active in the mouse embryonic cerebral cortex suggests sox/Pou cis-regulatory logics and heterogeneity of cortical progenitors. Cereb Cortex Oxford University Press. 2014;24:2822–34.

36. Briscoe J, Pierani A, Jessell TM, Ericson J. A homeodomain protein code specifies progenitor cell identity and neuronal fate in the ventral neural tube. Cell. 2000;101:435–45.

37. Muhr J, Andersson E, Persson M, Jessell TM, Ericson J. Groucho-mediated transcriptional repression establishes progenitor cell pattern and neuronal fate in the ventral neural tube. Cell. 2001;104:861–73.

38. Yamaguchi T, Hosono Y, Yanagisawa K, Takahashi T. NKX2-1/TTF-1: an enigmatic oncogene that functions as a double-edged sword for Cancer cell survival and progression. Cancer Cell Elsevier. 2013;23:718–23.

39. Saito R-A, Watabe T, Horiguchi K, Kohyama T, Saitoh M, Nagase T, et al. Thyroid Transcription Factor-1 Inhibits Transforming Growth Factor-β–Mediated Epithelial-to-Mesenchymal Transition in Lung Adenocarcinoma Cells. Cancer Res. Am Assoc Cancer Res. 2009;69:2783–91.

40. Boyer LA, Lee TI, Cole MF, Johnstone SE, Levine SS. Core transcriptional regulatory circuitry in human embryonic stem cells. Cell. 2005;122:947–56.

41. Takahashi K, Yamanaka S. Induction of pluripotent stem cells from mouse embryonic and adult fibroblast cultures by defined factors. Cell. 2006;126: 663–76.

42. Vierbuchen T, Ostermeier A, Pang ZP, Kokubu Y, Südhof TC, Wernig M. Direct conversion of fibroblasts to functional neurons by defined factors. Nature. 2010;463:1035–41.

43. McEvilly RJ, de Diaz MO, Schonemann MD, Hooshmand F, Rosenfeld MG. Transcriptional regulation of cortical neuron migration by POU domain factors. Science. 2002;295:1528–32.

44. Sugitani Y, Nakai S, Minowa O, Nishi M, Jishage K-I, Kawano H, et al. Brn-1 and Brn-2 share crucial roles in the production and positioning of mouse neocortical neurons. Genes & Development Cold Spring Harbor Lab. 2002; 16:1760–5.

45. Dominguez MH, Ayoub AE, Rakic P. POU-III transcription factors (Brn1, Brn2, and Oct6) influence neurogenesis, molecular identity, and migratory destination of upper-layer cells of the cerebral cortex. Cereb Cortex Oxford University Press. 2013;23:2632–43.

46. Lodato MA, Ng CW, Wamstad JA, Cheng AW, Thai KK, Fraenkel E, et al. SOX2 co-occupies distal enhancer elements with distinct POU factors in ESCs and NPCs to specify cell state. Barsh GS, editor. PLoS Genet. Public Libr Sci; 2013;9:e1003288.

47. Ambrosetti DC, Basilico C, Dailey L. Synergistic activation of the fibroblast growth factor 4 enhancer by Sox2 and Oct-3 depends on protein-protein interactions facilitated by a specific spatial arrangement of factor binding sites. Mol Cell Biol. Am Soc Microbiol. 1997;17:6321–9.

48. Nishimoto M, Fukushima A, Okuda A, Muramatsu M. The gene for the embryonic stem cell coactivator UTF1 carries a regulatory element which selectively interacts with a complex composed of Oct-3/4 and Sox-2. Mol Cell Biol . Am Soc Microbiol (ASM). 1999;19:5453–65.

49. Azim E, Jabaudon D, Fame RM, Macklis JD. SOX6 controls dorsal progenitor identity and interneuron diversity during neocortical development. Nat Neurosci NIH Public Access. 2009;12:1238–47.

50. Batista-Brito R, Rossignol E, Hjerling-Leffler J, Denaxa M, Wegner M, Lefebvre V, et al. The cell-intrinsic requirement of Sox6 for cortical interneuron development. Neuron. 2009;63:466–81.

51. Dumitriu B, Dy P, Smits P, Lefebvre V. Generation of mice harboring aSox6 conditional null allele. Genesis. 2006;44:219–24.

52. Xu Q, Tam M, Anderson SA. Fate mapping Nkx2.1-lineage cells in the mouse telencephalon. J Comp Neurol. 2008;506:16–29.

53. Osterwalder M, Barozzi I, Tissières V, Fukuda-Yuzawa Y, Mannion BJ, Afzal SY, et al. Enhancer redundancy provides phenotypic robustness in mammalian development. Nature. Nat Publ Group. 2018;489:57.

54. Dickel DE, Ypsilanti AR, Pla R, Zhu Y, Barozzi I, Mannion BJ, et al. Ultraconserved Enhancers Are Required for Normal Development. Cell. 2018; 172:491–499.e15.

55. Hoch RV, Lindtner S, Price JD, Rubenstein JLR. OTX2 transcription factor controls regional patterning within the medial ganglionic eminence and regional identity of the septum. Cell Rep. 2015;12:482–94.

13

Eph/Ephrin Signaling Controls Progenitor Identities In The Ventral Spinal Cord

Julien Laussu[1,2], Christophe Audouard[1], Anthony Kischel[1], Poincyane Assis-Nascimento[3], Nathalie Escalas[1], Daniel J. Liebl[3], Cathy Soula[1] and Alice Davy[1]* (iD)

Abstract

Background: In the vertebrate spinal cord, motor neurons (MN) are generated in stereotypical numbers from a pool of dedicated progenitors (pMN) whose number depends on signals that control their specification but also their proliferation and differentiation rates. Although the initial steps of pMN specification have been extensively studied, how pMN numbers are regulated over time is less well characterized.

Results: Here, we show that ephrinB2 and ephrinB3 are differentially expressed in progenitor domains in the ventral spinal cord with several Eph receptors more broadly expressed. Genetic loss-of-function analyses show that ephrinB2 and ephrinB3 inversely control pMN numbers and that these changes in progenitor numbers correlate with changes in motor neuron numbers. Detailed phenotypic analyses by immunostaining and genetic interaction studies between ephrinB2 and Shh indicate that changes in pMN numbers in ephrin mutants are due to alteration in progenitor identity at late stages of development.

Conclusions: Altogether our data reveal that Eph:ephrin signaling is required to control progenitor identities in the ventral spinal cord.

Keywords: Ephrins, Neural tube, Progenitors, Fate, Motor neurons, Sonic hedgehog, Mouse

Background

In vertebrates, motor neurons (MN) innervating skeletal muscles are born in the ventral neural tube, the future spinal cord, from a pool of progenitors located in the ventricular zone. As for other neuronal subtypes, the production of stereotyped numbers of MN requires the integration of different processes such as specification and proliferation of progenitors, followed by cell cycle exit and differentiation [1]. While these processes are common to the genesis of all neuronal subtypes throughout the central nervous system, one distinguishing feature of MN development is the fact that progenitor specification is dependent on their spatial organization within the neural tube. Indeed, the vertebrate neural tube is organized along its dorsoventral axis in different progenitor domains which first give rise to distinct neuronal subtypes and later on to subtypes of

glial cells. Combinatorial positional information provided by graded Sonic Hedgehog (Shh), Wnt, BMP and FGF signaling induces the regionalized expression of homeodomain and helix-loop-helix identity transcription factors (iTFs) in different progenitor domains [1]. For instance, progenitors of motor neurons (pMNs) express the iTF Olig2 while adjacent progenitors (p3) which give rise to v3 interneurons express the iTF Nkx2.2. Ventral patterning of the spinal cord, including specification of pMN and p3 progenitors, is controlled by the morphogen Sonic Hedgehog (Shh) produced by the notochord and the floor plate [2]. In addition to doses, different exposure times to Shh modulates the expression of these iTFs in progenitors, thus specifying the distinct progenitor identities [3, 4]. Specifically, the progressive emergence of a gene regulatory network (GRN) composed of three transcription factors- Pax6, Olig2 and Nkx2.2 whose expression is refined by cross-repressive interactions interprets graded Shh signaling, to control the size of the p3 and pMN progenitor domains [5, 6]. Although early steps of progenitor specification are fairly well characterized, mechanisms that ensure stereotypy in the

---

* Correspondence: alice.davy@univ-tlse3.fr
[1]Centre de Biologie du Développement (CBD), Centre de Biologie Intégrative (CBI), Université de Toulouse, CNRS, UPS, 118 Route de Narbonne, 31062 Toulouse, France
Full list of author information is available at the end of the article

size of progenitor domains as the tissue grows are less well understood. These mechanisms include maintenance of progenitor identities [4, 7, 8] as well as control of proliferation and differentiation rates that vary between progenitor types and over time [9]. In addition, mechanisms such as cell sorting have been shown to participate in defining and/or maintaining domain boundaries thus indirectly contributing to pattern progenitor domains [10–13].

Eph:ephrin signaling is a cell-to-cell communication pathway that has been implicated in numerous developmental processes [14, 15]. A distinctive feature of Eph:ephrin signaling is its ability to trigger forward signaling downstream of Eph receptors and reverse signaling downstream of ephrins. One of its major biological functions is to control cell adhesion and repulsion events in developing and adult tissues thus leading to the establishment and/or maintenance of axon tracts, tissue organization and patterning [16, 17]. In addition, Eph:ephrin signaling has been shown to control various aspects of neural progenitor development and homeostasis in the developing and adult mammalian cortex including self-renewal, proliferation, quiescence and differentiation [18]. In the developing spinal cord, the role of Eph:ephrin signaling has been prominently studied in post-mitotic neurons, specifically in axon guidance and fasciculation of MNs [19–21], as a consequence, virtually nothing is known on the function of this pathway in spinal progenitors. Here, we show that two B-class ephrins, ephrinB2 and ephrinB3 are differentially expressed in pMN and p3 progenitors. Loss of function analyses indicate that expression of ephrinB2 and ephrinB3 is not required for initial specification of these progenitors. However, at later developmental stages, expression of ephrinB2 and ephrinB3 is essential to maintain appropriate numbers of pMN and p3 progenitors. Interestingly, ephrinB2 and ephrinB3 mutants exhibit opposite phenotypes, matching their opposite differential expression patterns. Detailed analyses of ephinB2 mutants indicate that the change in pMN number is not due to a change in proliferation or differentiation rates. Rather, our data shows that *Efnb2* interacts with *Shh* to control the ratio between pMN and p3 progenitors. Lastly, loss of ephrinB3 -but not ephrinB2- leads to pMN and p3 progenitor intermingling. Altogether our data suggests that Eph:ephrin signaling plays a role in controlling progenitor identity.

Methods
Mice
Ephrin mutant mice were maintained in a mixed background and genotyped by PCR. The mouse lines Shh^{ko}, $Efnb3^{ko}$, $Efnb2^{lox}$ and $Efnb2^{GFP}$ have been described previously [22–24]. The *Olig2-Cre* mouse line [3] was maintained in a pure C57Bl6/J genetic background. For *Efnb2* cKO, control genotypes used in the study include $Efnb2^{lox/lox}$, $Efnb2^{lox/GFP}$, $Efnb2^{+/GFP}$ and $Efnb2^{+/GFP}$; *Olig2-Cre*. For *Efnb3* KO, control genotypes are always $Efnb3^{+/-}$. E0.5 is defined as the day on which a vaginal plug was detected.

In Situ Hybridization
In situ hybridization was performed using standard protocols on 70μm vibratome sections at brachial level. Antisense RNA probes labeled with digoxigenin were used to detect in vivo gene expression with a 72 h incubation time.

Immunostaining
All analyses for *Efnb2* cKO were performed on control and mutant littermates collected from at least two different litters. On the other hand, control and *Efnb3* mutant embryos were collected from independent litters. The number of embryo analyzed for each immunostaining and each developmental stage is indicated in the figure legends. To avoid bias in rostro-caudal axis, data was collected on thick vibratome sections covering the entire brachial region (600 μm). Antibody staining was performed following standard protocol on 70μm vibratome sections of mouse embryos at brachial level. For BrdU incorporation, pregnant dams were injected with BrdU (10mg/ml; 100mg/kg) with intraperitoneal injection. After 1 h, embryos were dissected in cold PBS and processed for subsequent immunostaining.

Antibodies used were: goat anti-Nkx2.2 (1/100, Santa Cruz Biotechnology); rabbit anti-Olig2 (1/1000, Sigma); mouse anti-Islet1/2, 39-4D5 (1/50, DSHB); rabbit anti-Foxp1 (1/200, Abcam), rabbit anti-P-H3 (1/1000, Millipore), rabbit anti-EphA4 (1/100, Santa Cruz Biotechnology), goat anti-EphB2 (1/50, R&D Systems), Tuj1 (1/1000, Covance). All secondary antibodies were from Jackson ImmunoResearch (1/1000).

Image processing and quantification
Images were collected on a Leica SP5 confocal microscope or Nikon eclipse 80i microscope for *in situ* hybridization data. Cell numbers were collected blindly on 5 vibratome sections ($n=25$ confocal Z-sections) per embryo and at least 2000 nuclei were recorded per embryo. The number of embryo analyzed for each immunostaining and each developmental stage is indicated in the figure legends. Acquisitions of nuclei 2D positions and semi quantitative analyses of fluorescence intensity were performed using Fiji [25]. Spatial distribution of progenitor subtypes was quantified using the R Project (http://www.r-project.org/), see Additional file 1: (Sup Code) for details on the code.

Statistical Analysis

For all analyses sample size was estimated empirically. Sample sizes are indicated in Figure legends and further details are provided in Additional file 2: Table S1. Statistical analyses were performed with GraphPad, using Mann-Whitney-Wilcoxon test or ANOVA, depending on the data set. $P<0.05$ was considered statistically significant.

Results

EphrinB2 and ephrinB3 exhibit restricted expression in progenitors of the ventral spinal cord.

A survey of members of the B-type Eph receptor family in the mouse ventral spinal cord (Fig. 1a) indicated that spinal progenitors co-express several EphB receptors, as well as EphA4, as shown by in situ hybridization (Fig. 1b-d) and immunofluorescence (Fig. 1e-g). Concerning B-type ephrin ligands, in situ hybridization at different developmental stages reveals that while *Efnb1* is not expressed at significant levels in progenitors of the ventral spinal cord (Fig. 1h-j), both *Efnb2* and *Efnb3* are expressed in subsets of these cells. More precisely, at all stages analyzed, *Efnb2* is expressed by progenitors located at an intermediate dorso-ventral position within the spinal cord, its expression never extending to the ventral-most region (Fig. 1k-m). Conversely, expression of *Efnb3* is highest in the ventral-most region of the spinal cord at all stages analyzed, with a lower expression extending more dorsally (Fig. 1n-p). Because *Efnb2* and *Efnb3* were expressed in distinct progenitor domains of the spinal cord, we asked whether these corresponded to progenitors with distinct identities, namely pMN progenitors expressing Olig2 and p3 progenitors expressing Nkx2.2. Since the expression of *Efnb2* in progenitors of the ventral neural tube detected by in situ hybridization was low, we took advantage of a reporter mouse line that expresses H2BGFP under the control of the *Efnb2* endogenous promoter [22]. The benefit of this reporter strategy is that H2BGFP accumulates in the nucleus thus highlighting low domains of expression and facilitating co-expression analyses. In accordance with in situ hybridization data, H2BGFP expression was detected in a restricted population of neural progenitors from E9.5 to E11.5 (Fig. 2a-d). Co-staining with Olig2 showed that the expression domain of *Efnb2* overlapped with the Olig2$^+$ (pMN) domain (Fig. 2a-l). Co-staining with Olig2 and Nkx2.2, the iTFs for pMN and p3 respectively, showed that the ventral boundary of *Efnb2* expression strictly corresponds to the p3/pMN boundary (Fig. 2m-p). Conversely, in situ hybridization for *Efnb3* followed by Olig2 immunostaining showed that the highest domain of *Efnb3* expression corresponds to Olig2$^-$ floor plate and p3 progenitors (Fig. 2q-s). Altogether, these expression analyses indicate that all progenitors of the ventral spinal cord co-express several Eph receptors and reveal that ephrinB2 and ephrinB3 are differentially expressed in pMN and p3 progenitors (Fig. 2t).

EphrinB2 controls the number of pMN and their progeny

Based on the expression of ephrinB2 in pMN but not p3 progenitors we hypothesized that it may be required for pMN development. We thus generated *Efnb2* loss-of-function mutant embryos and quantified the number of Olig2$^+$ progenitors at three different developmental stages. Since *Efnb2$^{-/-}$* (KO) embryos exhibit precocious lethality (E10.5) due to cardiovascular defects [26, 27] to analyze later stages of development we generated *Efnb2* conditional mutant embryos, using the *Olig2-Cre* mouse line (*Efnb2$^{lox/lox}$; Olig2-Cre* thereafter called cKO). At E9.5 and E10.5, no difference was observed in the number of Olig2$^+$ progenitors when comparing wild type and *Efnb2* KO or *Efnb2* cKO (Fig. 3a-d, g). On the contrary, at E11.5, the number of Olig2$^+$ progenitors was significantly decreased in *Efnb2* cKO (Fig. 3e-g), indicating that ephrinB2 is not required for initial pMN specification but is necessary at later stages to control the number of pMN progenitors. The decrease in the number of Olig2$^+$ progenitors between E10.5 and E11.5 which is observed in wild type embryos is partly driven by differentiation of these cells into MN [9], raising the possibility that the decrease in the number of pMN progenitors in absence of ephrinB2 could be due to increased differentiation. We thus assessed the number of pMN progeny in wild type and *Efnb2* mutant embryos. In the spinal cord, pMN first give rise to MN which settle in specific motor columns in the mantle zone and second, after the neuroglial transition, pMN give rise to oligodendrocyte precursors (OLP) that maintain Olig2 expression and migrate in the mantle zone. Immunostaining for Islet1/2 and Foxp1 to label MN showed that the reduction in pMN numbers correlates with a reduction in the total number of MN in E12.5 *Efnb2* cKO (Fig. 3h-j), which is not consistent with increased differentiation. To assess whether one subtype of MN was preferentially affected, we used different combination of Foxp1 and Islet1/2 to discriminate different motor columns. These quantifications showed that the reduction of total MN number does not correlate with reduction of one specific motor column, however, we observed that within this reduced pool of MN, slightly more LMCm MN were present in *Efnb2* cKO (Fig. 3k). Next we assessed the number of OLP by quantifying Olig2$^+$ nuclei in the mantle zone of E13.5 *Efnb2* cKO. Similar to what was observed for MN, loss of *Efnb2* in pMN correlates with a decrease in OLP numbers (Fig. 3l-p). Altogether, this data reveal that ephrinB2 is required to produce a stereotyped number of pMN and of their progeny by mechanisms likely independent of differentiation.

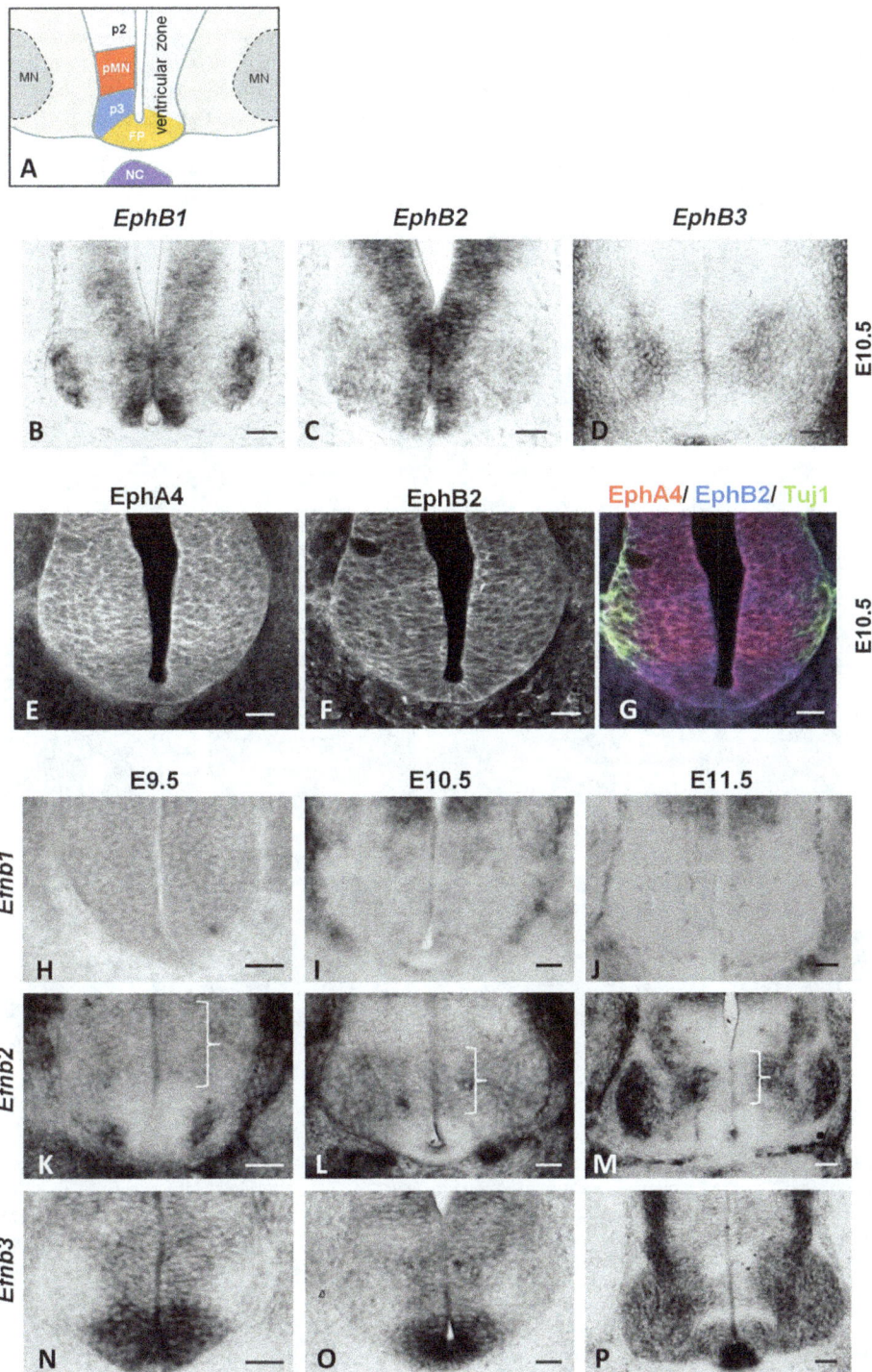

Fig. 1. Eph receptors and ephrins are expressed in progenitors of the ventral spinal cord. **a**. Schematic representation of the ventral spinal cord at E10.5. Progenitors are located in the ventricular zone, three progenitor domains are shown: p2, pMN and p3. Differentiated motor neurons (MN) are located laterally in the mantle zone. **b-d**. Expression of *EphB1* (**b**), *EphB2* (**c**) and *EphB3* (**d**) was monitored by in situ hybridization on transverse sections of E10.5 embryos. Scale bars: 50 μm. **e-g**. Transverse sections of E10.5 embryos were immunostained to detect EphA4 ((**e**), *red*), EphB2 ((**f**), *blue*) and differentiated neurons (Tuj1, green in (**g**)). Scale bars: 40 μm. (**h-p**). Expression of *Efnb1* (**h-j**), *Efnb2* (**k-m**) and *Efnb3* (**n-p**) was monitored by in situ hybridization on transverse sections of E9.5, E10.5 and E11.5 embryos, as indicated. Scale bars: 50 μm. Brackets indicate domains of *Efnb2* expression in progenitors. FP: floor plate, NC: notochord.

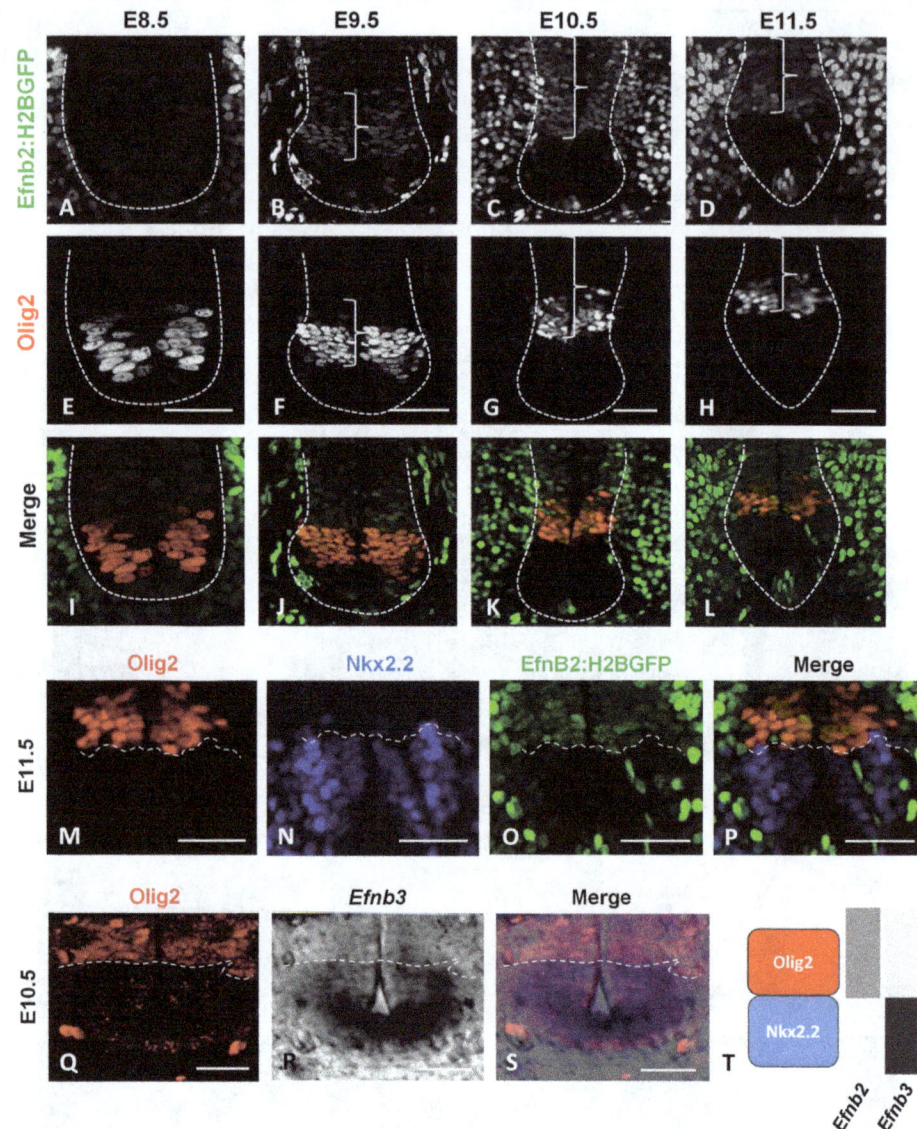

Fig. 2. EphrinB2 and ephrinB3 are expressed in complementary domains in progenitors of the ventral spinal cord. **a-l**. Transverse sections of *Efnb2^+/GFP* embryos at E8.5, E9.5, E10.5 and E11.5 (as indicated) were immunostained to detect Olig2 (**e-h**). Epifluorescence is shown on (**a-d**) and merged images are shown on (**i-l**). Scale bars: 50 μm. Dashed lines highlight the ventricular zone and brackets indicate domains of *Efnb2:H2BGFP* expression in progenitors. **m-p**. Transverse sections of *Efnb2^+/GFP* E11.5 embryos were immunostained to detect Olig2 (**m**) and Nkx2.2 (**n**). Epifluorescence is shown in (**o**) and a merged image is shown in (**p**). The dashed line marks the p3/pMN boundary. Scale bars: 50 μm. **q-s**. Transverse sections of wild type E10.5 embryos were processed for Olig2 immunostaining (**q**) and for *Efnb3* in situ hybridization (**r**). A merged image is shown in (**s**). The dashed line marks the p3/pMN boundary. Scale bars: 25 μm. T. Schematic representation of *Efnb2* and *Efnb3* expression in relation to pMN and p3 progenitors domains at E11.5.

Efnb2 interacts with *Shh* to control the ratio between pMN and p3 progenitors

To characterize the underlying causes of the decreased pMN number in ephrinB2 mutants, we first tested whether this reduction was due to altered rates of proliferation of pMN. We performed BrdU incorporation and immunostaining for Olig2 and quantified BrdU^+/Olig2^+ progenitors at two different developmental stages to monitor proliferation. At both stages, no difference in pMN proliferation was observed in *Efnb2* cKO compared to control embryos (Fig. 4a-f). We also assessed apoptosis and observed no change in the number of cleaved caspase positive pMN at E10.5 and E11.5 (data not shown). In addition, to confirm that the rate of pMN differentiation was unchanged in *Efnb2* cKO, we performed co-immunostaining for Olig2 and for the motor neuron (MN) marker Islet1/2 and quantified the fraction of Islet1/2^+ nuclei at the basal side of the ventricular zone (intermediate zone) which represent newborn MN. As expected, no difference was observed

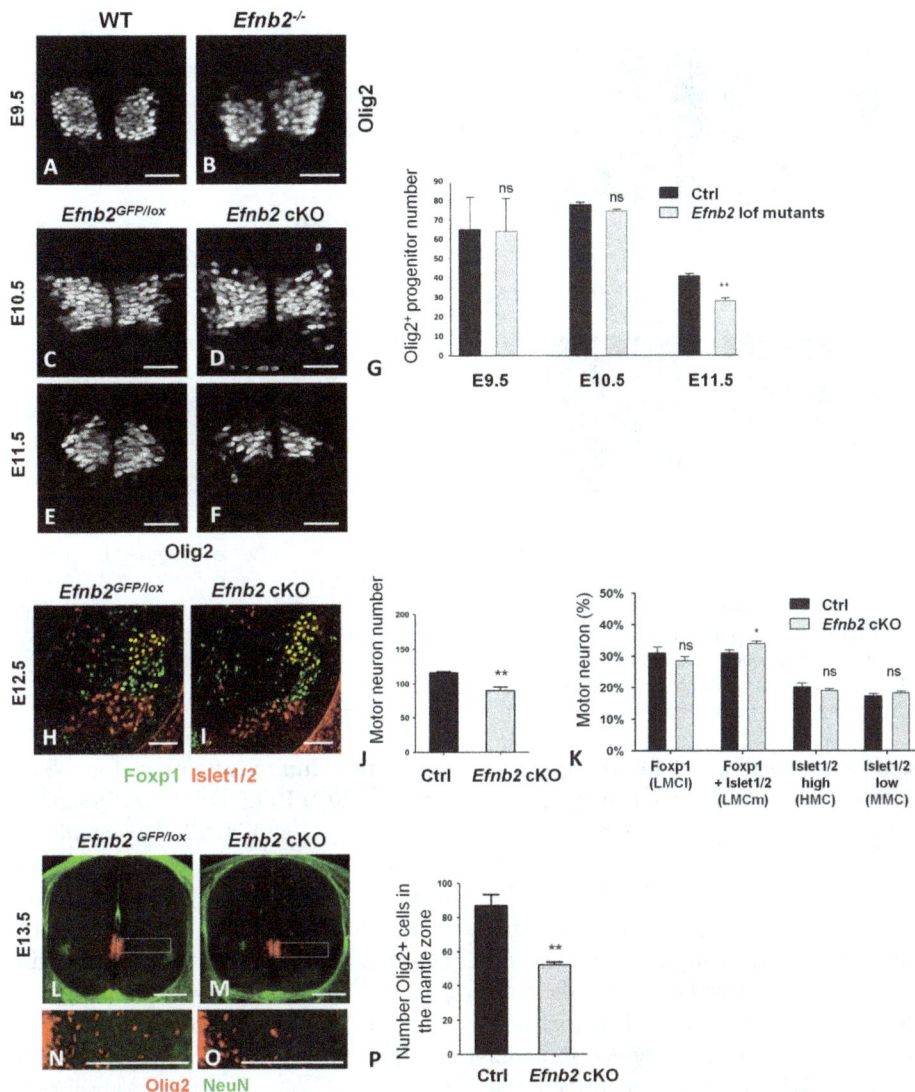

Fig. 3. EphrinB2 controls the number of pMN progenitors and their progeny. **a, b.** Transverse sections of wild type (**a**) and *Efnb2$^{-/-}$* (**b**) E9.5 embryos were immunostained to detect Olig2. **c, d.** Transverse sections of *Efnb2$^{lox/GFP}$* (**c**) and *Efnb2$^{lox/GFP}$;Olig2-Cre* (**d**) E10.5 embryos were immunostained to detect Olig2. **e, f.** Transverse sections of *Efnb2$^{lox/GFP}$* (**e**) and *Efnb2$^{lox/GFP}$;Olig2-Cre* (**f**) E11.5 embryos were immunostained to detect Olig2. **g.** The number of Olig2+ progenitors was quantified for all genotypes. Error bars indicate s.e.m. (*n*=3 embryos per genotype at E9.5; *n*=4 embryos per genotype at E10.5; *n*=5 embryos per genotype at E11.5); **$P<0.01$, ns= non significant (Mann-Whitney-Wilcoxon test). **h, i.** Transverse sections of E12.5 *Efnb2$^{lox/GFP}$* (**h**) and *Efnb2$^{lox/GFP}$; Olig2-Cre* (**i**) embryos were immunostained to detect Foxp1 (*green*) and Islet 1/2 (*red*). **j.** Quantification of the total number of motor neurons (Foxp1$^+$ and Islet 1/2$^+$) in both genotypes. **k.** Repartition of motor neurons in motor columns in both genotypes. Error bars indicate s.e.m. (*n*=6 embryos per group); *$P<0.05$; **$P<0.01$; ns= non significant (Mann-Whitney-Wilcoxon test). **l-o.** Transverse sections of E13.5 *Efnb2$^{lox/GFP}$* (**l, n**) and *Efnb2$^{lox/GFP}$; Olig2-Cre* (**m, o**) embryos were immunostained to detect Olig2 (*red*) and NeuN (*green*). **n, o** are zoomed areas indicated by a box in **m, n** respectively. **p.** Quantification of the total number of Olig2$^+$ cells in the mantle zone in both genotypes. Error bars indicate s.e.m. (*n*=4 embryos per group); **$P<0.01$ (Mann-Whitney-Wilcoxon test). Scale bars A-I: 50 μm; L-O: 200 μm.

between control and *Efnb2* cKO embryos (Fig. 4d, e, g). These results show that the reduction in pMN number in absence of ephrinB2 is not due to alteration in their rate of proliferation or differentiation.

An alternate possible cause for the decreased number of Olig2$^+$ progenitors at later stages of development could be that a fraction of progenitors wrongly acquire a non-pMN

identity after E9.5. To assess this possibility we quantified the number of Nkx2.2$^+$ progenitors in E11.5 *Efnb2* cKO embryos and observed that the decreased number of Olig2$^+$ progenitors was matched by an increased number of Nkx2.2$^+$ progenitors (Fig. 5a-c). Importantly, this was not due to an increase in the number of progenitors of mixed identity (expressing both iTFs) which was similar in

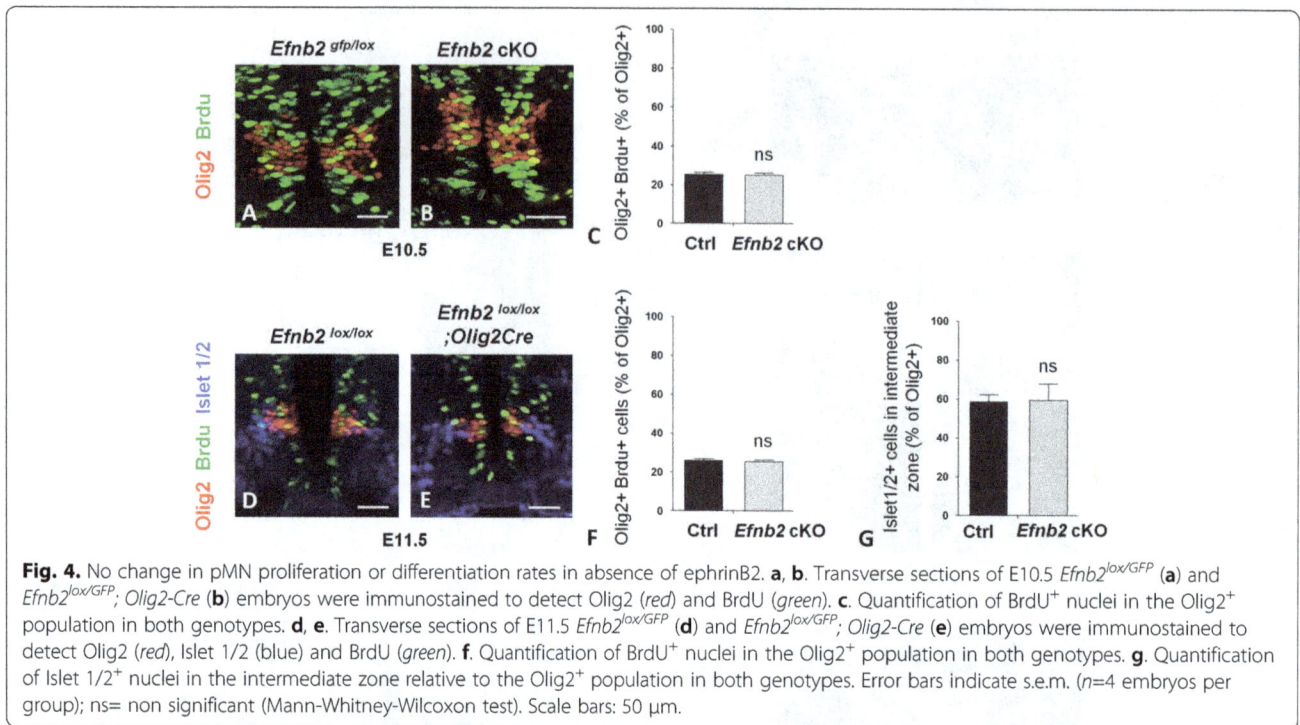

Fig. 4. No change in pMN proliferation or differentiation rates in absence of ephrinB2. **a, b**. Transverse sections of E10.5 $Efnb2^{lox/GFP}$ (**a**) and $Efnb2^{lox/GFP}$; Olig2-Cre (**b**) embryos were immunostained to detect Olig2 (red) and BrdU (green). **c**. Quantification of BrdU$^+$ nuclei in the Olig2$^+$ population in both genotypes. **d, e**. Transverse sections of E11.5 $Efnb2^{lox/GFP}$ (**d**) and $Efnb2^{lox/GFP}$; Olig2-Cre (**e**) embryos were immunostained to detect Olig2 (red), Islet 1/2 (blue) and BrdU (green). **f**. Quantification of BrdU$^+$ nuclei in the Olig2$^+$ population in both genotypes. **g**. Quantification of Islet 1/2$^+$ nuclei in the intermediate zone relative to the Olig2$^+$ population in both genotypes. Error bars indicate s.e.m. (n=4 embryos per group); ns= non significant (Mann-Whitney-Wilcoxon test). Scale bars: 50 μm.

control and *Efnb2* cKO embryos (Fig. 5c). Remarkably, the total number of pMN+p3 progenitors was also similar in control and *Efnb2* cKO embryos (Fig. 5a-c), strongly suggesting that in absence of ephrinB2, a fraction of progenitors wrongly acquire the p3 identity (Nkx2.2$^+$) at the expense of the pMN identity (Olig2$^+$). To challenge this interpretation, we tested for a potential genetic interaction between *Efnb2* and *Shh*, a key player in the specification of p3 and pMN identities [2]. First, we verified that *Shh* expression pattern was not changed in *Efnb2* mutants (Additional file 3: Figure S1). Next, we quantified the number of pMN and p3 progenitors in single *Efnb2* and *Shh* heterozygotes or in compound heterozygote embryos. While the number of Olig2$^+$ and Nkx2.2$^+$ progenitors in $Efnb2^{+/-}$ and $Shh^{+/-}$ heterozygous embryos was equivalent to wild type embryos, $Efnb2^{+/-}$; $Shh^{+/-}$ double heterozygous embryos exhibited a phenotype similar to *Efnb2* cKO embryos, with a decrease in Olig2$^+$ balanced by an increase in Nkx2.2$^+$ progenitors (Fig. 5d-h). These results establish that ephrinB2 and Shh interact genetically to control the ratio between pMN and p3 progenitors in the ventral spinal cord.

EphrinB3 inversely controls the ratio between pMN and p3 identities

The above data suggests that expression of ephrinB2 in pMN is required to impose the pMN identity (Olig2$^+$). As shown in Fig. 2, ephrinB3 is highly expressed in p3 progenitors (Fig. 2q-s). To test whether ephrinB3 plays a similar role in controlling p3 progenitor identity, we

performed immunostaining for Nkx2.2 and Olig2 in $Efnb3^{-/-}$ (KO) E11.5 embryos. Quantification of the number of Olig2$^+$ and Nkx2.2$^+$ progenitors showed that loss of *Efnb3* led to a decrease in the number of Nkx2.2$^+$ progenitors which was balanced by an increase in Olig2$^+$ progenitors (Fig. 6a-c). Importantly, the number of progenitors with a mixed identity and the total number of p3+pMN progenitors was unchanged in *Efnb3* KO compared to $Efnb3^{+/-}$ embryos (Fig. 6c), suggesting that a fraction of progenitors wrongly acquired the pMN at the expense of p3 identity in absence of ephrinB3. No change in progenitor numbers was observed at E9.5 (data not shown) and the increase in pMN number in *Efnb3* KO correlated with an increase in MN numbers (Additional file 3: Figure S2A-D). Interestingly, in addition to a change in the number of pMN and p3 progenitors, intermingling between these progenitors was observed in an increased fraction of sections from *Efnb3* KO compared to sections from $Efnb3^{+/-}$ embryos (Fig. 6b, d). To further quantify this phenotype, we measured surfaces encompassing all Olig2$^+$ or Nkx2.2$^+$ nuclei on multiple transverse sections of $Efnb3^{+/-}$ and *Efnb3* KO embryos and deduced their region of overlap (Fig. 6e, f). The surface of overlap between Olig2$^+$ and Nkx2.2$^+$ domains was increased in *Efnb3* KO compared to control embryos (Fig. 6e, f), confirming intermingling between Olig2$^+$ and Nkx2.2$^+$ progenitors in absence of ephrinB3. On the contrary, no overlap between Olig2$^+$ and Nkx2.2$^+$ domains was detected in *Efnb2* cKO (Additional file 3: Figure S3). Altogether,

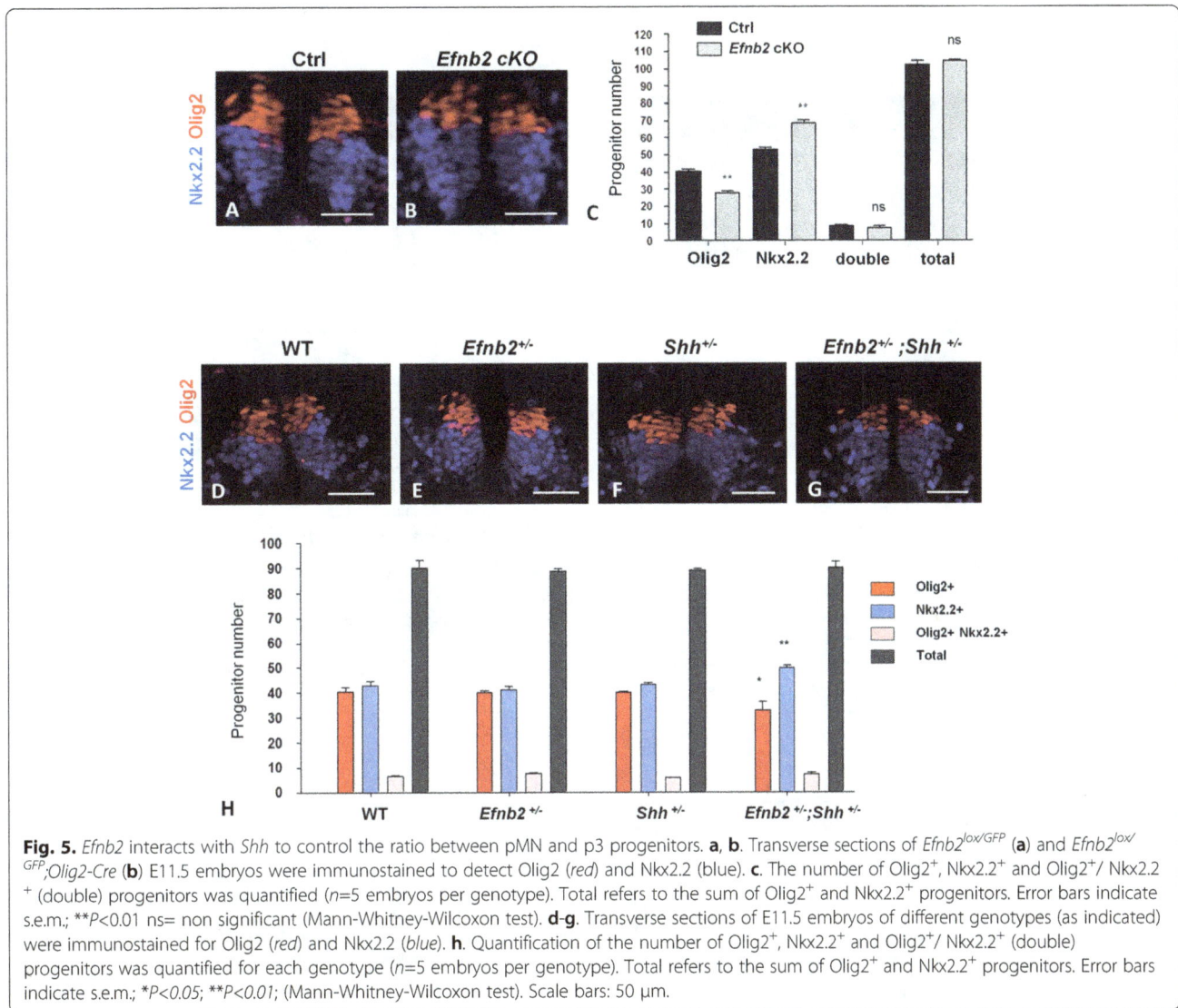

Fig. 5. *Efnb2* interacts with *Shh* to control the ratio between pMN and p3 progenitors. **a, b.** Transverse sections of *Efnb2^lox/GFP* (**a**) and *Efnb2^lox/GFP*;*Olig2-Cre* (**b**) E11.5 embryos were immunostained to detect Olig2 (*red*) and Nkx2.2 (blue). **c.** The number of Olig2$^+$, Nkx2.2$^+$ and Olig2$^+$/ Nkx2.2$^+$ (double) progenitors was quantified (*n*=5 embryos per genotype). Total refers to the sum of Olig2$^+$ and Nkx2.2$^+$ progenitors. Error bars indicate s.e.m.; **$P<0.01$ ns= non significant (Mann-Whitney-Wilcoxon test). **d-g.** Transverse sections of E11.5 embryos of different genotypes (as indicated) were immunostained for Olig2 (*red*) and Nkx2.2 (*blue*). **h.** Quantification of the number of Olig2$^+$, Nkx2.2$^+$ and Olig2$^+$/ Nkx2.2$^+$ (double) progenitors was quantified for each genotype (*n*=5 embryos per genotype). Total refers to the sum of Olig2$^+$ and Nkx2.2$^+$ progenitors. Error bars indicate s.e.m.; *$P<0.05$; **$P<0.01$; (Mann-Whitney-Wilcoxon test). Scale bars: 50 µm.

these results indicate that similar to ephrinB2, ephrinB3 is required to control the ratio between p3 and pMN progenitors and that in addition, ephrinB3 is required to maintain a sharp boundary between pMN and p3 progenitor domains.

Discussion

While early steps of ventral pMN specification have been extensively studied, highlighting the critical role of Shh, mechanisms that control the number of ventral progenitors over time are less well characterized. Here we show that Eph:ephrin signaling is required to precisely control the number of pMN (and p3) progenitors at late stages of development (after E9.5). It has been proposed previously that the modulation of p3 and pMN numbers after E9.5 is driven mainly by differentiation and/or proliferation, which vary over time and according to progenitor types [9]. Despite the fact that a number

of studies in the developing and adult cortex have shown a role for Eph:ephrinB signaling in controling the balance between proliferation and differentiation of neural progenitors in the cerebral cortex [18], our data unexpectedly show that changes in pMN progenitor numbers in ephrin mutants are not due to alterations of proliferation or differentiation rates.

Instead, our data indicate that ephrinB2 and ephrinB3 are respectively required to impose pMN and p3 identities at later stages of development (Fig. 7). What could be the underlying mechanisms? It has been shown previously that progenitor identity has to be actively maintained after initial specification. Indeed, mouse mutants in which Shh signaling is altered after ventral identities have been assigned exhibit a progressive loss of Olig2$^+$ progenitors (and to a lesser extend Nkx2.2$^+$ progenitors) indicating that continuous Shh signaling is required to maintain pMN (and p3) identity [4, 7, 8]. Maintenance

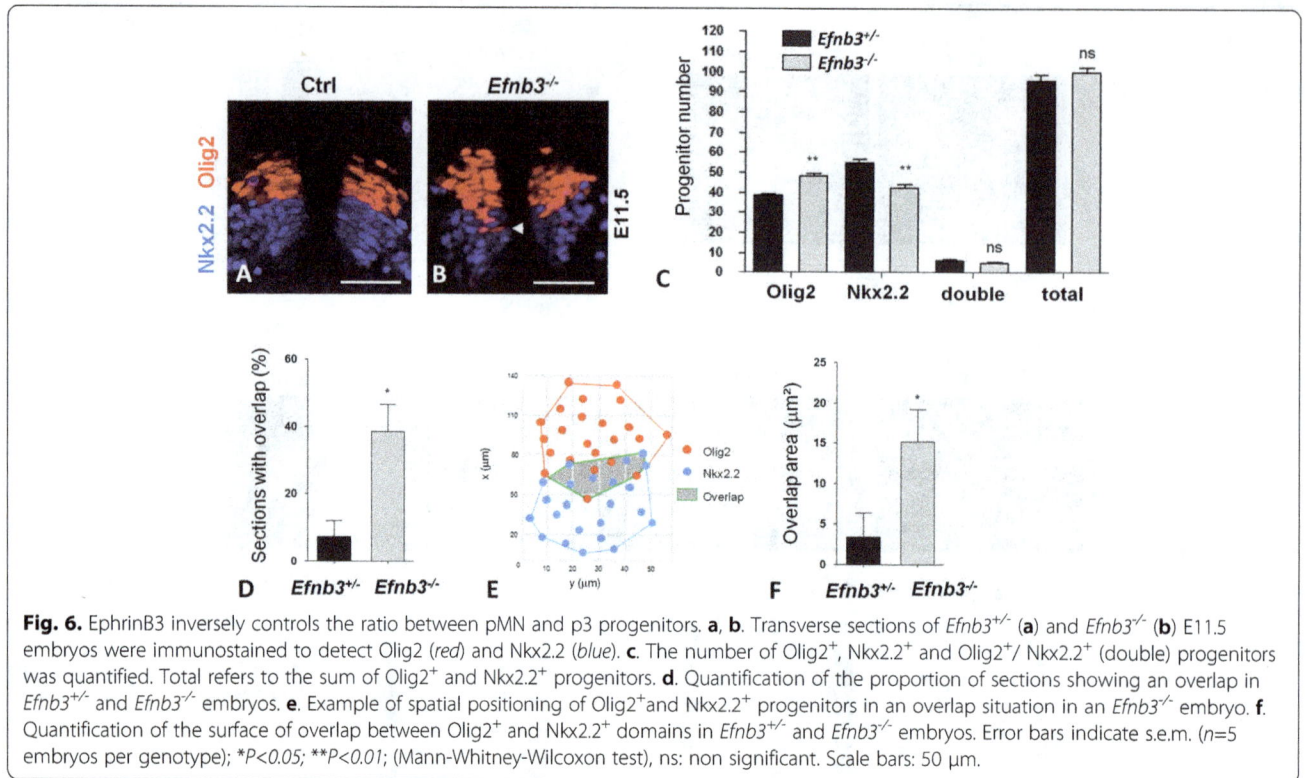

Fig. 6. EphrinB3 inversely controls the ratio between pMN and p3 progenitors. **a**, **b**. Transverse sections of *Efnb3⁺/⁻* (**a**) and *Efnb3⁻/⁻* (**b**) E11.5 embryos were immunostained to detect Olig2 (*red*) and Nkx2.2 (*blue*). **c**. The number of Olig2⁺, Nkx2.2⁺ and Olig2⁺/ Nkx2.2⁺ (double) progenitors was quantified. Total refers to the sum of Olig2⁺ and Nkx2.2⁺ progenitors. **d**. Quantification of the proportion of sections showing an overlap in *Efnb3⁺/⁻* and *Efnb3⁻/⁻* embryos. **e**. Example of spatial positioning of Olig2⁺and Nkx2.2⁺ progenitors in an overlap situation in an *Efnb3⁻/⁻* embryo. **f**. Quantification of the surface of overlap between Olig2⁺ and Nkx2.2⁺ domains in *Efnb3⁺/⁻* and *Efnb3⁻/⁻* embryos. Error bars indicate s.e.m. (*n*=5 embryos per genotype); *P<0.05; **P<0.01; (Mann-Whitney-Wilcoxon test), ns: non significant. Scale bars: 50 μm.

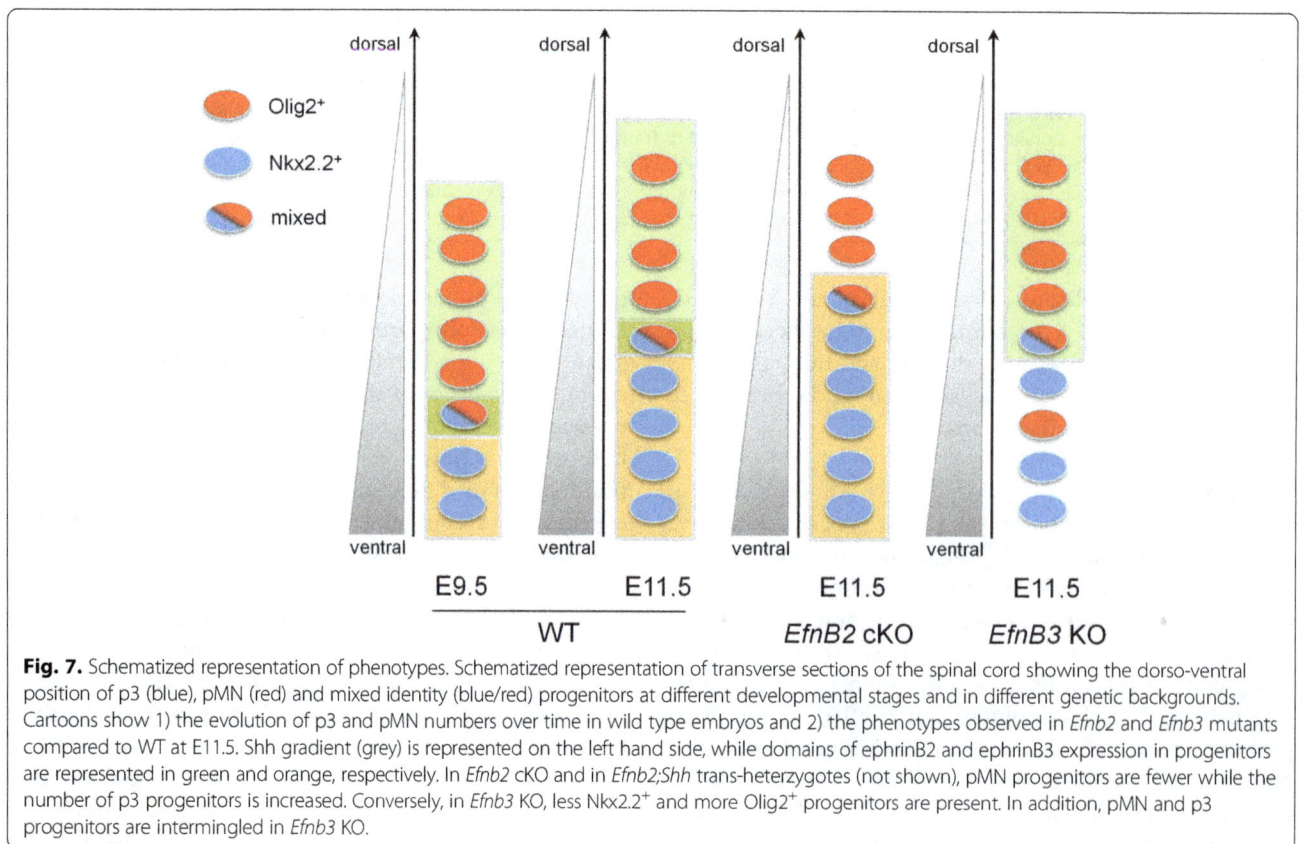

Fig. 7. Schematized representation of phenotypes. Schematized representation of transverse sections of the spinal cord showing the dorso-ventral position of p3 (blue), pMN (red) and mixed identity (blue/red) progenitors at different developmental stages and in different genetic backgrounds. Cartoons show 1) the evolution of p3 and pMN numbers over time in wild type embryos and 2) the phenotypes observed in *Efnb2* and *Efnb3* mutants compared to WT at E11.5. Shh gradient (grey) is represented on the left hand side, while domains of ephrinB2 and ephrinB3 expression in progenitors are represented in green and orange, respectively. In *Efnb2* cKO and in *Efnb2;Shh* trans-heterzygotes (not shown), pMN progenitors are fewer while the number of p3 progenitors is increased. Conversely, in *Efnb3* KO, less Nkx2.2⁺ and more Olig2⁺ progenitors are present. In addition, pMN and p3 progenitors are intermingled in *Efnb3* KO.

of identity could thus be one mechanism requiring co-operation between ephrins and Shh. However, we observed that the change in progenitor number in absence of ephrinB2 and ephrinB3 concerns only a small fraction of p3 and pMN progenitors, the majority of which maintain a correct identity in both ephrin mutants. An alternative possibility is thus that after E9.5, a fraction of progenitors requires cooperation between Shh and ephrins to commit to a specific fate. It is interesting to speculate that cells of mixed identity, which represent a small fraction of p3+pMN progenitors at all stages analyzed and are located close to the p3/pMN boundary, could be such a population susceptible to adopt one or the other identity depending on external signals. In cooperation with Shh signaling, EphrinB2 or ephrinB3 may tilt the balance in Olig2 and Nkx2.2 expression and due to the repressive regulatory loop between these iTFs, a shift in expression of one iTF would be amplified and result in commitment to a specific fate. In support to this, lineage tracing studies have shown that the majority of pMN progenitors derive from cells that transiently activate an enhancer for *Nkx2.2* supporting the notion that pMN and p3 progenitors share a common origin [12]. In addition, it has been shown that $Olig2^{-/-}$ embryos exhibit only a mild increase in the size of the $Nkx2.2^{+}$ domain [5], suggesting that only a small fraction of progenitors are competent to adopt a p3 fate even in complete absence of Olig2. Further, a similar shift in the ratio between $Nkx2.2^{+}$ and $Olig2^{+}$ progenitors has been described in $Tcf3^{-/-};Tcf4^{-/-}$ double mutants and this was linked to the role of Tcf3/4 in inhibiting Nkx2.2 expression in progenitors fated to become pMN [12]. Because Eph:ephrin signaling is a cell-to-cell signaling pathway, this function would be akin to the resolution of binary fates that has been described for Notch signaling in other neural contexts [28]. Of note, this role of ephrinB2 and ephrinB3 in progenitor identities is consistent with their expression patterns in pMN and p3 progenitors, respectively. However, ventral progenitors are in contact with newly generated neurons which also express ephrinB2 and ephrinB3, it is thus possible that the neuronal expression of these ligands may also contribute to maintain a correct ratio between p3 and pMN identities.

As a consequence of these changes in progenitor identities, *Efnb2* and *Efnb3* mutants exhibit opposite alterations in MN numbers at E12.5. It would be interesting to assess whether these changes are still present postnatally, however, postnatal changes in MN number may be due to distinct mechanisms, for instance a decrease in MN number associated with cell death at later stages than those analyzed here has been described in $EphA4^{-/-}$ mutants [29].

Traditionally, the role of Eph:ephrin signaling in specification processes has been linked to its function in boundary maintenance. For instance, a recent study has shown that loss of ephrinB2 in the developing cochlea leads to a switch in cell identity from supporting cell to hair cell fate and this was attributed to the mis-positioning of supporting cells into the hair cell layer [30]. No mis-positioning of p3 and pMN progenitors was observed in the *Efnb2* cKO mutants analyzed here. Whether excision of *Efnb2* in all neural tube progenitors would lead to a similar phenotype remains an open question. Here, we observed mis-positioning of progenitors only in ephrinB3 mutants although both ephrinB2 and ephrinB3 mutants exhibited changes in p3 and pMN progenitor ratio, indicating that resolution of identity is independent of mis-positioning. This is consistent with a growing number of published studies reporting a role for Eph:ephrin signaling in lineage commitment or cell fate maintenance via the modulation of intracellular signal transduction pathways and gene expression, independently of cell sorting at boundaries [31–36]. Another possibility, consistent with the genetic interaction between *Efnb2* and *Shh*, could be that ephrins impact on Shh signal transduction cascade as was recently described for Notch [37, 38]. In fact, genetic interaction between Shh and cell surface proteins has been reported previously and such studies identified Gas1, Cdo and Boc as components of the Shh signaling pathway [7, 39, 40]. In this context, it would be interesting to test for a genetic interaction between *Efnb3* and *Shh* in the control of p3 and pMN progenitor identity and positioning.

Conclusions

In conclusion, our study shows that ephrinB2 and ephrinB3 are required to control progenitor identities in the ventral spinal cord and suggests a role for Eph:ephrin signaling in refining morphogen-dependent tissue patterning.

Abbreviations

cKO: Conditional knock-out; h: Hour; kg: Kilogram; KO: Knock-out; mg: Milligram; ml: Milliliter; MN: Motor neurons; OLP: Oligodendrocyte precursors; Shh: Sonic hedgehog; WT: Wild type; μm: Micrometer

Acknowledgements

The Islet 1/2 antibody was obtained from the Developmental Studies Hybridoma Bank developed under the auspices of the NICHD and maintained by the University of Iowa, Iowa City, IA 52242. We thank Dr Novitch for sharing the *Olig2-Cre* mice. Dr Kania and Dr Henkemeyer provided some molecular reagents used in this study. We are grateful to Brice Ronsin for his help with confocal microscopy (TRI Imaging Core Facility) and to Marion Aguirrebengoa for her help with statistical analyses. We thank the ABC facility and ANEXPLO for housing mice. We are grateful for Sylvain Touret's help for writing the R code. We thank Eric Agius, Serge Plaza and Alain Vincent for critical reading of the manuscript.

Funding
Research in the Davy team is financed by the CNRS, by the Fondation ARC and by ANR (ANR-15-CE13-0010-01). JL received support from the French Ministère de l'Enseignement Supérieur et de la Recherche and from the Fondation pour la Recherche Médicale (FDT20140931010). DJL is funded by the Miami Project to Cure Paralysis and PAN by NIH/NINDS (NS089325).

Authors' contributions
JL planned, performed and analyzed experiments, and he participated in writing the manuscript; AK, CA and NE performed experiments; PA and DL collected and provided mutant embryos and revised the manuscript; CS provided scientific input on the project and revised the manuscript; AD supervised the project, planned the experiments, analyzed the data and wrote the manuscript. All authors read and approved the final manuscript.

Competing interests
The authors declare no conflict of interest.

Author details
[1]Centre de Biologie du Développement (CBD), Centre de Biologie Intégrative (CBI), Université de Toulouse, CNRS, UPS, 118 Route de Narbonne, 31062 Toulouse, France. [2]Present address: CRBM, 1919 route de Mende, 34293 Montpellier, France. [3]University of Miami Miller School of Medicine, The Miami Project to Cure Paralysis, 1095 NW 14th Terrace, Miami, FL R-48, USA.

References
1. Briscoe J, Novitch BG. *Regulatory pathways linking progenitor patterning, cell fates and neurogenesis in the ventral neural tube.* Philos Trans R Soc Lond B Biol Sci. 2008;**363**:57–70.
2. Dessaud E, McMahon AP, Briscoe J. *Pattern formation in the vertebrate neural tube: a sonic hedgehog morphogen-regulated transcriptional network.* Development. 2008;**135**:2489–503.
3. Dessaud E, et al. *Interpretation of the sonic hedgehog morphogen gradient by a temporal adaptation mechanism.* Nature. 2007;**450**(7170):717–20.
4. Dessaud E, et al. *Dynamic assignment and maintenance of positional identity in the ventral neural tube by the morphogen sonic hedgehog.* PLoS Biol. 2010;**8**(6):e1000382.
5. Balaskas N, et al. *Gene regulatory logic for reading the Sonic Hedgehog signaling gradient in the vertebrate neural tube.* Cell. 2012;**148**:273–84.
6. Cohen M, Briscoe J, Blassberg R. *Morphogen interpretation: the transcriptional logic of neural tube patterning.* Curr Opin Genet Dev. 2013;**23**(4):423–8.
7. Allen BL, Tenzen T, McMahon AP. *The Hedgehog-binding proteins Gas1 and Cdo cooperate to positively regulate Shh signaling during mouse development.* Genes Dev. 2007;**21**(10):1244–57.
8. Allen BL, et al. *Overlapping roles and collective requirement for the coreceptors GAS1, CDO, and BOC in SHH pathway function.* Dev Cell. 2011;**20**(6):775–87.
9. Kicheva A, et al. *Coordination of progenitor specification and growth in mouse and chick spinal cord.* Science. 2014;**345**(6204):1254927.

10. Wijgerde M, et al. *A direct requirement for Hedgehog signaling for normal specification of all ventral progenitor domains in the presumptive mammalian spinal cord.* Genes Dev. 2002;**16**:2849–64.
11. Lei Q, et al. *Transduction of graded Hedgehog signaling by a combination of Gli2 and Gli3 activator functions in the developing spinal cord.* Development. 2004;**131**:3593–604.
12. Wang H, et al. *Tcf/Lef repressors differentially regulate Shh-Gli target gene activation thresholds to generate progenitor patterning in the developing CNS.* Development. 2011;**138**:3711–21.
13. Xiong F, et al. *Specified neural progenitors sort to form sharp domains after noisy Shh signaling.* Cell. 2013;**153**:550–61.
14. Lisabeth EM, Falivelli G, Pasquale EB. *Eph Receptor Signaling and Ephrins.* Cold Spring Harb Perspect Biol. 2013;**5**:a009159.
15. Kania, A. and R. Klein, *Mechanisms of ephrin-Eph signalling in development, physiology and disease.* Nat Rev Mol Cell Biol. 2016;**17**:240–56.
16. Fagotto F, Winklbauer R, Rohani N. *Ephrin-Eph signaling in embryonic tissue separation.* Cell Adh Migr. 2014;**8**(4):308–26.
17. Cayuso, J., Q. Xu, and D.G. Wilkinson, *Mechanisms of boundary formation by Eph receptor and ephrin signaling.* Dev Biol. 2015;**401**:122–31.
18. Laussu J, et al. *Beyond boundaries: Eph/ephrin signaling in neurogenesis.* Cell Adh Migr. 2014;**8**:349–59.
19. Kao TJ, Kania A. *Ephrin-mediated cis-attenuation of Eph receptor signaling is essential for spinal motor axon guidance.* Neuron. 2011;**71**:76–91.
20. Luxey M, et al. *Eph/ephrin-B1 forward signaling controls fasciculation of motor and sensory axons.* Dev. Biol. 2013;**383**:264–74.
21. Luxey M, Laussu J, Davy A. *EphrinB2 sharpens lateral motor column division in the developing spinal cord.* Neural Dev. 2015;**10**:25.
22. Davy A, Soriano P. *Ephrin-B2 forward signaling regulates somite patterning and neural crest cell development.* Dev. Biol. 2007;**304**:182–93.
23. Grunwald IC, et al. *Hippocampal plasticity requires postsynaptic ephrinBs.* Nat. Neurosci. 2004;**7**:33–40.
24. Yokoyama N, et al. *Forward signaling mediated by ephrin-B3 prevents contralateral corticospinal axons from recrossing the spinal cord midline.* Neuron. 2001;**29**:85–97.
25. Schindelin J, et al. *Fiji: an open-source platform for biological-image analysis.* Nat Methods. 2012;**9**(7):676–82.
26. Adams RH, et al. *Roles of ephrinB ligands and EphB receptors in cardiovascular development: demarcation of arterial/venous domains, vascular morphogenesis, and sprouting angiogenesis.* Genes Dev. 1998;**13**:295–306.
27. Wang HU, Chen Z-F, Anderson DJ. *Molecular distinction and angiogenic interaction between embryonic arteries and veins revealed by ephrin-B2 and its receptor eph-B4.* Cell. 1998;**93**:741–53.
28. Cau E, Blader P. *Notch activity in the nervous system: to switch or not to switch?* Neural Dev. 2009;**4**:36.
29. Helmbacher F, et al. *Targeting of the EphA4 tyrosine kinase receptor affects dorsal/ventral pathfinding of limb motor axons.* Development. 2000;**127**:3313–24.
30. Defourny J, et al. *Cochlear supporting cell transdifferentiation and integration into hair cell layers by inhibition of ephrin-B2 signalling.* Nat Commun. 2015;**6**:7017.
31. Picco V, Hudson C, Yasuo H. *Ephrin-Eph signalling drives the asymmetric division of notochord/neural precursors in Ciona embryos.* Development. 2007;**134**:1491–7.
32. Stolfi A, et al. *Neural tube patterning by Ephrin, FGF and Notch signaling relays.* Development. 2011;**138**:5429–39.
33. Ashton RS, et al. *Astrocytes regulate adult hippocampal neurogenesis through ephrin-B signaling.* Nat. Neurosci. 2012;**15**:1399–407.
34. Haupaix N, et al. *p120RasGAP mediates ephrin/Eph-dependent attenuation of FGF/ERK signals during cell fate specification in ascidian embryos.* Development. 2013;**140**:4347–52.
35. Ottone C, et al. *Direct cell-cell contact with the vascular niche maintains quiescent neural stem cells.* Nat Cell Biol. 2014;**16**(11):1045–56.
36. Chen S, et al. *Interrogating cellular fate decisions with high-throughput arrays of multiplexed cellular communities.* Nat Commun. 2016;**7**:10309.
37. Stasiulewicz, M., et al., *A conserved role for Notch in priming the cellular response to Shh through ciliary localisation of the key Shh transducer, Smoothened.* Development. 2015.
38. Kong JH, et al. *Notch activity modulates the responsiveness of neural progenitors to sonic hedgehog signaling.* Dev Cell. 2015;**33**(4):373–87.
39. Martinelli DC, Fan CM. *Gas1 extends the range of Hedgehog action by facilitating its signaling.* Genes Dev. 2007;**21**:1231–43.
40. Tenzen T, et al. *The cell surface membrane proteins Cdo and Boc are components and targets of the Hedgehog signaling pathway and feedback network in mice.* Dev Cell. 2006;**10**:647–56.

14

Region-specific role of growth differentiation factor-5 in the establishment of sympathetic innervation

Gerard W. O'Keeffe[1,2†], Humberto Gutierrez[1,3†], Laura Howard[1†], Christopher W. Laurie[1†], Catarina Osorio[1,4], Núria Gavaldà[1,5], Sean L. Wyatt[1] and Alun M. Davies[1*]

Abstract

Background: Nerve growth factor (NGF) is the prototypical target-derived neurotrophic factor required for sympathetic neuron survival and for the growth and ramification of sympathetic axons within most but not all sympathetic targets. This implies the operation of additional target-derived factors for regulating terminal sympathetic axon growth and branching.

Results: Here report that growth differentiation factor 5 (GDF5), a widely expressed member of the transforming growth factor beta (TGFβ) superfamily required for limb development, promoted axon growth from mouse superior cervical ganglion (SCG) neurons independently of NGF and enhanced axon growth in combination with NGF. GDF5 had no effect on neuronal survival and influenced axon growth during a narrow window of postnatal development when sympathetic axons are ramifying extensively in their targets in vivo. SCG neurons expressed all receptors capable of participating in GDF5 signaling at this stage of development. Using compartment cultures, we demonstrated that GDF5 exerted its growth promoting effect by acting directly on axons and by initiating retrograde canonical Smad signalling to the nucleus. GDF5 is synthesized in sympathetic targets, and examination of several anatomically circumscribed tissues in *Gdf5* null mice revealed regional deficits in sympathetic innervation. There was a marked, highly significant reduction in the sympathetic innervation density of the iris, a smaller though significant reduction in the trachea, but no reduction in the submandibular salivary gland. There was no reduction in the number of neurons in the SCG.

Conclusions: These findings show that GDF5 is a novel target-derived factor that promotes sympathetic axon growth and branching and makes a distinctive regional contribution to the establishment of sympathetic innervation, but unlike NGF, plays no role in regulating sympathetic neuron survival.

Keywords: Sympathetic neuron, Axon growth, Innervation, GDF5

Background

Nerve growth factor (NGF) is the prototypical target-derived neurotrophic factor on which the foundations of neurotrophic theory are based [1]. In the developing peripheral nervous system, postganglionic sympathetic neurons and the majority of sensory neurons depend for their survival on a supply of NGF synthesized in their targets [2, 3]. While target-derived NGF plays no role in guiding axons to their targets during development [4], it acts locally on axon terminals within the target field to promote growth and branching within most but not all targets of NGF dependent neurons [5, 6]. This implies the operation of additional target-derived factors that regulate the terminal growth and branching of axons of NGF-dependent neurons in certain target tiisues.

Here we report that growth differentiation factor-5 (GDF5), a widely expressed member of the bone morphogenetic protein/growth differentiation factor (BMP/GDF) family which constitutes a collection of closely related proteins within the TGFβ superfamily [7], is a

---

* Correspondence: daviesalun@cf.ac.uk
†Equal contributors
[1]School of Biosciences, Cardiff University, Museum Avenue, Cardiff CF10 3AT, UK
Full list of author information is available at the end of the article

novel regulator of sympathetic axon growth, acting during the stage in development when the axon terminals of NGF-dependent sympathetic neurons of the superior cervical ganglion (SCG) neurons are growing and branching extensively in their targets in vivo. GDF5 has extensively characterized roles in chondrogenesis, joint formation, skeletal, tendon and ligament morphogenesis [8–10]. Several reports have also implicated GDF5 in neuronal development. GDF5 enhances the survival of embryonic midbrain dopaminergic neurons and promotes neurite outgrowth from these neurons in vitro [11, 12], it promotes the growth and elaboration of pyramidal cell dendrites in the embryonic hippocampus both in vitro and in vivo [13] and has a minor survival-promoting action on embryonic chicken dorsal root ganglion (DRG) neurons in vitro [14]. Here we report and characterize novel, physiologically relevant functions for GDF5 in sympathetic neuron development. We show that GDF5 promotes the growth and branching of sympathetic axons during a narrow window of postnatal development and functions as a novel target-derived regulator of sympathetic innervation in vivo that makes a distinctive regional contribution to the establishment of sympathetic innervation.

Results
GDF5 enhances neurite growth and branching from neonatal SCG neurons
GDF5 increased the size of the neurite arbors of newborn mouse (P0) SCG neurons cultured at low density in defined medium. It enhanced neurite arbor size of neurons cultured with saturating concentrations of NGF and promoted neurite growth from neurons cultured without NGF in medium containing the broad-spectrum caspase inhibitor Boc-D-FMK to prevent apoptosis of the neurons in the absence of NGF (Fig. 1a). Analysis of the neurite arbors of large numbers of neurons showed that GDF5 promoted highly significant increases in overall neurite length and the number of branch points in both the presence and absence of NGF (Fig. 1b). Dose response analysis revealed that the neurite growth-promoting effect of GDF5 reached saturation at 10 ng/ml (Fig. 1c).

Analysis of the influence of GDF5 on SCG neurons in cultures established over a range of ages revealed that the neurite growth enhancing effect of GDF5 was restricted to a narrow developmental window in the immediate postnatal period. Sholl analysis, which provides a graphic illustration of neurite length and branching with distance from the cell body, showed that the effect of GDF5 on neurite growth and branching was evident at P0 and P1 but not before or after this period (Fig. 1d). This contrasts with the neurite growth promoting effect of NGF, which is evident from the time the earliest

sympathetic axons reach their targets to well after the phase of programmed cell death [15–17]. In marked contrast to NGF, which promotes the survival of SCG neurons in addition to promoting neurite growth, GDF5 did not promote the survival of SCG neurons on its own and did not increase the number of neurons surviving with NGF (Fig. 1e). These results show that GDF5 enhances neurite growth from sympathetic neurons independently of NGF without affecting neuronal survival.

Because the neurites in short-term SCG cultures are exclusively axons [18], confirmed by absence of dendrite markers in SCG neurons cultured with or without GDF5 for 24 h (not shown), our findings suggest that GDF5 promotes axon growth and branching from SCG neurons independently of NGF without affecting neuronal survival over a narrow developmental window during the period when sympathetic axon terminals are growing and branching within their targets.

GDF5 acts locally on axon terminals to promote axon growth
To determine if, like NGF, GDF5 is capable of acting locally on axons to promote their growth, we cultured these neurons in microfluidic devices in which the cell bodies and axon terminals are grown in separate compartments (Fig. 2a). P0 SCG neurons were seeded into one compartment of a two-compartment device that contained NGF in both compartments. After 24 h incubation, maximal axon length in the axon compartment was quantified. Whereas supplementation of the axon compartment by GDF5 caused a highly significant increase in axon length compared to NGF alone, supplementation of the soma compartment by GDF5 did not enhance axon length compared to NGF alone (Fig. 2b-e). It was also clearly evident that addition of GDF5 to the axon compartment, but not the soma compartment, increased neurite density in the axon compartment (Fig. 2b-d). These data show that GDF5 acting locally on sympathetic axons, but not on neuronal soma, significantly increases axon growth

Expression of GDF5 receptors on developing SCG neurons
Members of the BMP/GDF family mediate their actions via a heterodimeric complex of type I and type II serine-threonine kinase receptors [19]. Among type I receptors, GDF5 binds most efficiently to BMPR1B expressed alone on cell lines but binds weakly to BMPR1A when co-expressed with ACVR2A (ActRII). Receptor reconstitution experiments in Mv1Lu epithelial cells have shown that GDF5 is able to transduce a signal via BMPR1B in combination with either ACVR2A or BMPR2 (BMPRII), but is also able to signal somewhat less effectively via BMPR1A in combination with ACVR2A [20].

Transcripts encoding BMPR1B, BMPR2, BMPR1A and ACVR2A were expressed in the developing SCG from

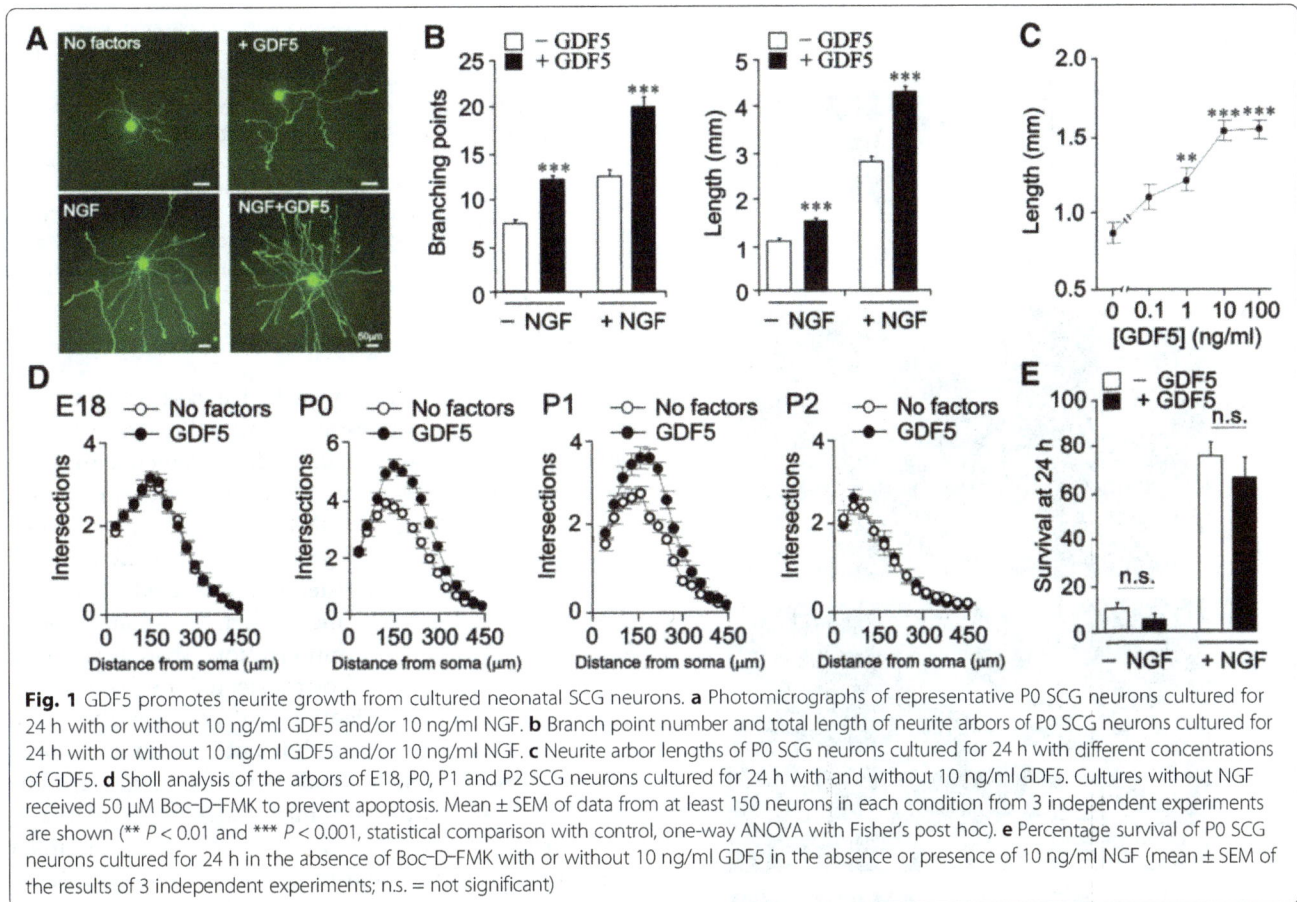

Fig. 1 GDF5 promotes neurite growth from cultured neonatal SCG neurons. **a** Photomicrographs of representative P0 SCG neurons cultured for 24 h with or without 10 ng/ml GDF5 and/or 10 ng/ml NGF. **b** Branch point number and total length of neurite arbors of P0 SCG neurons cultured for 24 h with or without 10 ng/ml GDF5 and/or 10 ng/ml NGF. **c** Neurite arbor lengths of P0 SCG neurons cultured for 24 h with different concentrations of GDF5. **d** Sholl analysis of the arbors of E18, P0, P1 and P2 SCG neurons cultured for 24 h with and without 10 ng/ml GDF5. Cultures without NGF received 50 μM Boc-D-FMK to prevent apoptosis. Mean ± SEM of data from at least 150 neurons in each condition from 3 independent experiments are shown (** $P < 0.01$ and *** $P < 0.001$, statistical comparison with control, one-way ANOVA with Fisher's post hoc). **e** Percentage survival of P0 SCG neurons cultured for 24 h in the absence of Boc-D-FMK with or without 10 ng/ml GDF5 in the absence or presence of 10 ng/ml NGF (mean ± SEM of the results of 3 independent experiments; n.s. = not significant)

E14 to at least P10, which spans the period over which SCG axons first reach their target tissues and sympathetic innervation is established. The expression profiles for *Bmpr1a* mRNA and *Acvr2a* mRNA (Fig. 3a) and *Bmpr1b* mRNA and *Bmpr2* mRNA (Fig. 3b) showed an overall small decrease from E14 to P10.

Immunocytochemistry revealed that antibodies to each receptor stained the neurites of virtually all P0 SCG neurons in culture (Fig. 3c to f). Cultures incubated with secondary antibody alone exhibited no background immunofluorescence (not shown). These studies suggest that receptor complexes containing BMPR1B and/or BMPR1A are available for mediating the neurite growth-promoting effects of GDF5.

GDF5 promotes retrograde canonical Smad signalling along SCG axons

In common with other members of the BMP/GDF family, GDF5 activates canonical Smad 1/5/8 signaling [21], which is required for GDF5 responsiveness in neurons [13]. To ascertain whether GDF5 could initiate retrograde Smad signaling to the nucleus, we first confirmed that GDF5 is able to activate Smads 1/5/8 in SCG neurons. Western blot analysis showed that GDF5 increased

Smad 1/5/8 phosphorylation in P0 SCG neurons as early as 5 minutes after GDF5 treatment (Fig. 4a). Immunocytochemistry using an antibody that recognizes phospho-Smad1/5/8 revealed that GDF5 promoted rapid nuclear accumulation of phospho-Smad1/5/8 in dissociated cultures of SCG neurons (Fig. 4b and c).

To assess retrograde Smad signaling, P0 SCG neurons were incubated for 12 h in compartment cultures containing NGF in both compartments before GDF5 was added to the axon compartment. After an hour, calcein-AM was added to the axon compartment to identify neurons with axons projecting into this compartment. The cultures were then fixed and stained for nuclear phospho-Smad-1/5/8. GDF5 treatment of sympathetic axons resulted in a highly significant increase in nuclear phospho-Smad1/5 immunoreactivity in neurons that projected axons into the axon compartment, but not in those neurons whose axons did not cross into this compartment (Fig. 4d and e). This demonstrates that GDF5 acting on sympathetic axons induced retrograde canonical Smad signaling along these axons, leading to nuclear accumulation of phospho-Smad proteins.

To test directly the importance of GDF5 receptor-dependent Smad activation and Smad-dependent gene

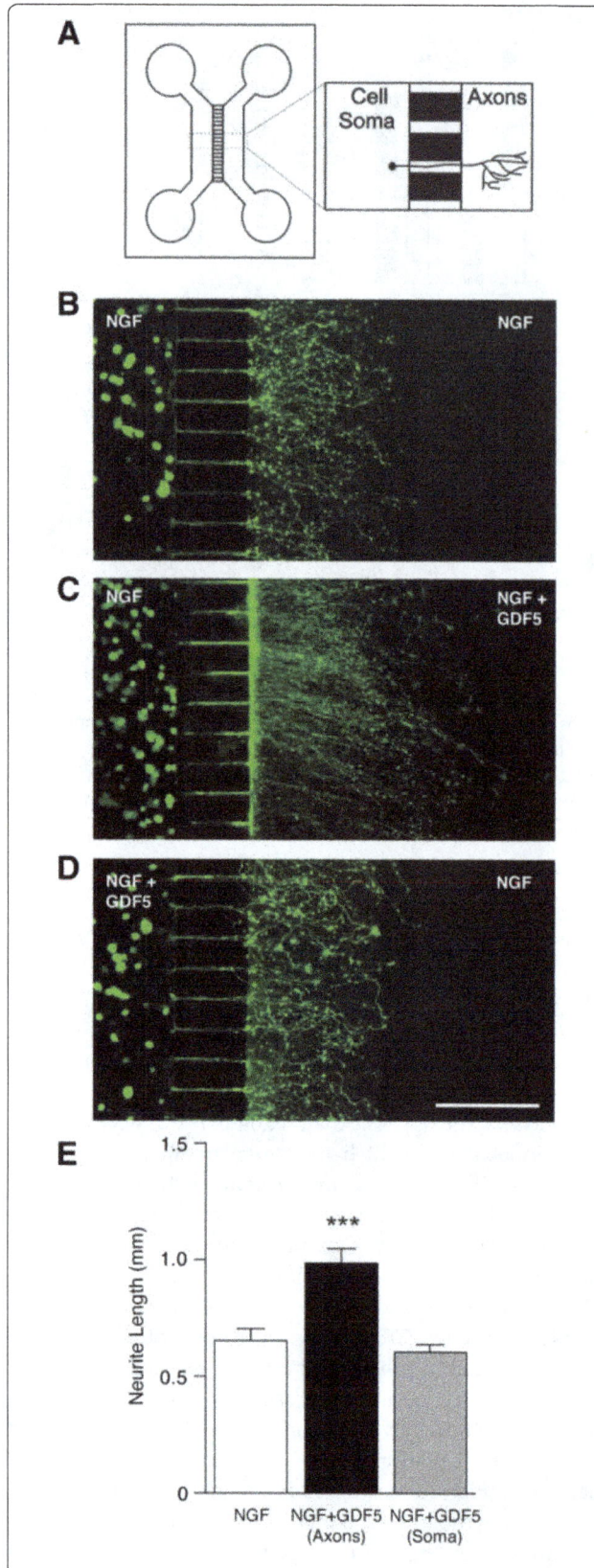

Fig. 2 GDF5 acts locally on axon terminals to promote axon growth. **a** Schematic illustration of the two-chamber microfluidic device. The inset shows a neuron with its cell body in the soma compartment on the left extending its axon arbor through a microchannel into the axon compartment on the right. **b-d** Photomicrographs of representative P0 SCG neurons cultured in defined medium for 24 h with 10 ng/ml NGF in both compartments (**b**), NGF in both compartments plus 10 ng/ml GDF5 in the axonal compartment (**c**) and NGF in both compartments plus 10 ng/ml GDF5 in the soma compartment (**d**). Scale bar = 200 μm. **e** Bar chart of axon length measurements in the axon compartment (*** $P < 0.0001$, statistical comparison with NGF alone, ANOVA)

transcription on neurite growth, we co-transfected P0 SCG neurons with a reporter construct in which GFP is under the control of Smad binding elements together with either a pcDNA plasmid that expresses a constitutively active BMPR-IB (caBMPR-IB) [22] or an empty pcDNA control plasmid. Quantification of the reporter signal 24 h after transfection revealed that the caBMPR-IB promoted a highly significant increase in Smad-dependent gene transcription that was completely prevented by a co-transfected decoy double-stranded DNA-oligonucleotide that contains the Smad consensus binding sequence but not by a control oligonucleotide with a scrambled sequence (Fig. 5a). The caBMPR-IB also promoted highly significant increases in neurite length (Fig. 5b), branch point number (Fig. 5c) and overall neurite arbor size and complexity (Fig. 5d and e) that were completely prevented by the Smad oligonucleotide decoy but not by the control oligonucleotide. There were no significant differences in the length and branching of the neurite arbors of neurons transfected with the control plasmid plus either decoy DNA or scrambled DNA (Fig. 5b-c).

GDF5 plays a distinctive role in establishing sympathetic innervation in vivo

To ascertain whether the increase in sympathetic axon growth and branching brought about by GDF5 in vitro contributes to the establishment of sympathetic innervation in vivo, we used tyrosine hydroxylase immunofluorescence to identify sympathetic fibers and quantify sympathetic innervation density in wild type mice and mice that are either heterozygous or homozygous for the $Gdf5^{bp}$ null mutation, a frame-shift mutation in the $Gdf5$ gene [23]. For this analysis, we studied the submandibular salivary gland, trachea and iris. While the terminal growth and branching of sympathetic axons in the submandibular salivary gland is dependent on NGF, the terminal ramification of sympathetic axons in the trachea occurs independently of NGF [5]. Our analysis was carried out at P10, which is after the period of development when GDF5 enhances neurite growth in vitro and is at a

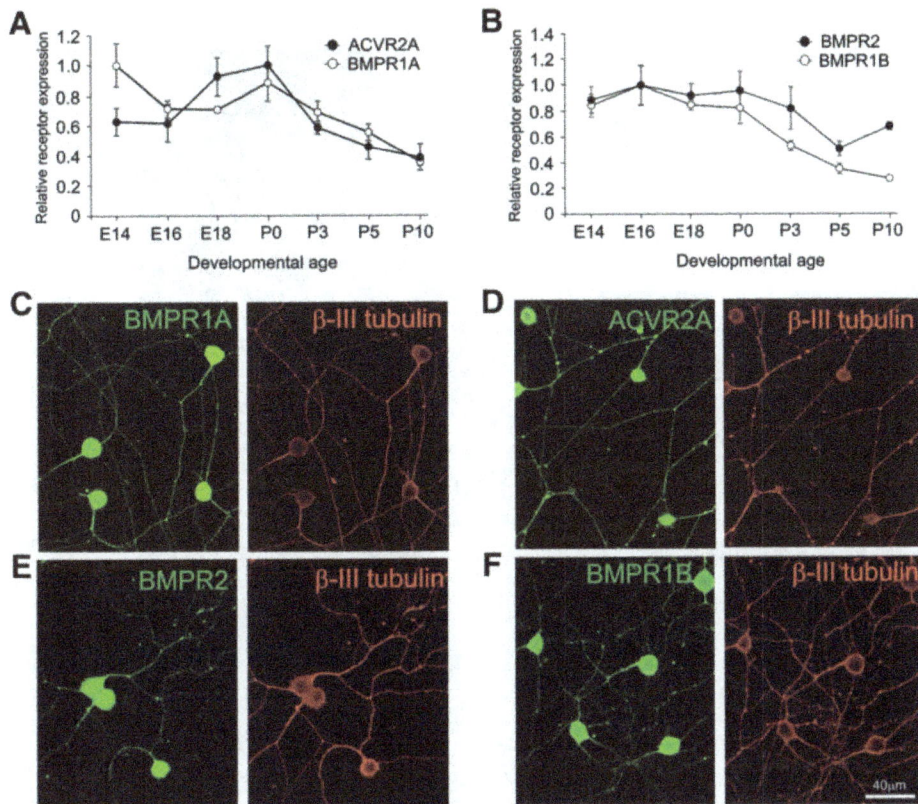

Fig. 3 Expression of GDF5 receptors. **a, b** Expression of transcripts encoding GDF5 receptors in the SCG at stages from E14 to P10 relative to the geometric mean of *Gapdh*, *Sdha* and *Hprt1* reference mRNAs (mean ± SEM, n = 3 per age). **a** Relative levels of *Bmpr1a* and *Acvr2a* mRNAs normalised to the peak of expression at E14 and P0, respectively. **b** Relative levels of *Bmpr1b* and *Bmpr2* mRNAs normalised to the peak of expression at E16. **c to f** Photomicrographs of representative P0 SCG neurons cultured for 24 h with NGF and double labelled for β-III tubulin and either BMPR1A (**c**), ACVR2A (**d**), BMPR2 (**e**) or BMPR1B (**f**). Scale bar = 40 μm

stage in vivo when the sympathetic innervation of these tissues has become well established.

Quantification of tyrosine hydroxylase immunofluorescence in tissue sections revealed marked, highly significant reductions in the iris of heterozygous and homozygous mice compared with wild type mice (Fig. 6a). The level of tyrosine hydroxylase immunoreactivity in the irides of heterozygous mice was intermediate between that of wild type and homozygous mice, indicative of a gene dosage effect. There was no significant reduction in the level of tyrosine hydroxylase immunoreactivity in the submandibular salivary gland of *Gdf5*[bp] mice compared with wild type mice (Fig. 6b). Because there are fewer sympathetic fibers in the trachea, we assessed innervation density by quantifying the density of tyrosine-hydroxylase-positive fibers in cleared whole-mount tissue preparations. This analysis revealed a statistically significant reduction in tyrosine hydroxylase-positive nerve fiber density in *Gdf5*[bp] mice compared with wild type mice (Fig. 6c). Figure 6d illustrates representative tyrosine hydroxylase-immunolabeled sections through the

irides of wild type mice and *Gdf5*[bp] mice, illustrating the clear decrease in sympathetic innervation density in the latter. To determine the site of GDF5 expression and to ascertain its relation to sympathetic fibers in the iris, we double labeled sections of the iris for tyrosine hydroxylase and GDF5. This showed prominent GDF5 immunoreactivity throughout the stroma and tyrosine hydroxylase-positive fibers ramifying within the stroma (Fig. 6e). GDF5 immunoreactivity was not observed in the irides of *Gdf5*[bp] mice, demonstrating the specificity of the anti-GDF5 antibody used (Fig. 6e). These observations show that GDF5 is expressed by cells in the target field. Figure 6f illustrates representative tyrosine hydroxylase-immunolabeled whole mounts of the trachea of wild type mice and *Gdf5*[bp] mice.

Neuron counts in the SCG at P5 and P10 revealed no significant differences between wild type mice and *Gdf5*[bp] mice at each age (Fig. 6g), suggesting that SCG neurons are not dependent on GDF5 for survival when sympathetic innervation is being established during the postnatal period. Taken together, these findings suggest

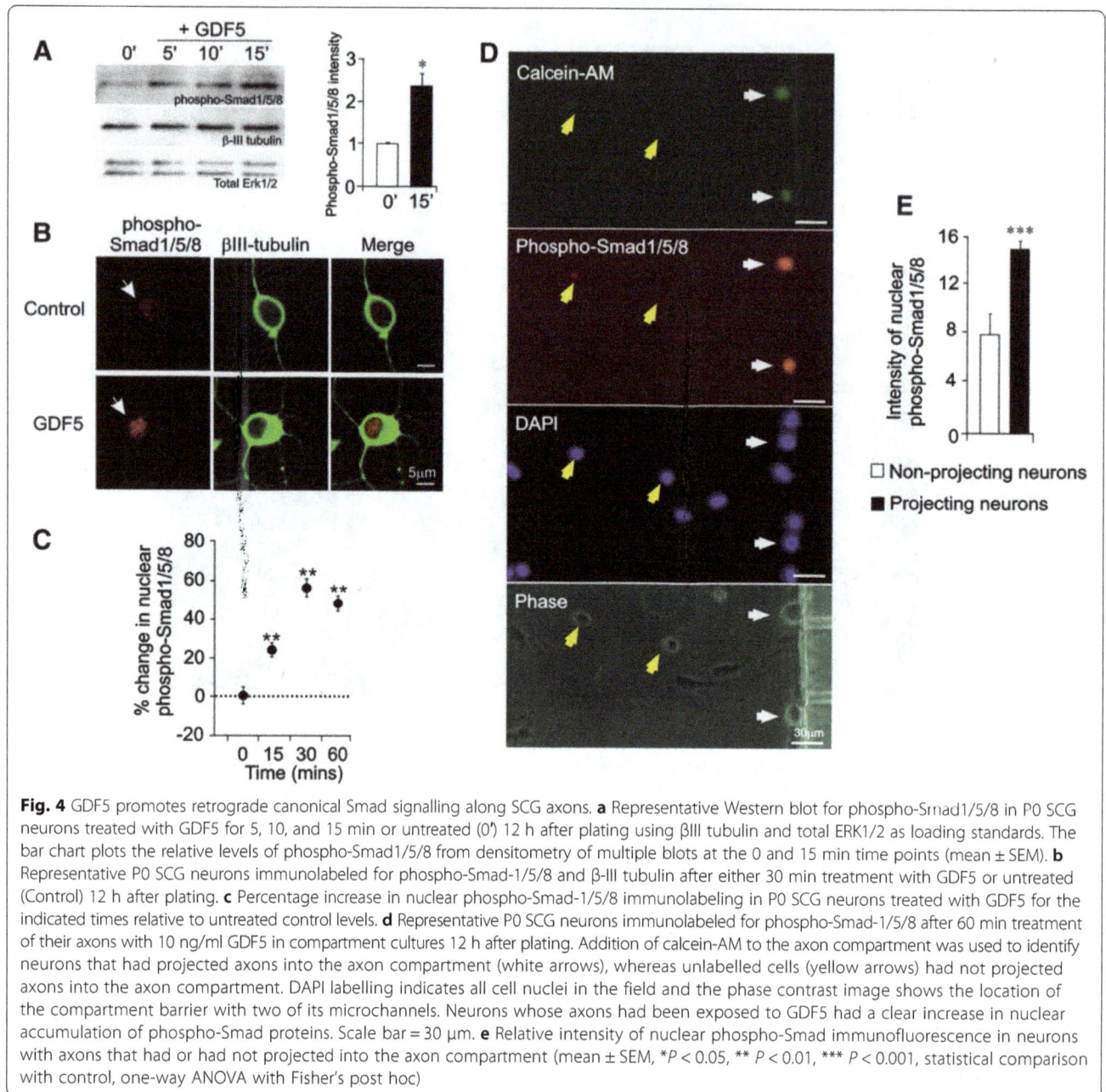

Fig. 4 GDF5 promotes retrograde canonical Smad signalling along SCG axons. **a** Representative Western blot for phospho-Smad1/5/8 in P0 SCG neurons treated with GDF5 for 5, 10, and 15 min or untreated (0') 12 h after plating using βIII tubulin and total ERK1/2 as loading standards. The bar chart plots the relative levels of phospho-Smad1/5/8 from densitometry of multiple blots at the 0 and 15 min time points (mean ± SEM). **b** Representative P0 SCG neurons immunolabeled for phospho-Smad-1/5/8 and β-III tubulin after either 30 min treatment with GDF5 or untreated (Control) 12 h after plating. **c** Percentage increase in nuclear phospho-Smad-1/5/8 immunolabeling in P0 SCG neurons treated with GDF5 for the indicated times relative to untreated control levels. **d** Representative P0 SCG neurons immunolabeled for phospho-Smad-1/5/8 after 60 min treatment of their axons with 10 ng/ml GDF5 in compartment cultures 12 h after plating. Addition of calcein-AM to the axon compartment was used to identify neurons that had projected axons into the axon compartment (white arrows), whereas unlabelled cells (yellow arrows) had not projected axons into the axon compartment. DAPI labelling indicates all cell nuclei in the field and the phase contrast image shows the location of the compartment barrier with two of its microchannels. Neurons whose axons had been exposed to GDF5 had a clear increase in nuclear accumulation of phospho-Smad proteins. Scale bar = 30 μm. **e** Relative intensity of nuclear phospho-Smad immunofluorescence in neurons with axons that had or had not projected into the axon compartment (mean ± SEM, *P < 0.05, ** P < 0.01, *** P < 0.001, statistical comparison with control, one-way ANOVA with Fisher's post hoc)

that GDF5 plays a tissue-selective role in establishing sympathetic innervation in vivo without affecting SCG neuron number.

Discussion

We have discovered and characterized novel and distinctive functions for GDF5 in the developing peripheral nervous system and show that these differ in several respects from the potential roles of GDF5 reported for other neurons. First, whereas GDF5 promotes the growth and branching of axons from sympathetic neurons, GDF5 promotes the growth and elaboration of dendrites but not axons from hippocampal pyramidal cells [13]. Second, whereas GDF5 neither promotes the survival of sympathetic neurons alone nor enhances the survival of these neurons in combination with NGF, GDF5 has a minor survival-promoting action on DRG neurons alone and enhances the survival-promoting action of NGF and NT3 in vitro [14]. GDF5 also promotes the survival of midbrain dopaminergic neurons in vitro [12] and is neuroprotective for these neurons exposed to toxic insults both in vitro [11, 24] and in vivo [25]. Third, whereas the effects of GDF5 on sympathetic neurons are restricted to a very narrow postnatal window of

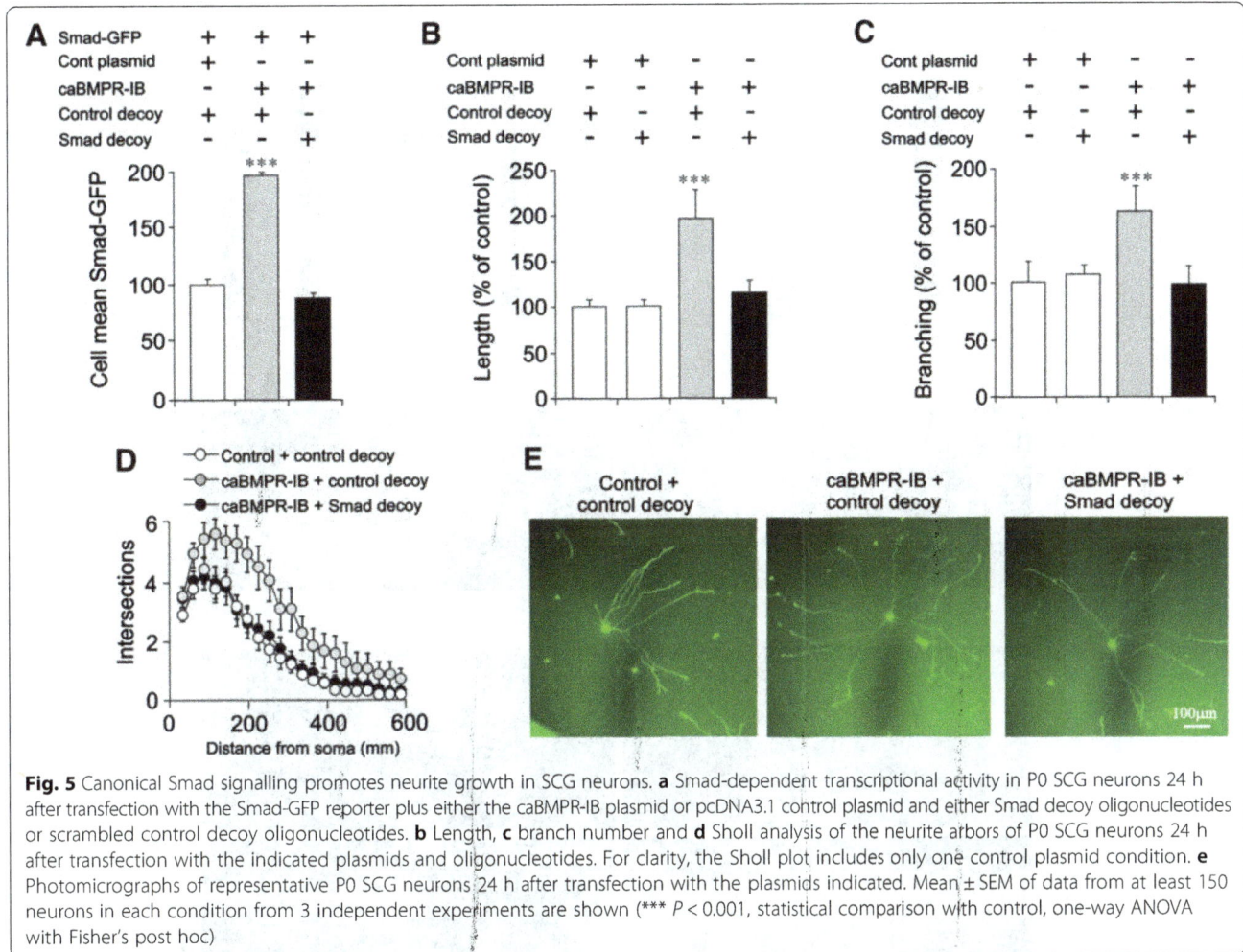

Fig. 5 Canonical Smad signalling promotes neurite growth in SCG neurons. **a** Smad-dependent transcriptional activity in P0 SCG neurons 24 h after transfection with the Smad-GFP reporter plus either the caBMPR-IB plasmid or pcDNA3.1 control plasmid and either Smad decoy oligonucleotides or scrambled control decoy oligonucleotides. **b** Length, **c** branch number and **d** Sholl analysis of the neurite arbors of P0 SCG neurons 24 h after transfection with the indicated plasmids and oligonucleotides. For clarity, the Sholl plot includes only one control plasmid condition. **e** Photomicrographs of representative P0 SCG neurons 24 h after transfection with the plasmids indicated. Mean ± SEM of data from at least 150 neurons in each condition from 3 independent experiments are shown (*** $P < 0.001$, statistical comparison with control, one-way ANOVA with Fisher's post hoc)

development, midbrain dopaminergic neurons remain responsive to GDF5 from embryonic stages into the adult [11, 12, 25]. Our current study together with previous work documents the multiple distinctive actions of GDF5 in the developing and mature nervous system.

In addition to GDF5, several other factors have been shown to enhance sympathetic axon growth and branching over restricted windows of development during the stage when sympathetic axons are ramifying extensively in their targets, without affecting neuronal survival. GDF5 and these other factors do not have redundant functions, but act by different mechanisms and have distinctive roles in establishing sympathetic innervation in vivo.

Both TNFR1 [26], acting via a TNF reverse signaling mechanism, and GDF5 act in a target-derived manner. TNFR1 and GDF5 are expressed in target tissues and act on sympathetic axon terminals to promote growth and branching. However, whereas studies of $Gdf5^{bp}$ mice reveal a distinctive regional requirement for GDF5 in vivo in the establishment of sympathetic innervation,

multiple tissues display defective sympathetic innervation in both $Tnfr1-/-$ and $Tnf-/-$ mice [25]. It is not clear why GDF5 plays a major role in establishing sympathetic innervation in the iris and to a lesser extent in the trachea, but not in the submandibular gland. Like TNFR1, GDF5 is widely expressed in multiple tissues, and the level of GDF5 is no higher in the iris than in the submandibular gland (data not shown). For this reason, the marked innervation defect in iris of $Gdf5^{bp}$ mice cannot be explained simply by regional differences in GDF5 expression and access of sympathetic axons to GDF5. Whether a subset of SCG neurons that innervate the iris and trachea respond to GDF5 in vivo, either because they are pre-specified to respond or because target-derived factors regulate GDF5 responsiveness, is an intriguing issue for future work. The trachea is the one tissue of the many analyzed whose sympathetic innervation is completely independent of NGF [5]. The small, though significant, decrease in the sympathetic innervation of the trachea of $Gdf5^{bp}$ mice shows that GDF5 makes a significant contribution to establishing

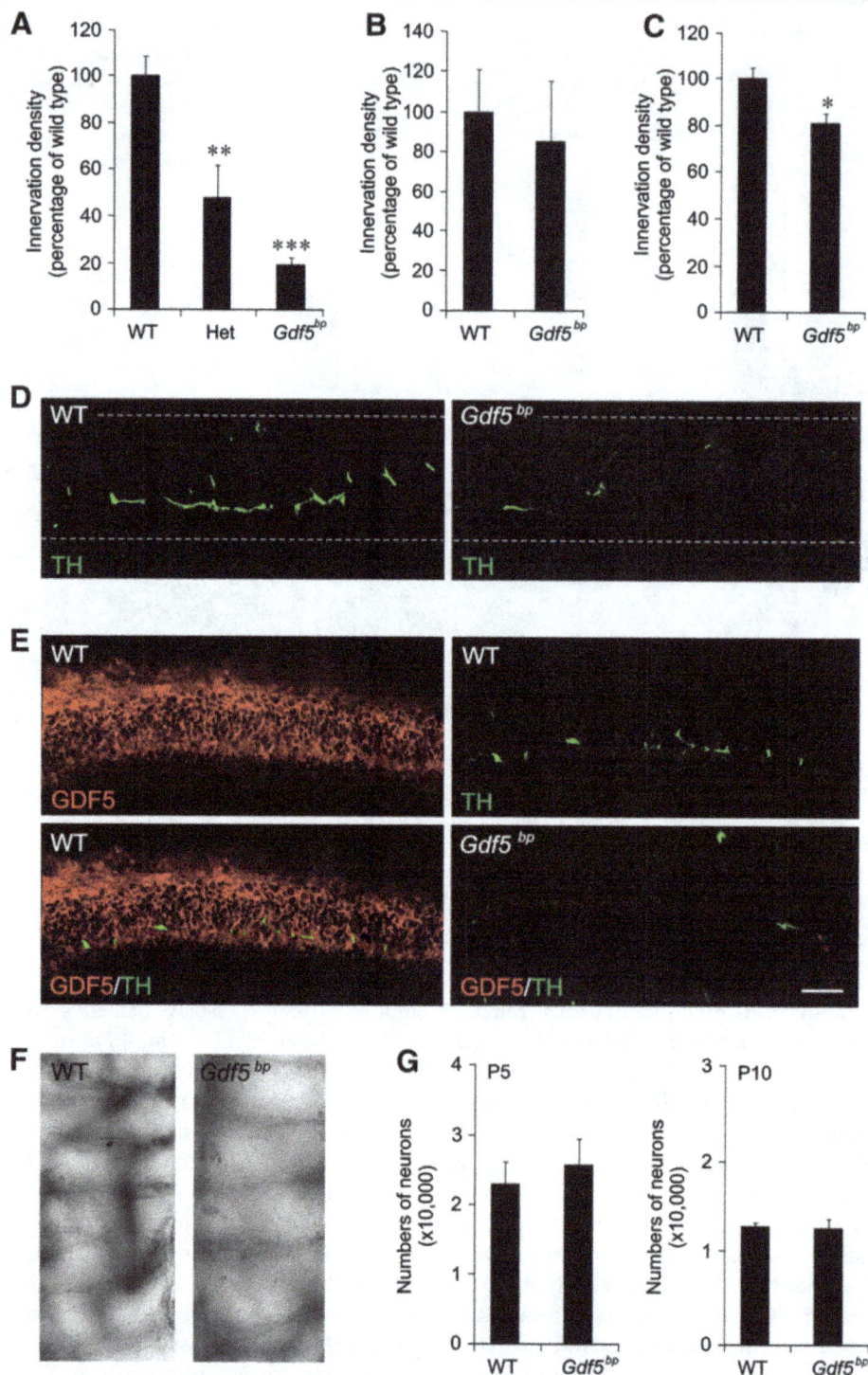

Fig. 6 Selective sympathetic innervation deficits in mice possessing the *Gdf5^{bp}* mutation. **a-c** Relative innervation density assessed by quantification of tyrosine hydroxylase-positive sympathetic fibres at P10 in the irides (**a**), submandibular glands (**b**) and trachea (**c**) of wild type mice (WT) and mice that are heterozygous (Het) or homozygous (*Gdf5^{bp}*) for the *Gdf5^{bp}* null mutation. The level of tyrosine hydroxylase staining is normalised to 100 for the tissue of wild type mice (mean ± SEM, *$P < 0.01$, **$P < 0.00001$, ***$P < 0.0000001$, statistical comparison with wild type, one-way ANOVA with Tukey HSD post hoc, $n = 10$ animals per genotype for the iris, $n = 5$ animal per genotype for the submandibular gland and the trachea). **d** Representative sections of the irides of P10 wild type and *Gdf5^{bp}* mice stained for tyrosine hydroxylase. The boundaries of the iris are indicated by the dashed lines. **e** Representative sections of the iris of a P10 wild type and *Gdf5^{bp}* mice double stained for GDF5 and tyrosine hydroxylase. Scale bar = 100 μm. **f** Representative whole mounts P10 wild type and *Gdf5^{bp}* mice stained for tyrosine hydroxylase. Scale bar = 100 μm. **g** Numbers of neurons in the SCG of P5 and P10 wild type and *Gdf5^{bp}* mice ($n = 3$ per genotype)

tracheal sympathetic innervation. The other factor or factors required for promoting the ramification of sympathetic fibres in this tissue remain elusive.

Like GDF5, GITR signaling and CD40 signaling enhance sympathetic axon growth during the immediate postnatal period without affecting neuronal survival and play roles in establishing sympathetic innervation in vivo [27, 28]. However, in contrast to the target-derived mode of action of GDF5, GITR signaling and CD40 signaling act by an autocrine mechanism. Also, in contrast to GDF5, which promotes sympathetic axon growth alone in the absence of NGF, stimulating these autocrine signaling loops in the absence of NGF does not promote sympathetic axon growth. Rather, these autocrine signaling loops enhance the axon growth-promoting actions of NGF [27, 28]. Despite modulating NGF responsiveness, $Cd40-/-$ mice, like $Gdf5^{bp}$ mice, display regional deficits in sympathetic innervation density [28]. This is because NGF negatively regulates the expression of both CD40 and its autocrine signaling partner CD40L, with the result that these proteins are only expressed at functionally relevant levels in low NGF-expressing tissues, which are those that are selectively hypo-innervated in $Cd40-/-$ mice [28].

HGF [29] and Wnt5a [30] are another two factors that enhance sympathetic axon growth by an autocrine mechanism during the stage of development when sympathetic axons are ramifying in their final targets. While this activity has only been reported for HGF in vitro, the importance of Wnt5a has been demonstrated in vivo in mice in which $Wnt5a$ is conditionally inactivated in sympathetic neurons. In these mice, sympathetic fibres reach their final targets, but display greatly reduced growth and terminal arborization in multiple tissues, which contrasts with the regional deficit observed in $Gdf5^{bp}$ mice.

Most SCG neurons are generated between E11.5 and birth [31, 32], the earliest sympathetic fibres reach SCG targets at E13 [33] and the density of sympathetic innervation of many tissues clearly increases between the late fetal and early postnatal period [5]. Thus, the brief window over which GDF5 enhances axon growth from SCG neurons appears to occur shortly after sympathetic axons have arrived at their target tissues and are ramifying within and refining connections in these tissues. GDF5 binds efficiently to BMPR1B and transduces a signal via BMPR1B in combination with either BMPR2 or ACVR2A. However, GDF5 also binds BMPR1A weakly when co-expressed with ACVR2A and transduces a signal in cell lines co-expressing BMPR1A and ACVR2A [20]. We show that SCG neurons express BMPR1A and ACVR2A as well as BMPR1B and BMPR2 during this brief window of GDF5 responsiveness. However, we find that transcripts for all receptors are expressed at similar

levels in the SCG for extended periods before and after the window of GDF5 responsiveness. This suggests that the timing of GDF5 responsiveness is unlikely to be due to changes in receptor expression. This contrasts with enhanced SCG axon growth brought about by activating TNF reverse signaling and by activating the extracellular Ca^{2+} sensitive receptor (CaSR). The developmental window of responsiveness of SCG neurons to TNFR1 and to elevated extracellular Ca^{2+} coincides with peaks in TNF [26] and CaSR expression [34]. Moreover, experimental elevation of CaSR expression after the normal peak of expression re-confers responsiveness to elevated extracellular Ca^{2+} [34]. Our current findings raise the possibility that the timing of GDF5 responsiveness might be due to developmental changes in GDF5 local signaling, retrograde GDF5 signaling or gene regulation.

GDF5 rapidly activates canonical Smad 1/5/8 signaling in hippocampal pyramidal cells and rat midbrain dopaminergic neurons, and this in turn is required for GDF5-promoted neurite growth and dendrite growth [13, 35]. Here we show that GDF5 also rapidly activates Smad 1/5/8 signaling in sympathetic neurons, and demonstrate using compartment cultures that treating sympathetic axons with GDF5 results in the rapid appearance of phospho-Smad immunoreactivity in the nucleus. This suggests that GDF5 induces retrograde Smad signaling. BMP4 also initiates retrograde Smad signaling along trigeminal sensory axons, and this plays a role in conveying spatial patterning information from the periphery in the developing trigeminal system [36]. Moreover, we show that decoy DNA encoding the Smad consensus binding sequence inhibits the enhanced axon growth associated with GDF5 receptor-dependent Smad activation, suggesting that Smad-dependent gene transcription enhances axon growth in developing sympathetic neurons. While these data suggest that retrograde Smad signaling to the nucleus is important for GDF5-promoted axon growth, compartment culture experiments show that GDF5 added to the axon compartment enhances axon growth, whereas GDF5 added to the soma compartment does not. This observation raises the possibility that retrograde Smad signaling alone is insufficient for GDF5-enhanced axon growth, but that local signaling is also required. This has parallels with other target-derived neurotrophic factors. For example, whereas retrograde NGF/TrkA signaling to the nucleus is required for NGF-promoted neuron survival, local TrkA-dependent signaling events in at the growth cone are required for axon growth promoted by NGF and NT3 [3, 37]. In future work it will be interesting to dissect the local signaling events required for GDF5-promoted axon growth.

Our current work demonstrates that GDF5 is one of a growing number of factors that promote, by a diversity of mechanisms, sympathetic axon growth and branching and have distinctive roles in establishing sympathetic innervation in vivo without affecting neuronal survival. In addition, factors expressed in target tissues such as RANKL inhibit sympathetic axon growth and branching, at least in vitro, without affecting neuronal survival [38]. In contrast, target-derived NGF performs the key dual roles of sustaining sympathetic neuron survival and promoting the growth and ramification of sympathetic axons in target tissues in vivo. Indeed, there is overwhelming evidence that the limited availability of NGF in different tissues governs the number of neurons that survive the phase of naturally occurring death to innervate these tissues [1]. Given this dual function, why are additional factors that regulate axon growth but not survival required? The most likely reason is that these additional factors permit regional adjustments in innervation density by the limited number of NGF-supported neurons that innervate particular tissues.

Conclusions

We have discovered and characterized novel and distinctive functions for GDF5 in the developing nervous system. GDF5 promotes the growth and branching of sympathetic axons independently of NGF without affecting sympathetic neuron survival during a brief window of postnatal development when sympathetic axons are ramifying within their targets. GDF5 is expressed in sympathetic targets, acts directly on sympathetic axons and initiates retrograde Smad signaling along these axons to the nucleus. In vivo, there is a distinctive regional requirement for GDF5 in the establishment of sympathetic innervation, being required in the iris, not in the submandibular gland and making a small, significant contribution to the trachea, whose innervation is independent of NGF. These findings extend our understanding of the physiology of GDF5 and provide a deeper understanding of the mechanisms that pattern sympathetic innervation during development.

Methods
Mice
C57BL6/J and brachypod ($Gdf5^{bp}$) mice were obtained from the Jackson Laboratory (Bar Harbor, Maine, USA). While $Gdf5^{bp}$ mice are recognized by their short limb phenotype, wild type and heterozygous mice are phenotypically indistinguishable and cannot be genotyped by standard PCR-based methods. To generate litters consisting of mice that are homozygous and heterozygous for the $Gdf5^{bp}$ mutation, a female $Gdf5^{bp}$ mouse was crossed with a male mouse that is heterozygous for the $Gdf5^{bp}$ mutation. Heterozygous male mice were identified as phenotypically normal mice that produced litters comprising phenotypically normal mice and $Gdf5^{bp}$ mice when crossed with $Gdf5^{bp}$ females. Age-matched wild

type mice were obtained by crossing C57BL6/J mice. All other studies were carried out on tissues obtained from CD-1 mice.

Real-time PCR quantification of mRNA levels
SCG were harvested from embryonic and postnatal mice. Because whole ganglia contain both neurons and satellite cells, the RNA used for these studies is derived from both cell types. Total RNA was isolated with the RNeasy Mini extraction kit (Qiagen, Germany) and was reverse transcribed with AffinityScript RT (Agilent). Reverse transcription (RT) reactions were amplified using the Brilliant III ultra-fast QPCR master mix (Agilent). QPCR assays for $Bmpr1a$, $Bmpr1b$, $Acvr2a$, $Bmpr2$ and the reference genes, $Gapdh$, $Sdha$ and $Hprt1$ used dual-labeled probes to detect PCR products. The forward and reverse primers were as follows: $Gapdh$, 5′-gagaaacctgccaagtatg-3′ and 5′-gggttgctgttgaagtc-3′; $Sdha$, 5′-ggaacactccaaaaacag-3′ and 5′-ccacagcatcaaattcat-3′; $Hprt1$, 5′-ttaagcagtacagccccaaaa tg-3′ and 5′-aagtctggcctgtatccaacac-3′; $Bmpr1a$, 5′-tacgca ggacaatagaat-3′ and 5′-aactatacagacagccat-3′; $Bmpr1b$, 5′-agtgtaataaagacctcca-3′ and 5′-aactacagacagtcacag-3′; $Bmpr2$, 5′-actagaggactggcttat-3′ and 5′-ccaaagtcactgataacac-3′; $Acvr2a$, 5′-cgccgtctttcttatctc-3′ and 5′-tgtcgccgtttatctt ta-3′. Dual labeled probes were: $Gapdh$, 5′- FAM-agacaa cctggtcctcagtgt-BHQ1-3′; $Sdha$, 5′-FAM-cctgcggctttc acttctct-BHQ1-3′; $Hprt1$, 5′-FAM-tcgagaggtcctttcaccagca ag-BHQ1-3′; $Bmpr1a$, 5′- FAM-tgagcacaaccagccatcg-BH Q1-3′; $Bmpr1b$, 5′-FAM-ccactctgcctcctctcaag-BHQ1-3′; $Bmpr2$, 5′-FAM-cacagaattaccacgaggaga-BHQ1-3′; $Acvr2a$, 5′-FAM-tgctcttcaggtgctatacttggc-BHQ1-3′. The PCR was performed (Mx3000P, Stratagene) for 40 cycles of 95 °C for 10 sec, and 60 °C for 30 sec. Standard curves were generated for every PCR run with each primer/probe set using serial five-fold dilutions of adult mouse brain RT RNA (Zyagen). $Bmpr1a$, $Bmpr1b$, $Bmpr2$ and $Acvr2a$ mRNAs were expressed relative to the geometric mean of the reference mRNAs.

Neuron cultures
Dissected SCG were trypsinized and the neurons were plated at very low density (~200 neurons per dish) in poly-ornithine/laminin-coated 35 mm tissue culture dishes (Greiner, Germany) in serum-free Hams F14 medium supplemented with 0.25 % Albumax I (Life Technologies, Paisley, UK) [39]. NGF (Calbiochem, UK), GDF5 (Biopharm, Germany) and the broad-spectrum caspase inhibitor Boc–D–FMK (Calbiochem, UK) were added as indicated.

Neuronal survival was estimated by counting the number of attached neurons within a 12 × 12 mm grid in the centre of each dish 2 h after plating and again after 24 h, and expressing the 24-h count as a percentage of the 2-h count [39]. Analysis of the size and complexity of neurite arbors was carried out 24 h after plating. The neurite arbors were labeled by incubating the neurons with the fluorescent vital dye calcein-AM (1:1000, Invitrogen, Paisley, UK). Images of neurite arbors were acquired by fluorescence microscopy and analyzed to obtain total neurite length, number of branch points and Sholl profiles [40].

For compartment cultures, the neurons were seeded in one compartment of a two compartment microfluidic device (Xona Microfludics, CA, USA) and the medium in both compartments was supplemented with 10 ng/ml NGF to promote the growth of axons in both compartments. 10 ng/ml GDF5 was added either to the axon compartment or the soma compartment at plating, and axon growth was assessed 24 h later following addition of the fluorescent vital dye Calcein-AM (Invitrogen) to the axonal compartment to label axons in this compartment. ImageJ was used to measure the lengths of the 10 longest axons per random field (distances to the 10 furthest growth cones from the compartment barrier) to obtain a mean measurement for each field. Means of these measurements were obtained from 7 separate random fields along the microfluidic barrier of each compartment culture.

For the retrograde signaling experiments, the neurons were incubated with 10 ng/ml NGF in both compartments for 12 h before 10 ng/ml GDF5 was added to the axon compartment, followed by addition of calcein-AM to identify which neurons had projected axons into the axonal compartment. Cultures where immediately fixed and stained for phospho-Smad, as described below.

Neuron transfection and reporter assays

SCG neurons were transfected as previously described [41] with the GFP-based Cignal Smad Reporter (SABiosciences, UK) and either an empty control plasmid or the caBMPR-IB plasmid together with either a Smad decoy (double stranded DNA oligonucleotide, 5′-gtacattgtc agtctagacataact-3′) prepared as described previously or a scrambled control decoy oligonucleotide (double stranded DNA oligonucleotide, 5′-atcataatttggaactgtagt ccg-3′). Reporter activity is expressed as the mean fluorescence intensity of individual cells as previously described [41].

Immunocytochemistry

Cultures were fixed in 4 % paraformaldehyde at room temperature for 10 min, washed with phosphate buffered saline (PBS) and blocked with 5 % bovine serum albumen (BSA) and 0.1 % TritronX-100 in PBS for 1 h at room temperature. The cells were incubated overnight with primary antibody in 1 % BSA at 4 °C. The following primary antibodies were used: rabbit polyclonal anti-BMPR1A (Abcam, Cambridge, UK, 1/200, catalogue number

ab38560), rabbit polyclonal anti-BMPR1B (Abcam, Cambridge, UK, 1/200, catalogue number ab175385), rabbit polyclonal anti-BMPR2 (Abcam, Cambridge, UK, 1/200, catalogue number ab124463), rabbit polyclonal anti-ACVR2A (Abcam, Cambridge, UK, 1/200, catalogue number ab96793), rabbit polyclonal anti-phospho-Smad1/5 (Ser463/465) (41D10) (Cell Signaling, Danvers, MA, USA, 1:100, catalogue number 9516) and β-III tubulin (Abcam, Cambridge, UK, 1:500, ab41489). After washing, the cultures were incubated with an Alexa-Fluor-labeled secondary antibody (1:500 Alexa Fluor 488 anti-rabbit, Life Technologies, UK, catalogue number A-1108 and 1:500 Alexa Fluor 594 anti-chicken, Abcam, Cambrdige, UK, catalogue number ab150172) for 1 h and counterstained with DAPI (Chemicon) where indicated. Quantification of nuclear staining of phospho-Smad1/5/8 was carried out as described [42].

Immunohistochemistry

The iris and submandibular salivary gland of wild type and mice that are heterozygous or homozygous for the GDF-5[bp] mutation were fixed in 4 % paraformaldehyde and 0.1 % TritonX-100 for 24 h and were cryoprotected in 30 % sucrose before freezing. 15 μm serial sections were blocked with 5 % BSA containing 0.1 % TritonX-100 in PBS for 1 h at room temperature, and then incubated for 18 h at 4 °C with a rabbit anti-tyrosine hydroxylase polyclonal antibody (Merck-Millipore, Dundee, UK, catalogue number AB152) diluted 1:200 in PBS with 1 % BSA together with or without anti-GDF5 (R&D systems, 1:50 or Biopharm GmBh, 1:100). The sections were washed and incubated with appropriate secondary antibodies (Alexa-Fluor, Invitrogen, 1:500). The density of tyrosine hydroxylase-positive sympathetic fibers was determined as described [26]. All imaging and quantification was carried out blind.

Whole-Mount preparations

Paraformaldehyde fixed tissue was processed to label tyrosine hydroxylase-positive sympathetic fibers by DAB-HRP staining followed by clearing in benzyl alcohol:benzyl benzoate as described previously [26]. To compare the extent of sympathetic nerve branching, a modified line-intercept method was used. Using ImageJ, a grid of 24 squares (4 × 6 squares, 158 μm side length per square) was aligned in a standard orientation on images of the trachea using the lateral axonal bundle entering the trachea as a guide. The number of fibre bundles intersecting the sides of squares in the grid was scored blind. Fibre density was estimated using the formula $\pi DI/2$, where D is the interline interval and I the mean number of intersections along one side of each square in the grid.

Quantification of neuron number in the SCG

Estimates of the numbers of neurons in the SCG of wild type and $Gdf5^{bp}$ mice were carried out by stereological analysis of 8 μm serial sections of the ganglia as described [25].

Western blotting

This was carried out as described [43]. Extracted proteins were transferred to PVDF membranes which were blocked with 5 % dried milk in PBS with 0.1 % Tween-20 and were incubated overnight with anti-phospho-Smad1/5/8 (1:1000; Cell Signaling), anti-β-III tubulin (1:10000; Promega) or anti-ERK1/2 (1:1000; Cell Signaling). The appropriate peroxidase-linked secondary antibody (1:2000; Promega) was used to detect each primary antibody on the blots and staining was visualized using ECL plus (Amersham).

Abbreviations

BMPR: bone morphogenetic protein receptor; BSA: bovine serum albumen; DRG: dorsal root ganglion; GDF5: growth differentiation factor-5; NGF: nerve growth factor; NT3: neurotrophin-3; PBS: phosphate buffered saline; SCG: superior cervical ganglion; TGFβ: transforming growth factor beta.

Competing interests

The authors declare that they have no competing interests.

Authors' contributions

GW, HG, LH and CL carried out the cell culture studies, LH, CL and CO quantified sympathetic innervation, NG did the Western analysis, SW did the qPCR and AMD supervised the work and wrote the manuscript. All authors read and approved the final manuscript.

Acknowledgements

This work was supported by a grant from the Wellcome Trust.

Author details

[1]School of Biosciences, Cardiff University, Museum Avenue, Cardiff CF10 3AT, UK. [2]Dept. Anatomy/Neuroscience and Biosciences Institute, UCC, Cork, Ireland. [3]Current address, School of Life Sciences, University of Lincoln, Brayford Pool, Lincoln LN6 7TS, UK. [4]Current address, MRC Centre for Developmental Neurobiology, King's College London, New Hunt's House, 4th Floor, Guy's Hospital Campus, London SE1 1UL, UK. [5]Current address, SOM Innovation Biotech SL, c/Baldiri Reixac 4, 08028 Barcelona, Spain.

References

1. Davies AM. Regulation of neuronal survival and death by extracellular signals during development. EMBO J. 2003;22:2537–45.
2. Huang EJ, Reichardt LF. Neurotrophins. roles in neuronal development and function. Ann Rev Neurosci. 2001;24:677–736.
3. Ye H, Kuruvilla R, Zweifel LS, Ginty DD. Evidence in support of signaling endosome-based retrograde survival of sympathetic neurons. Neuron. 2003;39:57–68.
4. Davies AM, Bandtlow C, Heumann R, Korsching S, Rohrer H, Thoenen H. Timing and Site of Nerve Growth-Factor Synthesis in Developing Skin in Relation to Innervation and Expression of the Receptor. Nature. 1987;326:353–8.
5. Glebova NO, Ginty DD. Heterogeneous requirement of NGF for sympathetic target innervation in vivo. J Neurosci. 2004;24:743–51.
6. Patel TD, Jackman A, Rice F, Kucera J, Snider WD. Development of sensory neurons in the absence of NGF/TrkA signaling in vivo. Neuron. 2000;25:345–57.
7. Rider CC, Mulloy B. Bone morphogenetic protein and growth differentiation factor cytokine families and their protein antagonists. Biochem J. 2010;429:1–12.
8. Mikic B. Multiple effects of GDF-5 deficiency on skeletal tissues. implications for therapeutic bioengineering. Ann Biomed Eng. 2004;32:466–76.
9. Lee J, Wikesjo UM. Growth/differentiation factor-5: pre-clinical and clinical evaluations of periodontal regeneration and alveolar augmentation. J Clin Periodontol. 2014;41:797–805.
10. Ratnayake M, Ploger F, Santibanez-Koref M, Loughlin J. Human chondrocytes respond discordantly to the protein encoded by the osteoarthritis susceptibility gene GDF5. PLoS One. 2014;9, e86590.
11. Krieglstein K, Suter-Crazzolara C, Hotten G, Pohl J, Unsicker K. Trophic and protective effects of growth/differentiation factor 5, a member of the transforming growth factor-beta superfamily, on midbrain dopaminergic neurons. J Neurosci Res. 1995;42:724–32.
12. O'Keeffe GW, Dockery P, Sullivan AM. Effects of growth/differentiation factor 5 on the survival and morphology of embryonic rat midbrain dopaminergic neurones in vitro. J Neurocytol. 2004;33:479–88.
13. Osorio C, Chacon PJ, Kisiswa L, White M, Wyatt S, Rodriguez-Tebar A, Davies AM. Growth differentiation factor 5 is a key physiological regulator of dendrite growth during development. Development. 2013;140:4751–562.
14. Farkas LM, Scheuermann S, Pohl J, Unsicker K, Krieglstein K. Characterization of growth/differentiation factor 5 (GDF-5) as a neurotrophic factor for cultured neurons from chicken dorsal root ganglia. Neurosci Lett. 1997;236:120–2.
15. Francis N, Farinas I, Brennan C, Rivas-Plata K, Backus C, Reichardt L, Landis S. NT-3, like NGF, is required for survival of sympathetic neurons, but not their precursors. Dev Biol. 1999;210:411–27.
16. Orike N, Thrasivoulou C, Wrigley A, Cowen T. Differential regulation of survival and growth in adult sympathetic neurons. an in vitro study of neurotrophin responsiveness. J Neurobiol. 2001;47:295–305.
17. Wyatt S, Piñon LGP, Ernfors P, Davies AM. Sympathetic neuron survival and TrkA expression in NT3-deficient mouse embryos. EMBO J. 1997;16:3115–23.
18. Lein P, Johnson M, Guo X, Rueger D, Higgins D. Osteogenic protein-1 induces dendritic growth in rat sympathetic neurons. Neuron. 1995;15:597–605.
19. Miyazono K, Kamiya Y, Morikawa M. Bone morphogenetic protein receptors and signal transduction. J Biochem. 2010;147:35–51.
20. Nishitoh H, Ichijo H, Kimura M, Matsumoto T, Makishima F, Yamaguchi A, Yamashita H, Enomoto S, Miyazono K. Identification of type I and type II serine/threonine kinase receptors for growth/differentiation factor-5. J Biol Chem. 1996;271:21345–52.
21. Massague J. TGF-beta signal transduction. Annu Rev Biochem. 1998;67:753–91.
22. Fujii M, Takeda K, Imamura T, Aoki H, Sampath TK, Enomoto S, et al. Roles of Bone Morphogenetic Protein Type I Receptors and Smad Proteins in Osteoblast and Chondroblast Differentiation. Mol Biol Cell. 1999;10:3010–818.
23. Lingor P, Unsicker K, Krieglstein K. Midbrain dopaminergic neurons are protected from radical induced damage by GDF-5 application. J Neural Transm. 1999;106:139–44.
24. Sullivan AM, Opacka-Juffry J, Hotten G, Pohl J, Blunt SB. Growth/differentiation factor 5 protects nigrostriatal dopaminergic neurones in a rat model of Parkinson's disease. Neurosci Lett. 1997;233:73–6.
25. Kisiswa L, Osorio C, Erice C, Vizard T, Wyatt S, Davies AM. TNFalpha reverse signaling promotes sympathetic axon growth and target innervation. Nature Neurosci. 2013;16:865–73.
26. O'Keeffe GW, Gutierrez H, Pandolfi PP, Riccardi C, Davies AM. NGF-promoted axon growth and target innervation requires GITRL-GITR signaling. Nature Neurosci. 2008;11:135–142.30.
27. McWilliams TG, Howard L, Wyatt S, Davies AM. Regulation of autocrine signaling in subsets of sympathetic neurons has regional effects on tissue innervation. Cell Rep. 2015;10:1443–9.
28. Yang XM, Toma JG, Bamji SX, Belliveau DJ, Kohn J, Park M, Miller FD. Autocrine hepatocyte growth factor provides a local mechanism for promoting axonal growth. J Neurosci. 1998;18:8369–81.
29. Ryu YK, Collins SE, Ho HY, Zhao H, Kuruvilla R. An autocrine Wnt5a-Ror signaling loop mediates sympathetic target innervation. Dev Biol. 2013;377:79–89.
30. Nishino J, Mochida K, Ohfuji Y, Shimazaki T, Meno C, Ohishi S, Matsuda Y, Fujii H, Saijoh Y, Hamada H. GFR alpha3, a component of the artemin receptor, is required for migration and survival of the superior cervical ganglion. Neuron. 1999;23:725–36.
31. Andres R, Forgie A, Wyatt S, Chen Q, De Sauvage FJ, Davies AM. Multiple effects of artemin on sympathetic neurone generation, survival and growth. Development. 2001;128:3685–95.
32. Korsching S, Thoenen H. Developmental changes of nerve growth factor levels in sympathetic ganglia and their target organs. Dev Biol. 1988;126:40–6.

33. Vizard T, O'Keeffe GW, Gutierrez H, Cos CH, Riccardi D, Davies AM. Regulation of axonal and dendritic growth by the extracellular calcium-sensing receptor. Nature Neurosci. 2008;11(135):285–91.

34. Hegarty SV, Collins LM, Gavin AM, Roche SL, Wyatt SL, Sullivan AM, O'Keeffe GW. Canonical BMP-Smad signalling promotes neurite growth in rat midbrain dopaminergic neurons. Neuromol Med. 2014;16:473–89.

35. Hodge LK, Klassen MP, Han BX, Yiu G, Hurrell J, Howell A, Rousseau G, Lemaigre F, Tessier-Lavigne M, Wang F. Retrograde BMP signaling regulates trigeminal sensory neuron identities and the formation of precise face maps. Neuron. 2007;55:572–86.

36. Kuruvilla R, Zweifel LS, Glebova NO, Lonze BE, Valdez G, Ye H, Ginty DD. A neurotrophin signaling cascade coordinates sympathetic neuron development through differential control of TrkA trafficking and retrograde signaling. Cell. 2004;118:243–55.

37. Gutierrez H, Kisiswa L, O'Keeffe GW, Smithen MJ, Wyatt S, Davies AM. Regulation of neurite growth by tumour necrosis superfamily member RANKL. Open Biol. 2013;3:120150.

38. Davies AM, Lee KF, Jaenisch R. p75-deficient trigeminal sensory neurons have an altered response to NGF but not to other neurotrophins. Neuron. 1993;11:565–74.

39. Gutierrez H, Davies AM. A fast and accurate procedure for deriving the Sholl profile in quantitative studies of neuronal morphology. J Neurosci Meth. 2007;163:24–30.

40. Gutierrez H, Hale V, Dolcet X, Davies AM. Nuclear factor kappa B signaling either stimulates or inhibits neurite growth depending on the phosphorylation status of p65/RelA. Development. 2005;132:1713–26.

41. Gutierrez H, O'Keeffe GW, Gavalda N, Gallagher D, Davies AM. Nuclear factor kappa B signaling either stimulates or inhibits neurite growth depending on the phosphorylation status of p65/RelA. J Neurosci. 2008;28:8246–56.

42. Gallagher D, Gutierrez H, Gavalda N, O'Keeffe G, Hay R, Davies AM. Nuclear factor-kappaB activation via tyrosine phosphorylation of inhibitor kappaB-alpha is crucial for ciliary neurotrophic factor-promoted neurite growth from developing neurons. J Neurosci. 2007;27:9664–9.

15

Prdm13 forms a feedback loop with Ptf1a and is required for glycinergic amacrine cell genesis in the *Xenopus* Retina

Nathalie Bessodes[1,2†], Karine Parain[2†], Odile Bronchain[2], Eric J. Bellefroid[1*] and Muriel Perron[2,3*] (iD)

Abstract

Background: Amacrine interneurons that modulate synaptic plasticity between bipolar and ganglion cells constitute the most diverse cell type in the retina. Most are inhibitory neurons using either GABA or glycine as neurotransmitters. Although several transcription factors involved in amacrine cell fate determination have been identified, mechanisms underlying amacrine cell subtype specification remain to be further understood. The Prdm13 histone methyltransferase encoding gene is a target of the transcription factor Ptf1a, an essential regulator of inhibitory neuron cell fate in the retina. Here, we have deepened our knowledge on its interaction with Ptf1a and investigated its role in amacrine cell subtype determination in the developing *Xenopus* retina.

Methods: We performed *prdm13* gain and loss of function in *Xenopus* and assessed the impact on retinal cell fate determination using RT-qPCR, in situ hybridization and immunohistochemistry.

Results: We found that *prdm13* in the amphibian *Xenopus* is expressed in few retinal progenitors and in about 40% of mature amacrine cells, predominantly in glycinergic ones. Clonal analysis in the retina reveals that *prdm13* overexpression favours amacrine cell fate determination, with a bias towards glycinergic cells. Conversely, knockdown of *prdm13* specifically inhibits glycinergic amacrine cell genesis. We also showed that, as in the neural tube, *prdm13* is subjected to a negative autoregulation in the retina. Our data suggest that this is likely due to its ability to repress the expression of its inducer, *ptf1a*.

Conclusions: Our results demonstrate that Prdm13, downstream of Ptf1a, acts as an important regulator of glycinergic amacrine subtype specification in the *Xenopus* retina. We also reveal that Prdm13 regulates *ptf1a* expression through a negative feedback loop.

Keywords: Retina, Amacrine cells, Subtype specification, Prdm13, Ptf1a

Background

The vertebrate retina is a suitable model system for studying neurogenesis. It comprises six classes of retinal cells organized in three cellular layers: retinal ganglion cells and displaced amacrine cells in the ganglion cell layer (GCL); bipolar, amacrine and horizontal cells as well as Müller glia in the inner nuclear layer (INL); rod and cone photoreceptors in the outer nuclear layer (ONL). These cell classes can be further divided into over more than 60

different subtypes of neurons. Amacrine cells belong to the most diverse class, with about 30 morphologically distinct subtypes [1, 2], and show a high molecular diversity [3]. Numerous cell fate determinants have been identified in the different classes of retinal cells [4–7]. Yet, the mechanisms by which retinal cell subtypes diversity is generated during development remain poorly understood.

Despite their broad morphological diversity, amacrine neurons are often divided in only two groups based on the expression of inhibitory glycine or γ-aminobutyric acid (GABA) neurotransmitters. These two subtypes have distinct birthdates, GABAergic amacrine cells being generated earlier than glycinergic ones [3, 8]. This suggests that different genetic programs are used to determine these cellular subtype identities. It is thus

* Correspondence: ebellefr@ulb.ac.be; muriel.perron@u-psud.fr
†Equal contributors
[1]ULB Neuroscience Institute (UNI), Université Libre de Bruxelles (ULB), B-6041 Gosselies, Belgium
[2]Paris-Saclay Institute of Neuroscience, CNRS, Univ Paris Sud, Université Paris-Saclay, UMR 9197- Neuro-PSI, Bat. 445, 91405 ORSAY Cedex, France
Full list of author information is available at the end of the article

important to examine cell-fate determination at the level of retinal cell subtypes. Some studies have addressed this issue and identified factors involved in amacrine subtype specification such as Neurod6, Bhlhb5 (Bhlhe22), Barhl2, Nr4a2, Islet-1 (Isl1), Ebf, [9–16]. We here focused our interest on the PRDM (PRDI-BF1 and RIZ homology domain) family of transcription factors.

PRDM proteins are characterised by a variable number of zinc-finger domains and a PR (PRDI-BF1-RIZ1) domain related to the SET (Su(var)3–9, Enhancer-of-zeste and Trithorax) domain found in a large group of histone methyltransferases [17, 18]. PRDM family members emerged as important regulators of neural development. In the retina, Prdm1 (Blimp1) was shown to specify photoreceptor over bipolar neuronal fate [19, 20]. Similarly to Isl1 and Bhlhb5, Prdm8 is part of the regulatory network governing bipolar cell development and amacrine cell diversity [21]. Interestingly, mutations in *prdm8* can cause human congenital stationary night blindness [21]. In the dorsal spinal cord, Prdm13 regulates neuronal diversity as a direct downstream target of Ptf1a (Pancreas Specific Transcription Factor, 1a) [22, 23]. Ptf1a is a bHLH (basic helix loop helix) transcription factor that determines inhibitory over excitatory neuronal identity in the spinal cord [24, 25], the cerebellum [26, 27] and the retina [28–33]. In the mouse retina, Prdm13 regulates subtype specification of amacrine cells, preferentially promoting GABAergic and glycinergic identities [34]. Mutations in human *prdm13* were recently found as causative of North Carolina macular dystrophy (NCMD) [35, 36]. NCMD is an autosomal dominant disease characterized by central macular defects that are present at birth, which shares phenotypic similarity with age-related macular degeneration [37]. This disorder was initially described in a family in North Carolina, but affected individuals have also been identified in Europe, Asia and South America.

In order to gain more insights into the role of Prdm13 in amacrine cells, we investigated the impact of *prdm13* gain and loss of function in the *Xenopus* retina. First, we found that *prdm13* is expressed in a subset of retinal progenitors and remains expressed in about 40% of amacrine cells, of GABA and glycinergic identity. We found that *prdm13* knockdown leads to a dramatic decrease in glycinergic amacrine cell genesis, while GABAergic cells remain largely unaffected. *Prdm13* overexpression promotes all amacrine cells, with a bias towards a glycinergic phenotype. We also provided evidence that in the retina, *Prdm13* also functions downstream of Ptf1a, and that it is subjected to negative autoregulation, likely due to its ability to repress *Ptf1a* expression. Together, this work highlights Prdm13 as a key determinant of glycinergic amacrine cell fate.

Methods

Xenopus laevis prdm13 expression construct

A *Xenopus laevis* cDNA clone containing the full *prdm13* open reading was amplified by RT-PCR using total RNA isolated from stage 40 tadpole eyes, using the following primers: forward 5′- GGAATTCCATGCATT GCAACAGGGCTC-3′ and reverse 5′-CCGCTCGAGT TAGGGTTCCTTGCTGCTTCCAG-3′. This led to the amplification of two distinct sequences (*prdm13–1* and *prdm13–2* GenBank BankIt submission ID: KY555727 and KY555728, respectively). These sequences were cloned into the EcoRI and XhoI restriction sites of the pCS2-Flag vector. In the present study, we worked with pCS2-Flag-*prdm13–2*, thereafter named pCS2-*prdm13*, since it encodes a protein showing the highest identity to the Prdm13 sequences characterised in other vertebrates.

Embryo culture, micro-injections and animal cap assays

Xenopus laevis embryos were obtained from adult frogs by hormone induced egg-laying and in vitro fertilization using standard methods and staged according to Nieuwkoop and Faber (1967). Synthetic mRNAs were made using Sp6 mMESSAGE mMACHINE (Ambion) and injected in a volume of 5 nl at a concentration of 25–50 pg/nl. Templates include pCS2-*prdm13* and previously described ones: pCS2-*ptf1a*-GR [38], pCS2-Flag-*mprdm13* (mouse *prdm13*, [23]), pCS2-*GFP* and pCS2-*lacZ* [39]. Standard control- and antisense-morpholino oligonucleotides (MO) were obtained from Genetools. We used *ptf1a*, *prdm13* and *prdm13*–5-mismatched (5 *mm*-MO) antisense morpholinos as previously described [23, 38]. Of note, the specificity of both *ptf1a* and *prdm13* MOs had already been demonstrated [23, 38]. All MO were injected in a volume of 5 nl and at a concentration of 50-100 μM. Embryos were injected at the two-cell stage in both blastomeres and either fixed or frozen at –80 °C at the indicated developmental stages. Embryos were co-injected with *GFP* mRNA as a tracer for the injection. Protein activity of Ptf1a-GR was induced by addition of 10 μM dexamethasone (Sigma) to the culture medium at the indicated stages.

For animal cap assays, 50-150 pg of in vitro synthesized mRNA (*ptf1a*-GR, *lacZ* or *mprdm13*) and 20 ng of MO (*prdm13*-MO, 5 *mm*-MO or control-MO) were microinjected into the animal region of each blastomere at the four-cell stage. Animal caps were dissected at the blastula stage (stage 9) and cultured in 1X Steinberg medium, 0.1% BSA until stage 26. Dexamethasone (10 μM) was added at stage 12 for Ptf1a-GR activation.

In vivo lipofection

pCS2-*GFP* and pCS2-*prdm13* were mixed with DOTAP liposomal reaction (Roche) in a 1:3 ratio and injected at stage 18 into the presumptive region of the retina as previously described [40, 41]. Embryos were fixed at stage 41 and cryostat sectioned (12 μm). GFP-positive cells were counted and cell types were identified based on their laminar position and morphology.

In situ hybridization and immunohistochemistry

Digoxigenin-labeled antisense RNA probes for *gad1* (also called *gad1.1*, [42]), *vglut1* (also called *slc17a7*, [43]), *glyt1* (also called *slc6a9*, [44]) and *prdm13* [23] were generated according to the manufacturer's instruction (Roche). Whole-mount in situ hybridization analysis of *Xenopus* embryos was performed as described [45]. For sections, embryos were agarose-embedded and vibratome-sectioned at 50 μm thickness. In situ hybridization at stage 42, double fluorescent in situ hybridizations or combination of in situ hybridization and immunofluorescent staining were performed on 12 μm cryostat sections following previously described procedures [46]. For EdU experiments, stage 28/30 or 42 tadpoles were incubated 3 h in a 1 mM EdU solution, then immediately fixed in 4% paraformaldehyde. In situ hybridization was first performed followed by Edu staining using the Click-iT EdU Alexa Fluor 488 Imaging Kit (Molecular Probes).

For immunofluorescent labelling, embryos were fixed in 4% paraformaldehyde/0.3% glutaraldehyde in 0.1 M phosphate buffer, pH 7.4 for 20 min. Then, they were cryoprotected with 30% (*w/v*) sucrose in PBS before cryosectioning (12 μm thickness). Immunolabeling was performed using rabbit anti-glycine (1:100, AB139, Millipore or 1:500, IG1001, Immunosolution), mouse anti-GFP (1:500, A11120, Molecular probes), rabbit anti-GABA (1:1000, 20,094, Immunostar), rabbit anti-calretinin (1:100, 7697, Swant) as primary antibodies, and anti-rabbit Alexa 594 (1:1000, A11012, Molecular Probes) or anti-mouse Alexa 488 (1:1000, A11001, Molecular Probes) as secondary antibodies. To improve the signal of the glycine antibody, an antigen retrieval method was performed as previously described [47]. Images were acquired on M2 Zeiss microscope with a digital camera AxioCam MRc and AxioVision Rel 7.8 software.

RT-qPCR analysis

Total RNA was extracted using the RNAspin Mini RNA isolation kit (GE Healthcare), cDNA was synthesized with the iScript™ cDNA synthesis kit (Biorad). Real time RT-qPCR reactions were performed in technical triplicates using the Step One Plus real Time PCR system (Applied biosystems) with Go Taq® qPCR Master Mix (promega) for SYBR Assay. *Xenopus gapdh* and *odc1* were used as reference genes. The following primers were used: *prdm13* (forward: 5'-CTGCCGACACAT GATGAAAAGG-3' and reverse: 5'-AGATTTTGGGG GAGGCAGAAAAG-3'); *ptf1a* (forward: 5'-CGGACT CCTTTGGTTCCAC-3' and reverse: 5'- CATTGGAAT

GATAAAGAGCGGG); *neurog2* (forward: 5'-GGCGCG TTAAAGCTAACAAC-3' and reverse: 5'-TTCGCTAA GAGCCCAGATGT-3'); *gapdh* (forward 5'-TAGTTG GCGTGAACCATGAG-3' and reverse 5'-GCCAAAGT TGTCGTTGATGA-3'); and *odc1* (forward: 5'- TTCTA CTCGAGCAGCATTTGG-3' and reverse: 5'-TTCAAA CAACATCCAGTCTCC-3'). For animal caps experiments, 40–50 embryos were used for each point. For retina experiments, 50–60 eyes were dissected for each point.

Results

Prdm13 is expressed in few progenitors and in a subset of amacrine cells during *Xenopus* retinogenesis

The spatial and temporal distribution of *prdm13* transcripts during *Xenopus laevis* retinogenesis was analysed by whole-mount in situ hybridization (Fig. 1a). *Prdm13* expression is detected in the presumptive eye region from stage 28 onwards. We confirmed on transversal sections that it is not detected in the optic vesicle at stage 25. At stage 28, the optic vesicle contains both proliferative progenitor cells and early born post-mitotic precursors. In order to assess in which cell population *prdm13* was expressed, we combined EdU labelling (to visualize cells in the S-phase of the cell cycle) with *prdm13* in situ hybridization (Fig. 1b). *prdm13* labelling was mainly detected in EdU-negative cells, suggesting that it is primarily expressed in post-mitotic retinal cells. Yet, we found 25.17% (±1.97, $n = 10$ sections, 305 cells) of double-labelled EdU/*prdm13* cells among the *prdm13*$^+$ cell population. From stage 33/34, *prdm13* expression is restricted to the INL of the retina and to the ciliary marginal zone (CMZ), where continuous neurogenesis occurs [48]. Within the CMZ, cells are spatially ordered, so that retinal stem cells reside in the most peripheral region, proliferating progenitor more centrally and postmitotic precursors in the most central region [49] (Fig. 1c). *prdm13* expression was not detected in the tip of the CMZ, suggesting that it is not expressed in retinal stem cells. In order to discriminate its expression in proliferative versus non-proliferative cells, we combined *prdm13* in situ hybridization and EdU labelling. We found double-labelled cells in the central region of the CMZ suggesting that at least a subset of proliferative progenitors express *prdm13* (Fig. 1d). At post-embryonic stage 42, in addition to this expression in the CMZ, the expression in the INL gets mostly restricted to the inner part of the layer. To further identify and quantify *prdm13* cell populations, we performed fluorescent in situ hybridization on retinal sections that allows assessing transcripts expression at a cellular resolution (Fig. 1e). We first quantified the distribution of *prdm13*$^+$ cells among the different layers of the retina (Fig. 1f). Most of *prdm13*$^+$ cells (87.8%) are localized in the inner part of the INL (two cell body rows), where most of the

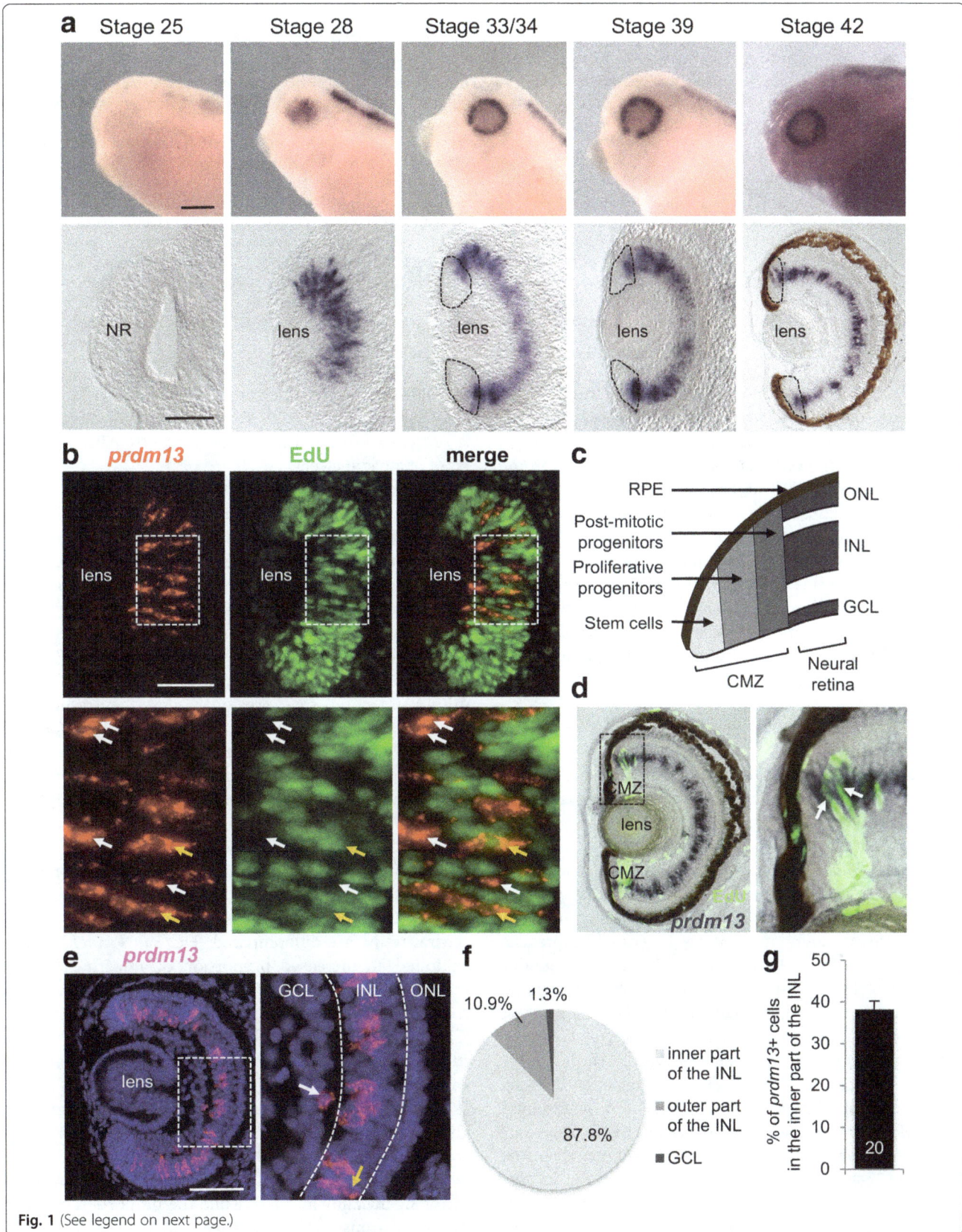

Fig. 1 (See legend on next page.)

(See figure on previous page.)
Fig. 1 *Prdm13* expression in the *Xenopus* retina. **a** Whole-mount in situ analysis of *prdm13* expression during embryogenesis, shown as lateral views of the embryo heads or as transversal retinal sections at the indicated stages. At stage 42, the in situ hybridization has been performed on retinal section. The brown colour is the retinal pigment epithelium. Dotted lines delineate the ciliary marginal zone (CMZ). **b** Stage 28/30 sections following *prdm13* in situ hybridization (red) and EdU incorporation assay (green). Below are enlargements of areas delineated with dotted lines. White arrows point to *prdm13*⁺/Edu⁻ cells while yellow arrows point to double labelled cells. **c** Schematic of a CMZ in the periphery of a *Xenopus* tadpole retina. **d** Stage 42 retinal section following *prdm13* in situ hybridization (dark blue) and EdU incorporation assay (green). Since EdU labels cells that are in the S-phase during the 3-h EdU pulse, not all proliferative cells are labelled, in particular the slowly cycling stem cells. Panel on the right is an enlargement of the area delineated with dotted lines. Arrows point to double labelled cells. **e** *Prdm13* fluorescent in situ hybridization (red) on stage 41 retinal section, counterstained with Hoechst to visualize nuclei (blue). Panel on the right is an enlargement of the white square. The white and yellow arrows point to *prdm13* positive cells localized in the ganglion cell layer (GCL), and the outer part of the inner nuclear layer (INL), respectively. Dotted lines delineate the three nuclear layers. **f** Pie chart showing the distribution of *prdm13*⁺ cells among the ganglion cell layer (GCL, 1.3 ± 0.5%), the inner part of INL (87.8 ± 1.3%) and the outer part of the INL (10.9 ± 1.3%). Data are presented as mean ± SEM, n = 20 sections. **g** Quantification of the percentage of *prdm13* positive cells among amacrine cells (defined by their localization in the inner part of the INL). Data are presented as mean ± SEM. Number of analysed sections is indicated in the bar. NR: Neural Retina, CMZ: ciliary marginal zone; RPE: Retinal Pigmented Epithelium, GCL: Ganglion Cell Layer, INL: Inner Nuclear Layer, ONL: Outer Nuclear layer. Scale bar represents 200 μm (whole mount), 100 μm (sections)

amacrine cells reside. Some (10.9%) are also found in the outer part (one cell body row), where cell bodies of bipolar, horizontal and Müller cells are located. Of note, scattered amacrine cells can occasionally be found in the outer part of the INL at this stage (as inferred from staining using amacrine cell markers, data not shown). Finally, a small percentage (1.3%) are located in the GCL. We then quantified the number of *prdm13*⁺ cells among the amacrine cell population (Fig. 1g). We found that 38,3% of amacrine cells are *prdm13* positive. Together, these data indicate that *prdm13* is expressed both in a small subset of retinal progenitors (in the optic cup and in the CMZ) and in about a third of amacrine cells.

Prdm13 is expressed in glycinergic and GABAergic amacrine cells

Amacrine cells are inhibitory neurons that mainly use GABA or glycine as neurotransmitters. To investigate in which amacrine cell subtypes *prdm13* is expressed, we first performed double fluorescent in situ hybridizations with *prdm13* and *gad1* (glutamate decarboxylase 1) as a marker for GABAergic neurons [42]. We found that 38% of *prdm13* cells within the INL were *gad1* positive (Fig. 2a,c). Interestingly, we found that among the *prdm13* expressing cells located in the GCL, 90% are *gad1*⁺, strongly suggesting that these cells are displaced amacrine cells. However, although unlikely, we cannot completely rule out that these are GABAergic ganglion cells as expression of GABA in retinal ganglion cells has been observed in some species [50, 51]. Besides, whether all displaced amacrine cells are GABAergic in *Xenopus* has not yet been determined. *prdm13*-positive cells that are localized in the GCL and are GABA-negative may thus be non-GABAergic displaced amacrine cells. We then combined *prdm13* in situ hybridization with anti-glycine or anti-calretinin immunostaining (Fig. 2b and data not shown). We found that 68% of *prdm13* cells were glycine⁺ while only 5% were calretinin⁺ (Fig. 2c). Of note, it has been shown in *Xenopus* retina

that 80–90% of calretinin positive amacrine cells are also GABAergic [52]. Together, these results show that *prdm13* is primarily expressed in glycinergic and GABAergic subtypes of amacrine cells.

Prdm13 overexpression promotes amacrine cell fate with a bias towards a glycinergic phenotype

To investigate the involvement of Prdm13 in neuronal specification within the retina, we first used a gain of function approach. As no cDNA containing the entire *Xenopus laevis prdm13* open reading frame was available, we cloned the full-length *prdm13* cDNA. We then overexpressed *prdm13* in 2-cell stage embryos through mRNA injections. As previously described, when the mouse *prdm13* mRNA was overexpressed in *Xenopus* embryos (*mprdm13*, [23]), we found that overexpressing *Xenopus prdm13* mRNA leads to gastrulation defects preventing subsequent analysis of retinal development (data not shown). We thus decided to overexpress *prdm13* only in a subset of retinal progenitors by in vivo lipofection in the eye field at stage 18. GFP expressing plasmid was co-transfected and used as a tracer to identify transfected cells at stage 41, when cells in the central retina are differentiated (Fig. 3a). *Prdm13* clones exhibited an increased proportion of amacrine cells at the expense of bipolar and Müller cells, compared to control retina from embryos lipofected with GFP alone (Fig. 3b). To know whether a particular amacrine cell subtype was favoured, we combined in vivo lipofection with anti-GABA or anti-glycine immunostaining (Fig. 3c). We found that the proportion of both GABAergic and glycinergic amacrine cells among lipofected cells is increased (Fig. 3d). However, the proportion of GABAergic neurons among the transfected amacrine cell population is not significantly affected, while the proportion of glycinergic neurons is higher than in controls (Fig. 3e). Together, these data suggest that Prdm13 acts cell autonomously in retinal precursors to promote GABAergic and

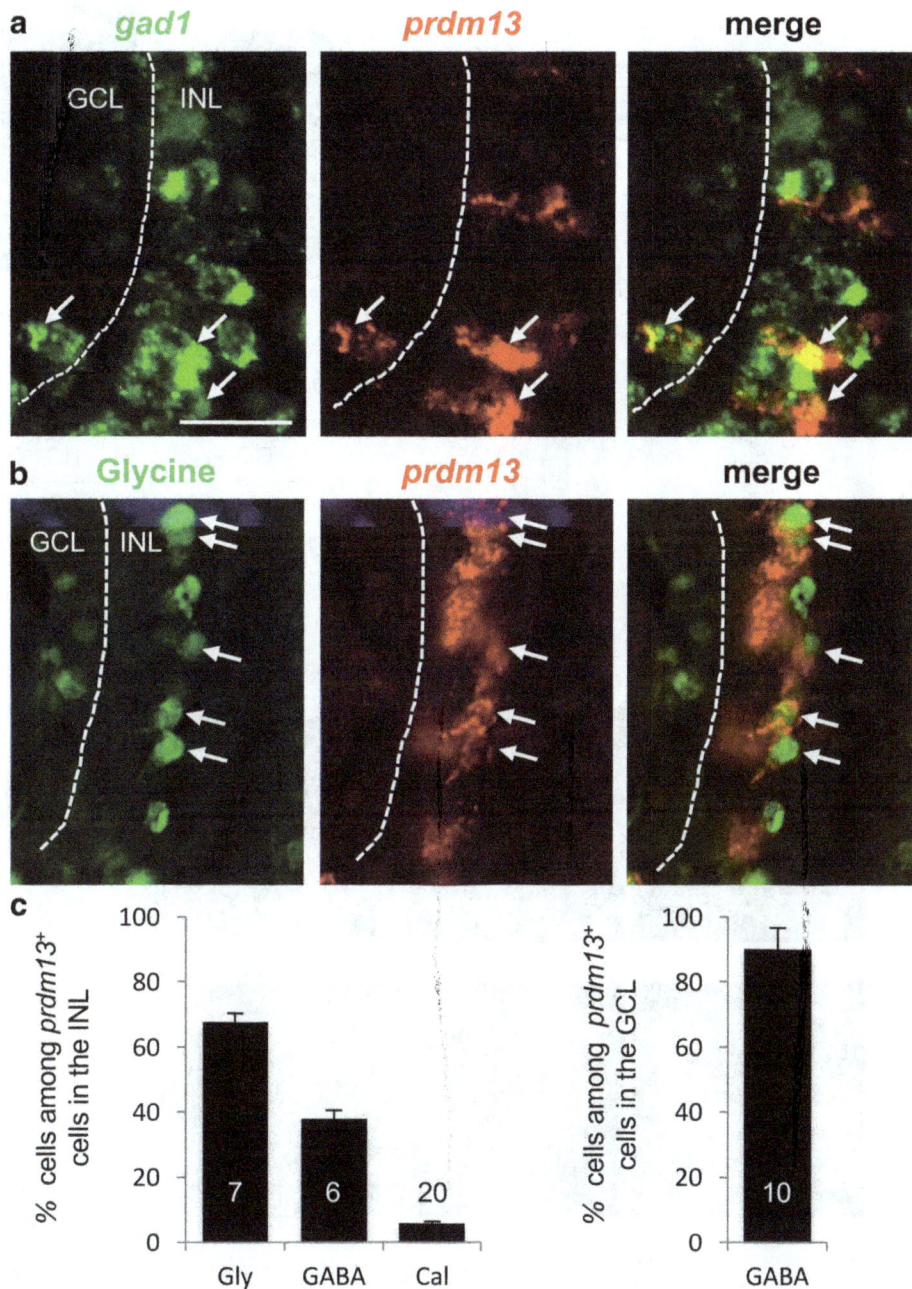

Fig. 2 *Prdm13* is expressed in glycinergic- and GABAergic-amacrine cells. **a** Double in situ hybridization with *prdm13* (red) and *gad1* (green) probes on stage 39/40 retinal section. **b** In situ hybridization with *prdm13* probe (red) coupled with anti-Glycine immunostaining (green) on stage 41/42 retinal section. Arrows point to double labelled cells. Dotted lines separate the GCL and the INL. **c** Quantification of the percentages of GABA (*gad1*+), Glycine (Gly) and Calretininin (Cal) amacrine cells among *prdm13*+ cells in the INL and in the GCL. Data are presented as mean ± SEM. Number of analysed sections is indicated in each bar. GCL: Ganglion Cell Layer, INL: Inner Nuclear Layer. Scale bar represents 25 μm

glycinergic amacrine cell genesis, with a bias towards a glycinergic phenotype.

Prdm13 loss of function leads to a decrease in glycinergic amacrine cell genesis

To address the potential requirement of Prdm13 in amacrine cell genesis, we performed loss of function experiments using a previously designed *prdm13* translation blocking morpholino antisense oligonucleotide (*prdm13*-MO, [23]) that targets both *Xenopus laevis* *prdm13* alloalleles. *Prdm13*-MO or a control-MO were injected in two blastomeres at two-cell stage, and retinal phenotypes were analysed by whole mount in situ hybridization at stage 41. As the knockdown of *prdm13*

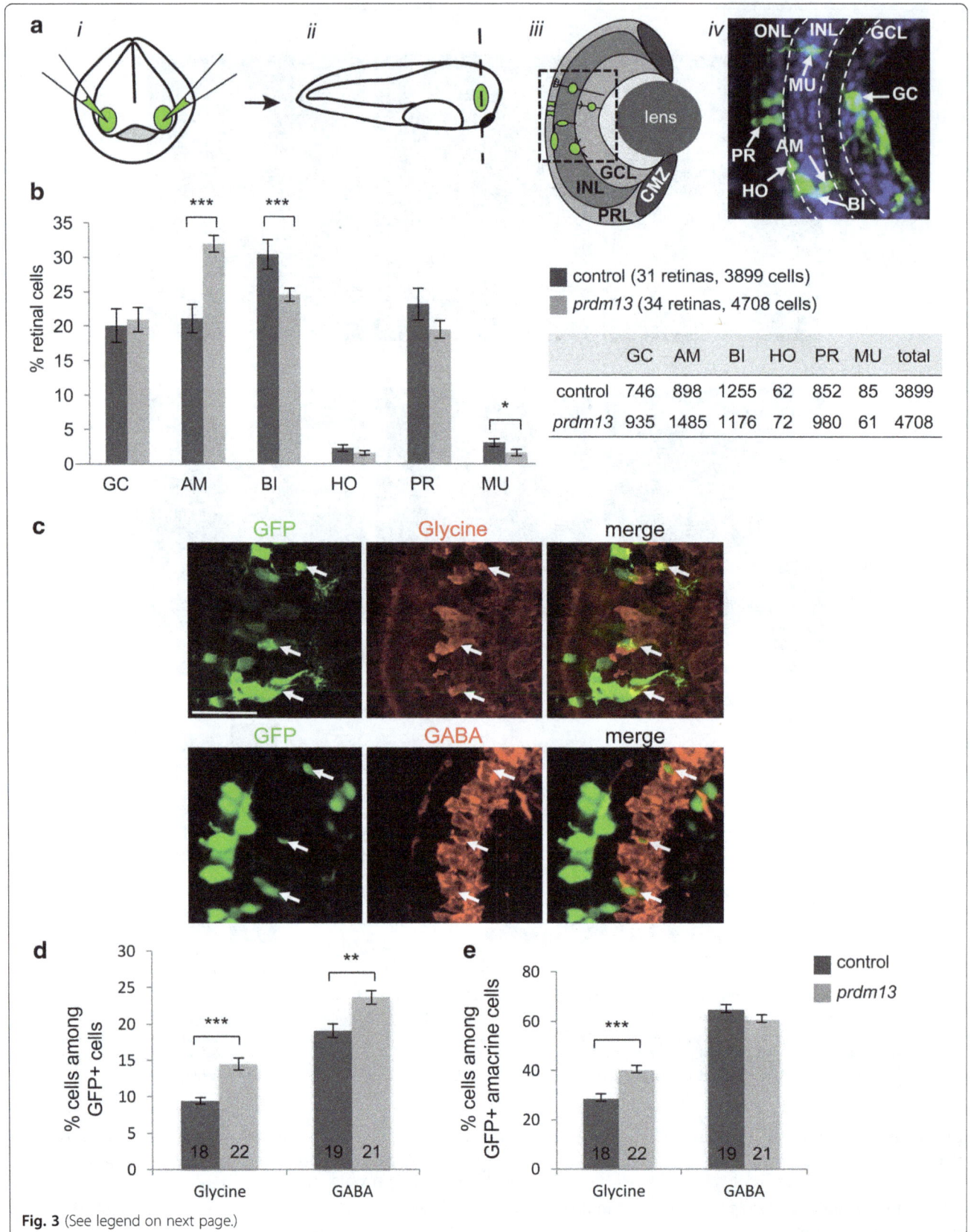

a

i, ii, iii, iv

b

% retinal cells (y-axis: 0 to 35)

GC, AM, BI, HO, PR, MU

*** (AM), *** (BI), * (MU)

■ control (31 retinas, 3899 cells)
■ prdm13 (34 retinas, 4708 cells)

	GC	AM	BI	HO	PR	MU	total
control	746	898	1255	62	852	85	3899
prdm13	935	1485	1176	72	980	61	4708

c

GFP   Glycine   merge

GFP   GABA   merge

d

% cells among GFP+ cells (y-axis: 0 to 30)

Glycine *** (18, 22), GABA ** (19, 21)

e

% cells among GFP+ amacrine cells (y-axis: 0 to 80)

Glycine *** (18, 22), GABA (19, 21)

■ control
■ prdm13

Fig. 3 (See legend on next page.)

Fig. 3 *Prdm13* overexpression promotes amacrine cells with a bias toward a glycinergic cell fate. **a** Illustration of the lipofection technique. *i* DNA is injected in the eye fields (green) of stage 18 embryos (frontal view). *ii* Retinas (green) are then sectioned (dashed line) at stage 41. *iii* Schema of a retinal section showing a clone of transfected cells (green) in the different retinal layers. *iv* Picture of a retinal section area (square in c) showing transfected cells (green). Nuclei are counterstained with Hoechst (blue). **b** Proportion of different retinal cell types in stage 41 *prdm13* lipofected and control embryos. The table indicates the absolute numbers of counted cells for each cell type. **c** Double-immunostaining with anti-GFP and anti-Glycine or anti-GABA antibodies on retinal sections of *prdm13* lipofected embryos. Arrows point to GFP positive cells that are Glycine or GABA-positive. **d,e** Quantification of GABA-positive and Glycine-positive cells among total GFP$^+$ cells (**d**) or among GFP$^+$ cells in the inner part of the INL where amacrine cells reside (**e**). Number of analysed retinas is indicated in each bar. GC: ganglion cells; AM: amacrine cells; BI: bipolar cells; HO: horizontal cells; PR: photoreceptor cells; MU: Müller cells. Values are given as mean ± SEM. * p-value <0,05; ** p-value <0,01; *** p-value <0,001 (Mann-Whitney test). Scale bar represents 50 μm

was previously shown to strongly upregulate *prdm13* expression in the dorsal neural tube [23], we first tested the effect of the injection of *prdm13*-MO on the expression of *prdm13* itself. We found that *prdm13*-MO injection leads to endogenous *prdm13* mRNA upregulation (Fig. 4a), indicating that Prdm13 also negatively regulates its expression in a feedback loop in the retina. Probes for *gad1*, *vglut1* (vesicular glutamate transporter 1, [42]), and *glyt1* (glycine transporter 1, [44]) were next used as markers of GABAergic, glutamatergic and glycinergic neurons, respectively. Whereas *vglut1* and *gad1* stainings were not affected by *prdm13*-MO injection, *glyt1* expression was dramatically reduced in the retina (Fig. 4a). This effect was quantified by immunostaining experiments using anti-glycine or anti-GABA antibodies (Fig. 4b-c). A significant decrease in the number of glycinergic cells following *prdm13*-MO injection was observed compared to control-MO injected embryos, while no effect was observed regarding GABAergic amacrine cell labelling. Together, these data reveal that *prdm13* knock-down impacts glycinergic, but not GABAergic amacrine cell genesis.

Prdm13 is a Ptf1a target in *Xenopus* retinal progenitor cells

Prdm13 is a direct target of Ptf1a in the dorsal neural tube [22, 23]. To determine the interaction between these two factors in the retina, we first investigated whether both genes are co-expressed in retinal cells, using double fluorescent in situ hybridizations (Fig. 5a). The percentage of double-labelled cells was then calculated at different stages of retinogenesis (Fig. 5b). At stage 33, about 50% of *prdm13*$^+$ cells are *ptf1a*$^+$, and vice versa. The percentage of *prdm13*$^+$ cells among *ptf1a*$^+$ cell population remains stable over the entire retina between stage 33 and stage 40 (50–70%). However, the number of *ptf1a*$^+$ cells among *prdm13* expressing cells progressively decreases from stage 33 to stage 40 as *ptf1a* expression gets restricted to the CMZ compartment. By stage 40 in the central retina, only 10% of *prdm13*$^+$ cells are still *ptf1a*$^+$. Thus, at all stages examined, some retinal cells express only *prdm13*, some only *ptf1a*, and some express both genes, consistent with a

possible genetic interaction in these cells. Moreover, the number of co-labelled cells might be higher if the analysis had been done at the protein level since Ptf1a protein may be retained in the cells after its mRNA downregulation.

Could Prdm13 be a Ptf1a target in a subset of retinal cells? *Prdm13* expression was shown to be lost in the mouse *ptf1a*$^{-/-}$ retina [34]. To further address this question in *Xenopus*, we performed *ptf1a* gain or loss of function experiments and analysed the impact on *prdm13* retinal expression at stage 41 (Fig. 5c). We used previously described MO to generate *ptf1a* knock-down embryos [30]. *Gad1* probe was used as a readout of *ptf1a*-MO activity, as *gad1* expression was previously shown to be regulated by Ptf1a [30]. In *ptf1a* morphants, *prdm13* expression was dramatically decreased in the retina. Of note, this was also the case for *glyt1* expression.

To overexpress *Ptf1a*, we injected at the two-cell stage mRNAs encoding a glucocorticoid inducible form of Ptf1a (Ptf1a-GR) [30]. Dexamethasone (dex) was added to the embryo culture medium at stage 21/22 in order to activate Ptf1a-GR at an early stage of retinogenesis. We confirmed that under such conditions *gad1* expression is strongly upregulated at stage 41, as expected from our previous work [30] (Fig. 5c). Surprisingly, *prdm13* expression was at that stage clearly decreased compared to the controls. Since our above data suggest that Prdm13 is required for glycinergic neuron genesis, we also examined *glyt1* expression and found that it is also reduced upon *ptf1a* overexpression.

Based on these unexpected observations, we further investigated the impact of *ptf1a* overexpression on *prdm13* at different stages of development. We found robust ectopic *prdm13* expression in the epidermis of embryos at stage 25 and stage 28 (Fig. 6a,b). Importantly, in transversal sections, a strong *prdm13* upregulation was also seen at both stages in the optic vesicle and optic cup (data not shown and Fig. 6c). However, the opposite effect, i.e. decrease in *prdm13* retinal expression, was obtained from stage 35 onwards (Fig. 6a-c). Since we saw above that Prdm13 negatively regulates its own expression, this data likely reveals a feedback control mechanisms. Together, our loss and gain of function

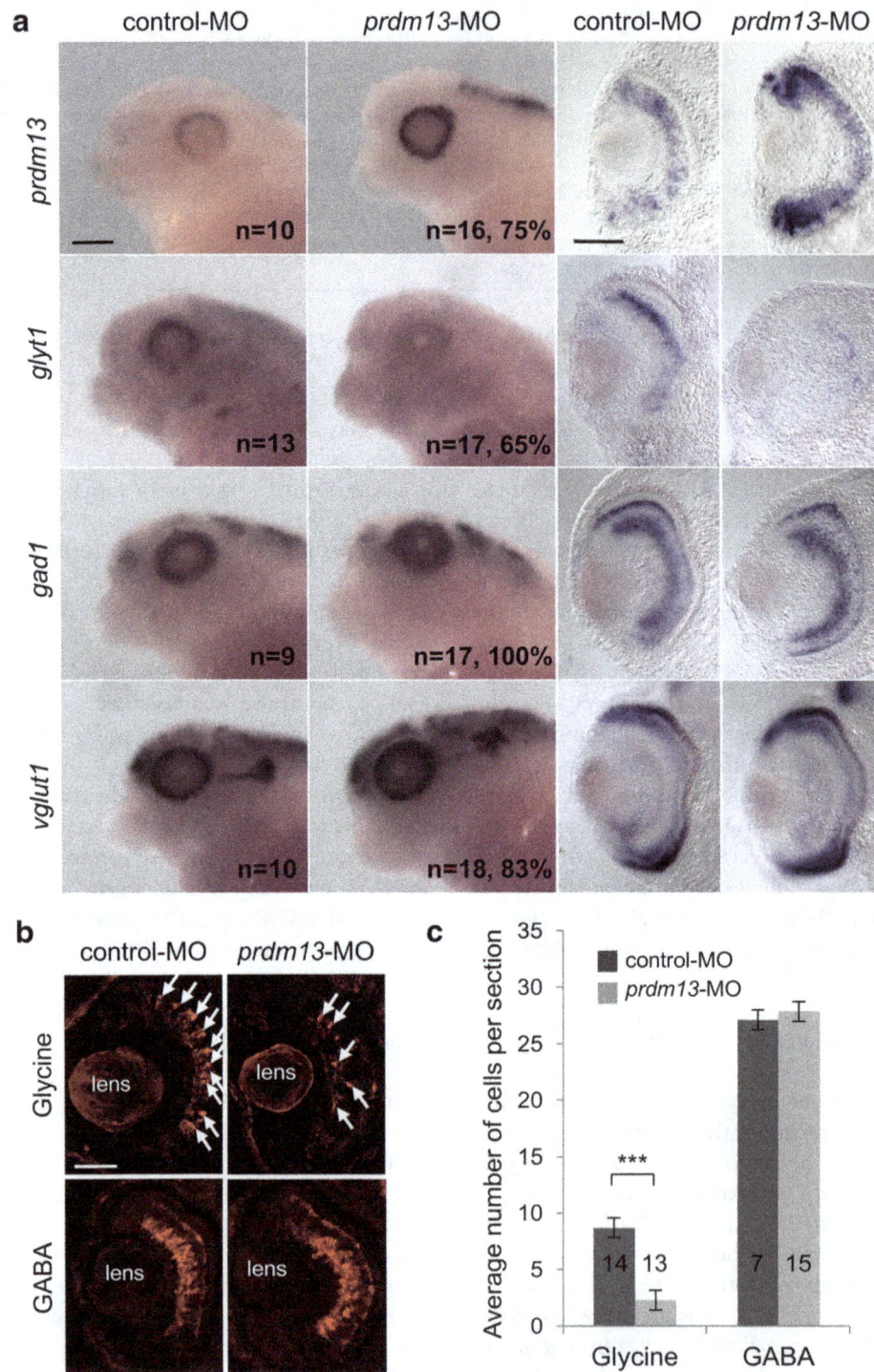

Fig. 4 *Prdm13* loss of function leads to a decrease in glycinergic but not GABAergic-amacrine cells. **a** Whole-mount in situ hybridization analysis of *prdm13*, *glyt1*, *gad1* and *vglut1* expression on stage 39/40 embryos injected with *prdm13*-MO or control-MO. Lateral views of the head and transversal sections of the retinas are shown. The number of analysed embryos and the percentage of embryos with represented phenotypes are indicated in each panel. **b** Stage 39/40 sections following GABA or Glycine-immunostaining on control-MO and *prdm13*-MO injected embryos. Arrows point to Glycine-positive cells. **c** Quantification of the average number of GABA- or Glycine-positive cells per section. Number of analysed sections is indicated in each bar. Data are presented as mean ± SEM. *p* < 0.001 (***) (Mann-Whitney test). Scale bars represent 200 μm (whole mount), 100 μm (sections)

Prdm13 forms a feedback loop with Ptf1a and is required for glycinergic amacrine cell genesis in the Xenopus...

225

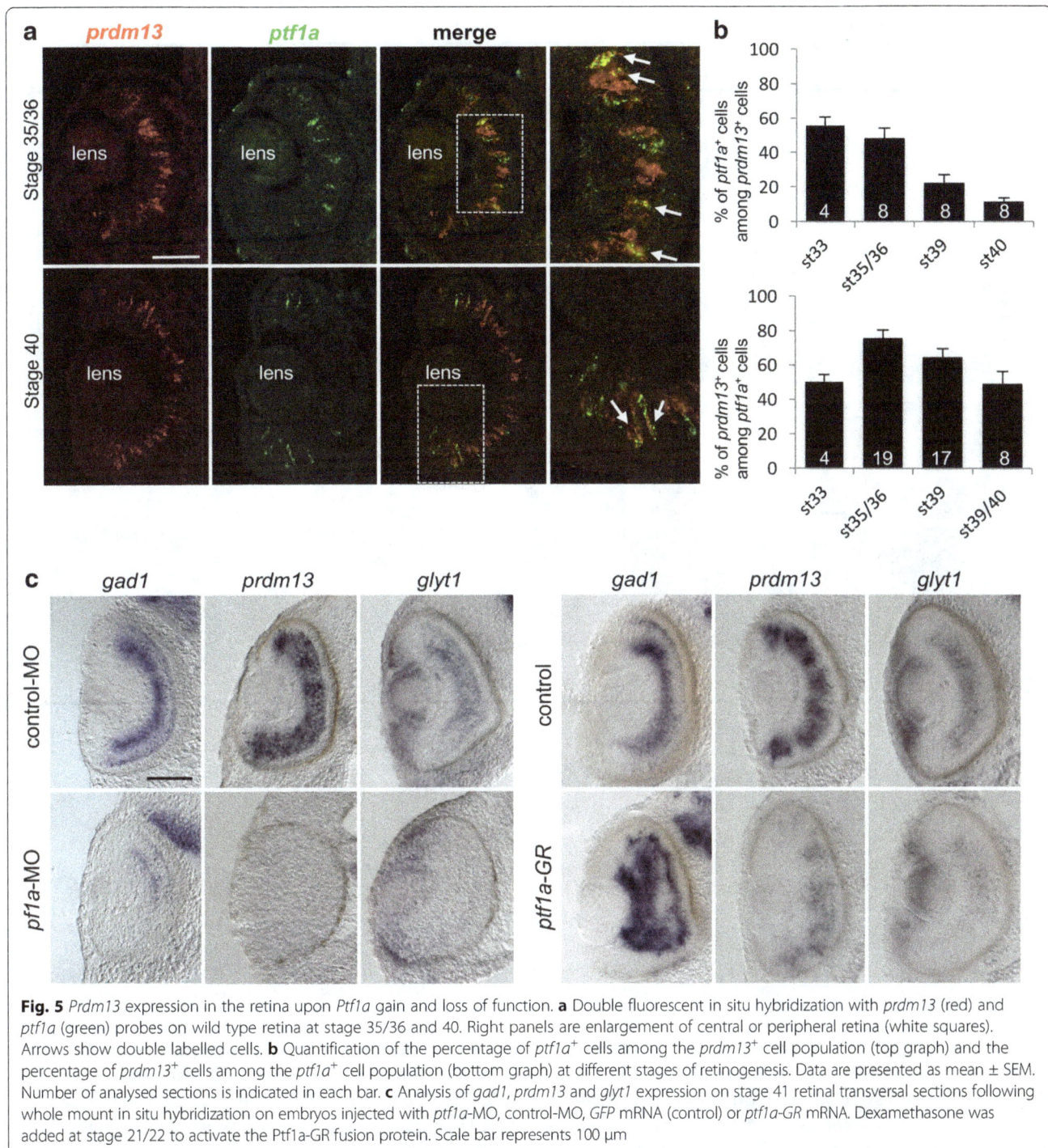

Fig. 5 *Prdm13* expression in the retina upon *Ptf1a* gain and loss of function. **a** Double fluorescent in situ hybridization with *prdm13* (red) and *ptf1a* (green) probes on wild type retina at stage 35/36 and 40. Right panels are enlargement of central or peripheral retina (white squares). Arrows show double labelled cells. **b** Quantification of the percentage of *ptf1a*+ cells among the *prdm13*+ cell population (top graph) and the percentage of *prdm13*+ cells among the *ptf1a*+ cell population (bottom graph) at different stages of retinogenesis. Data are presented as mean ± SEM. Number of analysed sections is indicated in each bar. **c** Analysis of *gad1*, *prdm13* and *glyt1* expression on stage 41 retinal transversal sections following whole mount in situ hybridization on embryos injected with *ptf1a*-MO, control-MO, *GFP* mRNA (control) or *ptf1a-GR* mRNA. Dexamethasone was added at stage 21/22 to activate the Ptf1a-GR fusion protein. Scale bar represents 100 μm

analysis suggest that *prdm13* is a target of Ptf1a in *Xenopus* retinal progenitor cells.

Prdm13 negatively regulates *Ptf1a* in a feedback loop

The results above indicate that *prdm13* in the retina is subjected to negative autoregulation (Fig. 4a). This regulation could be a direct autorepressive action of Prdm13 on its own promoter. Alternatively, it could be an indirect negative control of Prdm13 on the expression of its inducer, *ptf1a*. To test this hypothesis and given that Ptf1a induces its own expression [53], we examined the effect of Prdm13 gain and loss of function on *ptf1a* gene regulation in Ptf1a-GR overexpressing animal caps. Explants were treated with Dex at stage 10, cultured until stage 26 and analysed by RT-qPCR using 3'UTR *ptf1a* primers to specifically detect endogenous *ptf1a* mRNAs.

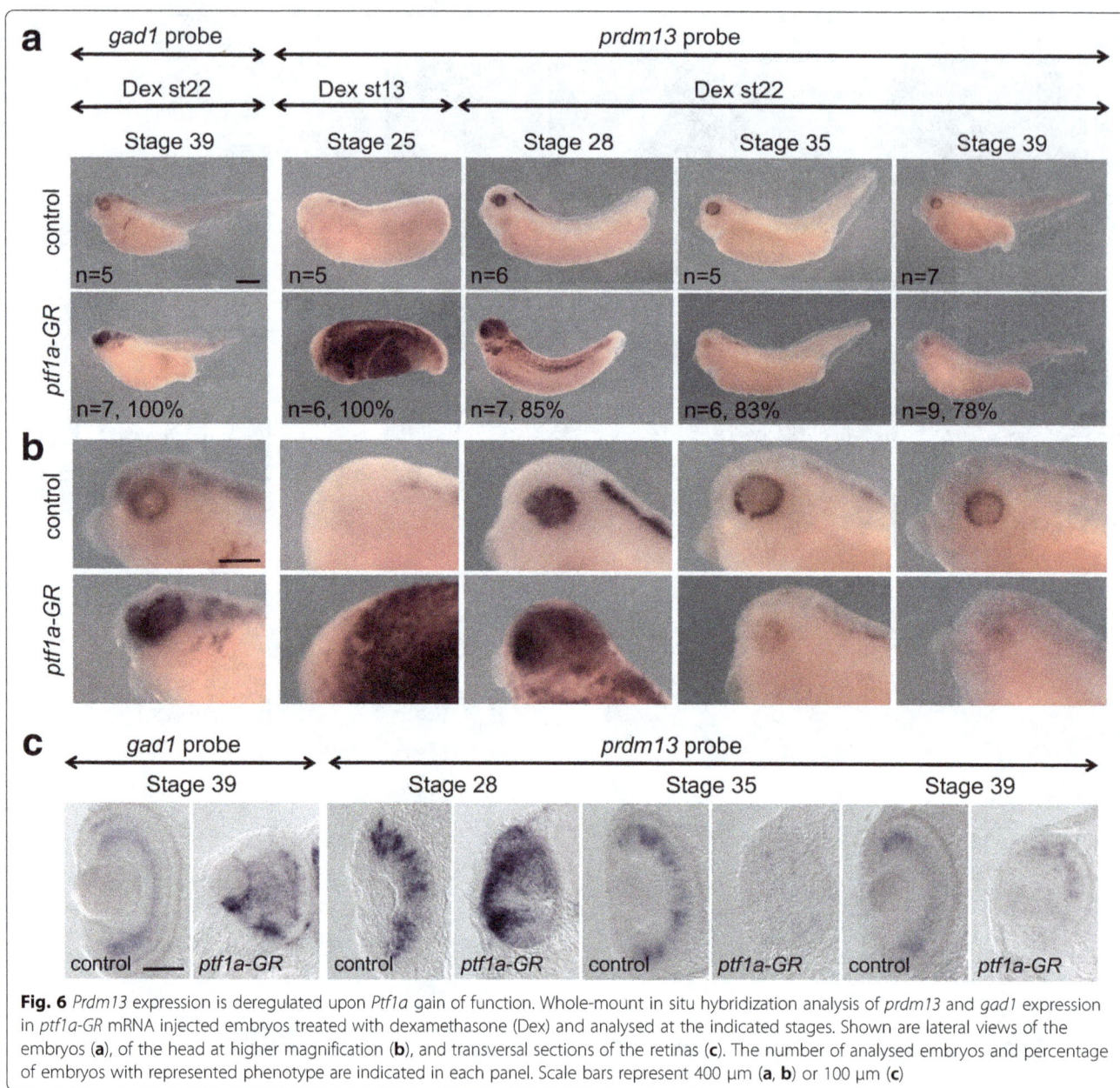

Fig. 6 *Prdm13* expression is deregulated upon *Ptf1a* gain of function. Whole-mount in situ hybridization analysis of *prdm13* and *gad1* expression in *ptf1a-GR* mRNA injected embryos treated with dexamethasone (Dex) and analysed at the indicated stages. Shown are lateral views of the embryos (**a**), of the head at higher magnification (**b**), and transversal sections of the retinas (**c**). The number of analysed embryos and percentage of embryos with represented phenotype are indicated in each panel. Scale bars represent 400 μm (**a**, **b**) or 100 μm (**c**)

As previously reported [53], we found that Ptf1a induces its own expression (Fig. 7a). Interestingly, this upregulation of *Ptf1a* expression was abolished following *Prdm13* overexpression. Overexpression of *lacZ*, which serves as a control, had no effect on Ptf1a auto-activation. Conversely, as observed for *prdm13* expression, a stronger upregulation of *ptf1a* was observed upon *prdm13* inhibition. Such increase in the expression of *ptf1a* was not observed with a control-MO or *5 mm*-MO. These results indicate that Prdm13 regulates Ptf1a in a negative feedback loop. To determine whether this mechanism also occurs during eye development, we analysed *ptf1a* expression at stages 39/40 by RT-qPCR in dissected eyes from *prdm13*-MO or control-MO injected embryos.

Both *prdm13* and *ptf1a* were upregulated in the retina of *prdm13*-MO injected embryos compared to controls (Fig. 7b). No such upregulation was observed for another bHLH gene, neurog2, that is expressed in retinal progenitors [49, 54]. Thus, Prdm13 appears to negatively retrocontrol *ptf1a* expression during retinogenesis.

Discussion

Amacrine cells are the most diverse class of neurons in the retina, with over 30 different subtypes. The genetic network governing the determination of these amacrine cell subtypes remains poorly known. In the current study, we found that the transcriptional regulator Prdm13 is expressed in subtypes of amacrine cells in the

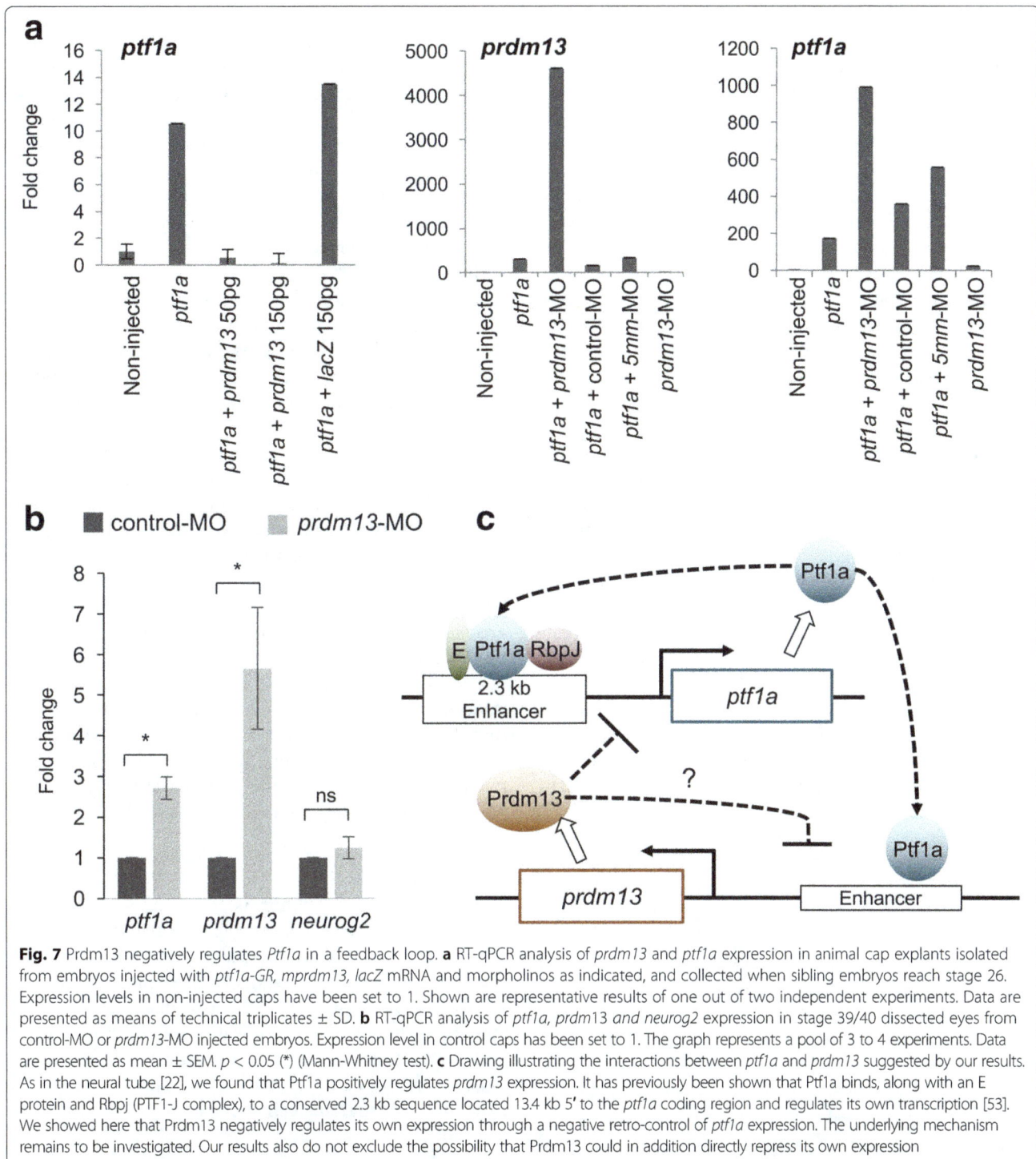

Fig. 7 Prdm13 negatively regulates *Ptf1a* in a feedback loop. **a** RT-qPCR analysis of *prdm13* and *ptf1a* expression in animal cap explants isolated from embryos injected with *ptf1a-GR, mprdm13, lacZ* mRNA and morpholinos as indicated, and collected when sibling embryos reach stage 26. Expression levels in non-injected caps have been set to 1. Shown are representative results of one out of two independent experiments. Data are presented as means of technical triplicates ± SD. **b** RT-qPCR analysis of *ptf1a, prdm13* and *neurog2* expression in stage 39/40 dissected eyes from control-MO or *prdm13*-MO injected embryos. Expression level in control caps has been set to 1. The graph represents a pool of 3 to 4 experiments. Data are presented as mean ± SEM. $p < 0.05$ (*) (Mann-Whitney test). **c** Drawing illustrating the interactions between *ptf1a* and *prdm13* suggested by our results. As in the neural tube [22], we found that Ptf1a positively regulates *prdm13* expression. It has previously been shown that Ptf1a binds, along with an E protein and Rbpj (PTF1-J complex), to a conserved 2.3 kb sequence located 13.4 kb 5′ to the *ptf1a* coding region and regulates its own transcription [53]. We showed here that Prdm13 negatively regulates its own expression through a negative retro-control of *ptf1a* expression. The underlying mechanism remains to be investigated. Our results also do not exclude the possibility that Prdm13 could in addition directly repress its own expression

Xenopus retina, in both glycinergic and GABAergic ones. Our gain of function analysis indicates that Prdm13 is an inducer of amacrine cells, with a bias towards a glycinergic destiny. *prdm13* knock-down prevents glycinergic cell genesis but does not significantly affect GABAergic amacrine cell specification. By combining studies in animal caps and in the retina, we also propose a regulatory

feedback loop between Prdm13 and Ptf1a where the latter would promote the expression of *Prdm13*, which would then negatively retro-controls *Ptf1a* expression.

It was shown in the mice that the major population of Prdm13+ amacrine cells express calbindin and calretinin, two calcium-binding proteins [34]. In *Xenopus* however, calbindin is a specific marker of cone photoreceptor cells, as it is in the human retina [55]. We therefore only tested co-expression between *prdm13* and calretinin. In *Xenopus*, calretinin expression is found mainly in bipolar cells, ganglion cells and only in few amacrine cells [52], while it is found in amacrine and ganglion cells in the mouse [56]. Our data revealed only few (5%) calretinin$^+$ cells among *prdm13*$^+$ population compared to 65% in the mouse [34]. Given that this calcium-binding protein labels different populations of retinal cells in different species, this apparent difference may not reveal significant difference regarding Prdm13 expression in amacrine cell subpopulations. More meaningfully, it was reported in the mouse retina that almost all of the Prdm13 amacrine cells are GABAergic (13.5%) or glycinergic (87.1%) [34]. We also found in the *Xenopus* retina that *prdm13* cells are primarily GABAergic (38%) and glycinergic (68%). In the mouse retina, it was reported that only rare *prdm13*$^+$ cells were proliferative cells, suggesting that *prdm13* is primarily expressed in postmitotic cells [34]. We investigated this issue at the level of *prdm13* mRNA. We also found that *prdm13* is mainly expressed in postmitotic cells. Yet, some *prdm13*$^+$ cells in the optic vesicle and in the CMZ were found to be EdU-positive, suggesting that a subset of retinal progenitors are expressing *prdm13* mRNA while still proliferating. As a whole, *prdm13* retinal expression in both species is similar.

GABAergic and glycinergic amacrine cells are reduced in *prdm13*$^{-/-}$ mouse retinas [34]. Our data revealed that only glycinergic amacrine cells are affected upon *prdm13* knockdown. This apparent discrepancy could highlight true differences between Prdm13 function in mouse and *Xenopus*. Alternatively, it could result from different experimental approaches since the *prdm13*$^{-/-}$ mouse is a null and we used a knockdown approach. Glycinergic amacrine cells may also be more sensitive to a reduction in Prdm13 protein level than GABAergic one. A CRISPR/Cas9 approach to target *prdm13* in *Xenopus* could contribute to address this hypothesis.

Our results indicate that Prdm13 negatively self-regulates its expression and that this may be due to a negative retro-control of Prdm13 on *ptf1a* expression. How Prdm13 negatively regulates *ptf1a* expression remains to be determined. Ptf1a levels have been shown to be regulated by autoregulation through the binding of Ptf1a, along with an E protein and Rbpj (the PTF1-J complex), to a conserved 2.3 kb sequence located 13.4 kb 5′ to the *ptf1a* coding region. This element has an enhancer activity in all *ptf1a* expression domains of the developing nervous system [53]. Therefore, one possibility is that Prdm13 negatively regulates *ptf1a* by blocking its autoregulation (Fig. 7c). This could be achieved through the enhancer element mentioned above for instance by preventing binding of the PTF1-J

complex. Since Prdm13 has been shown to form complexes by protein-protein interactions with bHLH factors such as Ascl1 [22], an alternative model would be that Prdm13 binds to *Ptf1a* and converts the PTF1-J complex from an activator to a repressor. Further experiments are required to decipher Prdm13 mode of action in *Ptf1a* regulation. Other transcription factors, such as Satb2, Ebf3 and Neurod6, have been described as key regulators of amacrine subtype diversity [9]. The precise integration of Prdm13 function to this genetic network remains to be investigated.

Using whole-genome sequencing, it has recently been discovered that mutations in human *PRDM13* gene are associated with NCMD, a Mendelian form of human macular disease [35]. NCMD was initially considered as a slowly progressive disease, with many phenotypic similarities to age-related macular degeneration, including an abnormal accumulation of drusen, atrophy of the retinal pigment epithelium and overlying photoreceptor cells, choroidal neovascularization and loss of central vision. However, 20 years later it was realized that it is actually a nonprogressive developmental disorder, with highly variable expressivity [57]. A complete duplication of the *prdm13* gene was discovered in one family with NCMD. From gain of function analysis in the mouse [34] and our data in *Xenopus*, it is expected that increased level of Prdm13 in patients would likely lead to impaired amacrine cell fate specification. However, how this leads to macular degeneration remains unknown. A better knowledge of Prdm13 function in retinal development and maintenance should help unravelling the mechanisms by which *prdm13* mutations cause macular dystrophies.

Conclusions

The present study confirms the important role of Prdm13 in amacrine cell subtype diversification downstream of Ptf1a. It also provides first evidence indicating that Prdm13 negatively regulates its expression, at least in part, by repressing Ptf1a in a feedback loop. Future studies, including the identification of its direct targets and partners, are required to determine how mechanistically Prdm13 control Ptf1a levels and promotes the generation of amacrine cell subtypes.

Abbreviations
bHLH: Basic helix loop helix; CMZ: Ciliary marginal zone; CRISPR: Clustered Regularly Interspaced Short Palindromic Repeats; DOTAP: N-[1-(2,3-Dioleoyloxy)propyl]-N,N,N-trimethylammonium methyl-sulfate; EdU: 5-éthynyl-2′-déoxyuridine; GABA: Gamma-Aminobutyric acid; gad1: Glutamate decarboxylase 1; GCL: Ganglion Cell Layer38; glyt1: Glycine transporter 1; INL: Inner Nuclear Layer; MO: Morpholino Oligonucleotide; NCMD: North Carolina macular dystrophy; ONL: Outer Nuclear Layer; PR: PRDI-BF1-RIZ1; PRDM: PRDI-BF1 and RIZ homology domain; Ptf1a: Pancreas Specific Transcription Factor, 1a; RT-qPCR: Reverse transcriptase-quantitative polymerase chain reaction; SET: Su(var)3–9, Enhancer-of-zeste and Trithorax

Acknowledgments
The authors would like to thank S. Kricha, S. Desiderio and S. Lourdel for technical assistance and C. Lioret for animal care.

Funding
This work was supported by a grant from the Walloon Region (First International project "EPIGENE") to E.B and M.P. Work in the M.P. laboratory was also supported by an ANR grant. N.B. was a Walloon region "First International" postdoctoral fellow.

Authors' contributions
NB, KP, EB and MP carried out the experiments and analysed the data. OB performed bioinformatics analysis. NB, KP, EB and MP wrote the manuscript. All authors read and approved the final manuscript.

Competing interests
The authors declare that they have no competing interests.

Author details
[1]ULB Neuroscience Institute (UNI), Université Libre de Bruxelles (ULB), B-6041 Gosselies, Belgium. [2]Paris-Saclay Institute of Neuroscience, CNRS, Univ Paris Sud, Université Paris-Saclay, UMR 9197- Neuro-PSI, Bat. 445, 91405 ORSAY Cedex, France. [3]Centre d'Etude et de Recherche Thérapeutique en Ophtalmologie, Retina France, Orsay, France.

References
1. MacNeil MA, Masland RH. Extreme diversity among amacrine cells: implications for function. Neuron. 1998;20:971–82.
2. MacNeil MA, Heussy JK, Dacheux RF, Raviola E, Masland RH. The shapes and numbers of amacrine cells: matching of photofilled with Golgi-stained cells in the rabbit retina and comparison with other mammalian species. J Comp Neurol. 1999;413:305–261.
3. Cherry TJ, Trimarchi JM, Stadler MB, Cepko CL. Development and diversification of retinal amacrine interneurons at single cell resolution. Proc Natl Acad Sci U S A. 2009;106:9495–500.
4. Bassett EA, Wallace VA. Cell fate determination in the vertebrate retina. Trends Neurosci. 2012;35:565–73.
5. Goetz JJ, Farris C, Chowdhury R, Trimarchi JM. Making of a retinal cell: insights into retinal cell-fate determination. Int Rev Cell Mol Biol. 2014;308:273–321.
6. Cepko C. Intrinsically different retinal progenitor cells produce specific types of progeny. Nat Rev Neurosci. 2014;15:615–27.
7. Boije H, MacDonald RB, Harris WA. Reconciling competence and transcriptional hierarchies with stochasticity in retinal lineages. Curr Opin Neurobiol. 2014;27:68–74.
8. Voinescu PE, Emanuela P, Kay JN, Sanes JR. Birthdays of retinal amacrine cell subtypes are systematically related to their molecular identity and soma position. J Comp Neurol. 2009;517:737–50.
9. Kay JN, Voinescu PE, Chu MW, Sanes JR. Neurod6 expression defines new retinal amacrine cell subtypes and regulates their fate. Nat Neurosci Nature Publishing Group. 2011;14:965–72.
10. Feng L, Xie X, Joshi PS, Yang Z, Shibasaki K, Chow RL, et al. Requirement for Bhlhb5 in the specification of amacrine and cone bipolar subtypes in mouse retina. Development. 2006;133:4815–25.
11. Huang L, Hu F, Feng L, Luo X-J, Liang G, Zeng X-Y, et al. Bhlhb5 is required for the subtype development of retinal amacrine and bipolar cells in mice. Dev Dyn. 2014;243:279–89.
12. Jiang H, Xiang M. Subtype specification of GABAergic amacrine cells by the orphan nuclear receptor Nr4a2/Nurr1. J Neurosci. 2009;29:10449–59.
13. Elshatory Y, Everhart D, Deng M, Xie X, Barlow RB, Gan L. Islet-1 controls the differentiation of retinal bipolar and cholinergic amacrine cells. J Neurosci. 2007;27:12707–20.
14. Jin K, Jiang H, Mo Z, Xiang M. Early B-cell factors are required for specifying multiple retinal cell types and subtypes from postmitotic precursors. J Neurosci Society Neurosci. 2010;30:11902–16.
15. Ding Q, Chen H, Xie X, Libby RT, Tian N, Gan L. BARHL2 differentially regulates the development of retinal amacrine and ganglion neurons. J Neurosci. 2009;29:3992–4003.
16. Mo Z, Li S, Yang X, Xiang M. Role of the Barhl2 homeobox gene in the specification of glycinergic amacrine cells. Development. 2004;131:1607–18.
17. Fog CK, Galli GG, Lund AH. PRDM proteins: important players in differentiation and disease. BioEssays. 2012;34:50–60.
18. Hohenauer T, Moore AW. The Prdm family: expanding roles in stem cells and development. Development. 2012;139:2267–82.
19. Brzezinski JA, Lamba DA, Reh TA. Blimp1 controls photoreceptor versus bipolar cell fate choice during retinal development. Development. 2010;137:619–29.
20. Katoh K, Omori Y, Onishi A, Sato S, Kondo M, Furukawa T. Blimp1 suppresses Chx10 expression in differentiating retinal photoreceptor precursors to ensure proper photoreceptor development. J Neurosci. 2010;30:6515–26.
21. Jung CC, Atan D, Ng D, Ploder L, Ross SE, Klein M, et al. Transcription factor PRDM8 is required for rod bipolar and type 2 OFF-cone bipolar cell survival and amacrine subtype identity. Proc Natl Acad Sci U S A. 2015;112:E3010–9.
22. Chang JC, Meredith DM, Mayer PR, Borromeo MD, Lai HC, Ou Y-H, et al. Prdm13 mediates the balance of inhibitory and excitatory neurons in somatosensory circuits. Dev Cell. 2013;25:182–95.
23. Hanotel J, Bessodes N, Thélie A, Hedderich M, Parain K, Van Driessche B, et al. The Prdm13 histone methyltransferase encoding gene is a Ptf1a-Rbpj downstream target that suppresses glutamatergic and promotes GABAergic neuronal fate in the dorsal neural tube. Dev Biol. 2014;386:340–57.
24. Glasgow SM, Henke RM, Macdonald RJ, Wright CVE, Johnson JE. Ptf1a determines GABAergic over glutamatergic neuronal cell fate in the spinal cord dorsal horn. Development. 2005;132:5461–9.
25. Huang M, Huang T, Xiang Y, Xie Z, Chen Y, Yan R, et al. Ptf1a, Lbx1 and Pax2 coordinate glycinergic and peptidergic transmitter phenotypes in dorsal spinal inhibitory neurons. Dev Biol. 2008;322:394–405.
26. Hoshino M, Nakamura S, Mori K, Kawauchi T, Terao M, Nishimura YV, et al. Ptf1a, a bHLH transcriptional gene, defines GABAergic neuronal fates in cerebellum. Neuron. 2005;47:201–13.
27. Pascual M, Abasolo I, Mingorance-Le Meur A, Martínez A, Del Rio JA, Wright CVE, et al. Cerebellar GABAergic progenitors adopt an external granule cell-like phenotype in the absence of Ptf1a transcription factor expression. Proc Natl Acad Sci U S A. 2007;104:5193–8.
28. Fujitani Y, Fujitani S, Luo H, Qiu F, Burlison J, Long Q, et al. Ptf1a determines horizontal and amacrine cell fates during mouse retinal development. Development. 2006;133:4439–50.
29. Nakhai H, Sel S, Favor J, Mendoza-Torres L, Paulsen F, Duncker GIW, et al. Ptf1a is essential for the differentiation of GABAergic and glycinergic amacrine cells and horizontal cells in the mouse retina. Development. 2007;134:1151–60.
30. Dullin J-P, Locker M, Robach M, Henningfeld K. A, Parain K, Afelik S, et al. Ptf1a triggers GABAergic neuronal cell fates in the retina. BMC Dev Biol. 2007;7:110.
31. Lelièvre EC, Lek M, Boije H, Houille-Vernes L, Brajeul V, Slembrouck A, et al. Ptf1a/Rbpj complex inhibits ganglion cell fate and drives the specification of all horizontal cell subtypes in the chick retina. Dev Biol Elsevier Inc. 2011;358:296–308.
32. Jusuf PR, Harris WA. Ptf1a is expressed transiently in all types of amacrine cells in the embryonic zebrafish retina. Neural Dev. 2009;4:34.
33. Jusuf PR, Almeida AD, Randlett O, Joubin K, Poggi L, Harris WA. Origin and determination of inhibitory cell lineages in the vertebrate retina. J Neurosci. 2011;31:2549–62.

34. Watanabe S, Sanuki R, Sugita Y, Imai W, Yamazaki R, Kozuka T, et al. Prdm13 regulates subtype specification of retinal amacrine interneurons and modulates visual sensitivity. J Neurosci. 2015;35:8004–20.

35. Small KW, DeLuca AP, Whitmore SS, Rosenberg T, Silva-Garcia R, Udar N, et al. North Carolina macular dystrophy is caused by Dysregulation of the retinal transcription factor PRDM13. Ophthalmology. 2016;123:9–18.

36. Weleber RG. Dysregulation of retinal transcription factor PRDM13 and North Carolina macular dystrophy. Ophthalmology. 2016;123:2–4.

37. Yang Z, Tong Z, Chorich LJ, Pearson E, Yang X, Moore A, et al. Clinical characterization and genetic mapping of North Carolina macular dystrophy. Vis Res. 2008;48:470–7.

38. Afelik S, Chen Y, Pieler T. Combined ectopic expression of Pdx1 and Ptf1a/p48 results in the stable conversion of posterior endoderm into endocrine and exocrine pancreatic tissue. Genes Dev. 2006;20:1441–6.

39. Turner DL, Weintraub H. Expression of achaete-scute homolog 3 in Xenopus embryos converts ectodermal cells to a neural fate. Genes Dev. 1994;8:1434–47.

40. Ohnuma S, Mann F, Boy S, Perron M, Harris WA. Lipofection strategy for the study of Xenopus retinal development. Methods. 2002;28:411–9.

41. Holt CE, Garlick N, Cornel E. Lipofection of cDNAs in the embryonic vertebrate central nervous system. Neuron. 1990;4:203–14.

42. Li M, Sipe CW, Hoke K, August LL, Wright MA, Saha MS. The role of early lineage in GABAergic and glutamatergic cell fate determination in Xenopus Laevis. J Comp Neurol. 2006;495:645–57.

43. Gleason KK, Dondeti VR, Hsia H-LJ, Cochran ER, Gumulak-Smith J, Saha MS. The vesicular glutamate transporter 1 (xVGlut1) is expressed in discrete regions of the developing Xenopus Laevis nervous system. Gene Expr Patterns. 2003;3:503–7.

44. Wester MR, Teasley DC, Byers SL, Saha MS. Expression patterns of glycine transporters (xGlyT1, xGlyT2, and xVIAAT) in Xenopus Laevis during early development. Gene Expr Patterns. 2008;8:261–70.

45. Parain K, Mazurier N, Bronchain O, Borday C, Cabochette P, Chesneau A, et al. A large scale screen for neural stem cell markers in Xenopus Retina. Dev Neurobiol. 2012;72:491–506.

46. Lea R, Bonev B, Dubaissi E, Vize PD, Papalopulu N. Multicolor fluorescent in situ mRNA hybridization (FISH) on whole mounts and sections. Methods Mol Biol. 2012;917:431–44.

47. Inoue D, Wittbrodt J. One for all-a highly efficient and versatile method for fluorescent immunostaining in fish embryos. PLoS One. 2011;6:e19713.

48. Fischer AJ, Bosse JL, El-Hodiri HM. The ciliary marginal zone (CMZ) in development and regeneration of the vertebrate eye. Exp Eye Res Elsevier Ltd. 2013;116:199–204.

49. Perron M, Kanekar S, Vetter ML, Harris WA. The genetic sequence of retinal development in the ciliary margin of the Xenopus eye. Dev Biol. 1998;199:185–200.

50. Sandell JH, Martin SC, Heinrich G. The development of GABA immunoreactivity in the retina of the zebrafish (brachydanio rerio). J Comp Neurol. 1994;345:596–601.

51. Fry KR, Chen NX, Glazebrook PA, Lam DM. Postnatal development of ganglion cells in the rabbit retina: characterizations with AB5 and GABA antibodies. Brain Res Dev Brain Res. 1991;61:45–53.

52. Gábriel R. Calretinin is present in serotonin- and gamma-aminobutyric acid-positive amacrine cell populations in the retina of Xenopus Laevis. Neurosci Lett. 2000;285:9–12.

53. Meredith DM, Masui T, Swift GH, MacDonald RJ, Johnson JE. Multiple transcriptional mechanisms control Ptf1a levels during neural development including autoregulation by the PTF1-J complex. J Neurosci. 2009;29:11139–48.

54. Nieber F, Pieler T, Henningfeld KA. Comparative expression analysis of the neurogenins in Xenopus Tropicalis and Xenopus Laevis. Dev Dyn. 2009;238:451–8.

55. Haley TL, Pochet R, Baizer L, Burton MD, Crabb JW, Parmentier M, et al. Calbindin D-28K immunoreactivity of human cone cells varies with retinal position. Vis Neurosci. 1995;12:301–7.

56. Haverkamp S, Müller U, Harvey K, Harvey RJ, Betz H, Wässle H. Diversity of glycine receptors in the mouse retina: localization of the α3 subunit. J Comp Neurol. 2003;465:524–39.

57. Small KW. North Carolina macular dystrophy, revisited. Ophthalmol. 1989;96:1747–54.

Permissions

All chapters in this book were first published in ND, by BioMed Central; hereby published with permission under the Creative Commons Attribution License or equivalent. Every chapter published in this book has been scrutinized by our experts. Their significance has been extensively debated. The topics covered herein carry significant findings which will fuel the growth of the discipline. They may even be implemented as practical applications or may be referred to as a beginning point for another development.

The contributors of this book come from diverse backgrounds, making this book a truly international effort. This book will bring forth new frontiers with its revolutionizing research information and detailed analysis of the nascent developments around the world.

We would like to thank all the contributing authors for lending their expertise to make the book truly unique. They have played a crucial role in the development of this book. Without their invaluable contributions this book wouldn't have been possible. They have made vital efforts to compile up to date information on the varied aspects of this subject to make this book a valuable addition to the collection of many professionals and students.

This book was conceptualized with the vision of imparting up-to-date information and advanced data in this field. To ensure the same, a matchless editorial board was set up. Every individual on the board went through rigorous rounds of assessment to prove their worth. After which they invested a large part of their time researching and compiling the most relevant data for our readers.

The editorial board has been involved in producing this book since its inception. They have spent rigorous hours researching and exploring the diverse topics which have resulted in the successful publishing of this book. They have passed on their knowledge of decades through this book. To expedite this challenging task, the publisher supported the team at every step. A small team of assistant editors was also appointed to further simplify the editing procedure and attain best results for the readers.

Apart from the editorial board, the designing team has also invested a significant amount of their time in understanding the subject and creating the most relevant covers. They scrutinized every image to scout for the most suitable representation of the subject and create an appropriate cover for the book.

The publishing team has been an ardent support to the editorial, designing and production team. Their endless efforts to recruit the best for this project, has resulted in the accomplishment of this book. They are a veteran in the field of academics and their pool of knowledge is as vast as their experience in printing. Their expertise and guidance has proved useful at every step. Their uncompromising quality standards have made this book an exceptional effort. Their encouragement from time to time has been an inspiration for everyone.

The publisher and the editorial board hope that this book will prove to be a valuable piece of knowledge for researchers, students, practitioners and scholars across the globe.

List of Contributors

Jo Begbie
Department of Physiology, Anatomy and Genetics, University of Oxford, Oxford, UK

Harry Clifford, Wilfried Haerty and Chris P. Ponting
Department of Physiology, Anatomy and Genetics, University of Oxford, Oxford, UK
MRC Functional Genomics, University of Oxford, Oxford, UK

Sebastian M. Shimeld
Department of Zoology, University of Oxford, Oxford, UK

Cedric Patthey
Department of Zoology, University of Oxford, Oxford, UK
Umeå Center for Molecular Medicine, Umeå University, Umeå, Sweden

Vladimir Vladimirovich Muzyka and Tudor Constantin Badea
Retinal Circuit Development and Genetics Unit, Building 6, Room 331B Center Drive, Bethesda, MD 20892–0610, USA

Matthew Brooks
Genomics Core, Neurobiology-Neurodegeneration and Repair Laboratory, National Eye Institute, NIH, Building 6, Room 331B Center Drive, Bethesda, MD 20892–0610, USA

Haley E. Brown and Timothy A. Evans
Department of Biological Sciences, University of Arkansas, Fayetteville, AR 72701, USA

Marie C. Reichert
Department of Biological Sciences, University of Arkansas, Fayetteville, AR 72701, USA
Present address: Intramural Research Training Program, National Human Genome Research Institute, Bethesda, MD 20892, USA

Marcela Lipovsek, Tanguy Lafont, Clemens Kiecker and Anthony Graham
Centre for Developmental Neurobiology, Kings College London, London SE1 1UL, UK

Thomas Butts
Centre for Developmental Neurobiology, Kings College London, London SE1 1UL, UK
School of Life Sciences, University of Liverpool, Liverpool L69 3BX, UK

Andrea Wizenmann
Institute of Clinical Anatomy and Cell Analysis, Department of Anatomy, University of Tübingen, Oesterbergstrasse 3, 72074 Tuebingen, Germany

Julia Ledderose
Institute of Clinical Anatomy and Cell Analysis, Department of Anatomy, University of Tübingen, Oesterbergstrasse 3, 72074 Tuebingen, Germany
Universitätsmedizin Berlin, NeuroCure - Institute of Biochemistry, ChariteCrossOver, Virchowweg, 610117 Berlin, Germany

Kavitha S. Rao and Melissa M. Rolls
Department of Biochemistry and Molecular Biology, The Pennsylvania State University, University Park, PA 16802, USA

José L. Juárez-Morales, Sofia A. Pezoa, Grace K. Vallejo, Samantha J. England and Katharine E. Lewis
1Department of Biology, Syracuse University, 107 College Place, Syracuse, NY 13244, USA

William C. Hilinski
Department of Biology, Syracuse University, 107 College Place, Syracuse, NY 13244, USA
Department of Neuroscience and Physiology, SUNY Upstate Medical University, 505 Irving Avenue, Syracuse, NY 13210, USA

Sarah de Jager and Claus J. Schulte
Department of Physiology, Development and Neuroscience, University of Cambridge, Downing Street, Cambridge CB2 3DY, UK

Rebecca L. Cunningham and Amy L. Herbert
Department of Developmental Biology, Washington University School of Medicine, St. Louis, MO 63110, USA

Breanne L. Harty and Kelly R. Monk
Department of Developmental Biology, Washington University School of Medicine, St. Louis, MO 63110, USA
Vollum Institute, Oregon Health and Science University, Portland, OR 97239, USA

Sarah D. Ackerman
Department of Developmental Biology, Washington University School of Medicine, St. Louis, MO 63110, USA
Institute of Neuroscience, University of Oregon, Eugene, OR 97403, USA

Jeremy Ng Chi Kei and Peter David Currie
Australian Regenerative Medicine Institute, Monash University, Clayton, VIC 3800, Australia

Patricia Regina Jusuf
Australian Regenerative Medicine Institute, Monash University, Clayton, VIC 3800, Australia
School of Biosciences, University of Melbourne, Parkville, VIC 3010, Australia

Bader Al-Anzi and Kai Zinn
Food and Nutrition Program, Environment and Life Sciences Research Center, Kuwait Institute for Scientific Research, 13109 Kuwait City, Kuwait
Division of Biology and Biological Engineering, California Institute of Technology, Pasadena, CA 91125, USA

Julien Le Friec and Valérie Dupé
Institut de Génétique et Développement de Rennes, Faculté de Médecine, CNRS UMR6290, Université de Rennes 1, IFR140 GFAS

Véronique David and Houda Hamdi-Rozé
Institut de Génétique et Développement de Rennes, Faculté de Médecine, CNRS UMR6290, Université de Rennes 1, IFR140 GFAS
Avenue du Pr. Léon Bernard, 35043 Rennes Cedex, France
Laboratoire de Génétique Moléculaire, CHU Pontchaillou, Rennes Cedex, France

Michelle Ware
Institut de Génétique et Développement de Rennes, Faculté de Médecine, CNRS UMR6290, Université de Rennes 1, IFR140 GFAS
Present address: Department of Physiology, Development and Neuroscience, University of Cambridge, Anatomy Building, Downing Street, CB2 3DY Cambridge, UK

Olga Y. Ponomareva and Mary C. Halloran
Department of Zoology, University of Wisconsin, 1117 West Johnson St., Madison, WI 53706, USA
Department of Neuroscience, University of Wisconsin, 1111 Highland Ave, Madison, WI 53705, USA
Neuroscience Training Program, University of Wisconsin, 1111 Highland Ave, Madison, WI 53705, USA
Medical Scientist Training Program, University of Wisconsin, 750 Highland Ave, Madison, WI 53705, USA

Kevin W. Eliceiri
Laboratory for Optical and Computational Instrumentation, University of Wisconsin, 1675 Observatory Dr, Madison, WI 53706, USA

Magnus Sandberg and John L. R. Rubenstein
Department of Psychiatry, UCSF Weill Institute for Neurosciences, University of California, San Francisco, San Francisco, CA 94143, USA

Leila Taher
Division of Bioinformatics, Department of Biology, Friedrich-Alexander Universität Erlangen-Nürnberg, 91054 Erlangen, Germany

Brian L. Black
Cardiovascular Research Institute, University of California, San Francisco, CA 94143, USA

Jianxin Hu
Cardiovascular Research Institute, University of California, San Francisco, CA 94143, USA
Present address: Biogen, Cambridge 02142, MA, USA

Alex S. Nord
Department of Psychiatry and Behavioral Sciences, University of California, Davis, Davis, CA 95817, USA
Department of Neurobiology, Physiology, and Behavior, University of California, Davis, Davis, CA 95616, USA

Christophe Audouard, Anthony Kischel, Nathalie Escalas, Cathy Soula and Alice Davy
Centre de Biologie du Développement (CBD), Centre de Biologie Intégrative (CBI), Université de Toulouse, CNRS, UPS, 118 Route de Narbonne, 31062 Toulouse, France

Julien Laussu
Centre de Biologie du Développement (CBD), Centre de Biologie Intégrative (CBI), Université de Toulouse, CNRS, UPS, 118 Route de Narbonne, 31062 Toulouse, France
Present address: CRBM, 1919 route de Mende, 34293 Montpellier, France

Poincyane Assis-Nascimento and Daniel J. Liebl
University of Miami Miller School of Medicine, The Miami Project to Cure Paralysis, 1095 NW 14th Terrace, Miami, FL R-48, USA

Eric J. Bellefroid
ULB Neuroscience Institute (UNI), Université Libre de Bruxelles (ULB), B-6041 Gosselies, Belgium

Nathalie Bessodes
ULB Neuroscience Institute (UNI), Université Libre de Bruxelles (ULB), B-6041 Gosselies, Belgium
Paris-Saclay Institute of Neuroscience, CNRS, Univ Paris Sud, Université Paris-Saclay, UMR 9197- Neuro-PSI, Bat. 445, 91405 ORSAY Cedex, France

Karine Parain and Odile Bronchain
Paris-Saclay Institute of Neuroscience, CNRS, Univ Paris Sud, Université Paris-Saclay, UMR 9197- Neuro-PSI, Bat. 445, 91405 ORSAY Cedex, France

Muriel Perron
Paris-Saclay Institute of Neuroscience, CNRS, Univ Paris Sud, Université Paris-Saclay, UMR 9197- Neuro-PSI, Bat. 445, 91405 ORSAY Cedex, France
Centre d'Etude et de Recherche Thérapeutique en Ophtalmologie, Retina France, Orsay, France

Index